Toxins and Other Harmful Compounds in Foods

Chemical and Functional Properties of Food Components Series

SERIES EDITOR

Zdzisław E. Sikorski

Toxins and Other Harmful Compounds in Foods
Edited by A. Witczak and Zdzisław E. Sikorski

Meat Quality: Genetic and Environmental Factors
Edited by Wiesław Przybylski and David Hopkins

Food Oxidants and Antioxidants: Chemical, Biological, and Functional Properties
Edited by Grzegorz Bartosz

Fermentation: Effects on Food Properties
Edited by Bhavbhuti M. Mehta, Afaf Kamal-Eldin and Robert Z. Iwanski

Methods of Analysis of Food Components and Additives, Second Edition
Edited by Semih Otles

Food Flavors: Chemical, Sensory and Technological Properties
Edited by Henryk Jelen

Environmental Effects on Seafood Availability, Safety, and Quality
Edited by E. Grazyna Daczkowska-Kozon and Bonnie Sun Pan

Chemical and Biological Properties of Food Allergens
Edited by Lucjan Jedrychowski and Harry J. Wichers

Chemical, Biological, and Functional Aspects of Food Lipids, Second Edition
Edited by Zdzisław E. Sikorski and Anna Kołakowska

Food Colorants: Chemical and Functional Properties
Edited by Carmen Socaciu

Mineral Components in Foods
Edited by Piotr Szefer and Jerome O. Nriagu

Chemical and Functional Properties of Food Components, Third Edition
Edited by Zdzisław E. Sikorski

Carcinogenic and Anticarcinogenic Food Components
Edited by Wanda Baer-Dubowska, Agnieszka Bartoszek and Danuta Malejka-Giganti

Toxins in Food
Edited by Waldemar M. Dąbrowski and Zdzisław E. Sikorski

Chemical and Functional Properties of Food Saccharides
Edited by Piotr Tomasik

Chemical and Functional Properties of Food Proteins
Edited by Zdzisław E. Sikorski

Toxins and Other Harmful Compounds in Foods

EDITED BY
Agata Witczak
Zdzisław E. Sikorski

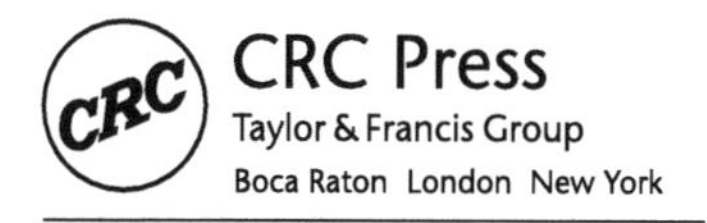

CRC Press is an imprint of the
Taylor & Francis Group, an informa business

CRC Press
Taylor & Francis Group
6000 Broken Sound Parkway NW, Suite 300
Boca Raton, FL 33487-2742

Printed on acid-free paper
Version Date: 20160901

International Standard Book Number-13: 978-1-4987-4852-0 (Hardback)

Library of Congress Cataloging-in-Publication Data

Names: Witczak, Agata. | Sikorski, Zdzisław E.
Title: Toxins and other harmful compounds in foods / Agata Witczak and Zdzisław E. Sikorski.
Description: Boca Raton : CRC Press, 2017. | Series: Chemical and functional properties of food components series
Identifiers: LCCN 2016029520| ISBN 9781498748520 (hardback : alk. paper) | ISBN 9781498748537 (e-book)
Subjects: LCSH: Foodborne diseases. | Phytotoxins. | Food contamination. | Food--Toxicology. | Food additives.
Classification: LCC QR201.F62 W58 2017 | DDC 615.9/54--dc23
LC record available at https://lccn.loc.gov/2016029520

Visit the Taylor & Francis Web site at
http://www.taylorandfrancis.com

and the CRC Press Web site at
http://www.crcpress.com

Printed and bound in the United States of America by
Edwards Brothers Malloy on sustainably sourced paper

Contents

Series Preface

Toxins and Other Harmful Compounds in Foods is the 20th volume in the CRC series of Chemical and Functional Properties of Food Components. The aim of this series is to present the actual state of knowledge on the contents, chemistry, and functionality of the main food constituents, on the methods of food analysis, as well as on the effects of the interactions of the components in various conditions of processing and storage on the sensory and biological properties of food products. These particular volumes are devoted to the individual components such as proteins, lipids, saccharides, colorants, and flavor compounds, to the effects of various environmental and breeding conditions on the quality of the raw materials (e.g., meat and seafood), to the factors affecting safety of foods, and to the role of crucial enzymatic and chemical reactions occurring during food storage, handling, and processing (e.g., hydrolysis, cross-linking, polymerization, or oxidation). The books are edited by renowned scientists according to strictly outlined rules. The individual chapters are prepared by specialists from Africa, Australia, Asia, Europe, and North America, who based them on their personal research and teaching experience, as well as on critical evaluation of the current literature. Because of the dedication of the authors, the chapters took several months to complete, and they present actual results of research.

Like other books in this series, *Toxins and Other Harmful Compounds in Foods* addresses some of the most pressing problems related to food economy and quality. It presents the occurrence of natural harmful chemical and biological factors in numerous raw materials, describes rational technological processes aimed at avoiding conditions and reactions leading to generation of toxic compounds, as well as adequate regulatory and control measures needed to produce safe food of high sensory quality.

Zdzisław E. Sikorski

Preface

Plants and animals have hardly been created intentionally to satisfy human needs for alimentation. Thus many of them contain not only proteins, lipids, saccharides, vitamins, other organic compounds, and mineral components valuable to people's nutrition, but also various chemical substances that fulfill different functions in the living plants or animals that otherwise may be toxic or harmful to humans. Furthermore, pathogenic micro-organisms, parasites, compounds generated due to processing, additives used illegally, and environmental pollutants occurring in food raw materials and products may pose a health hazard to the consumers. Research on the presence and properties of these harmful components/pollutants serves the purpose of minimizing the danger to human health. These hazards can be eliminated by limiting the maximal tolerable contents of the harmful elements and compounds, as well as by setting high standards of hygiene and rational processing parameters. The presently available methods make it possible to precisely analyze the composition of raw materials and products, enable the positioning of any particular components in the structure of the tissues, determine the concentration in the order of pg/g, speciation of pollutants, and running online effective control of the safety of food. The information presented in this volume should help the reader to understand the real hazards related to the presence and toxicity of harmful compounds in food raw materials and products. Sound knowledge on the occurrence and effects of toxins and other harmful compounds may help all those involved in the production, processing, and distribution of food to decrease the incidents of food-borne poisonings and help the educated consumers to rationally select their food products on the market.

The main idea of this book has been to present up-to-date knowledge on the occurrence, structure, and properties of harmful components in foods, the mode of action of these compounds in the human organism, on the possibilities to detect them, and on the procedures applied to eliminate the health hazards caused by food toxins and other noxious constituents. The chapters have been written by renowned specialists on food chemistry, toxicology, and microbiology. The information available in current world literature has been critically evaluated and presented in a very concise and user-friendly form. In most chapters, only the pertinent bibliographic sources have been cited, although the large number of new developments in some areas of research made it difficult to keep the lists of references really short.

The first chapter presents the factors that affect the health hazards caused by food toxins and other harmful compounds. Chapters 2 through 4 deal with the occurrence and effects of natural toxins of plant origin and marine phycotoxins. Chapter 5 describes the health hazards caused by biogenic amines that are found predominantly in fish and fermented products. Mycotoxins and bacterial toxins are discussed in Chapters 6 and 7. Pollution of foods as a result of human activities and environmental effects is presented in Chapters 8, 9, 11, 12, 14, and 17. The role of phytoestrogens and allergens, as well as the epidemiological and medical impact of contamination by viruses' transmission via food and water, is discussed in Chapters 10, 13, and 15. The risks and benefits of processing are presented in Chapter 16. The methods of detection of harmful compounds and the international regulations established to control harmful food contaminations are presented in Chapters 18 and 19.

As the editors of this volume, we acknowledge with thanks the valuable contributions of the authors. Our thanks are especially due to those colleagues who prepared their chapters ahead of time, thus giving the editors a chance to check the material thoroughly.

We dedicate this volume to all people working in the whole food chain whose efforts serve the purpose of increasing food safety.

Agata Witczak and Zdzisław E. Sikorski
Szczecin and Gdańsk, Poland

Editors

Agata Witczak, PhD, DSc, earned her BS and MS at the Technical University, Szczecin, Poland, her PhD at the Agricultural University, Szczecin, and her DSc at the West Pomeranian University of Technology (ZUT), Szczecin. She serves as a vice dean for the quality of education, and for the field of study of management of food safety and quality, at the Faculty of Food Sciences and Fisheries, ZUT. She is a member of the American Chemical Society and the Polish Society of Food Technologists, and an expert at the Sectorial Centre of Competence for the Food Industry at the Regional Centre for Innovation and Technology Transfer, ZUT. She is a chemist and toxicologist who researches persistent organic pollutants (POPs) in environmental and food safety studies. Dr. Witczak is involved in the risk assessment from xenobiotics distribution and transfer in the environment. She evaluates the effects of technological processes, including culinary processing, on POPs content in foodstuff. She is an author/coauthor of more than 70 original papers in Polish and international journals, and a coauthor of a number of unpublished works made for industrial entities and environmental protection units. She also reviews articles for prestigious magazines. Dr. Witczak is a member of the Committee of Analytical Chemistry, the Polish Academy of Sciences.

Zdzisław E. Sikorski, PhD, DSc, earned his BS, MS, PhD, and DSc at the Gdańsk University of Technology (GUT), and *Dr honoris causa* at the Agricultural University, Szczecin, Poland. He is a fellow of the International Academy of Food Science and Technology and an honorary professor emeritus of GUT. He gained industrial experience in breweries, fish-, meat-, and vegetable-processing plants, and on a deep-sea fishing trawler. He was the founder, professor, and head of the Department of Food Chemistry and Technology, GUT, served there 5 years as dean of the Faculty of Chemistry, was chairman of the Committee of Food Technology and Chemistry of the Polish Academy of Sciences, chaired the scientific board of the Sea Fisheries Institute in Gdynia, and was an elected member of the Main Council of Science and Tertiary Education in Poland. He also worked for several years as a postdoc/researcher/professor at Ohio State University, Columbus; CSIRO in Hobart, Australia; DSIR in Auckland, New Zealand; and National Taiwan Ocean University, Keelung, Taiwan. His research was focused mainly on food smoking and freezing and functional properties of food proteins. He is an author/coauthor of 210 journal papers, published 19 books, wrote 18 chapters on marine food science and food chemistry for other books, and holds several patents.

Contributors

Hassan Abdel-Gawad
Chemical Industries Division
National Research Centre
Giza, Egypt

Joanna Bober
Department of Medical Chemistry
Pomeranian Medical University in Szczecin
Szczecin, Poland

Perng-Kuang Chang
USDA-ARS
Southern Regional Research Center
New Orleans, Louisiana

Daniel Cook
USDA Agricultural Research Service Poisonous Plant Research Laboratory
Logan, Utah

Waldemar Dąbrowski
Department of Applied Microbiology and Biotechnology
West Pomeranian University of Technology
Szczecin, Poland

Stefaan De Henauw
Ghent University
Department of Public Health
Ghent, Belgium

Shilpi Gupta Dixit
All India Institute of Medical Sciences
Jodhpur, Rajasthan, India

Alicja Dłubała
Department of Applied Microbiology and Biotechnology
West Pomeranian University of Technology
Szczecin, Poland

Tine Fierens
Unit of Environmental Risk and Health
Flemish Institute for Technological Research (VITO NV)
Belgium

Grażyna Gałęzowska
Department of Environmental Toxicology
Medical University of Gdańsk
Gdańsk, Poland

Benedict T. Green
USDA Agricultural Research Service Poisonous Plant Research Laboratory
Logan, Utah

Gustaaf M. Hallegraeff
Institute for Marine and Antarctic Studies (IMAS)
University of Tasmania
Hobart, Australia

Izabela Helak
Department of Applied Microbiology and Biotechnology
West Pomeranian University of Technology
Szczecin, Poland

Sui-Sheng T. Hua
USDA-ARS
Western Regional Research Center
Albany, New York

Sevim Köse
Faculty of Marine Sciences
Karadeniz Technical University
Trabzon, Turkey

Roman Kotłowski
Department of Microbiology
Gdańsk University of Technology
Gdańsk, Poland

Elżbieta Kucharska
Department of Human Nutrition
West Pomeranian University of Technology
Szczecin, Poland

Błażej Kudłak
Department of Analytical Chemistry
Gdańsk University of Technology
Gdańsk, Poland

Stephen T. Lee
USDA Agricultural Research Service Poisonous Plant Research Laboratory
Logan, Utah

Jacek Namieśnik
Department of Analytical Chemistry
Gdańsk University of Technology
Gdańsk, Poland

Jeffrey Palumbo
USDA-ARS
Western Regional Research Center
Albany, New York

Kip E. Panter
USDA Agricultural Research Service Poisonous Plant Research Laboratory
Logan, Utah

Mikołaj Protasowicki
West Pomeranian University of Technology
Szczecin, Poland

Zdzisław E. Sikorski
Department of Food Chemistry, Technology, and Biotechnology
Gdańsk University of Technology
Gdańsk, Poland

Isabelle Sioen
Ghent University
Ghent, Belgium

Stefan S. Smoczyński
University of Warmia and Mazury in Olsztyn
Olsztyn, Poland

Arnout Standaert
Unit of Environmental Risk and Health
Flemish Institute for Technological Research (VITO NV)
Belgium

Hanna Staroszczyk
Department of Chemistry, Technology, and Food Biotechnology
Gdańsk University of Technology
Gdańsk, Poland

Maciej Tankiewicz
Department of Environmental Toxicology
Medical University of Gdańsk
Gdańsk, Poland

Mirja Van Holderbeke
Unit of Environmental Risk and Health
Flemish Institute for Technological Research (VITO NV)
Belgium

Kevin D. Welch
USDA Agricultural Research Service
Poisonous Plant Research Laboratory
Logan, Utah

Monika Wieczerzak
Department of Food Chemistry, Technology, and Biotechnology
Gdańsk University of Technology
Gdańsk, Poland

Agata Witczak
Department of Toxicology
West Pomeranian University of Technology
Szczecin, Poland

Lidia Wolska
Department of Environmental Toxicology
Medical University of Gdańsk
Gdańsk, Poland

Barbara Wróblewska
Polish Academy of Sciences
Olsztyn, Poland

1 Problems of Food Safety

Waldemar Dąbrowski and Agata Witczak

CONTENTS

1.1 INTRODUCTION

Knowledgeable consumers expect not only high sensory quality of food, but also need the elimination of risks from frequently dangerous microbial, biological, and chemical contamination. Microbial contamination results from negligence during the transport, storage, and production stages, as well as from genetic variability and metabolic flexibility of micro-organisms. An example of such flexibility is the bacterium *Escherichia coli*. These micro-organisms were characterized many years ago as human and animal commensals or pathogens. They were categorized into 6 groups and 190 serotypes. In 2011, a new strain of *E. coli* occurred in Germany—a highly pathogenic, enteroaggregative strain of serotype O104:H4 that caused an outbreak involving 3842 cases of human infections, including 51 deaths. The disease resulted from the consumption of contaminated sprouted fenugreek seeds (Beutin and Martin 2012). More than 800 people infected had symptoms of hemolytic uremic syndrome, which may lead to loss of kidney functions. Apart from Germans, there were also residents of other countries, especially France, Denmark, and Sweden, among the infected people. The contaminated seeds were probably imported from Egypt. The major causes of the outbreak were globalization of raw materials, lack of adequate hygienic standards in mass production, and international migrations of people.

Chemical contamination may also result from negligence during production, but its major cause is the widespread chemicalization of the natural and human environment. Improvements in analytical and diagnostic methods, including meta-analysis, cohort studies, and randomization, enable detection of previously unknown hazards and causes of human health disorders. Improved analytical methods, including the introduction of high-performance gas and liquid chromatography, in particular coupled with mass spectrometry, enable detection of compounds that were undetectable by conventional analytical methods. For example, some foods regarded as strongly healthy have been found to contain hazardous compounds such as 3-monochloropropane-1,2-diol in soya sauces or carbamates in pickled products.

Today most hazardous chemicals penetrate human organisms via the alimentary tract, and inadequate nutrition is regarded among the major pathogenic factors.

1.2 CHANGES IN FOOD PRODUCTION AND NUTRITION

Changes in food production involve the following:

- Concentration of production in factories of increasing processing efficiency
- Changed production methods
- Increased number and more types of products
- Increased number and more types of unconventional foods (from other regions of the world)

Increased production efficiency in a food-processing factory contributes to increased production, which significantly increases the number of consumers, and thus enlarges the risk from any production negligence. The consolidation of dairy plants in Poland (creamery and cheese-making industry) may be cited as an example. Currently, there are nearly 250,000 consumers to one creamery.

Changes in production methods concern various aspects, for example, changed sterilization methodology, where technologies of high-pressure, high-voltage electric impulses, or light impulses are introduced instead of thermal sterilization. Another example of threat associated with changes in production methods is hydroponic production of sprouts. In 1996, 6,000 children from Sakai, Japan, got infected after eating radish sprouts contaminated by enterohemorrhagic *E. coli* of 0157:H7 serotype. A similar big outbreak triggered by sprouts contaminated by *E. coli* 0104:H4 occurred in Germany in 2011. According to Meathead Goldwyn, "raw sprouts may be the riskiest food in the world" (http://amazingribs.com/blog/raw_sprout_are_risky.html).

Ready-to-eat food products are growing in number and variety. Such foods usually require heating before serving. In the case of dumplings, the most appropriate procedure is processing in boiling water. Consumers, however, usually prefer microwave heating, which does not fully prevent the risk of infection with some kinds of pathogens (Szymczak and Dąbrowski 2015).

On the market, there are more and more food products from all over the world. Surimi crabsticks or Japanese sushi have become quite widespread. Their production on Asiatic markets is usually combined with centuries-long tradition. However, starting their mass production in distant countries may be hazardous. Recently in Europe, a red rice appeared, also called "red koji," "red Chinese rice," or "red mold rice." This rice has been produced in China for centuries, with the use of molds *Monascus purpureus*. As early as in the fifteenth century, Chinese pharmacopeia described health-promoting properties of this rice, as it regulates consumers' lipid metabolism due to the presence of monacolin—a precursor of statins. However, some *Monascus* strains produce citrinin, an extremely harmful hepatonephrotoxin, which may produce dramatic health effects in consumers when the control of import is inadequate.

1.3 THE GLOBALIZATION OF FOOD PRODUCTION

Globalization is a process of changes in societies and economies, leading to an increasing interrelationship and integration of countries, societies, economies, and cultures. This integration applies to economic issues in particular. In Europe, it was initiated by establishing the European Free Trade Association (EFTA) in 1960. A free trade area among EFTA member states was formed in 1968. In 1992, the European Economic Community (EEC) and EFTA reached an agreement and formed a common free trade area for all goods. This agreement entered into force on January 1, 1994, and established the European Economic Area. In 1980, the United Nations Convention on Contracts for the International Sale of Goods (CISG) was signed in Vienna, which is a multilateral international treaty on the rules of international sale of goods. Until 2010, the convention had been ratified by 77 states. These agreements promote, among others, international food trade, which is also facilitated by opened boarders in the European Union (EU), the Customs Union abolishing customs duties within the EU, and the rapid development of road, sea, and air transport. All this strongly influences the development of the food industry and related food safety, as well as increasingly complex cross-border flows of raw materials and finished products (Hawkes 2006). Areas previously free from some hazards are currently exposed to the import of foods, often from different climate zones, contaminated by unknown types of micro-organisms. This poses an additional risk, especially for children, for example, due to the occurrence of viral diarrhea of unknown origin. Closer attention is also paid to adequate conditions of transportation and storage, especially considering the long logistic chains. A classic example of improper production and transportation was the case when in 1960 more than 100,000 turkeys on poultry farms in England died as a result of intoxication by feed contaminated by an aflatoxin from imported peanuts.

1.4 CHANGES IN PUBLIC HEALTH AND DIETARY HABITS

Health condition of a society is proportional to its wealth. The wealthier a society is, the more valued is human health and life (http://www.who.int/health-accounts/ghed/en/). These theses can be based not only on data on the expenditures of individual countries on disease prevention and treatment, but also on the comparison of infant mortality and average life expectancy. This stimulates medicine development and contributes to continuous introduction of new drugs. The effects are not only positive, but also negative. Among negative ones, there is suppressed immunity in patients due to frequent use of anticancer and immunosuppressive drugs. These medicines are widely used in therapies against cancer, autoimmune diseases, and allergies, as well as in patients after an organ transplant. As a result of the pharmacotherapy, there are an increasing number of people with suppressed immunity, for which an infection with even trivial micro-organisms may be life threatening. Therefore, even micro-organisms of low pathogenicity, when present in food, may pose a health risk. Moreover, the progress of civilization increases the number of allergic people. Previously, natural selection eliminated a large part of the population with this genetic predisposition. Asthmatic children usually died as a result of secondary pneumonia. Currently, they reach the reproductive age, and for both parents with allergies, the likelihood of having an allergic child increases by 20%–30%. Food allergies affect 4%–6% of children and 2%–3% of adults (Sicherer and Samson 2014). For these people, even trace amounts of allergens in food can be of dramatic consequences. The fact has been imposing increasingly rigorous "allergic hygiene" standards upon food manufacturers, so that finally a food allergy hazard analysis and critical control points (HACCP) system has been developed.

Increased risk for human health from food consumption is also associated with changing life styles, consumption patterns, and dietary habits. We live faster and differently. Many people eat out, which is a consequence of working time duration, and sometimes also of travel-to-work time. At home, a large number of families have made drastic changes in their dietary habits. Excessive amounts of crisps, chips, and other junk foods and beverages excessively sweetened with glucose–fructose syrup are consumed. As a result, a massive increase in obesity has occurred among the people of developed countries, followed by an increase in diabetes and cardiovascular diseases. Certain foods, for example, harden vegetable fats containing trans-fatty acids, which are formed during the partial hydrogenation of vegetable oils. Trans-fats double the risk of breast cancer and increase the level of bad cholesterol, low-density lipoprotein (LDL), which translates into an increased risk of atherosclerotic diseases. Denmark and Canada, in an attempt to solve this problem, require food manufacturers to report data on trans-fat content in their products on product labels and to reduce the content.

1.5 XENOBIOTICS IN THE ENVIRONMENT AND FOOD

Food safety should be a guarantee that no adverse effects occur in the human body after food ingestion. Over the centuries, humans have learned to avoid certain plant and animal species—recognized as inedible or even poisonous (Wilcock et al. 2004). Potential contaminants in foodstuff may be of a natural origin (e.g., bacterial and fungal toxins, amygdalin, and solanine) or may be absorbed from the polluted environment (e.g., nitrates (V), nitrates (III), heavy metals—lead, cadmium, mercury, residues of fertilizers and pesticides, dioxins, phthalates, and residues of veterinary drugs). Contaminants that accumulate in the organisms are considered as the most dangerous. A wide use of antibiotics in animal husbandry also became a serious problem, as it contributed to the transfer of antibiotic resistance from animals to humans. Significant sources of food contamination also include substances formed during technological processing and storage. This group consists of mycotoxins, nitrosamines, acrolein, epoxides, and other compounds.

Another group of food contaminants consists of foreign substances introduced to food products during technological processing. The group includes cleaning agents, preservatives, sweeteners, dyers, and chemical contaminants passing to food from the packaging and equipment.

A majority of chemical contaminants detected in foods are difficult or even impossible to avoid. These include certain metals, nitrates, *N*-nitroso compounds, pesticides, dioxins, dibenzofurans, PAHs, and other polyhalogenated polycyclic aromatic compounds. An important group is constituted by halogenated aromatic hydrocarbons, classified as persistent organic pollutants (POPs).

Some of the substances mentioned earlier (pesticide residues, dioxins, polychlorinated biphenyls, and other POPs) have been detected for many years in both aquatic and terrestrial environment worldwide, which is reflected in their constant, although gradually decreasing, presence in food.

1.6 CONCLUSIONS

Food safety, according to the Food and Agriculture Organization, is an important component of food security, that is, physical and economical access to food for each resident. Ensuring food safety is closely related to minimizing the risk of any side effects in the human body.

Food safety is an area of increasing global interest because of its direct impact on human health. Safe food is food that comes from a clean, unpolluted natural environment. Since 1960s, health hazards have been regarded not only in terms of microbiological, but also chemical food contamination. Currently, health quality and safety of food are among the most important criteria for consumers' assessment of food. For this reason, food quality assessment covers not only functional, sensory, esthetic, and hygienic aspects, but also the content of foreign chemicals (xenobiotics) in the product that may endanger human safety.

As shown in numerous studies, incorrect culinary or technological processing or improper storage may result in the formation of toxic compounds in foods, including acrolein, nitrosamines, and mycotoxins.

The most dangerous risks associated with the majority of xenobiotics are their carcinogenicity, teratogenicity, and endocrine-disrupting activity.

Among numerous chemical hazardous to human health, the leading ones are some of the natural substances, for example, mycotoxins, as well as anthropogenic compounds, which are environmental pollutants, or deliberately used chemicals, or by-products in various processes, for example, dioxins, dibenzofurans, pesticides, polychlorinated biphenyls, nitrates, and heavy metals.

At present, the problem of food contamination has become an important issue for food processing companies. It is reflected in the introduction of a "farm-to-table" system, which enables the control of the product since the very moment of raw materials harvesting, and further at all stages of production. Drawbacks to modern food production also include an extended way from raw materials to finished products, resulting from the phenomenon of globalization and multistage production of foods, for example, convenience foods.

Worth emphasizing is the fact that the occurrence of some groups of toxic compounds (pharmaceuticals, pesticides, additives, and preservatives) in food may be avoided or reduced to an acceptable level, provided that food security systems (e.g., HACCP, good manufacturing practice, and good hygiene practice) are appropriately implemented and used. A greater concern for food safety is also reflected in the introduction of increasingly stringent standards on acceptable levels of toxic chemicals in various types of foods.

At present, some risk is indicated with indiscriminate use of pesticides. Another important problem concerns malpractices in crop protection, usually resulting from disregarding the recommendations for proper use, which poses health risk to humans and animals. The size of population exposed to pesticides is difficult to estimate.

The most frequent effects include gastrointestinal dysfunctions, such as loss of appetite, nausea, dysgeusia, and vomiting, and also neurological disorders, such as headaches, dizziness, impaired balance, and hyperactivity (Gilden et al. 2010). Prenatal exposure to organophosphate pesticides may also significantly contribute to lower birth weights and decreased gestational ages (Rauch et al. 2012).

According to Sanghi et al. (2003), even low-dose exposures to chlorpyrifos during pregnancy and just after birth may inhibit DNA synthesis and reduce the number of neuronal cells in certain parts of the brain. It is suspected that even low-level exposure to chlorpyrifos early in life may adversely affect the function of the nervous system later in life.

Consumer education and reliable information on food composition from food manufacturers have become highly important because of potential hazards that may occur in both raw materials and processed food products.

REFERENCES

Beutin, L. and A. Martin. 2012. Outbreak of Shiga Toxin-Producing *Escherichia coli* (STEC) O104:H4 Infection in Germany Causes a Paradigm Shift with Regard to Human Pathogenicity of STEC Strains. *Journal of Food Proteins* 75(2): 408–418.

Gilden, R.C., K. Huffling, and B. Sattler. 2010. Pesticides and Health Risks. *Journal of Obstetric, Gynecologic, & Neonatal Nursing* 39(1): 103–110.

Hawkes, C. 2006. Uneven Dietary Development: Linking the Policies and Processes of Globalization with the Nutrition Transition, Obesity and Diet-Related Chronic Diseases. *Globalization and Health* 2: 4.

Rauch, S.A., J.M. Braun, D.B. Barr, A.M. Calafat, J. Khoury, M.A. Montesano, K. Yolton, and B. Weight. 2012. Associations of Prenatal Exposure to Organophosphate Pesticide Metabolites with Gestational Age and Birth Weight. *Environmental Health Perspectives* 120(7): 1055–1060.

Sanghi, R., M.K.K. Pillai, T.R. Jayalekshmi, and A. Nair. 2003. Organochlorine and Organophosphorus Pesticide Residues in Breast Milk from Bhopal, Madhya Pradesh, India. *Human & Experimental Toxicology* 22(2): 73–76.

Sicherer, S.H. and H.A. Sampson. 2014. Food Allergy: Epidemiology, Pathogenesis, Diagnosis, and Treatment. *Journal of Allergy and Clinical Immunology* 133(2): 291–307.

Szymczak B. and W. Dąbrowski. 2015. Effect of Filling Type and Heating Method on Prevalence of *Listeria species* and *L. monocytogenes* in dumplings produced in Poland. *Journal of Food Science* 80(5): M1060–M1065.

Wilcock, A., M. Pun, J. Khanona, and M. Aung. 2004. Consumer Attitudes, Knowledge and Behaviour: A Review of Food Safety Issues. *Trends in Food Science & Technology* 15: 56–66.

2 Natural Toxins of Plant Origin (Phytotoxins)

Kevin D. Welch, Stephen T. Lee, Daniel Cook, Benedict T. Green, and Kip E. Panter

CONTENTS

2.1 INTRODUCTION

Natural toxins, and specifically those produced by plants, have multiple and diverse functions that can either be detrimental or beneficial to both animals and humans. It has been argued for decades that many of these compounds serve as a defense mechanism to protect plants against herbivory, predation, or disease (reviewed by Wink 1999). Secondary compounds can protect a plant in various ways by imparting bitterness or causing discomfort or some other negative cue to inhibit herbivory, or it may be overtly toxic thus killing the predator, debilitating it, or causing an inherent aversion to the plant.

Plant secondary compounds may have other significant survival roles such as signals to attract insects, birds, or other animals to enhance pollination and/or seed dispersal. In addition to any potential functions, secondary compounds may concomitantly serve a physiologic function such as protection against UV light or frost, or provide a function of nitrogen transport and storage. In several instances, compounds can serve multiple functions in the same plant. Anthocyanins or monoterpenes can be insect attractants in flowers, but are insecticidal and antimicrobial at the same time in leaves (Wink 1999). Similarly, insects and other organisms have evolved with plants, thereby utilizing the protective mechanism of the plant. For example, a relationship between milkweeds and the Monarch butterfly demonstrates such a relationship between a plant and an insect (Harborne 1993). The larvae of the Monarch butterfly feed on milkweeds and accumulate cardenolides. Birds feeding on the caterpillar, pupa or adult, will vomit and subsequently become averted and thus avoid the Monarch butterflies. There are numerous other examples whereby plants, insects, large herbivores, and other organisms play an intertwined role in nature's balance. Multiple functions are typical of plant compounds and do not contradict in any way their main role as chemical defense and signal-induction compounds. If a trait serves multiple functions in a given plant or animal, it is more likely to survive the rigors of natural selection.

In general, plant parts that are important for survival and reproduction, such as flowers and seeds, will concentrate defense compounds. Consequently, compounds may be more rapidly synthesized or stored at certain stages of critical growth, that is, buds, young tissue, or seedlings. Many of these plant species rely on secondary compounds during early growth phase or seed phase, yet the vegetative and mature stages are protected by mechanical or morphological adaptations. Although plants have a limited capacity to replace or regenerate parts that are eaten, diseased, or damaged, secondary compounds are of major importance to promote survival.

The capacity for open growth and regeneration, which is prominent in perennials, allows for a margin of tolerance toward herbivores and microbes. While the role of secondary compounds in plant evolution is significant for survival, the impact on the health and wellbeing of man and animals may be beneficial or deleterious.

Over 100,000 secondary compounds have been identified including alkaloids, glycosides, proteins, polypeptides, amines and nonprotein amino acids, organic acids, alcohols, polyacetylenes, resinous toxins, and mineral toxins. For thousands of years, man has used some of these compounds as flavors, dyes, fragrances, insecticides, hallucinogens, nutritional supplements, animal or human poisons, and therapeutic/pharmaceutical agents. Volumes have been written on the natural toxins of plants. While the negative impact of plant toxins on livestock and humans has been the most publicized, the diversity of these toxins and their potential as new pharmaceutical agents for the treatment of diseases in humans and animals has received widespread interest in modern society. Scientists are actively screening plants from all regions of the world for bioactivity and potential pharmaceuticals for the treatment or prevention of many diseases. This chapter will focus on plants and their toxins that have been researched at the USDA-Agricultural Research Service, Poisonous Plant Research Laboratory (PPRL) in Logan, Utah, with casual mention of other relevant toxins affecting animals and humans.

2.2 ALKALOIDS

2.2.1 Introduction

An alkaloid is a basic, nitrogen-containing compound generally found in higher plants. Pelletier (1983) suggested that an alkaloid is a cyclic compound containing nitrogen in a negative oxidation state, which is of limited distribution in living organisms. Pelletier's definition includes alkaloids with nitrogen as part of a heterocyclic system and extracyclic bound nitrogen.

Several thousand alkaloids have been identified and characterized in plants. Over 20% of higher plant families contain alkaloids, thus alkaloids are the most ubiquitous and significant class of plant toxins (Blackwell 1990). Although alkaloids have been suggested to be waste byproducts of plant metabolism, they may play a role in binding ionic nitrogen needed by seedlings. Alkaloids were initially associated with members of the plant kingdom, but more and more alkaloid compounds are being discovered in micro-organisms, fungi, marine invertebrates, insects, and higher animals (Roberts and Wink 1998). Many of these alkaloids have led to the discovery of new pharmaceuticals and the treatment of disease in man and animals.

Bitter alkaloids may have evolved a universal role in plant chemical defense as a feeding deterrent. Quinine, strychnine, and brucine are extremely bitter alkaloids. However, there are little data on animal/plant relationships that show bitterness is the only controlling factor in preventing herbivore ingestion of poisonous plants. There are many examples of animals eating plants that, in human terms, are "bitter as gall." Wink et al. (1993) partially disproved the bitterness theory in a feeding trial with geese, in which the birds avoided essential oils but tolerated bitter alkaloids.

2.2.2 Piperidine Alkaloids

Piperidine alkaloids are widely distributed in nature, mostly in plants, but also in lower animals such as Nemertine worms. Of the hundreds of piperidine alkaloids known, most are derived by 1 of 3 biosynthetic pathways in the plant using the building blocks of lysine, acetate, or mevalonate as precursors (reviewed by Panter and Keeler 1989). The common nucleus of all piperidine alkaloids is the piperidine ring (Figure 2.1). Some of the more simple-structured piperidines follow the lysine and acetate pathways, while the more complex ones use mevalonate. Acetate-derived piperidine alkaloids are common in nature in plants and lower animals. For example, the simple piperidines in poison hemlock, gamma-coniceine and coniine, are acetate pathway derived. Likewise, anabaseine, also acetate pathway derived and a known tobacco alkaloid, has been identified as a poison gland product of *Aphaenogaster* ants and various 2,6-disubstituted piperidine alkaloids have been isolated from the fire ant (*Solenopsis saevissima*), in which these alkaloids function as attractants (Roberts and Wink 1998). More than 100 different alkaloids (many of them piperidine) have been isolated from neotropical frogs of the *Dendrobatidae* family, and others have been identified in numerous microorganisms.

The piperidine alkaloids are historically significant because of the ancient Greek practice of executing criminals with poison-hemlock tea. Early literature refers to human poisoning more frequently than animal poisoning. Even today, accidental human poisonings occasionally occur; however, most current reports involve ingestion by livestock species. A human incident was reported by Frank et al. (1995) in which a 6-year-old boy and his father were successfully treated for accidental poison-hemlock poisoning. After ingesting young poison-hemlock leaves, the boy became unresponsive and was then hospitalized. After plant identification and appropriate hospital treatment, the boy recovered completely. One of the most famous historical accounts of poison hemlock is the execution of the philosopher Socrates, who was sentenced to death by drinking hemlock tea after he was convicted of introducing new divinities into the philosophy of that day. A historical account of Socrates' death was published by Daugherty (1995).

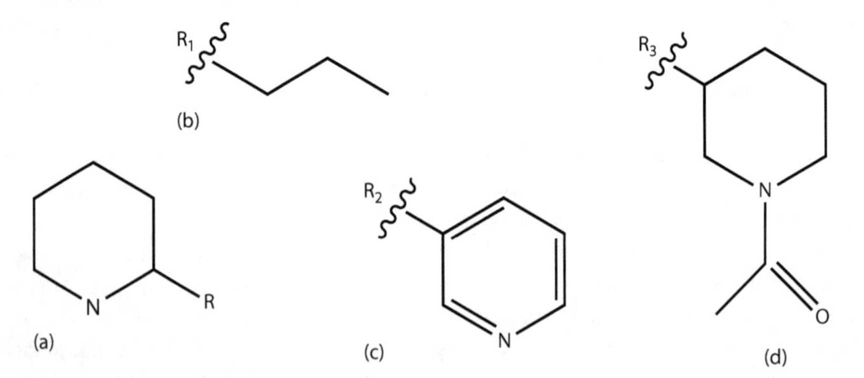

FIGURE 2.1 Piperidine ring (a) and three functionalities of three carbons or larger that impart teratogenic activity, that is, coniine (R_1), anabasine (R_2), and ammodendrine (R_3), respectively b, c, d.

In ancient times, *Conium* seed was collected green, dried, and stored to be used medicinally as a sedative. The dried leaf and juice of *Conium maculatum* were listed in pharmacopoeias of London and Edinburgh from 1864 to 1898, and the last official record appeared in Great Britain in the British Pharmaceutical Codex of 1934. Interest in the medicinal value of poison hemlock has declined because of the unpredictability of its effects. The unpredictability is now understood as the toxin profile, and concentration in the plant and green seed can vary dramatically because of environmental factors or even diurnally. Poison hemlock also has historical significance to researchers because coniine was the first alkaloid discovered in 1827 and first synthesized in 1886 (Landenburg 1886; reviewed by Panter and Keeler 1989).

Poison hemlock contains three major and five minor alkaloids. The toxicity and teratogenic effects of the three major alkaloids from poison hemlock have been compared (Figure 2.2). Gamma-coniceine usually predominates in early vegetative stages of plant growth, and coniine and *N*-methyl coniine usually predominate in seed and mature plant. Gamma-coniceine is the precursor to all the other poison-hemlock alkaloids. Gamma-coniceine is 7–8 times more toxic in a mammalian bioassay compared to coniine, which is 1.5–2 times more toxic than *N*-methyl coniine (Figure 2.2). The pharmacological activity is similar among these alkaloids but varies in potency because of structural differences. Pharmacological studies with *Conium* alkaloids have demonstrated that they act as stereoselective nicotinic acetylcholine receptor agonists (Lee et al. 2013). Peripheral actions on smooth muscle are initiated by ganglionic stimulation and subsequent receptor desensitization, which explains some of the early clinical signs of stimulation to the gastrointestinal (GI) tract and urinary system. Spinal reflexes are later blocked, which has been attributed to the increased membrane permeability to potassium ions. Pharmacologically, the properties of all three alkaloids are very similar, except gamma-coniceine is more stimulatory to autonomic ganglia and *N*-methyl coniine has a greater desensitizing effect (Fodor and Colasanti 1985).

The teratogenic effects of poison hemlock are well known and have been described in cattle, sheep, goats, and pigs (Panter et al. 1999; Green et al. 2013a). Numerous field cases of poisoning and subsequent malformations have been reported. The mechanism of action, susceptible stages of pregnancy, and detailed descriptions of the teratogenic effects have been reviewed by Panter et al. (2013b) and Green et al. (2013a, 2013b).

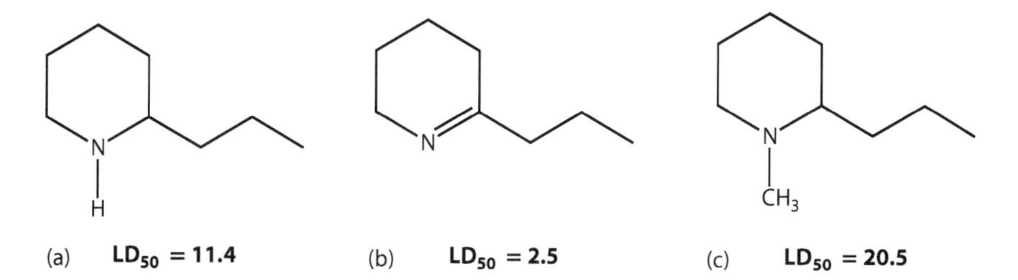

FIGURE 2.2 Three piperidine alkaloid teratogens from *Conium maculatum* (poison-hemlock) with accompanying LD_{50} as determined in a mouse bioassay: coniine (a), gamma-coniceine (b), and *N*-methyl coniine (c).

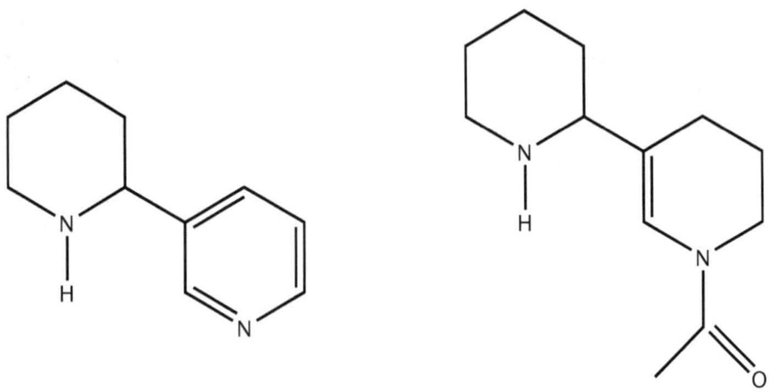

(a) $LD_{50} = 1.6$ (b) $LD_{50} = 134.4$

FIGURE 2.3 Piperidine teratogens from *Nicotiana glauca* (anabasine [a]) and *Lupinus formosus* (ammodendrine [b]).

In addition to poison-hemlock alkaloids, *Nicotiana* species and certain lupine species also contain potent toxic and teratogenic piperidine alkaloids (Figure 2.3). All teratogenic piperidine alkaloids have certain structural characteristics that are required for induction of birth defects. The molecular structure includes a piperidine ring with a side chain of at least three carbons or larger attached to the ring adjacent to the nitrogen atom (Figure 2.1). The structural characteristics were first proposed by Keeler and Balls (1978), and all experiments since that time have supported this theory. The structural requirement for teratogenicity is thought to occur because the alkaloids bind to the nicotinic acetylcholine receptors of the neuromuscular junction. Fetal clinical effects include a significant reduction in fetal movement during critical stages of gestation. Just as fetal movement helps prevent skeletal contracture malformations, fetal movement is critical in the prevention of cleft palate. The stage of gestation when the fetus is exposed to alkaloids is related to the type of malformation manifested. Malformations are the same and the mechanism of action is the same for all piperidine alkaloids possessing structural characteristics as discussed above.

In addition to lupines, poison hemlock, and *Nicotiana* spp., other plant species of the genera *Genista*, *Prosopis*, *Lobelia*, *Cytisus*, *Sophora*, *Pinus*, *Punica*, *Duboisia*, *Sedum*, *Withania*, *Carica*, *Hydrangea*, *Dichroa*, *Cassia*, *Ammondendron*, *Liparia*, and *Colidium* contain potentially toxic and teratogenic piperidine alkaloids. Many plant species or varieties from these genera may be included in animal and human diets (Keeler and Crowe 1984).

2.2.3 Quinolizidine Alkaloids

Quinolizidine alkaloids are mainly found in genera of the Fabaceae (Legume) family, a large and commercially important family that contains hundreds of quinolizidine alkaloids. More than 150 quinolizidine alkaloids have been structurally identified and characterized in lupines alone (Kinghorn and Balandrin 1984). Significant genera containing quinolizidine alkaloids include *Lupinus*, *Laburnum*, *Cytisus*, *Thermopsis*, and *Sophora*. Most of these genera contain the teratogen anagyrine (Figure 2.4).

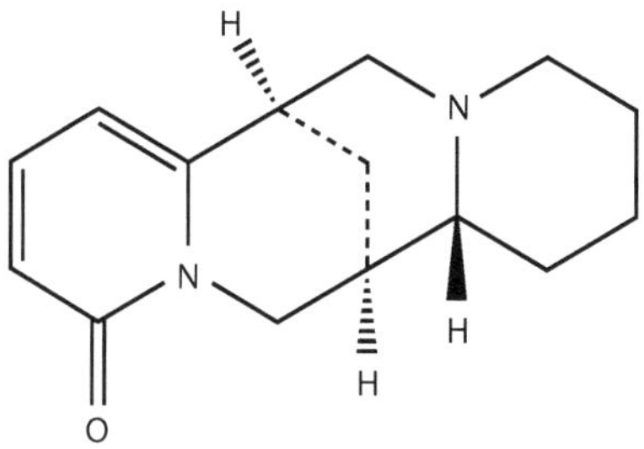

FIGURE 2.4 Teratogenic quinolizidine alkaloid anagyrine from *Lupinus* spp.

The common structural feature of quinolizidine alkaloids is a decalin ring system with a nitrogen atom at one vertex. Often a second or third nitrogen atom is incorporated into additional six-membered rings. Bicyclic, tricyclic, tetracyclic, and even more complex alkaloids with 5–10 rings have been characterized (Keeler 1989).

Lupinus spp. (lupines) contain both quinolizidine and piperidine alkaloids that are toxic and teratogenic. Eighteen western US lupine species have been reported to contain the teratogen anagyrine (Figure 2.4), with 14 of these containing teratogenic levels (Davis and Stout 1986). Two species, *L. formosus* and *L. arbustus*, contain teratogenic levels of the piperidine alkaloid ammodendrine (Figure 2.4; Panter et al. 1998). Lupine alkaloids are produced by leaf chloroplasts and are translocated via the phloem and stored in epidermal cells and in seeds (Wink et al. 1995).

Quinolizidine alkaloid content and profile varies between lupine species and in individual plants depending on environmental conditions, season of the year, and stage of plant growth (Wink and Carey 1994). Alkaloid content (per gram of plant) may be highest during early growth stages, decreasing through the bud stage, and concentrating in the flowers and maturing seeds. Seed pods contain high protein levels and high concentrations of alkaloids.

The effects of site and elevation on alkaloid content have been described by Carey and Wink (1994). Total alkaloid content decreases as elevation increases and was shown to be six times higher in plants at 2,700 m versus plants collected at 3,500 m. This phenomenon persisted even when seedlings from the highest and lowest elevations were grown under identical greenhouse conditions, thus suggesting evolutionary differences genetically.

2.2.3.1 Mechanism of Action

The proposed mechanism of action for lupine-induced malformations and cleft palate in cattle has been elucidated using a goat model. Using ultrasound imaging, Panter et al. (1990) hypothesized that the mechanism for induced contracture defects and cleft palate involves a chemically induced reduction in fetal movement much as one would expect with a sedative, neuromuscular blocking agent, or anesthetic. The proposed mechanism of action was supported by experiments using radio ultrasound where a direct relationship was recorded between reduced fetal activity and severity of contracture-type skeletal defects and cleft palate in sheep and goats (Panter et al. 1990; Weinzweig et al. 2008). Further research suggests that this inhibition of fetal movement must be over a protracted period of time during specific stages of gestation.

2.2.3.2 Biomedical Application

The establishment of appropriate animal models for biomedical application is essential if new techniques and procedures are to be applied to human conditions. The syndrome of plant-induced cleft palate and contracture skeletal malformations in livestock (crooked calf syndrome) is the same whether it is induced by *Lupinus*, *Conium*, or *Nicotiana* spp. Likewise, the malformations are described as the same in cattle, sheep, goats, and pigs. A small ruminant (goat) model was developed primarily to study the mechanism of action of "crooked calf syndrome." However, interest in the induced congenital cleft palate and the goat model led to biomedical applications (Panter et al. 2000a; Weinzweig et al. 2006).

Cleft palates induced by toxic plants in the goat model closely mimic the human cleft condition (Weinzweig et al. 1999a, 1999b). This model is also useful for histological comparison of the prenatal and postnatal repaired cleft palate and comparison of craniofacial growth and development. Therefore, the goat model provides an ideal congenital model to study the etiology of cleft palate in humans, for development of fetal surgical techniques *in utero*, and to compare palate histology after prenatal or postnatal repair. The biomedical application of these plants and the specific animal model selected has evolved over time and occurred because of the discovery of certain specific biological effects in the goat and their relationship with similar conditions in humans (Panter et al. 2000b; Weinzweig et al. 2008).

Recent research has focused on the privileged period of fetal scarless healing and development of *in utero* surgical procedures to repair human cleft palates early in gestation. To emphasize the significance of this research, Jeff Weinzweig stated, "Children born with cleft palate often undergo a series of operations to correct the ensuing deformities, only the first of which is the actual palate repair at the age of 6–12 months. For many children, speech remains a major problem as well as craniofacial development. Our goal, of course, is to eliminate the need for any of these reconstructive procedures by performing the cleft palate repair *in utero*. Never, more than now, in the age of fetal surgery has this been a real possibility. Despite this, what is truly exciting is that we now have a congenital goat model of cleft palate as well as the model of *in utero* cleft repair." Therefore, the biomedical value of the goat model using *N. glauca* plant or anabasine-rich extracts to induce cleft palates has been applied to human medicine (Weinzweig et al. 2008).

While fetal surgical intervention in life-threatening circumstances has been demonstrated, the role of fetal intervention (surgery) in the treatment of non-life-threatening congenital anomalies remains a source of much debate. Recently, Weinzweig et al. (2002) described and characterized a congenital model for cleft palate in the goat, presented the methodology and techniques used to successfully repair congenital cleft palates *in utero*, and demonstrated successful scarless palatal healing and development after repair. This model closely simulates the etiopathogenesis of the human anomaly. Thus, *in utero* cleft palate repair early in gestation (on or before day 85 in the goat) is feasible and results in scarless healing of the soft and hard palates. Furthermore, this congenital cleft palate goat model is highly reproducible, with little variation representing an ideal animal model.

In summary, this research has significant implications in the management of fetal cleft palates in humans and application in the study of the etiology and treatment for agricultural research. Understanding periods of fetal susceptibility, elucidating teratogenic plants and toxins there from, and understanding mechanisms of action will provide information to limit the adverse effects of these plant toxins.

2.2.4 Steroidal Alkaloids and Steroidal Glycoalkaloids

Steroidal alkaloids and steroidal glycoalkaloids are common toxins found in the Liliaceae and Solanaceae families, respectively. *Veratrum* spp. (false hellebore) and *Zigadenus* spp. (death camas) from the lily family, and *Solanum* spp. (nightshades, potato, eggplant, and Jerusalem cherry) and *Lycopersicon* (tomato) from the Solanaceae family are reported to be toxic and some are teratogenic (Gaffield and Keeler 1994). Over 1,100 steroidal alkaloids have been characterized, and toxicity information is known for many of these. These alkaloids are generally divided into solanum and veratrum or jerveratrum classes based on structural features and biological activity. Table 2.1 illustrates the relative potency of 13 of these alkaloids in a hamster bioassay (Gaffield and Keeler 1994).

2.2.4.1 Solanum Glycoalkaloids

Solanum spp. are distributed worldwide and have been responsible for numerous cases of livestock and human poisoning. Because of their importance as food plants, particularly the potato, there have been numerous studies done to assess the distribution and concentration of glycoalkaloids in different plant parts.

TABLE 2.1
Steroidal Alkaloids Found in *Veratrum* spp. and *Solanum* spp. with their Relative Teratogenic Potency, as Determined in a Hamster Assay

Alkaloid	Teratogenicity
Tomatidine	0
Tomatine	1
5α,6-Dihydrosolasodine	4
Solasodine	6
5α,6-Dihydrosolanidine	10
α-Solanine	35
Solanidine	35
Cyclopamine	35
5α,6,12β,13α-Tetrahydrojervine	40
22*S*,25*R*-Solanidanes	50
α-Chaconine	50
12β,13α-Dihydrojervine	60
Jervine	100

Source: Gaffield, W. and R.F. Keeler, *Pure Appl. Chem.*, 66, 2407–2410, 1994.

The chemistry of the potato, including tubers, vines, and sprouts, has been reported by Sharma and Salunkhe (1989). For example, the flesh of the tuber is the lowest at 12–50 μg/g, followed by the skins at 300–600 μg/g, the leaves at 400–1,000 μg/g, and sprouts and flowers at 2,000–5,000 μg/g (values represented as total glycoalkaloid). As would be expected, the photosynthesizing parts contain the highest concentration of the glycoalkaloids, and for this reason, vines and the green and sprouted potatoes are usually removed from the human food supply. However, these green culled potatoes, and occasionally the vines, are fed to livestock, especially when regional feed sources have become scarce. Sometimes this practice has caused severe poisoning and death.

The structural features of the solanum alkaloids are based on two primary skeletal configurations; (1) solanidane, with or without glycoside functionalities as featured by the toxic and teratogenic steroidal alkaloids α-chaconine and α-solanine with the indolizidine type E-F ring (Figure 2.5a) or (2) the spirosolane configuration represented by the nonteratogenic alkaloids tomatine or tomatidine with spirofused E and F rings (Gaffield and Keeler 1994; Figure 2.5b). Both classes are represented by alkaloids with or without glycoside functionality. A number of *Solanum* spp. have caused poisoning in livestock. *Solanum fastigiatum*, *S. kwebense*, and *S. dimidiatum* have induced cerebellar degeneration in cattle including progressive degeneration and vacuolation of Purkinje cells (Cheeke 1998). The lesions appear as a lysosomal storage disease similar to that caused by locoweeds. These plants contain the solanidane-type alkaloids with the indolizidine configuration of the E-F rings like that found in locoweeds (Figure 2.5b; see indolizidine section).

Little data have been reported on the alkaloid profiles or concentrations of the wild *Solanum* spp. (nightshades). Livestock poisoning has been reported from black

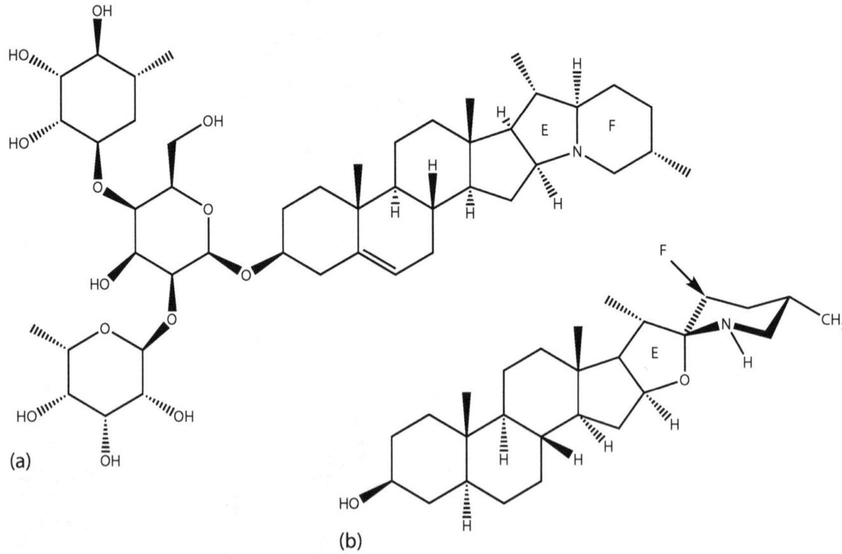

FIGURE 2.5 Two steroidal alkaloids from *Solanum* spp., that is, one with teratogenic activity (α-chaconine [a]) and the nonteratogenic alkaloid tomatidine (b).

nightshade (*S. nigrum*), climbing nightshade (*S. dulcamara*), and silverleaf nightshade (*S. eleagnifolium*). Clinical effects from ingestion of these species include gastrointestinal upset and associated problems such as diarrhea and reduced feed intake. A neurological effect from the inhibition of acetylcholinesterase has also been reported (reviewed by Beasley 1997).

Other plants of the nightshade family contain atropine-like toxins, including *Atropa belladonna* (deadly nightshade), *Hyoscyamus niger* (black henbane), and *Datura stramonium* (Jimson weed) that are anticholinergic, blocking the muscarinic receptors. Atropine and atropine-like alkaloids are discussed in a later section in this chapter.

2.2.4.2 Veratrum and Zigadenus Alkaloids

Steroidal alkaloids found in the Liliaceae family, primarily *Veratrum* and *Zigadenus*, have been responsible for large losses in livestock. Human and livestock deaths have occurred from accidental ingestion of death camas (Panter et al. 1987). Thousands of lambs have died or been destroyed because of *Veratrum*-induced malformations, most notably a craniofacial defect called cyclopia (Binns et al. 1965; James 1999). Tracheal stenosis, skeletal malformations, and early embryonic death are also common (Keeler and Young 1986), along with abnormalities in placentation (Welch et al. 2012b). *Zigadenus* has caused overt poisoning in sheep and cattle although no teratogenic effects have been reported.

The steroidal alkaloids in *Veratrum* and *Zigadenus* are divided into two classes: the jerveratrum and ceveratrum types (Figure 2.6a,b). These alkaloids have a

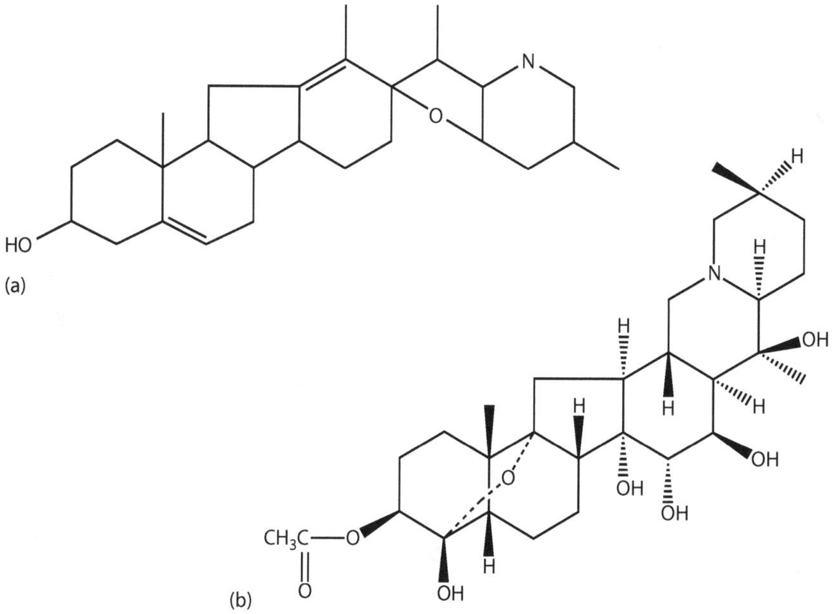

FIGURE 2.6 The steroidal alkaloid teratogen cyclopamine (a) from *Veratrum* spp. and the nonteratogenic alkaloid zygacine (b) from *Zigadenus* spp.

modified cyclopentanoperhydrophenanthrene ring structure (steroid skeleton) with C-nor-D-homo with a contracted C-ring and an expanded D-ring (Gaffield 2000). Jerveratrum alkaloids have alkamines with one, two, or three oxygen atoms, and occur as such or as monoglycosides. Ceveratrum alkaloids have seven, eight, or nine oxygens, and occur as free alkamines or esters of simple aliphatic or aromatic acids. They do not occur as glycosides. Several structural variations around the nitrogen portion of the veratrum alkaloids are found in the plant including the highly bioactive teratogens jervine, cyclopamine, and the glucose glycoside cycloposine.

2.2.4.2.1 Veratrum Alkaloids

Jerveratrum alkaloids were responsible for multiple congenital defects in sheep when pregnant ewes grazed *Veratrum* plants during specific stages of gestation (Keeler 1986; Welch et al. 2009). Because of the *Veratrum*-induced anomalies and their relationship to human conditions, the steroidal alkaloids have become important tools or probes to study developmental processes involving craniofacial, limb, and foregut morphogenesis. During gastrulation, the embryo undergoes several morphogenetic events that lead to differentiation of the three primary germ layers: the gut (endoderm); the muscles, bones, and connective tissue (mesoderm); and the skin and nervous tissue (ectoderm; reviewed by Gaffield 2000).

The Sonic hedgehog gene and the Hedgehog (Hh) family of secreted proteins play key roles in developmental processes ranging from bone morphogenesis to neurological differentiation (reviewed by Gaffield 2000). Sonic hedgehog directs the intercellular signals between germ layers at the time of differentiation and was shown to be responsible for the induction of the cyclopic malformation in sheep from *Veratrum*. The link between *Veratrum*-induced cyclopia in sheep and the inhibition of the Sonic hedgehog gene pathway resulted from research on mouse embryos that lacked functional copies of Sonic hedgehog that caused several forms of holoprosencephaly (Chiang et al. 1996; Maity et al. 2005). Subsequently, cyclopamine and jervine were shown to specifically inhibit the Sonic hedgehog gene pathway causing the various forms of holoprosencephaly (Cooper et al. 1998). Sonic hedgehog also regulates other processes controlled by genes downstream and is intimately involved in the development of limbs, skin, eye, lung, teeth, nervous system, and differentiation of sperm and cartilage (Hammerschmidt et al. 1997).

2.2.4.2.2 Zigadenus Alkaloids

Zigadenus spp. (death camas) contain several steroidal alkaloids of the ceveratrum type (with 7, 8, or 9 oxygens, and the nitrogen incorporated into a quinolizidine ring; Figure 2.6b). The most known alkaloids are zygacine and zygadenine (Welch et al. 2011). While the alkaloids are similar in structure to *Veratrum* alkaloids, they are not thought to be teratogenic and they impart a different clinical toxicosis. All parts of the plant, especially the bulb, are toxic. The alkaloids decrease blood pressure, slow heart rate, and may cause pulmonary congestion before death (Welch et al. 2013). Poisoning generally occurs in sheep, but cattle, horses, pigs, and humans have all been poisoned (Panter et al. 1987).

2.2.4.2.3 Potential Biomedical Applications of Cyclopamine

A variety of diseases and clinical disorders result from mutations in the human Sonic hedgehog gene and associated pathways. Hedgehog is known to regulate downstream genes called Patched, Smoothened, or Gli (Hammerschmidt et al. 1997; Rimkus et al. 2016). Since cyclopamine selectively inhibits the hedgehog pathway, it makes perfect sense that *Veratrum* alkaloids (cyclopamine) could provide tools or probes to investigate hedgehog-associated diseases in humans. Among the associated diseases are not only holoprosencephaly and various tumors, but also several forms of polydactyly that are derived from genetic defects in hedgehog network genes. Holoprosencephaly syndrome in humans is relatively common in early embryogenesis, occurring in 1 of 250 spontaneous abortions and 1 in 16,000 live births (Matsunaga and Shiota 1977). Cyclopamine's ability, both to induce holoprosencephaly in experimental animals and to strongly inhibit Sonic hedgehog signal transduction, offers the potential to enhance understanding of human brain and spinal cord development at the cellular and molecular levels (Gaffield and Keeler 1996). Other genetic disorders have been associated with the hedgehog gene and the downstream genes (Patched, Smoothened, or Gli) that are positively or negatively regulated by the hedgehog proteins (reviewed by Gaffield et al. 2000). For example, Patched, Smoothened, and Gli have been implicated in basal cell nervous syndrome, rhabdomyosarcoma, medulloblastomas, and primitive neuroectodermal tumors. These genes are regulated downstream from Sonic hedgehog. In addition, Patched mutations have been identified in breast carcinoma, a meningioma, esophageal squamous carcinoma, and trichoepithelioma. Activating mutations in Smoothened are often found in sporadic basal cell carcinomas and primitive neuroectodermal tumors. Cyclopamine or its derivatives, because of their ability to regulate hedgehog genes, have been proposed as potential mechanism-based therapeutic agents for the treatment of tumors arising from the disruption of components of the hedgehog pathway. Hedgehog inhibitors such as cyclopamine might be effective in controlling the onset or progression of certain lesions or disease states in non-pregnant adults because of the low toxicity of drug levels that are effective in blocking Sonic hedgehog (Taipale et al. 2000). Several pharmaceutical companies have investigated the potential of cyclopamine, or other Sonic hedgehog pathway inhibitors, as a therapy for several types of cancer. The US FDA has approved two inhibitors of Sonic hedgehog signaling pathway for the treatment of adults with metastatic basal cell carcinoma, or with locally advanced basal cell carcinoma that has recurred following surgery or who are not candidates for surgery, and who are not candidates for radiation (Rimkus et al. 2016), with promising initial results (Basset-Seguin et al. 2015).

Cyclopamine also interferes with cholesterol metabolism that results in decreased cholesterol synthesis and the accumulation of late biosynthetic intermediates. Cyclopamine was evaluated as an inhibitor of multi-drug resistance in tumor cells. Intrinsic or acquired resistance of tumor cells to cytotoxic drugs is a major cause of failure of chemotherapy. Both cyclopamine and the spirosolane alkaloid tomatidine from tomatoes act as potent and effective chemosensitizers in multidrug resistant cells (Lavie et al. 2001). Therefore, plant steroidal alkaloids such as cyclopamine and tomatidine, or their analogs, may serve as chemosensitizers in combination with chemotherapy and conventional cytotoxic drugs for treating multi-drug-resistant cancers.

Pancreatic development in the embryo was enhanced upon exposure to cyclopamine. Cyclopamine inhibition of Sonic hedgehog signaling apparently permits the expansion of portions of the endodermal region of the foregut where Sonic hedgehog signaling does not occur, resulting in pancreatic differentiation in a larger area of the foregut endoderm (Kim and Melton 1998), thus providing a tool in the treatment of pancreatic diseases and development of cell-replacement therapies or an artificial pancreas.

2.2.4.3 Norditerpenoid Alkaloids

Over 40 norditerpenoid alkaloids have been reported in species of larkspurs; toxicity data in a mammalian system for 25 of these have been reported by the PPRL (reviewed by Panter et al. 2002). The commonality among all the wild larkspur species is the presence of norditerpenoid alkaloids. These alkaloid toxins are of three general classes based on chemical structural features: (1) the lycoctonine type; (2) the 7,8-methylene-dioxylycoctonine (MDL) types (deltaline); and (3) the *N*-(methylsuccinimido)-anthranoyllycoctonine (MSAL) types (MLA) (Figure 2.7a–c). These distinct structural features have been correlated to their toxic activity. The MSAL type alkaloids (Figure 2.7c) and, in particular, methyllycaconitine (MLA), nudicauline (NUD), and 14-deacetynudicauline (14-DAN), are the toxic alkaloids responsible for the majority of poisonings by larkspurs (Welch et al. 2015a). Deltaline (Figure 2.7b) of the MDL type, though much less toxic, is prevalent in most larkspur populations, and if present in high-enough concentrations, will exacerbate the toxic effects of the MSAL alkaloids (Welch et al. 2012a). Deltaline by itself would not be a significant threat to livestock, unless toxic levels of the MSAL alkaloids are present (Cook et al. 2011). The lycoctonine type alkaloids (Figure 2.7a) are the least toxic and are found in variable concentrations in larkspurs.

The norditerpenoid alkaloids are potent neuromuscular poisons in mammals, acting at the post-synaptic neuromuscular junction. Clinical signs of larkspur poisoning in cattle include respiratory depression, tremors in locomotor muscles, failure of voluntary muscular coordination, and collapse (Green et al. 2009). Variations in

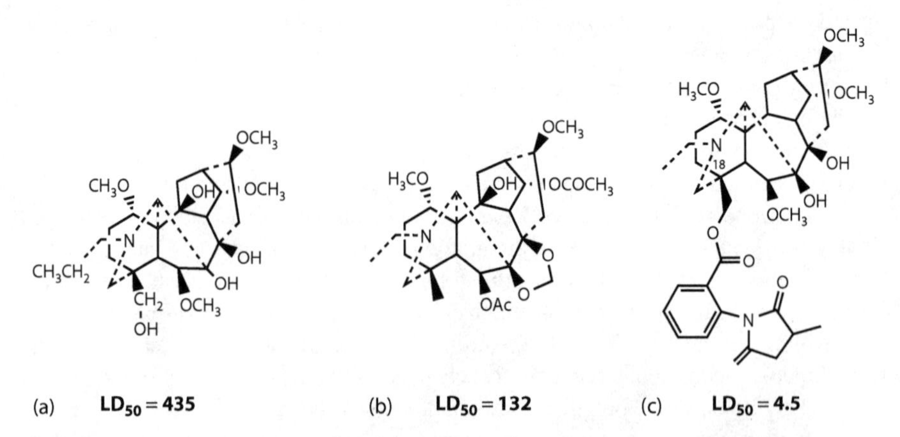

FIGURE 2.7 Norditerpenoid alkaloids from larkspurs including lycoctonine (lycoctonine type), deltaline (MDL type), and methyllycaconitine (MSAL type) with accompanying LD_{50}.

structural features of each norditerpenoid alkaloid can exacerbate or reduce toxicity. While the mechanism of action of the norditerpenoid alkaloids involves blocking of neuromuscular transmission at the nicotinic acetylcholine receptors, relative toxicity of individual alkaloids is observed to change with variations in the structural characteristics of the alkaloids (Dobelis et al. 1999). In comparison with the lycoctonine and MDL-type alkaloids, the high toxicity of the three MSAL-type alkaloids (NUD, 14-DAN, and MLA) can be associated with the presence of a methylsuccinylanthranoyl ester at C18 (Figure 2.7c). Removal of the ester functionality from MLA, thereby forming lycoctonine (Figure 2.7a), eliminates the neuromuscular activity.

The larkspur species are generally divided into three categories: (1) tall larkspurs (*D. barbeyi*, *D. occidentale*, *D. glaucescens*, *D. brownii*, and *D. glaucum*), 1–2 m in height, generally growing in moist high-mountain habitats above 2,400 m; (2) intermediate larkspurs (*D. geyeri*; plains larkspur), 0.6–1 m tall and present on the short-grass prairies of Wyoming, Colorado, and Nebraska; and (3) low larkspurs (*D. andersonii* and *D. nuttallianum*), which generally grow on the desert/semi-desert, foothill, or low mountain ranges and are less than 0.6 m tall (Nielsen and Ralphs 1987; Majak et al. 2000). However, the risk that larkspurs pose can vary tremendously between different populations of the same species of larkspur due to differences in their norditerpenoid alkaloid profiles (Cook et al. 2009a).

2.2.4.4 Pyrrolizidine Alkaloids

Pyrrolizidine alkaloids (PA) are common in three plant families, that is, Fabaceae (*Crotalaria* spp.), Asteraceae (*Senecio* spp.), and Boraginaceae (*Amsinckia*, *Borago*, *Cynoglossum*, *Echium*, *Heliotropium*, and *Symphytum*). There are over 1,200 *Senecio* spp. throughout the world, with many containing toxic PAs (Cheeke 1998). Over 250 species of *Senecio* are endemic to South Africa (Kellerman et al. 1988), 128 spp. to Brazil (Habermehl et al. 1988), and over 200 to Chile (Smith and Culvenor 1981). PA poisoning is a worldwide problem in animals and humans, and is a significant impediment to international trade because of contaminated or potentially contaminated animal feeds and human foods (Huxtable and Cooper 2000; Edgar and Smith 2000). PA can enter the human food chain via contaminated grains, milk, honey, eggs, and other foods or herbal products. In 1992, the German Federal Health Bureau established intake limits for PAs. Regulations specified that 0.1 microgram was the maximum daily amount of hepatotoxic PAs and their N-oxides from herbal plants or plant extracts. Prescribing herbal products containing PAs to pregnant or lactating women is strictly prohibited. Intake limitations and restrictions of use have created trade restrictions with various countries.

Human poisonings have been common throughout the world and numerous cases have been reported (Huxtable and Cooper 2000). These cases are generally veno-occlusive disease, manifest as abdominal distention due to ascitic fluid. Pulmonary disease, vertigo, and vomiting have also been reported. Human cases of 1 or 2, or up to 50 or 60, are common, but larger death losses have been reported, such as over 3,900 in Tajikistan in 1993 and 7,200 in Afghanistan in 1976 from *Heliotropium*, several hundred in the West Indies from *Crotalaria* and *Senecio* in 1954, and over 200 in Uzbekistan in 1950 from *Trichodesma* are reported. Some PAs and the pyrroles are carcinogenic (Brown et al. 2015).

Recent research at the PPRL provided chemical profiles of three plants with significant impact on humans (Colegate et al. 2005; 2012; 2014b). Comfrey (*Symphytum officianale*) is a common herbal product used by people, Sun Hemp (*Crotalaria juncea*) is increasingly used as a green manure in crop rotations, and *Echium plantagineum* is a noxious species with impact on honey quality. A recent study completed at the PPRL compared the toxicity of an alkaloid extract from a commercially available comfrey product with two pure alkaloids, lycopsamine and intermedine, in a chicken model (Brown et al. 2015; Colegate et al. 2014a). The alkaloid extract was more toxic than either lycopsamine or intermedine, suggesting that risk of using the comfrey product is unacceptable. Exposure to DHPAs may be intentional, such as use of comfrey products, or it may be unintentional from contamination of bread, pastries, cereal grains, honey products, eggs, milk, or other food products. As part of this overall research approach, Brown et al. (2014) demonstrated the utility of a heterozygous p53 knockout mouse model for screening DHPAs for carcinogenicity. Brown's group used riddelliine as the test DHPA and dosed p53 mice at different amounts and over multiple time periods ranging from 14 days to 12 months. The most common neoplasm was hepatic hemangiosarcoma and tumors developed in a time- and dose-dependent manner. Another common lesion observed was angiectasis.

Structurally, PAs contain two fused five-member rings with a nitrogen at one of the vertices (necine base; Figure 2.8a) and one or more branched carboxylic acids attached as esters to one or two of the necine hydroxyl groups (Figure 2.8a–c). The PAs in toxic plants are of three general classes, that is, monoesters, noncyclic diesters, and cyclic diesters. Most hepatotoxic PAs are esters of the base retronecine or heliotridine, and diastereomers of each other with opposing configuration at the C7 position of the pyrrolizidine nucleus (Figure 2.8b). Cyclic diesters (Figure 2.8c) are the most toxic, noncyclic diesters are of intermediate toxicity, and monoesters least toxic (Cheeke 1998). The heliotridine esters are more reactive than the retronecine esters.

For PAs to be toxic, there are certain key structural features necessary, that is, a double bond in the 1, 2 position of the PA nucleus and branching in the ester group. The PAs that are more easily hydrolyzed by esterases produce less toxic pyrroles upon liver activation. However, PAs with more branching in the side chains produce more toxic pyrroles because hydrolysis is hindered, allowing the PA to get to the liver where toxic activation occurs. These toxic pyrroles are powerful alkylating agents

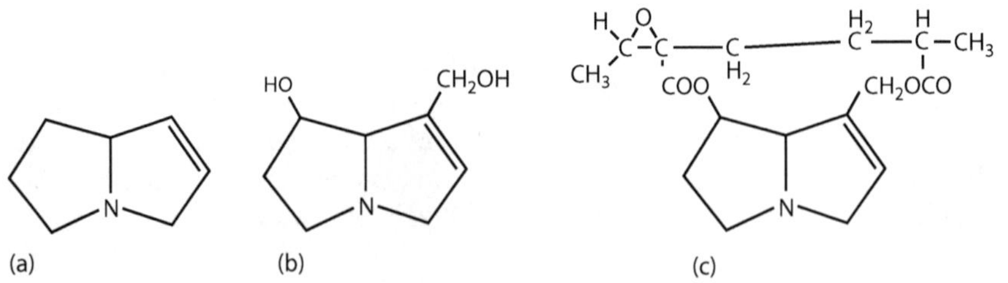

FIGURE 2.8 Pyrrolizidine alkaloid toxins including the pyrrolizidine nucleus, a less toxic monoester, and a highly toxic cyclic diester.

and will react with many tissues. Small amounts of pyrroles may escape hepatic circulation and can cause lesions in the lungs, heart, kidneys, GI tract, or brain. Minimal toxic activation of some PAs may occur in these tissues, although the level of microsomal enzyme activity in these tissues is not fully understood. Damage from PAs found in *Senecio*, *Heliotropium*, and *Echium* is generally confined to the liver, while *Crotalaria* intoxication induces significant pulmonary lesions.

A recent case of cattle poisoning from *Amsinckia* in Arizona stimulated the analytical evaluation of the implicated plants and a follow-up survey of herbarium specimens (Colegate et al. 2013; 2014b). Ten herbarium specimens collected between 1889 and 2013, and two PPRL *Amsinckia* collections, one from the poisoning case in Arizona and the other from rangelands in Washington State where no poisoning is reported, were evaluated for dehydropyrrolizidine alkaloids (DHPA) and their N-oxides. In brief, DHPAs were detected in all specimens examined ranging from 1 to 4,000 μg/g of plant. The plants from Arizona contained much higher levels of DHPAs compared to the plants from Washington State, partially, if not totally, explaining the difference in toxicity of the two populations.

The hepatotoxic element of PA toxicosis in cattle often has a latent period between ingestion and manifestation of the disease. The PA found in the plant is generally not toxic, but requires metabolic activation in the liver by microsomal enzymes to the reactive pyrrole or pyrrolic dehydroalkaloids (DHAs; Figure 2.9). Once the toxic pyrrole is formed, it binds to DNA (crosslinks) and is believed to remain in the liver or hepatic circulation, further exacerbating liver disease. Metabolism and toxicity of PAs were reviewed by Huxtable and Cooper (2000). While PAs are primarily liver toxins, there are PAs that are extrahepatic

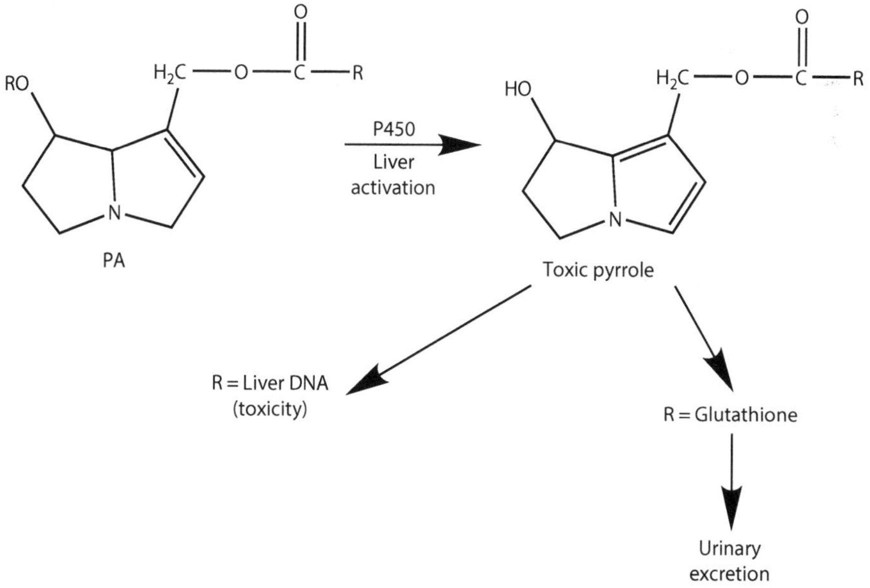

FIGURE 2.9 Metabolic activation of the pyrrolizidine alkaloid via the liver to the toxic pyrrole (liver bound and highly toxic) and the glutathione conjugate (excretion metabolite).

in their pathology. Pulmonary, neurological, and other organ damage have been reported, but it is not clear whether it results from toxic metabolism in those tissues or from circulating toxic pyrroles that have escaped the hepatic circulation after activation. Acute poisonings have been reported in experimental settings where relatively high single doses have been administered. Acute poisonings are not of the hepatic type, but rather involve pulmonary function and neurological function which are seldom observed in the field or with chronic poisoning. Occasionally, acute poisoning has been diagnosed in humans eating highly contaminated foods or when pregnant women drink comfrey tea containing high levels of PAs.

Ingestion of relatively low amounts of PAs daily over weeks or months will often not result in any outward clinical signs of poisoning. However, pathologically, the hepatocytes will gradually enlarge, bile ducts will proliferate, and lobular atrophy will occur. Central and sublobular veins are often occluded by fibrous tissue. The large hepatocytes (megalocytosis) are generally pathogneumonic for PA poisoning. Hepatocyte enlargement is generally accompanied by an absence of cell division (antimitotic activity). PA poisoning continues to be a significant problem in the USA and throughout the world.

2.2.4.5 Indolizidine and Polyhydroxy Alkaloids

Indolizidine alkaloids are defined by an indane ring system, with nitrogen at one vertex as represented by the locoweed toxin swainsonine (Figure 2.10). Since swainsonine's discovery in the late 1970s and early 1980s, first by Colegate et al. (1979) from the Darling pea (*Swainsona*) in Australia and then by Molyneux and James (1982) in the *Astragalus* and *Oxytropis* locoweeds, many other glycosidase-inhibitory alkaloids have been discovered (Molyneux et al. 2002). In Australia, Darling pea poisoning was called "peastruck", and in the USA, a similar disease called "locoism" has been induced by ingestion of *Astragalus* spp. and *Oxytropis* spp. Initially, only represented by swainsonine, the broader class of compounds called "polyhydroxy alkaloids" now includes indolizidine, pyrrolizidine, and tropane alkaloids, and some of the pyrrolidine and piperidine analogs. Because of similar biological activity and chemical features (all contain multiple hydroxyl groups), these alkaloids are often discussed together as polyhydroxy alkaloids.

Interest in swainsonine was high from the outset as its potent and specific inhibition of α-mannosidase was key in explaining the mechanism of action of certain

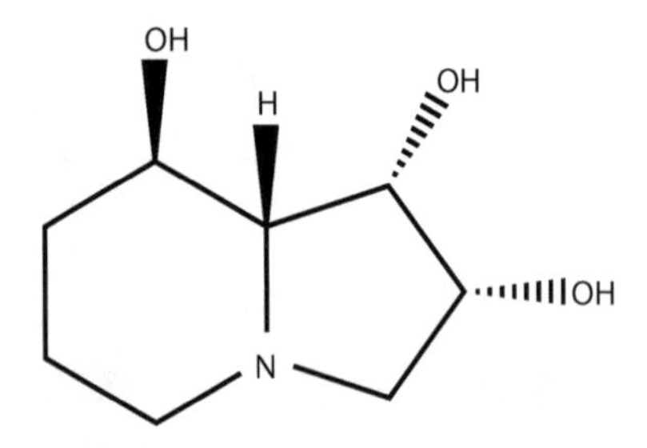

FIGURE 2.10 The indolizidine alkaloid toxin, swainsonine (a potent inhibitor of α-mannosidase), responsible for locoweed toxicosis.

genetic disorders and the plant-induced locoism in livestock. Since swainsonine's discovery, it has been used as a biochemical tool for studying numerous biochemical processes in the cell such as glycoprotein processing and synthesis, glycoprotein modification and storage, specific glycoprotein disorders, T-lymphocyte function, and cancer metastasis (reviewed by James et al. 2004).

Similarly, discovery of other polyhydroxylated indolizidine alkaloids, which possess glycosidase inhibitory properties such as castanospermine and lentiginosine, and their derivatives have been reported (Molyneux et al. 1991). Castanospermine, the major alkaloid in Moreton Bay chestnut (*Castanospermum australe*), has also been associated with livestock poisoning. Castanospermine is a potent competitive inhibitor of β-glucocerebrosidase and lysosomal α-glucosidase and, like swainsonine, interferes with glycoprotein processing, although in a slightly different way. Interest in castanospermine was stimulated when it was discovered to inhibit tumor growth, viral replication, and human immunodeficiency virus (HIV) syncytium formation (reviewed by Roitman and Panter 1995). An epimer of castanospermine, 6-epicastanospermine, is a potent inhibitor of amyloglucosidase but does not inhibit β-glucosidase or α or β-mannosidase. These alkaloids have a high degree of specificity for individual enzymes, yet they differ only slightly in chemical structure.

A second pair of dehydroxyindolizidine alkaloids (also epimers of each other) was isolated from locoweeds. Lentiginosine is a potent inhibitor of amyloglucosidase, but the 2-epilentiginosine epimer is not, thus demonstrating again the unique specificity of these compounds to inhibit only specific enzymes. Lentiginosine and its epimer are present in some locoweeds as minor components, but they are potent inhibitors of cellular enzyme function and most likely contribute to the emaciated condition of animals severely poisoned on locoweed.

Only species of *Astragalus* and *Oxytropis* that contain swainsonine are true locoweeds. Since the discovery of swainsonine as the toxin in locoweeds in 1982, many species of *Astragalus* and *Oxytropis* in the USA, South America, and China have been confirmed as locoweeds (Molyneux et al. 1994). Recently, swainsonine was isolated from a member of the morning-glory family (*Ipomoea carnea*), which has been responsible for a locoweed-like syndrome in sheep and goats in Australia and South Africa. In addition to swainsonine, *A. lentiginosus* contains minor amounts of the N-oxide derivative, and lentiginosine and 2-epilentiginosine, two structurally related dihydroxy alkaloids that undoubtedly contribute to the reported toxicoses.

Swainsonine is not a plant-derived secondary metabolite, but is produced by an endophyte associated with all swainsonine-containing *Astragalus*, *Oxytropis*, and *Swainsona* species investigated to date (Baucom et al. 2012; Grum et al. 2013). Endophytes associated with the swainsonine-containing legumes belong to *Alternaria* spp. Section *Undifilum* (Pryor et al. 2009; Lawrence et al. 2016). Swainsonine concentrations differ among species, populations, and individuals within a population (Ralphs et al. 2008, Cook et al. 2009b). For a thorough review of the relationship between swainsonine and endophyte in the various plant taxa, one is referred to Cook et al. (2014).

The isolation of swainsonine from *Swainsona* species resulted from the observation that the poisoning induced in livestock by these plants was biochemically, morphologically, and clinically similar to the genetic disease "mannosidosis," which, like locoism, results from an insufficiency of the enzyme α-mannosidase. It was, therefore, hypothesized that the toxin was an inhibitor of α-mannosidase. This enzyme was used as a probe for bioactivity and ultimately the separation and purification of the active compound (Dorling et al. 1978; Colegate et al. 1979). The chemical structure of swainsonine is not complex and has many similarities to the simple sugar mannose, which it mimics. It suppresses the action of the enzyme α-mannosidase, which is essential for proper functioning of all animal cells. The enzyme trims sugar molecules from complex, but abnormal, molecules known as glycoproteins within the cell. Once the correct number of sugars have been trimmed, the smaller molecules can be targeted for other functions. Failure of the trimming process results in an accumulation of complex molecules within the cell, resulting in vacuolation. After a sufficient number of cells have been damaged from over-accumulation of these compounds, signs of poisoning appear. Since all cells depend on proper functioning of α-mannosidase, many different organs can be damaged, including the brain, heart, liver, pancreas, thyroid, and reproductive system (Stegelmeier et al. 1999).

Like simple sugars, swainsonine is water soluble and therefore distributed to many parts of the body. It is rapidly excreted, primarily in the urine, but in lactating animals, a portion of it is transferred to the milk (James and Hartley 1977). This fast excretion rate suggests that occasional consumption of locoweeds for short periods is unlikely to have serious effects, but continuous consumption, even at low levels, results in poisoning.

By recognizing swainsonine as an inhibitor of α-mannosidase, and its ability to interact with receptor sites for mannose substrates on the enzyme, other structurally similar alkaloids were proposed to have similar properties. One such alkaloid, castanospermine, was isolated from seeds of the Moreton Bay chestnut (*Castanospermum australe*), an Australian rainforest tree. The leguminous seeds, which litter the ground beneath the trees, are toxic to livestock. When tested, castanospermine was found to be a potent inhibitor of α- and β-glucosidase, enzymes that are essential for glycoprotein processing, especially in digestion. The discovery of the biochemical activity of this alkaloid suggested a close analogy to locoweed poisoning, although the signs of poisoning are different with pronounced gastrointestinal disturbances and no discernable neurological damage.

A chemical analysis of *C. australe* seeds resulted in the identification of several structurally related indolizidine alkaloids, differing from castanospermine only in the orientation of specific hydroxyl groups around the ring system. These include some pyrrolizidine alkaloids, which were named australines. These alkaloids inhibited α- and β glucosidases to a greater or lesser extent, but were present at significantly lower levels than castanospermine. The identification of swainsonine, castanospermine, and australine, together with isomers differing in their stereochemistry, suggests that other similar compounds capable of mimicking sugars might exist in nature as glycosidase inhibitors (Molyneux et al. 1994)

A syndrome in livestock occurs with respect to *Ipomoea* species, which have been found to poison sheep in Australia and goats in Africa (Molyneux et al. 1995). The analysis of *I. calobra* and *I. polpha* from Queensland showed that these plants contained not only calystegines B2 and C1 but also swainsonine. An analogous pattern of alkaloids was detected in *I. carnea* from Mozambique (de Balogh et al. 1999). Ipomoea species are also associated with a fungal endophyte that belongs to the order Chaetothyriales that produces swainsonine but not the calystegines (Cook et al. 2013). The toxicity of these plants results from the effect of the toxins on at least three different enzymes, and many of the symptoms (neurological) have been correlated with locoism induced by α-mannosidase inhibition and GI dysfunction exacerbated by inhibition of α-galactosidase and β-glucosidase.

The fundamental cellular function of glycoprotein processing is that it affects glycoproteins that are involved in numerous essential physiological functions, especially cell-cell recognition reactions critical to pathogenesis, inflammation, parasitism, development, cell adhesion, and symbiosis. The polyhydroxy alkaloids exhibit a diversity of biological effects, including insecticidal, herbicidal, antimicrobial, and therapeutic activity. The discovery and isolation of many of the alkaloids have been a result of observations of the ultimate clinical effects which result from the consumption by animals of plants containing these bioactive compounds.

2.2.4.5.1 Biomedical Applications

There are genetic diseases in man and animals that occur as a result of inhibition of glycoprotein-processing enzymes (reviewed by James et al. 2004). These diseases are collectively known as lysosomal storage diseases. The animal diseases, genetic or induced, have counterparts in humans. For example, (1) Pompe's disease is a generalized glycogenosis caused by a deficiency of the lysosomal enzyme α-1,4-glycosidase resulting in abnormal storage of glycogen in skeletal muscles, heart, liver, and other organs; (2) Gaucher's disease is a chronic familial deficiency of a glucocerebroside-cleaning enzyme resulting in abnormal storage of cerebrosides in reticuloendothelial cells and characterized by spenomegaly, hepatomegaly, skin pigmentation, pinqueculae of the scleras, and bone lesions; (3) Fabry's disease (*angiokeratoma corporis diffusum universale*) is an inherited disorder of glycolipid metabolism due to a deficiency of a ceramide trihexosidase-cleaving enzyme; (4) genetic mannosidosis has been described in man, Angus cattle, and Murray Gray cattle, and is characterized by a deficiency of α-mannosidase leading to storage of excess mannose-rich oligosaccharides in lysosomes. Pathologically, there is vacuolation of reticuloendothelial cells in the liver and lymph nodes, pancreatic exocrine cells, and neurons. Affected cattle are ataxic, uncoordinated, fail to thrive, and die in the first year of life. Locoweed poisoning mimics exactly the genetic mannosidosis. Thus, the availability of specific inhibitors (plant toxins) of these enzymes provides a mechanism for induction of phenocopies of these genetic diseases in animal models. As an example, feeding experiments with castanospermine in rats resulted in vacuolation of hepatocytes, and skeletal myocytes and glycogen accumulation, consistent with Pompe's disease. Young rats treated with swainsonine developed axonal dystrophy in the CNS as a consequence of lysosomal storage of incompletely processed mannosides, which has a parallel in genetic mannosidosis and locoweed poisoning. Experiments using the indolizidine alkaloids described and other alkaloids have the potential to provide useful information for early diagnosis and possible methods of intervention to interrupt the progression of such diseases.

Although mammalian toxicity of the polyhydroxy alkaloids is an obvious concern with regard to their medicinal implications, the capability to disrupt the general cellular function of glycoprotein processing leads to the expectation that these compounds should have therapeutic potential for the treatment of various disease states. Although many drug candidates have significant toxicity, it is well recognized that an appropriate dose-response relationship can often be achieved, which minimizes harmful side effects. Moreover, adverse effects, such as the neurological damage caused by swainsonine, often develop quite slowly and appear to be reversible if ingestion of the alkaloid is terminated, as would be the situation with most drug regimens. Investigation of these alkaloids for therapeutic potential has so far concentrated on four major disease states, namely the treatment of cancer, inhibition of metastasis, anti-viral treatments, and anti-parasitic therapy. Structurally related compounds have also been investigated as anti-diabetic drugs.

Swainsonine has received particular attention as an anti-metastatic agent, and this effect has been shown to be due to enhancement of natural killer T-cells to cancerous cells. *In vivo* experiments with mice have shown that animals provided with drinking water containing 3 μg/ml swainsonine for 24 hours prior to injection with B16-F10 murine melanoma cells had an 80% reduction in pulmonary colonization. Pharmacokinetic studies indicate that the levels of alkaloid and period of administration would be insufficient to produce neurological damage. It has been suggested that post-operative metastasis of tumor cells in humans could be suppressed by intravenous administration of the alkaloid prior to and following surgery. Administration of swainsonine in clinical trials in humans with advanced malignancies showed that lysosomal α-mannosidases and Golgi mannosidase II were inhibited and improvement in clinical status occurred.

Castanospermine suppresses the infectivity of a number of retro viruses, including the HIV responsible for AIDS. This effect is a direct consequence of glycoprotein processing inhibition, resulting in changes in the structure of the glycoprotein coat of the virus. Cellular recognition of the host is prevented and syncytium formation is suppressed. In spite of this effect, the alkaloid suffers from the disadvantage that it is highly water soluble and therefore rapidly excreted. This limitation has been partially dealt with by optimization to give a lipophilic derivative. This has undergone clinical trials against AIDS in humans, either alone or in combination with AZT, with the only significant side effect being gastrointestinal disturbances, as might be predicted (Dennis et al. 1993).

The ability of polyhydroxy alkaloid glycosidase inhibitors to prevent cellular recognition has resulted in their use in studies of clinical situations where suppression of an immune response would be desirable, or for use against parasitic diseases. *In vivo* experiments have shown that castanospermine can be used as an immunosuppressive drug, promoting heart and renal allograft survival in rats. Parasitic diseases may also be controlled by altering cellular recognition processes. Swainsonine has been demonstrated to inhibit the association of *Trypanosoma cruzi* (the cause of Chagas' disease) with the host cell by formation of defective mannose-rich oligosaccharides on the cell surface. Castanospermine provides protection against cerebral malaria by preventing adhesion of *Plasmodium falciparum* to infected erythrocytes. Polyhydroxy alkaloids have considerable potential for treatment of a variety of disease states in humans and animals. The challenge to using them as commercial drugs is to minimize their toxicity and enhance the specificity of their beneficial effects.

2.2.4.6 Tropane Alkaloids

Tropane alkaloids are primarily found in the Solanaceae family and include Jimson weed (*Datura stramonum*), henbane, (*Hyoscyamus niger*), mandrake (*Mandragora*), *Atropa belladonna* (deadly nightshade), *Brugmansia* spp., and *Solandra* spp. They also appear in other plant families including Convolvulaceae, Brassixcaceae, Protaceae, Euphorbiaceae, Moraceae, Oleaceae, Rhizophoraceae, and Erythroxylaceae. *Brugmansia* is native to the Andes Mountains and is very similar to *Datura* spp.; at one time, both were included in *Datura* and have in common the given name "angel's trumpet" because of the large, pendulous, trumpet-like, five-toothed flowers. Jimson weed, as are most plants containing the tropane alkaloids, is unpalatable to animals although poisoning of most classes of livestock and humans have been reported in the literature (Kingsbury 1964; Burrows and Tyrl 2013). Ingestions of fresh plant material, contaminated hay or silage and seeds, have produced toxicoses. Clinical signs in animals and humans include intense thirst, restlessness, pupillary dilation, increased heart rate, dyspnea, dry mucous membranes, aberrant behavior, and death. In cattle, bloat may occur and in horses, colic.

Species of *Datura*, *Hyoscyamus*, and other tropane-containing genera are of more risk to humans than animals. These plants and their seeds have been used for religious or social functions with ritualistic emphasis. Numerous cases of bizarre and often aggressive behavior have been reported in people using seeds or teas from these plants (Burrows and Tyrl 2013). As recently as October 2003, a report appeared at *CNN.com* of four teens that ate Jimson weed seeds. All hallucinated and had to be hospitalized. Two were sedated and placed on life support to prevent danger to themselves and others. This same press release reported that the Centers for Disease Control and Prevention recorded 1,072 poisonings, including one death, in 2002 from Jimson weed and similar plants.

The tropane alkaloids are divided into two main groups (Figure 2.11a,b): the Solanaceous tropane alkaloids including atropine, scopolamine, hyoscyamine, and norhyoscyamine (Figure 2.11a), and the coca tropane alkaloids including cocaine (Figure 2.11b), cinnamoylcocaine, ecgonine, and other coca derivatives (Harborne and Baxter 1996). Calystegins are a class of tropane alkaloids that have received recent interest because of their potent enzyme inhibition, as discussed in the indolizidine section of this chapter.

Calystegin B2 was first isolated from *Calystegia sepium* and given the name calystegin. It has also been isolated from field bindweed (*Convolvulus arvensis*). Calystegins resemble the indolizidine alkaloids, swainsonine and castanospermine, and are potent inhibitors of glycoprotein enzymes (Molyneux et al. 1993). Calystegin C1 is a potent and specific inhibitor of β-glucosidase; calystegin B1 and B2 inhibit α-galactosidase and β-glucosidase. Whether calystegins are important toxins to humans and animals is yet to be fully determined, but a condition in horses characterized by colic, weight loss, intestinal thickening and fibrosis, and vascular sclerosis has been linked to tropane alkaloids in field bindweed (*C. arvensis*; Knight and Walter 2001).

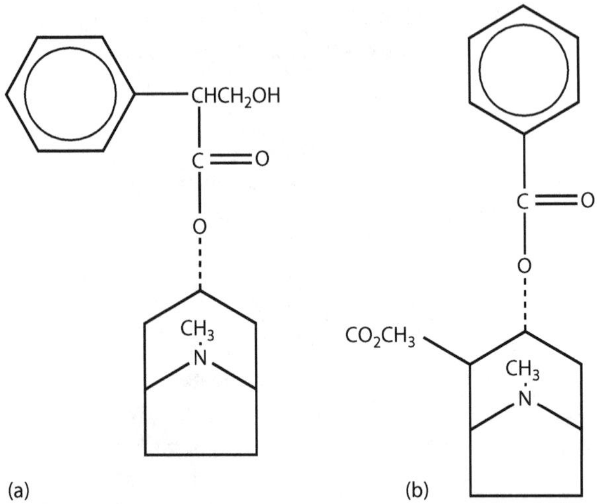

FIGURE 2.11 Two common tropane alkaloids in *Solanum* spp., atropine (*Datura*) and Cocaine (*Erythroxylon coca*).

2.3 GLYCOSIDES

2.3.1 Introduction

Glycosides are the second most ubiquitous and important group of plant toxins after alkaloids (see reviews by Cheeke 1998; Knight and Walter 2001; Burrows and Tyrl 2013). Glycosides are defined as two-part molecules containing a noncarbohydrate moiety (aglycone) joined by an ether bond to a carbohydrate functionality like D-glucose. The nonsugar portion of the glycoside (aglycone) is often the active portion that imparts toxicity and is released through enzymatic action when the plant tissue is damaged. Glycosides are relatively nontoxic when the two parts of the molecule are connected; however, hydrolysis in the GI tract of animals, especially ruminants, liberates the aglycone, resulting in toxicity. There are many different classes of glycosides including cyanogenic, steroidal, nitropropanol, calcinogenic, estrogenic, coumarin, goitrogenic, and others. Vicine from fava beans, carboxyatractyloside from cocklebur, and anthraquinones in senna and *Aloe* spp. are also glycosides.

2.3.2 Cyanogenic Glycosides

The cyanogenic glycosides occur in many plant genera and species including *Prunus* (wild cherry), *Hydrangea*, *Sambucus* (elderberry), *Linum* (flax), *Sorghum* (sorghum, sudangrass, and johnsongrass), *Manihot* (cassava), and *Bambusa* (bamboo). The aglycone is cyanide or hydrogen cyanide (HCN), referred to as prussic acid. Cyanide is cytotoxic, blocking activity of specific enzymes (cytochrome oxidase) at the terminal stage of the cellular respiratory pathway (Cheeke 1998; Knight and Walter 2001). When cytochrome oxidase is blocked, ATP production stops, the cellular organelles in tissue cease to function, and death is rapid. Labored breathing (dyspnea), excitement, gasping, staggering, convulsions, and coma are clinical effects. The mucous membranes and blood are bright cherry red as oxygen is supplied to the tissues but cannot be used. Cherry red blood is diagnostic for cyanide poisoning.

Cyanide is readily hydrolyzed from the sugar in ruminants or in plants that have been damaged through wilting, frost, trampling, bruising, drought, or chewing. Cellular damage in the plant brings the nontoxic glycoside in contact with the cytosolic enzymes (glucosidases and lyases) that are responsible for the rapid release of free HCN. Ruminant micro-organisms also contain these enzymes, and the reaction is optimum at neutral pH. Therefore, ruminants are more susceptible to cyanogenic glycoside poisoning than nonruminants because of rapid liberation of free cyanide. This potent cellular toxin acts very quickly and, if high-enough doses are ingested, death quickly occurs from cyanosis and asphyxia.

There is a chronic form of cyanide poisoning manifest in humans as a neurological disease called tropical ataxic neuropathy. This has been reported in the tropics of West Africa, where cassava is a dietary staple. Clinical effects are the result of demyelinization of the optic, auditory, and peripheral nerve tracts. Goiter is also frequently reported and results from interference of iodine transport by thiocyanate formation as a detoxification product. In animals, chronic cyanide ingestion also causes degeneration of the nerve tracts resulting in posterior ataxia, urinary incontinence, and cystitis, and can cause birth defects (arthrogryposis) in the fetus. Urinary incontinence and cystitis (equine sorghum cystitis-ataxia syndrome) are common in horses fed sudan grass hay or sorghum fodder for long periods of time. The cystitis-ataxia syndrome results from demyelinization of the peripheral nerves caused by the lathyrogen, T-glutamyl β-cyanoalanine, a metabolite of cyanide glycoside conversion. The lathyrogen interferes with neurotransmitter activity in peripheral nerves and the central nervous system. Animals may slowly recover if the source of the toxic aminonitrile is removed before nerve damage becomes too severe (Knight and Walter 2001).

Cyanide is readily detoxified in the animal as all animal tissues contain the thiosulfate sulfurtransferase enzyme rhodanese. Rhodanese readily converts cyanide to the thiocyanate, which is excreted in the urine.

$$\underset{\text{Thiosulfate}}{S_2O_3^{2-}} + CN^- \xrightarrow{\text{rhodanese}} \underset{\text{Thiocyanate}}{SO_3^{2-} + SCN}$$

Acute poisoning occurs only when the detoxification mechanism is overwhelmed. This reaction is enhanced by giving sodium thiosulfate and sodium nitrate as 20% solutions in a 3:1 ratio intravenously and is a recommended antidote for acute cyanide poisoning. It is the thiocyanate metabolite that causes chronic disease when cyanide forage is ingested over an extended period of time.

2.3.3 Steroidal/Triterpenoid Glycosides

2.3.3.1 Cardiac Glycosides

Toxic cardiac glycosides are found in 11 plant families and more than 34 genera (Knight and Walter 2001). There are two groups of glycosides in plants—cardenolides and bufadienolides—both affecting cardiac function. The cardenolides are the best understood of the two and comprise toxins containing the parent glycosides of digitalis such as digoxin and digitoxin. Bufadienolides are similar to the cardenolides but differ in the functionality at C-17 on the D ring. Bufadienolides are prevalent in South African plant species and are more important in plant poisoning of livestock than the cardenolides (Botha et al. 1998). They are found in three genera of Crassulaceae (*Cotyledon*, *Tylecodon*, and *Kalanchoe*). *Kalanchoe* spp. are popular garden and house plant varieties, and can be a significant threat to children and pets.

The dogbane family (Apocynaceae) comprises 180–200 genera including *Apocynum*, *Strophanthus*, *Nerium*, *Pentalinon*, and others, of which there are over 1,500 species that contain cardiac glycosides. There are three general types of intoxications caused by members of the Apocynaceae family: GI irritation, neurotoxicity, and cardiotoxicoses. The most toxic species are those that produce the cardenolides. These glycosides, like glycosides in general, are composed of an aglycone, the cardiotoxic portion, and one or more sugars. While the sugars do not cause toxicity, they can alter potency depending on which sugar is present by enhancing absorption and metabolism.

Some of the most well-known cardenolides include digitoxin from *Digitalis purpurea* (foxglove), convallarin from *Convallaria* (lily-of-the-valley), ouabain from *Strophanthus* and *Acokanthera*, many digitoxin-like cardenolides from *Asclepias* (milkweeds), and cardiotoxic genins from *Nerium* (oleander; Knight and Walter 2001).

The cardiotoxic activity of glycosides is due to inhibition of ATPase transport and to the increase of myocardial contractility in the same manner as the digitalis pharmaceuticals. Cardiac glycosides given in therapeutic doses can increase the contractility of the heart muscle and slow the heart rate, thereby regulating cardiac output in patients suffering from acute or congestive heart failure. Toxic doses (often only slightly higher than therapeutic) may cause depression, excess salivation, vomiting, diarrhea, weakness, bradycardia, cardiac arrhythmia, and cardiac arrest and death.

2.3.3.2 Sapogenic Glycosides

Plants of the Liliaceae family are common sources of steroidal saponins. Sapogenic glycosides are not as toxic as the cardenolides. Saponins contain a polycyclic sapogenin or aglycone (steroid or triterpenoid) and a side chain of sugars attached by an ether bond. Ingestion of saponins often results in gastric irritation and GI upset. Saponins are soap-like substances that cause profuse foaming, producing a distinctive honey-combed, stable foam when shaken in an aqueous solution. This same action will cause bloat in ruminants. Saponins are widely distributed in plants and are particularly important in animal nutrition and especially prevalent in forage legumes. They are bitter compounds and may decrease palatability and feed intake, for example, exhibiting growth-depressing properties in poultry and swine. Saponins are not readily absorbed into the blood stream but once the aglycone is absorbed, hemolysis may occur. Some saponins, such as those in *Yucca schidigera*, have beneficial effects in animals and are used as feed additives (Cheeke 1998).

2.3.4 Nitropropanol Glycosides

Many *Astragalus* species, such as timber milk vetch (*Astragalus miser*, thus the name miserotoxin), Emory milk vetch (*A. emoryanus*), and crown vetch (*Coronilla* spp.), are toxic because of the nitropropanol glycosides of 3-nitro-1-propanol (3-NPOH) and 3-nitropropionic acid (3-NPA; Majak and Pass 1989). These compounds, especially 3-NPOH, are acutely toxic, producing methemoglobinemia. The glycosides of 3-NPOH are of greater toxicologic importance in livestock than those of 3-NPA. *A. canadensis* and *A. falcatus* are known to contain high levels of 3-NPA and are very toxic. Cattle are more susceptible to *Astragalus* nitro poisoning than sheep. Miserotoxin, which is the β-D-glucoside of 3-nitro-1-propanol, is the most important 3-NPOH type. Other 3-NPA derivatives include cibarian, corollin, coronarian, coronillin, and karakin. These parent compounds are hydrolyzed to the free aglycones 3-NPA and 3-NPOH by esterases and β-glucosidases in the rumen or gut of herbivores. They are both readily absorbed: 3-NPOH more rapidly than 3-NPA and also more toxic. 3-NPA is of lesser toxicologic importance because it is more readily degraded in the digestive tract before absorption.

2.3.5 Calcinogenic Glycosides

Calcinogenic glycoside-containing plants include *Cestrum diurnum*, *S. malacoxylon*, and *Trisetum flavescens* (Knight and Walter 2001). The toxin is a glycoside of 1,25-dihyroxycholecalciferol, which is hydrolyzed to the active vitamin D_3. The consumption of these plants by cattle and horses results in excessive calcium absorption and the calcification of soft tissues such as tendons, arteries, and kidneys. There is about 30,000 IU equivalent of Vitamin D_3 per kg of plant material, resulting in increased calcium absorption and increased calcium-binding protein. The glycoside in *C. diurnum* is less water soluble than the glycoside in *S. malacoxylon*, and therefore, causes less extensive calcification of soft tissues. The resulting dystrophic calcification is especially noticeable in the horse as manifested by bony prominences on the legs, face, and so on, tense abdominal muscles, stiffness with a noticeable short choppy gait, reluctance to move, and eventual recumbency and death. There may be pain upon palpation of tendons and ligaments. *Cestrum* spp. and *S. malacoxylon* also contain cardenolides that may induce similar cardiotoxicity as ouabain. There are other glycosides in some of these species including carboxyparquin and parquin, which are responsible for hepatic necrosis. These are closely related to the carboxyatractylosides found in cocklebur seedlings.

2.3.6 Estrogenic Glycosides (Isoflavones, Coumestans)

Estrogenic glycosides include isoflavones and coumestans in plants that exhibit estrogenic activity. Many of these phytoestrogens are also phenolics. These phytoestrogens induce reproductive dysfunction in animals that graze them for long periods of time. Phytoestrogens are particularly important in subterranean clover (*Trifolium subterran*) and red clover (*T. pratense*), with a history of causing infertility in sheep (clover disease; Cheeke 1998). Sheep that graze subterranian clover pastures do not exhibit normal seasonal breeding cycles or estrus cycles, and develop cystic ovaries. Wethers exhibit teat enlargement when chronically exposed to phytoestrogens. Fertility returns once ewes are removed from clover pastures, although long-term reduction in fertility has been reported in flocks repeatedly affected season after season. The phytoestrogens (isoflavones) contain a flavone nucleus. Examples of isoflavones are genistein, formononetin, and coumestrol, all with potent estrogenic activity. Soybean isoflavones are a concern in human nutrition because of their estrogenic benefits.

2.3.7 Coumarin Glycosides

Coumarin glycosides are found throughout the plant kingdom (Burrows and Tyrl 2013). Seeds of *Aesculus glabra* (Ohio buckeye) contain the coumarin esculin, which is a mild neurotoxin. Sweet clovers (*Melilotus* spp.) contain coumarins that are considered harmless unless moldy conditions exist in which fungal activity produces the double coumarin dicoumarol. Dicoumarol is a powerful anticoagulant that causes internal hemorrhage and was responsible for extensive losses in the 1920s in cattle in the Midwest and Canada. A benefit to human medicine is the dicoumarol medications (Coumadin7; Warfarin Sodium, etc.) used to thin blood and control clotting in patients with cardiovascular disease. A Warfarin (dicoumarol) derivative is the main ingredient in some rodenticides used as rat and mouse poisons (DeconJ). Other coumarin-related compounds include furans found in moldy sweet potatoes and the furan coumarin complexes (furanocoumarins) in parsnip leaves (psoralens). They are photo-reactive compounds (primary photosensitizers) exacerbating sunburn to psoralen-exposed skin.

2.3.8 Goitrogenic Glycosides

Goitrogens decrease production of thyroid hormones by inhibiting their synthesis by the thyroid gland. Consequently, the thyroid enlarges to compensate for reduced thyroxin output, producing a goiter. These compounds are collectively called glucosinolates and are commonly found in *Brassica* spp. such as broccoli, kale, cabbage, cauliflower, and rape (Cheeke 1998). The glucosinolates are hydrolyzed by glucosinolases to β-D-glucose and derivatives of the aglycone including isothiocyanates, nitriles, and thiocyanates. The glucosinolate enzymes are released from plant tissues by chewing and by rumen microflora activity. Glucosinolates (mustard oil glycosides) are common in the *Brassica* family and are mild gastrointestinal irritants if ingested in excess. The thiocyanates and isothiocyanates may interfere with iodine metabolism and contribute to thyroid gland enlargement (goiters). Recent research has shown that glucosinolates found in cruciferous vegetables are degraded into isothiocyanates with strong inhibitory properties for phase I enzymes and inducers of phase II enzymes with strong potential as cancer chemopreventors (Zhang and Talalay 1998).

2.3.9 Other Glycosides

Anthraquinone glycosides found in senna (*Cassia fistulosa*) and *Aloe* spp. have been included in some commercial cathartics. Vicine is a glycoside in fava beans (*Vicia faba*), and it causes hemolytic anemia in people who have a genetic deficiency of glucose-6-phosphate dehydrogenase activity in their red blood cells. Fava beans are grown as a protein supplement for livestock. A glycoside called carboxyatractyloside has been identified as the toxin in cocklebur (*Xanthium strumarium*). The toxin is in high concentration in seeds and cotyledons, but rapidly diminishes as true leaves develop. Carboxyatractyloside produces hepatic lesions, convulsions, and severe hypoglycemia, which is thought to be the result of uncoupling of oxidative phosphorylation. In the USA, pigs seem to be the livestock most frequently poisoned. Signs of toxicity include depression, reluctance to move, nausea, vomiting, weakness and prostration, dyspnea, paddling, convulsions, coma, and death. Severe hypoglycemia occurs when normal blood glucose levels drop 10-fold, thus causing sudden death (Cheeke 1998).

2.4 PROTEINACEOUS COMPOUNDS, POLYPEPTIDES, AND AMINES

2.4.1 Proteinaceous Compounds

Proteins are generally not thought of as overtly toxic but are considered to be a group of beneficial compounds that are essential building blocks of cells and cellular function in plants and animals. However, there are numerous examples of harmful protein toxins found in nature, that is, bacterial toxins, insect and snake venoms, and toad and fish toxins. The number of harmful or toxic proteinaceous substances occurring naturally in plants is relatively small, especially when compared to alkaloidal or glycoside groups. However, there are proteinaceous plant toxins of significance because of their potent cellular toxicity and for their research potential in "molecular neurosurgery." These toxic lectins include ricin from *Ricinus communis* (castor bean), abrin from *Abrus precatorius* (rosary pea or precatory bean), modeccin from *Adenia digitata*, volkensin from *Adenia volkensii*, and saporin from *Saponaria officinalis*. These lectins are potent cytotoxins acting as proteolytic enzymes, thus preventing protein synthesis at the cellular level (ribosomes; Wiley 2000). Ricin and abrin are extremely toxic if ingested, and a few seeds chewed up and ingested can be fatal. Both toxins are more toxic when injected. The minimum lethal dose of ricin is 0.00000001% of body weight. These plant toxins have been used to make highly selective neural lesions for animal modeling to study neurodegenerative diseases such as Alzheimer's and Parkinson's disease (Wiley 2000).

2.4.2 Polypeptides

Toxic polypeptides are found in several species of fungi belonging to the *Amanita* genera (Powell 1990). *Amanita phalloides* (death cap) and its close relatives contain the cyclopeptides amatoxin, phallotoxin, and phalloidin. These toxins interfere with RNA-polymerase, thereby inhibiting protein synthesis. Cellular degeneration occurs in the intestines, liver, kidney, and heart. *Amanita* is the genus of mushroom most often involved in fatal mushroom poisoning in humans. Blue-green algae (cyanobacter) also contains cyclopeptides that cause GI tract upset and liver damage in cattle. This is a common problem in livestock in late summer or early fall after significant algae bloom (Beasley 1997).

2.4.3 Amines

Toxic amines are common in the *Lathyrus* genera (vetches and sweet peas), mistletoe berries (*Phorandendron* spp.), and *Leucaena* spp. The toxic amines in *Lathyrus* cause degeneration of motor tracts of the spinal cord, resulting in paralysis and even death. The condition called lathyrism was common in certain human populations before the discovery of the cause and identification of the toxins. The toxins are derivatives of aminopropionitrile. In mistletoe, the toxins are phenylethylamine and tyramine. Clinical signs of poisoning include acute GI tract inflammation, decreased blood pressure, and cardiovascular collapse. *Leucaena* spp. contain mimosine, which is degraded to 3-hydroxy-4(1H)-pyridone (3,4-DHP; see next section for more detail). *Leucaena*, while toxic to unadapted ruminants, is a good source of protein and minerals for many livestock species in some countries. However, *Leucaena* ingested at 50% or more of the diet will depress growth, cause hair loss, and reduce reproductive performance. Mimosine is a toxin that animals may become adapted to, and ruminal adaptation can be transferred from animal to animal, suggesting a specific set of rumen organisms are capable of detoxifying this amine.

2.5 NONPROTEIN AMINO ACIDS

Almost 300 nonprotein amino acids have been isolated from or identified in plants. Of these, about 20 have been implicated in toxicoses in humans and animals (Hegarty 1978; Cheeke 1998). Hypoglycin A from the fruit of *Blighia sapida*, a tree that grows in Jamaica and Africa, causes hypoglycemia and vomiting in animals and humans. Fatalities have occurred, which was attributed to a sudden drop in blood sugar. The lathyrogenic amino acids include β-N-(γ-L-Glutamyl) aminopropionitrile from the sweet pea (*Lathyrus odoratus*) and α-Amino-β-oxyalylaminopropionic acid, diaminobutyric acid, and oxalyl diaminopropionic acid from the flat pea (*L. sylvestris*). The lathyrogenic amino acids are responsible for a disease complex called lathyrism. The complex has been divided into two diseases with differing etiology: (1) osteolathyrism, characterized by skeletal abnormalities and (2) neurolathyrism, characterized as a neurological disease affecting humans, horses, and cattle.

Mimosine is a toxic amino acid, structurally similar to tyrosine, in *Mimosa pudica* and *Leucaena leucocophala*, both legumes. *Leucaena* is a pan-tropical shrub legume and an important pasture plant in the tropics and sub-tropics. In St. Croix, USA Virgin Islands, *Leucaena* is a significant grazing plant for sheep and cattle in the region (personal communication 2001). It is a vigorous, rapidly growing, drought-tolerant, palatable, and high-yielding plant, and its leaves contain from 25% to 35% crude protein. Little or no toxicoses are reported in ruminants where they have become adapted to the plant. This adaptation is from ruminal organisms that can degrade the mimosine and mimosine-metabolites 3,4-DHP (3-hydroxy-4(IH)-pyridone) and 2,3-DHP (2,3-dihydroxy pyridine) to nontoxic products. The mimosine degrading microflora have been artificially transferred from resistant goats to susceptible cattle, thus imparting the ability to degrade mimosine to the cattle. Nonruminants are more sensitive to mimosine, apparently because of the lack of degrading microflora (Cheeke 1998).

Mimosine toxicoses include hair loss in horses, cattle and laboratory animals, and fleece loss in sheep. Cataracts and reproductive problems have also been reported in rodent models. Prolonged ingestion of *Leucaena* by cattle in northern Australia resulted in low weight gains, hair loss, and goiter. The effects of leucaena and mimosine on nonruminants can be reduced to some extent by diet supplementation with ferrous sulfates. Mimosine forms a complex with iron, which is excreted in the feces. Zinc supplementation has reduced the toxicity in cattle, and it is believed that copper and zinc ions bind more strongly to mimosine than most other amino acids.

2.6 ORGANIC ACID TOXINS

This class of compounds is relatively rare in plants but is significant when livestock poisoning is considered. The most common example is the oxalic acid and its soluble salts, sodium oxalate and potassium acid oxalate. Plants known to contain toxic levels of oxalate include *Halogeton glomeratus*, a range plant introduced into Nevada, Idaho, and Utah, which was responsible for extensive losses in sheep in the desert areas of those states in the mid-1900s (James 1978; Young et al. 1999). Other plants of the *Atriplex*, *Bassia*, *Chenopodium*, *Salsola*, *Rumex*, *Oxalis*, and *Spinacia* genera also contain soluble oxalates, although generally not in concentrations considered toxic. The clinical signs of poisoning are associated with hypocalcemia as the oxalate generally binds blood calcium. This may result in the presence of calcium oxalate crystals present in the walls of the gut, blood vessels, and certain organs such as the kidneys. Other plants including jack-in-the-pulpit, dumbcane, and caladium contain oxalate crystals as the solid form in plant tissues. These household plants can cause tissue damage and inflammation to the mouth, tongue, and lips if eaten and are considered dangerous for children and pets (Beasley 1997).

2.7 ALCOHOLS/POLYACETYLENES

Although few alcohol-based toxins are naturally occurring in plants, there are two groups of significant importance to man and animals. The first is the cicutoxin-like compounds (long chain diols) found in water hemlock (*Cicuta* spp.; cicutoxin) of North America and *Oenanthe* spp. (oenanthotoxin) of Europe (King et al. 1985). The second is the benzofuran ketone (tremetone) class of toxins found in white snakeroot (*Ageratina altissima*) of the Midwestern USA and rayless goldenrod (*Isocoma pluriflora*) of the Southwestern USA (Cheeke 1998). Both are highly toxic to both humans and animals, and numerous poisonings have occurred.

The cicutoxin-like compounds are known for their extreme and violent toxicity. There are other plant species that contain these polyacetylene type compounds; however, none is as toxic as cicutoxin and oenanthotoxin. These species include *Falcaria vulgaris*, *Sium sisarum*, *Carum carvi*, *Aegopodium podagraria*, and *Daucus carota*. *Daucus carota* is the common carrot, and it contains a similar cicutoxin-like compound, caratotoxin, but is less toxic than cicutoxin. Caratotoxin is found in minute amounts in carrots and is not considered a human health concern (Crosby and Aharonson 1967).

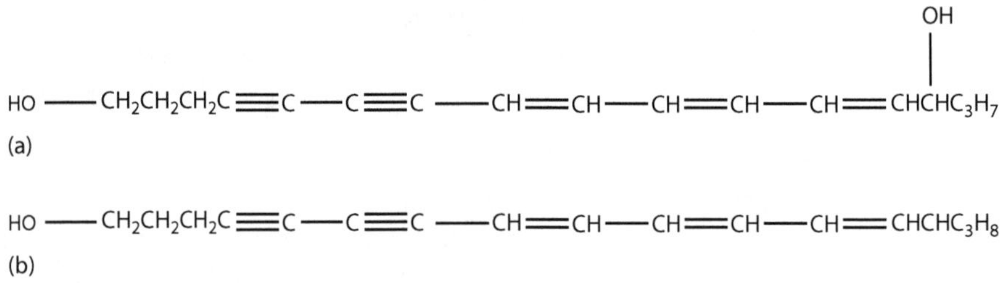

$$HO{-}CH_2CH_2CH_2C{\equiv}C{-}C{\equiv}C{-}CH{=}CH{-}CH{=}CH{-}CH{=}CH\underset{}{\overset{OH}{\overset{|}{C}}}HC_3H_7$$

(a)

$$HO{-}CH_2CH_2CH_2C{\equiv}C{-}C{\equiv}C{-}CH{=}CH{-}CH{=}CH{-}CH{=}CHCHC_3H_8$$

(b)

FIGURE 2.12 Two nitrogen-free toxins from *Cicuta* spp., that is, the highly toxic cicutoxin and the less toxic cicutol.

The diols (cicutoxin and oenanthotoxin, $C_{17}H_{22}O_2$) are C-17 complex linear structures containing two trienes and three dienes in differing orders and are the most toxic, whereas the alcohol derivatives ($C_{17}H_{22}O$) are relatively nontoxic (Figure 2.12a,b). Eleven similar polyacetylene compounds have been described in *Cicuta virosa* in Europe. While toxicity has not been determined for each of these compounds, the diols are believed to be the most dangerous. The toxic diols are unstable when exposed to air, thus making detection in tissue samples for diagnostic purposes difficult. These compounds are found throughout the plant, with greater concentrations in immature green seed and tubers (Panter et al. 2011).

Clinically, cicutoxin causes grand mal seizures and death in its victims. The mechanism of action is at the CNS level, causing seizures resembling those induced by picrotoxin from the East Indies shrub *Anamirta coculus.* The pharmacologic action of picrotoxin is the noncompetitive antagonism of $GABA_A$ receptors (Green et al. 2015). In the mammalian central nervous system, GABA and the $GABA_A$ receptors provide inhibitory neural tone in the central nervous system. Cicutoxin blockade of the $GABA_A$ receptors inhibits GABA central nervous system tone, causing seizures observed in poisoned people and animals (Schep et al. 2009). No appreciable effect is seen until the dose is high enough to induce seizures (narrow threshold). The signs of poisoning for cicutoxin are similar. In a cell culture model, the benzodiazepine midazolam reversed the actions of an aqueous extract of water hemlock, suggesting that it may be effective in preventing seizures and death from plant poisoning by water hemlock (Green et al. 2015).

For many years, it was believed that the tubers and early growth immature plants of water hemlock were the most toxic. However, more recently, the PPRL reported a case of death losses in cattle after ingesting green seed heads from *Cicuta douglasii* (Panter et al. 2011). Subsequent research confirmed the toxicity in a rodent model and, in fact, determined that the green seeds were as toxic as the tubers on a weight basis and two cicuctol-like compounds were the most prevalent compounds in the seed and were believed to be the toxins responsible for the toxicity (Panter et al. 2011).

Pathologic lesions are skeletal and heart muscle damage, with accompanying elevation in serum enzymes. Lesions result from strong muscular contractions during repeated seizure activity. Administration of pentobarbital therapy before or at the beginning of seizures will prevent grand mal seizures, pathological changes, and death. The powerful and rapid action of cicutoxin requires quick action to prevent death.

Even at lethal doses, treatment can be very successful with anticonvulsants, especially barbiturates. Treatment is required within minutes of poisoning to avoid death.

The second alcohol toxin of significance is tremetol, the toxin found in white snakeroot in the east through the Midwestern USA and rayless goldenrod in the Southwestern USA. Tremetol is an oily extract of the plant and was first associated with the toxic effects and named appropriately by Couch in 1927. Tremetol is a mixture of methyl ketone benzofuran derivatives including tremetone, dehydrotremetone, and hydroxytremetone (Beier and Norman 1990).

Diseases referred to as "trembles" in cattle and "milk sickness" in humans have significant historical interest because of large losses to cattle and humans as the settlers moved into the Midwest USA during the nineteenth century (reviewed by Burrows and Tyrl 2013). The disease was especially severe in the Mississippi and Ohio River valleys, Indiana, Illinois, Kentucky, North Carolina, Ohio, and Tennessee. In areas of Indiana and Ohio, one-fourth to half of all the deaths in the early 1800s were attributed to milk sickness. Abraham Lincoln's mother (Nancy Hanks Lincoln), many of her relatives and neighbors, and their animals died during an epidemic of milk sickness in 1818 in Pigeon Creek, Indiana. Hindustan Falls, a thriving settlement on the White River of southern Indiana, fell victim to what was referred to at the time as a mysterious malady. Much of the livestock and a substantial portion of the human population died of what is now known to be white snakeroot poisoning. The settlement was abandoned, although the cause at the time was yet unknown. While not confirmed that white snakeroot (*A. altissima*) was the cause until 1910, it was suggested in the 1830s by Anna Pierce and John Rowe, but ignored.

2.8 RESINOUS AND PHENOLIC COMPOUNDS

2.8.1 Phenolic Compounds

Generally these compounds are diverse and often chemically unrelated. As diverse as the chemical nature is, so is the diversity of their effects in mammals when ingested or when physical contact is made. One of the most familiar phenolic compounds is tetrahydrocannabinol (THC), the active ingredient in marijuana (*Cannabis sativa*). Over 60 cannabinoids have been isolated from *C. sativa* (Knight and Walter 2001). Although initially introduced into the USA as a fiber-producing plant for making rope, the practice ended in the 1950s. Because of the euphoric effect this plant has when people smoke the leaves and the street value determined by the illicit drug market, more potent biotypes of *Cannabis* have been selected in tropical countries for importation into the USA. Grades of marijuana cultivated in other parts of the world have high potency, and the female parts from the flowers of Arabian cannabis are known specifically as hashish. While legalization of marijuana in the USA is still being debated, the medicinal uses to treat various diseases such as glaucoma, chemotherapeutic-induced nausea during cancer treatment, and antibacterial effects are well documented (Physician's Desk Reference, PDR for Herbal Medicines 2000).

Tannins are polyhydroxyphenolic toxins found in the oak (*Quercus*) family (Cheeke 1998; Knight and Walter 2001). About 60 oak species grow in North America in a wide range of habitats. Two common species in Western USA associated with livestock poisoning are scrub oak (*Quercus gambelii*) and shinnery oak (*Q. havardii*). These species contain gallotannins, which are hydrolyzed in the rumen of cattle to smaller active compounds including gallic acid, pyrogallol, and resorcinol. Most severe lesions occur in the kidneys, liver, and GI tract. In small quantities, rumen microflora can detoxify tannins and it is when this detox mechanism is overwhelmed that poisoning occurs. Goats and wild ruminants are able to detoxify tannic acid because they have a tannin-binding protein in their saliva that prevents toxicosis. Goats have been used effectively for brush control to slow the spread of oak. Oak is poisonous at all stages of growth but buds, new growth, and green acorns are especially toxic. Cattle, sheep, pigs, and horses are susceptible to oak poisoning. Clinical signs of poisoning will vary depending on the amount eaten. Signs begin with depression, feed refusal, and intestinal stasis, progressing to abdominal pain, dehydration, diarrhea or constipation, and death 5–7 days later. Pathologically, liver necrosis, kidney necrosis, hemorrhagic gastroenteritis, and marked elevation in serum liver enzymes occur.

Other significant phenolic resin compounds include the mixture of urushiol variants, immunogenic compounds causing severe dermatitis from the *Rhus* spp. (poison ivy, poison oak, and poison sumac). Hypericin from St. John's wort is another phenolic compound with multiple rings and multiple double bonds. This compound readily absorbs UV light and is a primary photosensitizing agent that will result in severe sunburn in species that either ingest the plant or come in contact with plant dust or leaf extracts.

Gossypol is a phenolic compound found in the pigment glands of cottonseed (*Gossypium* spp.; Yu et al. 1993). In addition to gossypol, there are 15 other phenolic compounds in cotton seed. Cotton seed is used for oil production and leftover meal for livestock feed. During the oil extraction process, processors leave most of the gossypol in the meal by heat treating, which causes gossypol to bind to the meal. In animal feeding, the main concern is free gossypol, as the bound compound is physiologically inactive. Research studies concluded that diets containing 200 µg/g or less of free gossypol as cotton seed meal were safe for Holstein calves. At 400 µg/g, there was an increase in cardiovascular and lung lesions, leading to increased calf losses. Mature beef cows can be safely fed cottonseed meal as the entire protein supplement as this is generally kept relatively low, whereas dairy cows should not receive more than 3.6 kg per head per day (reviewed by Cheeke 1998). Ruminants are more tolerant to gossypol than nonruminants because of further protein binding in the rumen. The biological effects of gossypol are cumulative, with toxicosis being manifest abruptly after prolonged feeding of cottonseed meal to nonruminants, especially pigs. Gossypol reacts with minerals, especially iron. If fed to laying hens, egg yolks turn green because of the gossypol/iron complex that transfers to the egg protein. Anemia is one of the clinical signs of poisoning because of iron deficiency due to the complexing of iron with gossypol. Gossypol-induced lesions include edema, liver damage, ascites, cardiovascular lesions, and kidney damage. Gossypol has gained interest in society as a male contraceptive because of its infertility properties, yet does not reduce libido. Sperm counts are depressed and spermatozoa are immotile. Extensive damage has been shown to occur to the germinal epithelium in bulls and rams, thus cottonseed meal should only be fed at low levels or not at all during the breeding season. Testosterone levels in growing bulls are not affected by gossypol, but testicular morphology changes occurred.

Other phenolic compounds of commercial importance include the terpenoids including mono-, di-, tri-, and sesquiterpenes. While most of these are used as essential oils, fragrances, and flavors in various products, they are toxins in certain species. For example, the sesquiterpene lactones of the *Centaurea* species cause an irreversible Parkinson's-like condition in horses called nigro-pallidal encephalomalacia. This is a lethal condition and the prognosis for recovery is grave; in most cases, affected horses should be euthanized before ever reaching the terminal stages.

2.8.2 Pine Needle Abortion

A significant group of resin compounds (labdane resin acids) with biological activity in cattle have been identified in pine, juniper, and other related species. Cattle grazing ponderosa pine needles, lodgepole pine needles, Monterey cypress, and juniper species are known to abort their calves, especially when grazed in the last trimester of pregnancy (Gardner and James 1999) with no apparent effect on estrus (Welch et al. 2015b). The labdane resin acid, isocupressic acid, was isolated from ponderosa pine needles and determined to be the putative abortifacient in cattle (Gardner et al. 1994; Figure 2.13a). Other derivatives and metabolites have now been identified with known abortifacient activity (Figure 2.13b,c). Research has demonstrated that there is variation in the concentration of labdane acids in both ponderosa pine and western juniper trees between different geographic locations (Cook et al. 2010; Welch et al. 2015c).

Twenty-three other tree and shrub species found throughout the western and southern states were analyzed for ICA (Gardner and James 1999). Significant levels (>0.5% dry weight of the needles) were detected in *Pinus jefferyi* (Jeffrey pine),

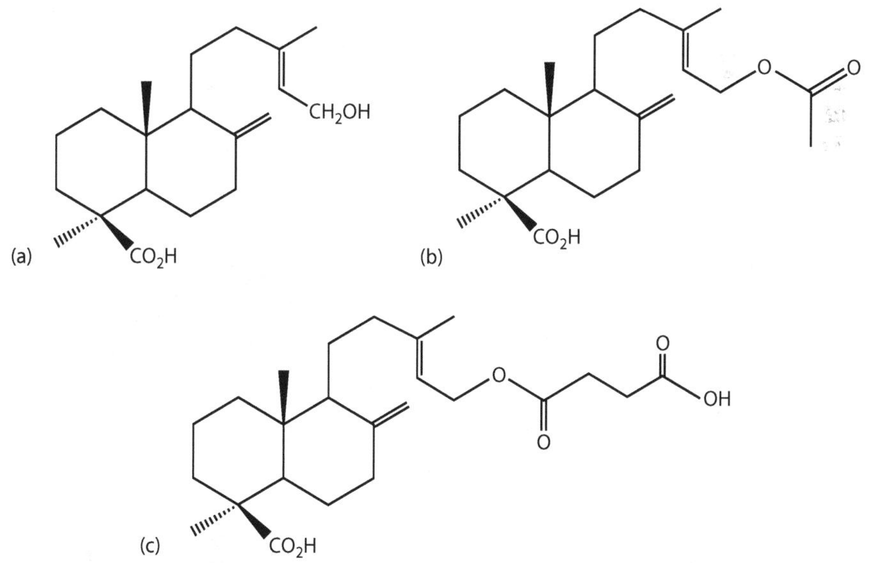

(a) CH_2OH CO_2H

(b) O O CO_2H

(c) O O O OH CO_2H

FIGURE 2.13 Three labdane resin acid compounds (isocupressic acid and the acetyl and succinyl derivatives) found in certain pine, juniper, and cypress trees that are abortifacient in late term pregnant cattle.

P. contorta (lodgepole pine), *Juniperus scopulorum* (Rocky Mountain juniper), and *J. communis* (common juniper), and from *Cupressus macrocarpa* (Monterey cypress) from New Zealand and Australia.

Toxicoses from pine needles have been reported in field cases, but are rare and have only occurred in pregnant cattle. No toxicity other than abortion in cattle has been demonstrated from ICA or ICA derivatives. However, the abietane-type resin acids in ponderosa pine needles (concentrated in new growth pine tips) have been shown to be toxic but not abortifacient at high doses when administered orally to cattle, goats, and hamsters. Pathological evaluations of intoxicated animals include nephrosis, edema of the central nervous system, myonecrosis, and gastroenteritis (Stegelmeier et al. 1996). While abietane-type resin acids may contribute to the occasional toxicoses reported in the field, they do not contribute to the abortions.

2.9 MINERAL TOXINS

Mineral toxins are rather unique and probably unrelated to the plant protection theories reviewed in the introduction. These are minerals or metals that the plant usually takes up because of soil conditions and the mineral being in high concentration in the root zones of plants. Occasionally, plants can take up lethal quantities of mineral toxins such as selenium. While selenium is an essential micro nutrient, in excess it is toxic, causing a host of chronic and acute disease conditions. Chronic and acute poisoning can result when livestock and wildlife ingest plants containing a few μg/g up to many thousands of μg/g selenium. Livestock and wildlife can be exposed to high selenium forages where high soil selenium exists naturally or due to human activity. While acute selenium poisoning from plants is rare, it can occur and was recently the cause of large sheep losses on mining reclamation sites. While most acute selenium poisoning has been attributed to indicator plants such as *Astragalus* and some asters, there are a number of species that are known to take up selenium in toxic levels when selenium is available in the soil. Species of the Brassica family, aster family, and legume family are known to accumulate large levels of selenium. These species also act as selenium pumps drawing selenium from lower soil profiles to the surface where grasses and other shallow-rooted forbs can take up levels of selenium that are toxic. Some plant species taking up large quantities of selenium include *Medicago* (alfalfa; 1,100 μg/g), *Grindelia nana* (gum weed; >6,000 μg/g), *Aster eatonii* (aster; >4,000 μg/g), and *Symphyotrichum* spp. (>6,500 μg/g; Hall, J., unpublished data, 2003). It was determined that as little as 30–60 g of fresh aster plant containing over 4,000 μg/g selenium was enough to be lethal to sheep grazing in this area. It was also observed that the sheep preferred the aster and gum weed over the alfalfa.

Interestingly, grazing behavior is much different among livestock and wildlife species. For example, acute poisoning and death losses in sheep and cattle have occurred on mining reclamation sites where high-selenium soils were used from reclamation projects. Acute death losses in sheep occurred when hungry sheep were unloaded near a reclamation site and grazed young growing aster plants. The aster plants contained 1,000s of μg/g selenium (Davis et al. 2013a). While cattle are less likely to graze forbs as sheep do, acute poisoning in cattle would be expected less frequently, and in fact, that is the case. However, an unusual case of acute poisoning and death losses in cattle was reported recently, wherein cattle grazed mature aster plants containing 1,000s of μg/g of selenium (Davis et al. 2012).

Chronic selenium poisoning is more common and is frequently reported in cattle and horses. Horses are very sensitive to excess selenium in the diet, and lose hair and develop severe hoof lesions. The form of selenium ingested is important as the organic forms are more bio-available than the inorganic forms, which also impact toxicity (Davis et al. 2013a; 2013b). Sheep are more tolerant and fewer cases of chronic poisoning are reported in sheep. While it is unknown how high-selenium forages impact wildlife, a recent study in elk demonstrated that elk can differentiate between alfalfa pellets containing different levels of selenium (Pfister et al. 2015). Interestingly, the elk always selected the pellets with the least amount of selenium when multiple concentrations were offered in a cafeteria pen trial. Sheep and cattle were less discriminating and only when cattle became sick on the pellets did they stop eating the selenium pellets. Clinical effects include hair, tail, and mane losses, hoof growth abnormalities, and reproductive problems in some species. Davis et al. (2014) reported a method using hair from horses' manes and tails to evaluate long-term selenium exposure in horses grazing pastures where soil selenium is high. Briefly, a horse's tail is naturally about three feet long and grows at about one inch per month. Davis cut tail hair into one inch increments and analyzed each segment for selenium concentration. Interestingly, the selenium exposure over a three-year period could be evaluated and the precise location where the horses grazed could be retrospectively determined. The analytical results of this study showed selenium levels in the horse's tail hair in a sine wave pattern over the three-year period and accurately determined when horses were exposed to high selenium in feed or water and when the animals were removed from those pastures (Davis et al. 2014).

Other striking examples of plants that take up minerals or heavy metals can be found in plants growing on similar mine tailing sites. For example, sheep fescue (*Festuca ovina*) and fine bent (*Agrostis tenuis*) rapidly colonized tailings of heavy metal mining (Harborne 1988). *Agrostis* spp. can successfully grow on soils containing as much as 1% lead. Plants have the ability to rapidly adapt to different soil conditions; however, the mechanism for adaptation is not fully understood. Phytochelatins were discovered in the 1980s. While the exact role of these phytochelatins in heavy metal detoxification in plants is not fully understood, the fact remains that these chelatins provide a plant mechanism whereby metals enter the root system and are transported to the vegetative portions of the plant. *Deschampsia caespitosa* accumulates zinc; *Hybanthus floribundus* accumulates nickel and is an indicator plant for soil nickel and can accumulate up to 22% of its ash as nickel. *Eriogonum ovalifolium* is an indicator of silver deposits in Montana, and certain *Astragalus* species are indicators of selenium and uranium in western states. *Phacelia sericea* accumulates gold as the cyanide derivative up to 21 ng/g gold in leaves. *Leptospermum scoparium* is a chromium accumulator and *Anthoxanthum odoratum* accumulates lead. While frequent cases of selenium poisoning from plant uptake from the soil have been reported, no documented cases of poisoning from silver, lead, gold, and chromium have been reported (Harborne 1988). Molybdenum concentration can be unusually high in forages growing on soils where there is a naturally high content in the soils. Molybdenum/Copper ratios (1:2) are important in animal health, especially in sheep.

Molybdenum toxicoses in cattle from plant ingestion have been reported to cause depigmentation of the hair, anemia, depressed growth, and bone disorders. While plants may adapt to and grow on soils containing high levels of metals, accumulation of those metals into vegetative parts of the plant makes them potentially toxic.

2.10 CONCLUSION

Paracelsus is famously quoted as saying that all substances are poisonous, only the dose differentiates between a poison and a remedy. The same can be said about natural toxins found in human food stuffs. Consumption of too much of any food stuff, together with its natural toxins, can be harmful. In this chapter, we have covered some of the more visible natural toxins. However, the natural toxins discussed in this chapter are only a few in comparison to what is found in nature and has been reported in the literature. Entire volumes have been dedicated to individual classes of compounds (Kingsbury 1964; Cheeke 1998; Knight and Walter 2001; Burrows and Tyrl 2013). Poisonous plant research is going on in many university and government laboratories throughout the world. Research provides new information and tools to better manage livestock grazing systems, thus reducing losses and enhancing animal product quality. Additional spin-off benefits from research on poisonous plants include the development of animal models for the study of human diseases, new techniques and technologies for diagnosis and treatment of livestock poisoning, development of antibody-based diagnostic tools (ELISAs), novel treatments (chemotherapeutic agents), the discovery of new bioactive compounds, and improved livestock management strategies to enhance animal and human health.

ACKNOWLEDGMENTS

The authors thank Ms. Terrie Wierenga for technical and editorial assistance in preparation of the manuscript.

REFERENCES

Baucom, D., M. Romero, R. Belfon, and R. Creamer. 2012. Two new species of *Undifilum*, the swainsonine producing fungal endophyte, from *Astragalus* species of locoweed in the United States. *Botany* 90:866–875.

Basset-Seguin, N., A. Hauschild, J.J. Grob, R. Kunstfeld, B. Dréno, L. Mortier et al. 2015. Vismodegib in patients with advanced basal cell carcinoma (STEVIE): A pre-planned interim analysis of an international, open-label trial. *The Lancet Oncology* 16, 729–736.

Blackwell, W.H. 1990. *Poisonous and Medicinal Plants*. Englewood Cliffs, NJ: Prentice Hall.

Beasley, V. 1997. A systems affected approach to veterinary toxicology. Reference notes for toxicology. Champaign, IL: University of Illinois Press.

Beier, R.C. and J.O. Norman. 1990. The toxic factor in white snakeroot: Identity, analysis and prevention. *Human Vet. Toxicol.* 32:81–88.

Binns, W., J.L. Shupe, R.F. Keeler, and L.F. James. 1965. Chronological evaluation of teratogenicity in sheep fed *Veratrum californicum*. *J. Am. Vet. Med. Assoc.* 147:839–842.

Botha, C.J., J.J. Van der Lugt, G.L. Erasmus, T.S. Kellerman, R.A. Schultz, and R. Vleggaar. 1998. Krimpsiekte, a paretic condition of small stock poisoned by bufadienolide-containing plants of the Crassulaceae in South Africa. In *Toxic Plants and Other Natural Toxicants*, eds. T. Garland and A.C. Barr, pp. 407–412. Wallingford, CT: CAB International.

Brown, A.W., B.L. Stegelmeier, S.M. Colegate et al. 2015. The comparative toxicity of a reduced, crude comfrey (*Symphytum officinale*) alkaloid extract and the pure, comfrey-derived pyrrolizidine alkaloids, lycopsamine and intermedine in chicks (*Gallus gallus domesticus*). doi:10.1002/jat.3205.

Brown, A.W., B.L. Stegelmeier, S.M. Colegate, K.E. Panter, E.L. Knoppel, and J.O. Hall. 2014. Heterozygous p53 knockout mouse model for dehydropyrrolizidine alkaloid-induced carcinogenesis. *J. Appl. Toxicol.* doi:10.1002/jat.3120.

Burrows, G.E. and R.J. Tyrl. 2013 *Toxic Plants of North America*, 2nd ed. Hoboken, NJ: Wiley-Blackwell.

Carey, D.B. and M. Wink. 1994. Elevational variation of quinolizidine alkaloid contents in a lupine (*Lupinus argenteus*) of the Rocky Mountains. *J. Chem. Ecol.* 20: 849–857.

Cheeke, P.R. 1998. *Natural Toxicants in Feeds, Forages, and Poisonous Plants.* Danville, IL: Interstate Publishers.

Chiang, C., Y. Litingtung, E. Lee et al. 1996. Cyclopia and defective axial patterning in mice lacking sonic hedgehog gene function. *Nature* 383: 407–413.

Colegate, S.M., J.A. Edgar, A.M. Knill, and S.T. Lee. 2005. Solid Phase extraction and LCMS profiling of pyrrolizidine alkaloids and their N-oxides: A case study of *Echium Plantagineum. Pytochemical Anal.* 16: 108–119.

Colegate, S.M., P.R. Dorling, and C.R. Huxtable. 1979. A spectroscopic investigation of swainsonine: An α-mannosidase inhibitor isolated from *Swainsona canescens. Aust. J. Chem.* 32: 2257–2264.

Colegate, S.M., D.R. Gardner, J.M. Betz, and K.E. Panter. 2014a. Semi-automated separation of the epimeric dehydropyrrolizidine alkaloids lycopsamine and intermedine: Preparation of the *N*-oxides and NMR comparison with rinderine and echinatine. *Phytochem. Anal.* 25:429–438.

Colegate, S.M., D.R. Gardner, R.J. Joy, J.M. Betz, and K.E. Panter. 2012. Dehydropyrrolizidine alkaloids, including monoesters with an unusual esterifying acid, from cultivated *Crotalaria juncea* Sun Hemp CV. 'Tropic Sun'. *J. Agric. Food Chem.* 60: 3541–3550.

Colegate, S.M., D.R. Gardner, T.Z. Davis, S.L. Welsh, J.M. Betz, and K.E. Panter. 2013. Identification of a lycopsamine-N-oxide chemotype of *Amsinckia intermedia. Biochem. Syst. Ecol.* 48: 132–135.

Colegate, S.M., S.L. Welsh, D.R. Gardner, J.M. Betz, and K.E. Panter. 2014b. Profiling of dehydropyrrolizidine alkaloids and their N-oxides in herbarium-preserved specimens of *Amsinckia* species using HPLC-esi(+) MS. *J. Agric. Food Chem.* 62: 7382–7392.

Cook, D., D.R. Gardner, J.A. Pfister et al. 2009a. The biogeographical distribution of duncecap larkspur (*delphinium occidentale*) chemotypes and their potential toxicity. *J. Chem. Ecol.* 35: 643–652.

Cook, D., D.R. Gardner, J.A. Pfister et al. 2010. Differences in ponderosa pine isocupressic acid concentrations across space and time. *Rangelands* 32: 14–17.

Cook, D., B.T. Green, K.D. Welch et al. 2011. Comparison of the toxic effects of two duncecap larkspur (*delphinium occidentale*) chemotypes in mice and cattle. *Amer. J. Vet. Res.* 72: 706–714.

Cook, D., W.T. Beaulieu, I.W. Mott et al. 2013. Production of the alkaloid swainsonine by a fungal endosymbiont of the Ascomycete order Chaetothyriales in the host *Ipomoea carnea. J. Agric. Food Chem.* 61: 3797–3803.

Cook, D., D.R. Gardner, and J.A. Pfister. 2014. Swainsonine-containing plants and their relationship to endophytic fungi. *J. Agric. Food Chem.* 62: 7326–7334.

Cook, D., D.R. Gardner, M.H. Ralphs, J.A. Pfister, K.D. Welch, and B.T. Green. 2009b. Swainsonine concentrations and endophyte amounts of *Undifilum oxytropis* in different plant parts of *Oxytropis sericea. J. Chem. Ecol.* 35: 1272–1278.

Cooper, M.K., J.A. Porter, K.E. Young et al. 1998. Teratogen-mediated inhibition of target tissue response to shh signaling. *Science* 280: 1603–1607.

Crosby, D.G. and N. Aharonson. 1967. The structure of carotatoxin, a natural toxicant from carrot. *Tetrahedron* 23: 465–472.

Daugherty, C.G. 1995. The death of Socrates and the toxicology of hemlock. *J. Med. Biography* 3: 178–182.

Davis, A.M. and D.M. Stout. 1986. Anagyrine in western American lupines. *J. Range Manage.* 39: 29–30.

Davis, T.Z., B.L. Stegelmeier, B.T. Green et al. 2013a. Evaluation of the respiratory elimination kinetics of selenate and se-methylselenocysteine after oral administration in lambs. *Res. Vet. Sci.* 95: 1163–1168.

Davis, T.Z., B.L. Stegelmeier, K.D. Welch et al. 2013b. Comparative oral dose toxicokinetics of selenium compounds commonly found in selenium accumulator plants. *J. Anim. Sci.* 91: 4501–4509.

Davis, T.Z., B.L. Stegelmeier, and J.O. Hall. 2014. Analysis in horse hair as a means of evaluating selenium toxicoses and long-term exposures. *J. Agric. Food Chem.* 62: 7393–7397.

Davis, T.Z., B.L. Stegelmeier, K.E. Panter et al. 2012. Toxicokinetics and pathology of plant-associated acute selenium toxicosis in steers. *J. Vet. Diagn. Invest.* 24: 319–327.

de Balogh, K.K.I.M., A.P. Dimande, J.J. vander Lugt, R.J. Molyneux, T.W. Naude, and W.G. Welmans. 1999. A lysosomal storage disease induced by *Ipomoea carnea* in goats in Mozambique. *J. Vet. Diagn. Invest.* 11: 266–273.

Dennis, J.W., S.L. White, A.M. Freer, and D. Dime. 1993. Carbonoyloxy analogs of the anitmetastatic drug swainsonine. Activation in tumor cells by esterases. *Biochem. Pharmacol.* 46: 1459–1466.

Dobelis, P., J.E. Madl, J.A. Pfister, G.D. Manners, and J.P. Walrond. 1999. Effects of *Delphinium* alkaloids on neuromuscular transmission. *J. Pharmacol. Exp. Ther.* 291: 538–546.

Dorling, P.R., C.R. Huxtable, and P. Vogel. 1978. Lysosomal storage in *Swainsona* spp. toxicosis: An induced mannosidosis. *Neuropathol. Appl. Neurobiol.* 4: 285–295.

Edgar, J.A. and L.W. Smith. 2000. Transfer of pyrrolizidine alkaloids into eggs: Food safety implications. In *Natural and Selected Synthetic Toxins: Biological Implications*, eds. A.T. Tu and W. Gaffield, pp. 118–128. Washington, DC: American Chemical Society.

Fodor, G.B. and B. Colasanti. 1985. The pyridine and piperidine alkaloids: Chemistry and pharmacology. In *Alkaloids: Chemical and Biological Perspectives*, vol. 3, ed. S. Pelletier, 3–91. New York: John Wiley and Sons.

Frank, B.S., W.B. Michelson, K.E. Panter, and D.R. Gardner. 1995. Ingestion of poison-hemlock (*Conium maculatum*). *West. J. Med.* 163: 573–574.

Gaffield, W. 2000. The *Veratrum* alkaloids: Natural tools for studying embryonic development. In *Studies in Natural Products Chemistry,* vol. 23, ed. Atta-ur-Rahman, pp. 563–589. Amsterdam, the Netherlands: Elsevier Science.

Gaffield, W., J.P. Incardona, R.P. Kapur, and H. Roelink. 2000. Mechanistic investigation of *Veratrum* alkaloid-induced mammalian teratogenesis. In *Natural and Selected Synthetic Toxins: Biological Implications*, eds. A.T. Tu and W. Gaffield, pp. 173–187. Washington, DC: American Chemical Society.

Gaffield, W. and R.F. Keeler. 1994. Structure-activity relations of teratogenic natural products. *Pure and Appl. Chem.* 66: 2407–2410.

Gaffield, W. and R.F. Keeler. 1996. Steroidal alkaloid teratogens: Molecular probes for investigation of craniofacial malformations. *J. Toxicol. Toxin Rev.* 15: 303–326.

Gardner, D.R. and L.F. James. 1999. Pine needle abortion in cattle: Analysis of isocupressic acid in North American Gymnosperms. *Phytochem. Anal.* 10: 1–5.

Gardner, D.R., R.J. Molyneux, L.F. James, K.E. Panter, and B.L. Stegelmeier. 1994. Ponderosa pine needle-induced abortion in beef cattle: Identification of isocupressic acid as the principal active compound. *J. Agric. Food Chem.* 42: 756–761.

Green, B.T., J.A. Pfister, D. Cook et al. 2009. Effects of larkspur (*Delphinium barbeyi*) on heart rate and electrically evoked electromyographic response of the external anal sphincter in cattle. *Amer. J. Vet. Res.* 70: 539–546.

Green, B.T., C. Goulart, K.D. Welch et al. 2015. The non-competitive blockade of gabaa receptors by an aqueous extract of water hemlock (*Cicuta douglasii*) tubers. *Toxicon* 108: 11–14.

Green, B.T., S.T. Lee, K.D. Welch, and K.E. Panter. 2013a. Plant alkaloids that cause developmental defects through the disruption of cholinergic neurotransmission. *Birth Defects Res.earch Part C* 99: 235–246.

Green, B.T., K.D. Welch, K.E. Panter, and S.T. Lee. 2013b. Plant toxins that affect nicotinic acetylcholine receptors: A review. *Chem. Res. Toxicol.* 26: 1129–1138.

Grum, D.S., D. Cook, D. Baucom et al. 2013. Production of the alkaloid swainsonine by a fungal endophyte in the host *Swainsona canescens*. *J. Nat. Prod.* 76: 1984–1988.

Habermehl, G.G., W. Martz, C.H. Tokarnia, J. Dobereiner, and M.C. Mendez. 1988. Livestock poisoning in South America by species of the *Senecio* plant. *Toxicon* 26: 275–286.

Hammerschmidt, M., A. Brook, and A.P. McMahon. 1997. The world according to hedgehog. *Trends Genet.* 13: 14–21.

Harborne, J.B. 1988. *Introduction to Ecological Biochemistry*, 3rd ed. London: Academic Press.

Harborne, J.B. 1993. *Introduction to Ecological Biochemistry*, 4th ed. London: Academic Press.

Harborne, J.B. and H. Baxter. 1996 *Dictionary of Plant Toxins*. New York: John Wiley and Sons.

Hegarty, M.P. 1978. Toxic amino acids of plant origin. In *Effects of Poisonous Plants on Livestock*, eds. R.F. Keeler, K.R. VanKampen, and L.F. James, pp. 575–585. New York: Academic Press.

Huxtable, R.J. and R.A. Cooper. 2000. Pyrrolizidine alkaloids: Physicochemical correlates of metabolism and toxicity. In *Natural and Selected Synthetic Toxins: Biological Implications*, eds. A.T. Tu and W. Gaffield, pp. 100–117. Washington, DC: American Chemical Society.

James, L.F. 1978. Oxalate poisoning in livestock. In *Effects of Poisonous Plants on LivestockI*, eds. R.F. Keeler, K.R. Van Kampen, and L.F. James, pp. 139–145. New York: Academic Press.

James, L.F. 1999. Teratological research at the USDA-ARS Poisonous Plant Research Laboratory. *J. Nat. Toxins* 8: 63–80.

James, L.F. and W.J. Hartley. 1977. Effects of milk from animals fed locoweed in kittens, calves, and lambs. *Amer. J. Vet. Res.* 38: 1263–1265.

James, L.F., K.E. Panter, W. Gaffield, and R.J. Molyneux. 2004. Biomedical applications of poisonous plant research. *J. Agric. Food Chem.* 52: 3211–3230.

Keeler, R.F. 1986. Teratology of steroidal alkaloids. In *Alkaloids: Chemical and Biological Perspectives*, ed. S.W. Pelletier, pp. 389–425. New York: John Wiley and Sons.

Keeler, R.F. 1989. Quinolizidine alkaloids in range and grain lupins. In *Toxicants of Plant Origin, Vol I Alkaloids*, ed. P.R. Cheeke, pp. 133–168. Boca Raton, FL: CRC Press.

Keeler, R.F. and L.D. Balls. 1978. Teratogenic effects in cattle of *Conium maculatum* and conium alkaloids and analogs. *Clin. Toxicol.* 12: 49–64.

Keeler, R.F. and M.W. Crowe. 1984. Teratogenicity and toxicity of wild tree tobacco, *Nicotiana glauca* in sheep. *Cornell Vet.* 74: 50–59.

Keeler, R.F. and S. Young. 1986. When ewes ingest poisonous plants: The teratogenic effects. *Vet. Med. Food Anim. Pract.* May: 449–454.

Kellerman, T.S., J.A.W. Coetzer, and T.W. Naude. 1988. *Plant Poisonings and Mycotoxicoses of Livestock in Southern Africa.* Cape Town: Oxford University Press.

Kim, S.K. and D.A. Melton. 1998. Pancreas development is promoted by cyclopamine, a hedgehog signaling inhibitor. *Proc. Natl. Acad. Sci.* 95: 13036–13041.

King, L.A., M.J. Lewis, D. Parry, P.J. Twitchett, and E.A. Kilner. 1985. Identification of oenanthotoxin and related compounds in hemlock water dropwort poisoning. *Human Toxicol.* 4: 355–364.

Kinghorn, A.D. and M.F. Balandrin. 1984. Quinolizidine alkaloids of the Leguminosae: Structural types, analysis, chemotaxonomy and biological activities. In *Alkaloids: Chemical and Biological Perspectives*, ed. S.W. Pelletier, pp. 105–148. New York: John Wiley and Sons.

Kingsbury, J.M. 1964. *Poisonous Plants of the United States and Canada*. Englewood Cliffs, NJ: Prentice Hall.

Knight, A.P. and R.G. Walter. 2001. *A Guide to Plant Poisoning of Animals in North America*. Jackson: Teton NewMedia.

Landenburg, H. 1886. Research with the synthesis of coniine. *Chem. Ber.* 19: 439–441.

Lavie, Y., T. Harel-Orbital, W. Gaffield, and M. Liscovitch. 2001. Inhibitory effect of steroidal alkaloids on drug transport and multidrug resistance in human breast cancer cells. *Anticancer Res.* 21: 1189–1194.

Lawrence, D.P., F. Rotondo, and P.B. Gannibal. 2016. Biodiversity and taxonomy of the pleomorphic genus *Alternaria*. *Mycol. Prog.* 15: 1–22.

Lee, S.T., B.T. Green, K.D. Welch, G.T. Jordan, Q. Zhang, K.E. Panter et al. 2013. Stereoselective potencies and relative toxicities of gamma-coniceine and N-methylconiine enantiomers. *Chem. Res. Toxicol.* 26: 616–621.

Maity, T., N. Fuse, and P. A. Beachy. 2005. Molecular mechanisms of sonic hedgehog mutant effects in holoprosencephaly. *Proc. Natl. Acad. Sci. USA* 102: 17026–17031.

Majak, W., R.E. McDiarmid, J.W. Hall, and W. Willms. 2000. Alkaloid levels of a tall larkspur species in southwestern Alberta. *J. Range Manage.* 53: 207–210.

Majak, W. and M.A. Pass. 1989. Aliphatic nitrocompounds. In *Toxicants of Plant Origin. II. Glycosides*, ed. P.R. Cheeke, pp. 143–159. Boca Raton, FL: CRC Press.

Matsunaga, E. and K. Shiota. 1977. Holoprosencephaly in human embryos: Epidemiologic studies of 150 cases. *Teratology* 16: 261–272.

Molyneux, R.J., D.R. Gardner, L.F. James, and S.M. Colegate. 2002. Polyhydroxy alkaloids: Chromatographic analysis. *J. Chromatogr. Anal.* 967: 57–74.

Molyneux, R.J. and L.F. James. 1982. Loco Intoxication: Indolizidine alkaloids of spotted locoweed (*Astragalus lentiginosus*). *Science* 216: 190–191.

Molyneux, R.J., L.F. James, K.E. Panter, and M.H. Ralphs. 1991. Analysis and distribution of swainsonine and related polyhydroxyindolizidine alkaloids by thin layer chromatography. *Phytochem. Anal.* 2: 125–129.

Molyneux, R.J., L.F. James, M.H. Ralphs, J.A. Pfister, K.E. Panter, and R.J. Nash. 1994. Polyhydroxy alkaloid glycosidase inhibitors from poisonous plants of global distribution: Analysis and identification. In *Plant-Associated Toxins: Agricultural, Phytochemical and Ecological Aspects*, eds. S.M. Colegate and P.R. Dorling, pp. 107–112. Wallingford, CT: CAB International.

Molyneux, R.J., R.A. McKenzie, B.M. O'Sullivan, and A.D. Elbein. 1995. Identification of the glycosidase inhibitors swainsonine and calystegine B_2 in Weir vine (*Ipomoea* sp. Q6 [aff. calobra]) and correlation with toxicity. *J. Nat. Prod.* 58: 878–886.

Nielsen, D.B. and M.H. Ralphs. 1987. Larkspur economic considerations. In *Ecology and Economic Considerations of Poisonous Plants*, eds. L.F. James, M.H. Ralphs, and D.B. Nielsen, pp. 119–129. Boulder, CO: Westview Press.

Panter, K.E., T.D. Bunch, R.F. Keeler, D.V. Sisson, and R.J. Callan. 1990. Multiple congenital contractures (MCC) and cleft palate induced in goats by ingestion of piperidine alkaloid-containing plants: Reduction in fetal movement as the probable cause. *Clin. Toxicol.* 28: 69–83.

Panter, K.E., D.R. Gardner, L.F. James, B.L. Stegelmeier, and R.J. Molyneux. 2000a. Natural toxins from poisonous plants affecting reproductive function in livestock. In *Natural and Selected Synthetic Toxins: Biological Implications*, eds. A.T. Tu and W. Gaffield, pp. 154–172. ACS Symposium Series 745, Washington, DC: American Chemical Society.

Panter, K.E., D.R. Gardner, and R.J. Molyneux. 1998. Teratogenic and fetotoxic effects of two piperidine alkaloid-containing lupines (*L. formosus* and *L. arbustus*) in cows. *J. Nat. Toxins* 7: 131–140.

Panter, K.E., D.R. Gardner, B.L. Stegelmeier, K.D. Welch, and D. Holstege. 2011. Water hemlock poisoning in cattle: Ingestion of immature Cicuta maculata seed as the probable cause. *Toxicon* 57: 157–161.

Panter, K.E., C.C. Gay, R. Clinesmith, and T.E. Platt. 2013a. Management practices to reduce lupine-induced crooked calf syndrome in the Northwest. *Rangelands* 35: 12–16.

Panter, K.E., L.F. James, and D.R. Gardner. 1999. Lupines, poison-hemlock and *Nicotiana* spp: Toxicity and teratogenicity in livestock. *J. Nat. Toxins* 8: 117–134.

Panter, K.E. and R.F. Keeler. 1989. Piperidine alkaloids of poison hemlock (*Conium maculatum*). In *Toxicants of Plant Origin, Vol I Alkaloids*, ed. P.R. Cheeke, 109–132. Boca Raton, FL: CRC Press.

Panter, K.E., G.D. Manners, B.L. Stegelmeier et al. 2002. Larkspur poisoning: Toxicology and alkaloid structure-activity relationships. *Biochem. Syst.ematics Ecol.* 30: 113–128.

Panter, K.E., M.H. Ralphs, R.A. Smart, and B. Duelke. 1987. Death camas poisoning in sheep: A case report. *Vet. Human Toxicol.* 29: 45–48.

Panter, K.E., J. Weinzweig, D.R. Gardner, B.L. Stegelmeier, and L.F. James. 2000b. Comparison of cleft palate induction by *Nicotiana glauca* in goats and sheep. *Teratology* 61: 203–210.

Panter, K.E., K.D. Welch, D.R. Gardner, and B.T. Green. 2013b. Poisonous plants: Effects on embryo and fetal development. *Birth Defects Research Part C* 99: 223–234.

Pelletier, S.W. 1983. The nature and definition of an alkaloid. In *Alkaloids: Chemical and Biological Perspectives,* vol. 1, ed. S.W. Pelletier, pp. 1–31. New York: Wiley.

Pfister, J.A., T.Z. Davis, J.O. Hall et al. 2015. Elk (*Cervus canadensis*) preference for feeds varying in selenium concentration. *J. Anim. Sci.* 93: 3690–3697.

Powell, M.J. 1990. Poisonous and medicinal fungi. In *Poisonous and Medicinal Plants*, ed. W.H. Blackwell, pp. 71–110. Englewood Cliffs, NJ: Prentice Hall.

Pryor, B.M., R. Creamer, R.A. Shoemaker, J. McClain-Romero, and S. Hambleton. 2009. *Undifilum*, a new genus for endophytic *Embellisia oxytropis* and parasitic *Helminthosporium bornmuelleri* on legumes. *Botany* 87: 178–194.

Ralphs, M.H., R. Creamer, D. Baucom et al. 2008. Relationship between the endophyte *Embellisia* spp. and the toxic alkaloid swainsonine in major locoweed species (*Astragalus* and *Oxytropis*). *J. Chem. Ecol.* 34: 32–38.

Rimkus, T.K., R.L. Carpenter, S. Qasem et al. 2016. Targeting the sonic hedgehog signaling pathway: Review of smoothened and gli inhibitors. *Cancers* 8. doi:10.3390/cancers8020022.

Roberts, M.F. and M. Wink. 1998. *Alkaloids: Biochemistry, Ecology, and Medicinal Applications.* New York: Plenum Press.

Roitman, J.N. and K.E. Panter. 1995. Livestock poisoning caused by plant alkaloids. In *The Toxic Action of Marine and Terrestrial Alkaloids*, ed. M.S. Blum, pp. 53–124. Fort Collins, CO: Alaken.

Schep, L.J., R.J. Slaughter, G. Becket, and D.M. Beasley. 2009. Poisoning due to water hemlock. *Clin. Toxicol. (Phila.* 47: 270–278.

Sharma, R.P. and D.K. Salunkhe. 1989. Solanum glycoalkaloids. In *Toxicants of Plant Origin, Vol I Alkaloids*, ed. P.R. Cheeke, pp. 179–236. Boca Raton, FL: CRC Press.

Smith, L.W. and C.C.J. Culvenor. 1981. Plant sources of hepatotoxic pyrrolizidine alkaloids. *J. Nat. Prod.* 44: 129–152.

Stegelmeier, B.L., D.R. Gardner, L.F. James, K.E. Panter, and R.J. Molyneux. 1996. The toxic and abortifacient effects of Ponderosa pine. *Vet. Pathol.* 33: 22–28.

Stegelmeier, B.L., L.F. James, K.E. Panter et al. 1999. The pathogenesis and toxicokinetics of locoweed (*Astragalus* and *Oxytropis* spp.) poisoning in livestock. *J. Nat. Toxins* 8: 35–45.

Taipale, J., J.K. Chen, M.K. Cooper et al. 2000. Effects of oncogenic mutations in Smoothened and Patched can be reversed by cyclopamine. *Nature* 406: 1005–1009.

Weinzweig, J., K.E. Panter, M. Pantaloni et al. 1999a. The fetal cleft palate: I. Characterization of a congenital model. *Plast. Reconstr. Surg.* 103: 419–428.

Weinzweig, J., K.E. Panter, M. Pantaloni et al. 1999b. The fetal cleft palate: II. Scarless healing after *in utero* repair of a congenital model. *Plast. Reconstr. Surg.* 104: 1356–1364.

Weinzweig, J, K.E. Panter, J. Patel, D.M. Smith, A. Spangenberger, and M.B. Greeman. 2008. The fetal cleft palate: V. Elucidation of the mechanism of palatal clefting in the congenital caprine model. *Plast. Reconstr. Surg.* 121(4): 1328–1334.

Weinzweig, J., K.E. Panter, J. Seki, M. Panteloni, A. Spangenberger, and J.S. Harper. 2006. The fetal cleft palate: IV. Midfacial growth and bony palatal development following in utero and neonatal repair of the congenital caprine model. *Plast. Reconstr. Surg.* 118(1): 81–93.

Weinzweig, J., K.E. Panter, A. Spangenberger, J.S. Harper, R. McRae, and L.E. Edstrom. 2002. The fetal cleft palate: III. Ultrastructural and functional analysis of palatal development following *in utero* repair of the congenital model. *Plast. Reconstr. Surg.* 104: 2355–2362.

Welch, K.D., B.T. Green, D.R. Gardner et al. 2015a. The effect of administering multiple doses of tall larkspur (delphinium barbeyi) to cattle. *J. Anim. Sci.* 93(8): 4181–4188.

Welch, K.D., B.T. Green, D.R. Gardner et al. 2012a. The effect of 7, 8–methylenedioxylycoctonine-type diterpenoid alkaloids on the toxicity of tall larkspur (*Delphinium* spp.) in cattle. *J. Anim. Sci.* 90: 2394–2401.

Welch, K.D., B.T. Green, D.R. Gardner et al. 2013. The effect of low larkspur (*Delphinium* spp.) co-administration on the acute toxicity of death camas (*Zigadenus* spp.) in sheep. *Toxicon* 76C: 50–58.

Welch, K.D., K.E. Panter, D.R. Gardner et al. 2011. The acute toxicity of the death camas (*zigadenus* species) alkaloid zygacine in mice, including the effect of methyllycaconitine coadministration on zygacine toxicity. *J. Anim. Sci.* 89: 1650–1657.

Welch, K.D., K.E. Panter, S.T. Lee et al. 2009. Cyclopamine-induced synophthalmia in sheep: Defining a critical window and toxicokinetic evaluation. *J. Appl. Toxicol.* 29: 414–421.

Welch, K.D., K.E. Panter, B.L. Stegelmeier et al. 2012b. Veratrum-induced placental dysplasia in sheep. *Int. J. Poisonous Plant Res.* 2: 54–62.

Welch, K.D., C. Parsons, D.R. Gardner et al. 2015b. Evaluation of the seasonal and annual abortifacient risk of western juniper trees on oregon rangelands. *Rangelands* 37: 139–143.

Welch, K.D., C.A. Stonecipher, D.R. Gardner et al. 2015c. The effect of western juniper on the estrous cycle in beef cattle. *Res. Vet. Sci.* 98: 16–18.

Wiley, R.G. 2000. Molecular neurosurgery: Using plant toxins to make highly selective neural lesions. In *Natural and Selected Synthetic Toxins: Biological Implications*, eds. A.T. Tu and W. Gaffield, pp. 194–203. Washington, DC: American Chemical Society.

Wink, M. 1999. *Functions of Secondary Metabolites and Their Exploitation in Biotechnology: Annual Plant Reviews*, vol. 3. Boca Raton, FL: CRC Press.

Wink, M. and D.B. Carey. 1994. Variability of quinolizidine alkaloid profiles of *Lupinus argenteus* (Fabaceae) from North America. *Biochem. Syst. Ecol.* 22: 663–669.

Wink, M., M.A. Hofer, M. Bilfinger, E. Englert, M. Martin, and D. Schneider. 1993. Geese and plant dietary allelochemicals-food palatability and geophagy. *Chemoecology* 4:93–107.

Wink, M., C. Meibner, and L. Witte. 1995. Patterns of quinolizidine alkaloids in 56 species of the genus Lupinus. *Phytochemistry* 38: 139–153.

Young, J.A., P.C. Martinelli, R.E. Eckert, and R.A. Evans. 1999. *Halogeton: A history of mid-20th Century range conservation in the Intermountain Area.* USDA-ARS Publication Number 1553.
Yu, F., T.N. Barry, P.J. Moughan, and G.F. Wilson. 1993. Condensed tannin and gossypol concentrations in cottonseed and in processed cottonseed meal. *J. Sci. Food Agric.* 63: 7–15.
Zhang, Y. and P. Talalay. 1998. Mechanism of differential potencies of isothiocyanates as inducers of anticarcinogenic phase 2 enzymes. *Cancer Res.* 58: 4632–4639.

3 Mushroom Toxins

Roman Kotłowski

CONTENTS

3.1 INTRODUCTION

The importance and nutritional value of edible mushrooms often is an interesting subject of public discussions. There are strong supporters of mushrooms, which they value for their flavor and nutritional value. There are also their opponents who argue that the consumption of mushrooms may result in indigestion, allergies, and other harmful effects on health. It is no secret that despite the fact that mushrooms are known all over the world and mushroom picking is a popular form of pastime, they continue to pose a threat to human health and even life. This is most often due to mistaken identification of species by amateur mushroom pickers, leading to serious problems.

The synthesis of toxins in poisonous mushrooms occurs using ribosomes or in biochemical pathways. In the first case, cyclopeptide toxins such as amatoxins, phallotoxins, and most probably virotoxins (Hallen et al. 2007) are produced and post-translationary enzymatically modified. In the second type of synthesis, different enzymes involved are responsible for toxins' biosynthesis in biochemical pathways. The death cap and its white variants most commonly cause fatal poisonings of mushroom pickers. This is due to the presence of cyclopeptides such as amatoxins and phallotoxins. Amatoxins are about 10–20 times more toxic than phallotoxins. The structure of amatoxins includes amino acid sequences Ile-Trp-Gly-Ile-Gly-Cys-Asn-Pro (α-amanitin) or Ile-Trp-Gly-Ile-Gly-Cys-Asp-Pro (β-amanitin), cyclized by "head-to-tail" peptide bonds, and the connection between Trp and Cys residues. Further differentiation between amatoxins (α-, γ-, β-, ε-amanitin, amanin, amanullin, amanullinic acid, proamanullin, and amanin amide—occur only in *Amanita virosa*) is the different distributions of the specific substituents: -H, -OH, and -NH_2. Peptides are post-translationary cyclized (Luo et al. 2014) to form biologically active toxins (Figure 3.1) present in mushrooms (Sgambelluri et al. 2014). The mode of action of α-amanitin relies on strong affinity to the catalytic site of RNA polymerase II

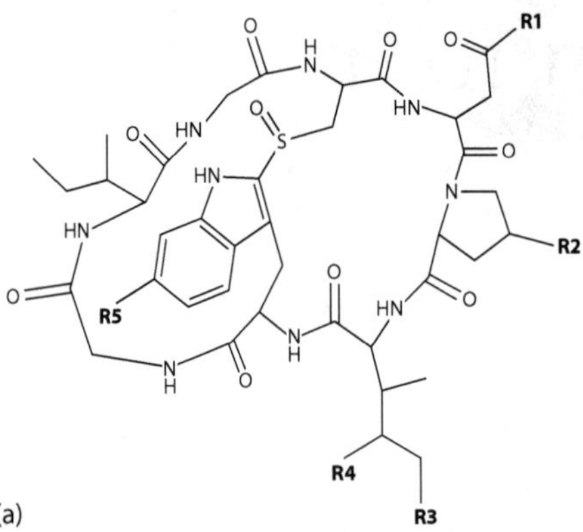

Compound	R1	R2	R3	R4	R5
α-amanitin	NH_2	OH	OH	OH	OH
amaninamide	NH_2	OH	OH	OH	H
γ-amanitin	NH_2	OH	OH	H	OH
amanullin	NH_2	OH	H	H	OH
proamanullin	NH_2	H	H	H	OH
β-amanitin	OH	OH	OH	OH	OH
amanin	OH	OH	OH	OH	H
ε-amanitin	OH	OH	OH	H	OH
amanullinic acid	OH	OH	H	H	OH

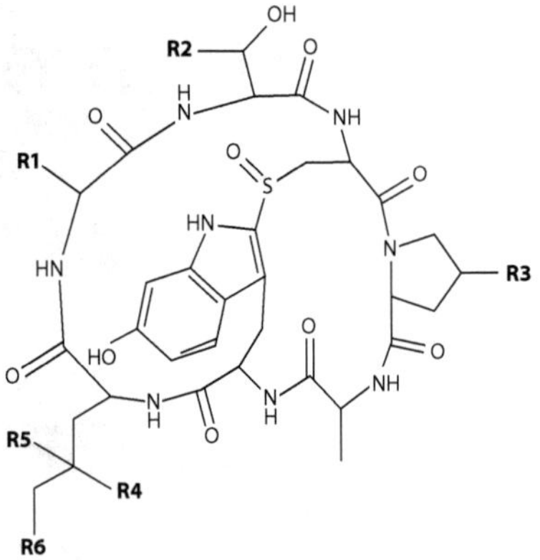

Compound	R1	R2	R3	R4	R5	R6
phallisin	CH_3	CH_3	OH	OH	OH	OH
phalloidin	CH_3	CH_3	OH	H	OH	OH
phalloin	CH_3	CH_3	OH	H	OH	H
prophalloin	CH_3	CH_3	H	H	OH	H
phallisacin	$CH(CH_3)_2$	COOH	OH	OH	OH	OH
phallacidin	$CH(CH_3)_2$	COOH	OH	H	OH	OH
phallacin	$CH(CH_3)_2$	COOH	OH	H	OH	H

Sgambelluri et al., 2014

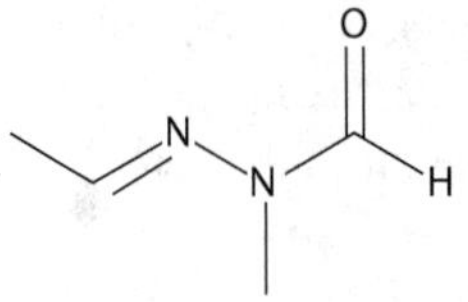

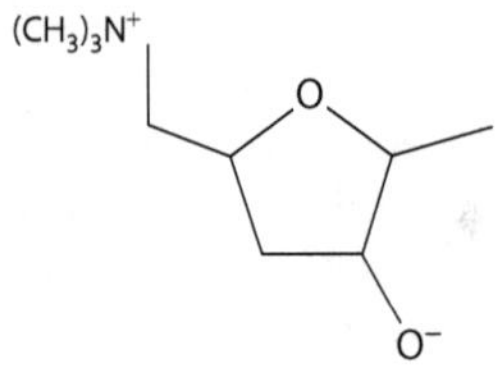

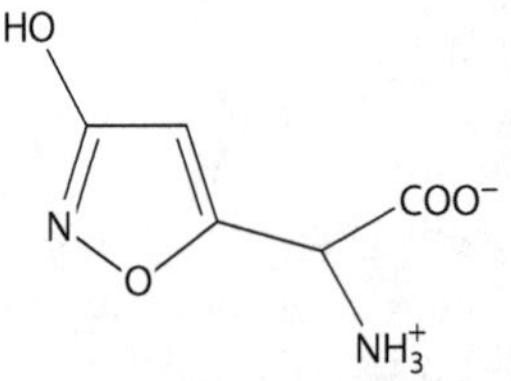

FIGURE 3.1 The structures of (a) α-amanitin, (b) phalloidin, (c) gyromitrin, (d) muscarin, (e) ibotenic acid, (f) coprin. *(Continued)*

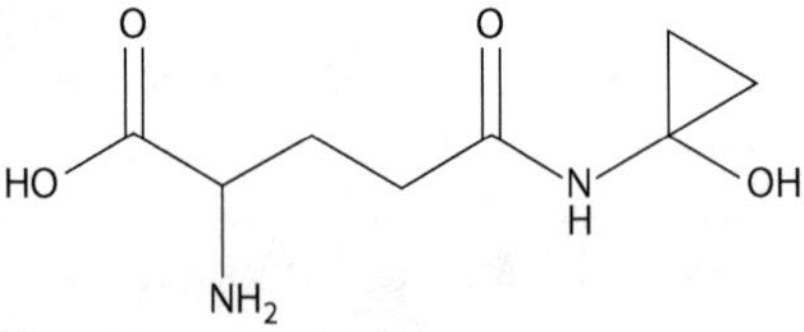

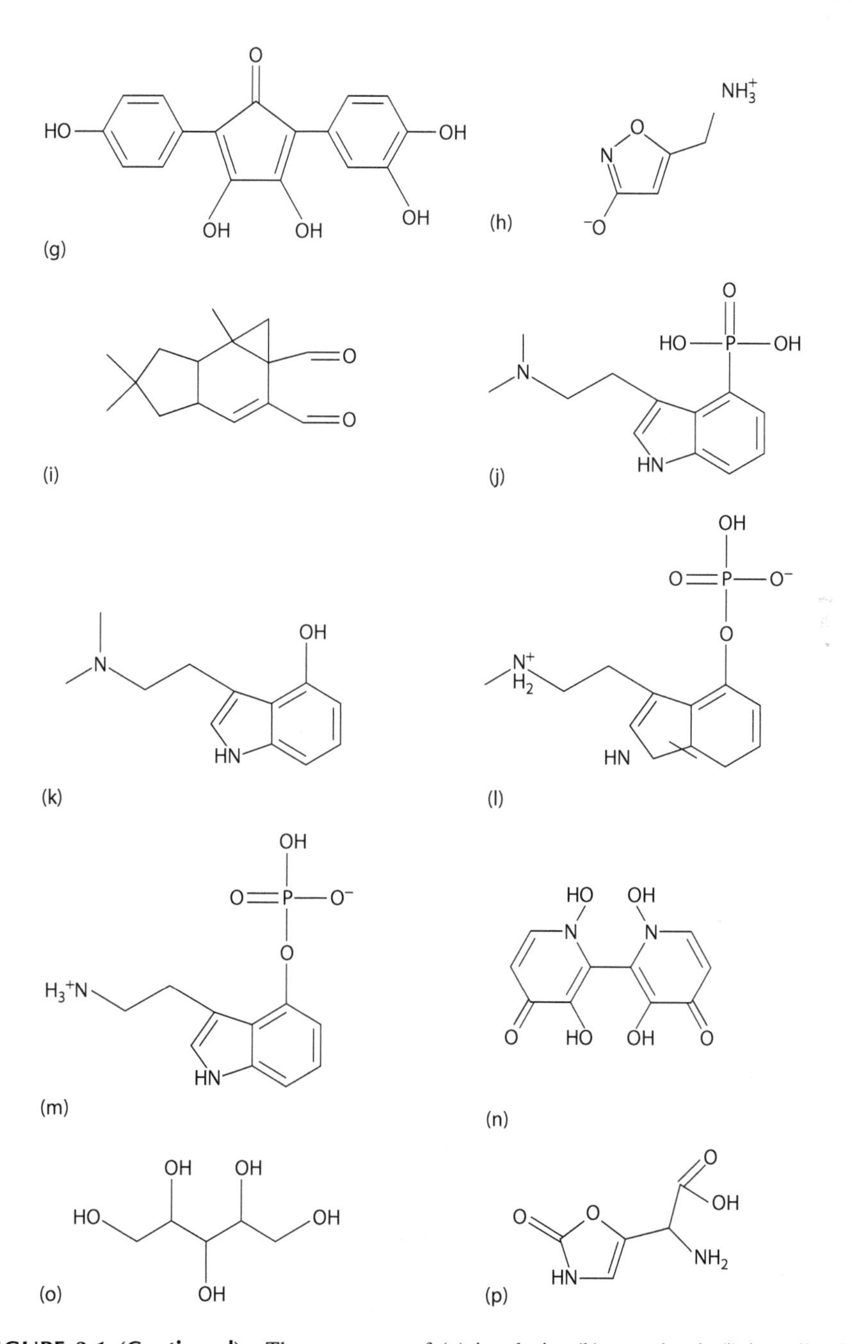

FIGURE 3.1 (Continued) The structures of (g) involutin, (h) muscimol, (i) isovelleral, (j) psilocybin, (k) psilocin, (l) baeocystin, (m) norbaeocystin, (n) orlleanin, (o) arabitol and (p) muscazone.

(Bushnell et al. 2002). Phallotoxins include toxins such as phalloin, phalloidin (most toxic), phallisin, phallacin, phallacidin, and phallisacin. Another isolated compound, prophalloin, is virtually harmless. These compounds, similar to amatoxins, differ in the arrangement of the following substituents: -H, -OH, $-CH_3$, $-CH(CH_3)_2$, and -COOH. They are structurally related to amatoxins, although they are shorter by one amino acid residue. Cyclopeptide toxins cause irreversible liver and other organ damage.

The edible species most similar to the death cap are yellow knight (*Tricholoma equestre*) and green-cracking Russula (*Russula virescens*). The false death cap (*Amanita citrina*) is considered an inedible species or slightly toxic. However, it has a very strong resemblance to the deadly poisonous death cap, and its white variety is not suitable for consumption. One highly toxic *Amanita* species is the panther cap. It includes such toxins as ibotenic acid and muscimol (Chilton and Ott 1976), which act on the central nervous system causing hallucinations. Ingestion of this fungus also causes diarrhea and vomiting.

Another poisonous species of mushrooms is the funeral bell, often confused with sheathed wood tuft (*Kuehneromyces mutabilis*), owing its name to its growth in the form of colonies on the wood of dead trees. This species also produces amatoxins (Enjalbert et al. 2004). *Inocybe rubescens* is a species producing muscarine, which can cause nausea, vomiting, lacrimation, diarrhea, and breathing disorders. *Gyromitra esculenta* is often confused with the edible morel (*Morchella esculenta*). This species is toxic because it contains gyromitrin (List and Luft 1968), which causes gastrointestinal disturbances and damage to the liver, spleen, kidneys, and eyes. Another poisonous mushroom is the fool's webcap, a lethal species producing orellanine (Grzymala and Fiksinski 1960), which damages the kidneys. The toxicity of the naked brim cap manifests itself when the body begins to produce antibodies against its own blood cells. Consequently, this may lead to impaired blood flow to vital organs. A commonly confused mushroom is the sickener, confused with the edible *Russula paludosa*. It is not a highly poisonous mushroom but after ingestion of even small amounts, it causes abdominal pain, nausea, and vomiting. Very rare is the poisonous species Satan's Bolete (*Boletus satanas*). The species is strictly protected. Eating it, especially in the raw state, causes severe gastrointestinal symptoms. The toxicity of this species is probably associated with the presence of bolesatine, a glycoprotein (Kretz et al. 1991). The common ink cap (*Coprinopsis atramentaria*) is dangerous to the human body only while consuming alcohol. Coprine produced by this species blocks the metabolism of ethanol, leading to acetaldehyde poisoning. The main toxic component of the fly agaric is ibotenic acid. Ingestion of this mushroom can cause diarrhea, vomiting, shortness of breath, and slower pulse.

In recent years, there has been increased interest in hallucinogenic mushrooms—the so-called "magic mushrooms"—which contain narcotic substances. So far about 80 species of mushrooms containing substances having narcotic properties have been described. These are mainly species belonging to the genera *Psilocybe*, *Panaeolus*, and *Gymnopilus*, as well as some species of the genus *Inocybe*, *Conocybe*, *Stropharia*, and *Pluteus*, and several species of fly agaric, including the fly agaric (*Amanita muscaria*) and the panther cap (*Amanita pantherina*). Their popularity stems from the fact that access to hallucinogenic mushrooms in many countries is relatively easy. Another "advantage" is their low price. According to the law, possession and trade of mushrooms containing narcotics is a crime. Therefore, accurate identification of species of mushrooms that contain toxic substances, also those illegal, is very important for the purposes of legal and medical proceedings.

3.2 THE NUMBER OF CASES OF MUSHROOM POISONING

The best-documented data for mushroom poisonings come from the United States. From the graph shown in Figure 3.2, the average number of registered cases of intoxication by hallucinogenic mushrooms in the United States is about 715 ± 138. However, the annual number of intoxications with hallucinogenic mushrooms is decreasing in recent years. In contrast, the number of registered cases of poisonings with mushrooms that produce cyclopeptide toxins will remain at a level slightly below 50 cases per year. Statistical data on the number of existing mushroom poisonings without specification on the toxin types in Poland in the same period between 1999–2015 is oscillating around 200 ± 160 cases. Poland is representing European countries where gathering mushrooms is a popular habit and higher prevalence of mushroom poisonings is reported in comparison to Western European countries.

3.3 MORPHOLOGY

For proper selection of treatment, the poisonous mushroom species ingested by a patient must be identified quickly. However, the process of cooking and digestion in the human body makes it impossible to maintain the original shape of the fungus.

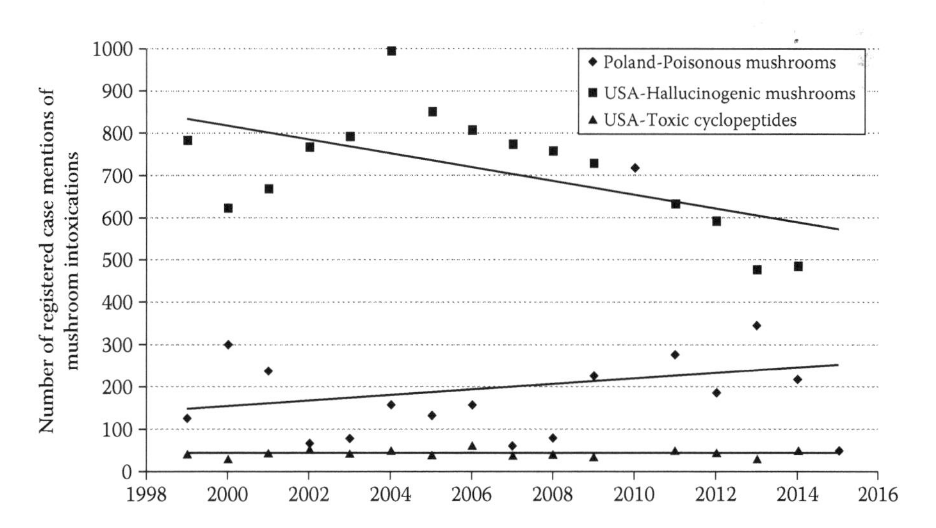

FIGURE 3.2 Annual number of registered case mentions of mushroom intoxications in the USA from hallucinogenic mushrooms and mushrooms producing poisonous cyclopeptides, and number of mushroom poisonings without specification on the toxin types in Poland.

Even an experienced mycologist may have problems performing morphological analysis of such samples. Problems with identification may result from the large similarity of spores of different species. The standard method for identifying species of mushrooms is morphological analysis, which includes macroscopic and microscopic tests. Macroscopic analysis consists in determining the characteristic color, size, and structure of mushrooms. Prolonged and painstaking microscopic examination is primarily based on a comparison of the appearance of spores and measuring the length and width, which does not always bring satisfactory results. Usually, identification is made more difficult by the too low number of spores in the secretions of the stomach, highly degraded material, or the presence of fat droplets that are easily mistaken for death cap spores. In view of the difficulties encountered during morphological analysis, it is necessary to find a new improved method of species identification, independent of morphology. It seems the detection of genetic material in samples submitted for testing is the most reliable basis of diagnosis.

3.4 PHYLOGENETIC ANALYSIS

Taxonomic studies give a better understanding of the phylogenetic relationships between basidiomycetes. The phylogenetic similarity between species of poisonous mushrooms, for the sequences ITS1, 5,8S, and ITS2, are shown in Figure 3.3. The most dangerous and the most commonly mistaken species of poisonous mushrooms are the death cap (*Amanita phalloides*), its white varieties destroying angel (*Amanita virosa*) and fool's

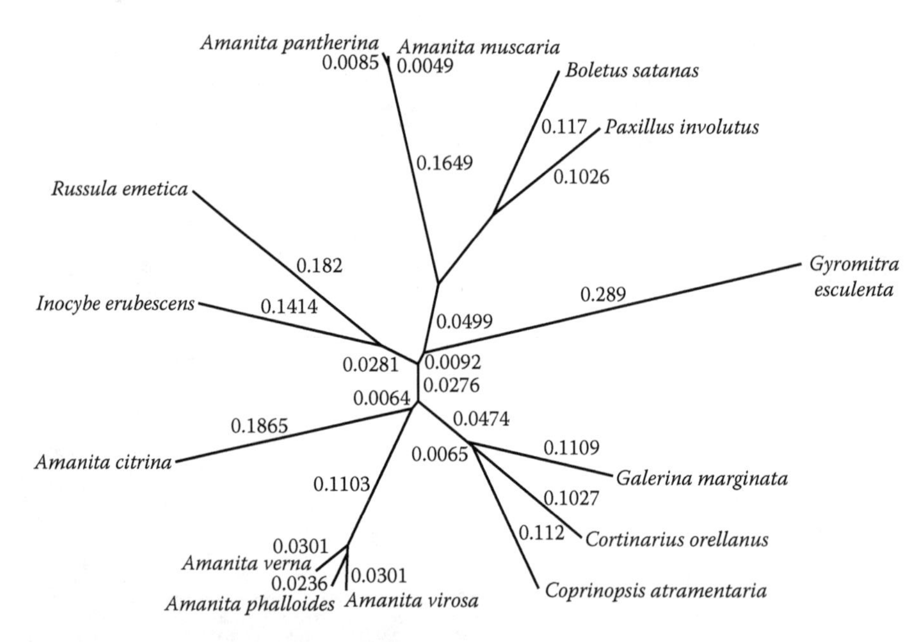

FIGURE 3.3 The phylogenetic similarity of poisonous mushrooms selected within the sequences ITS1, 5,8S, and ITS2. The numbers indicate the degree of relatedness of DNA sequences. A level close to 0 denotes almost identical DNA sequences, and a total value close to 1 reveals unrelated DNA sequences.

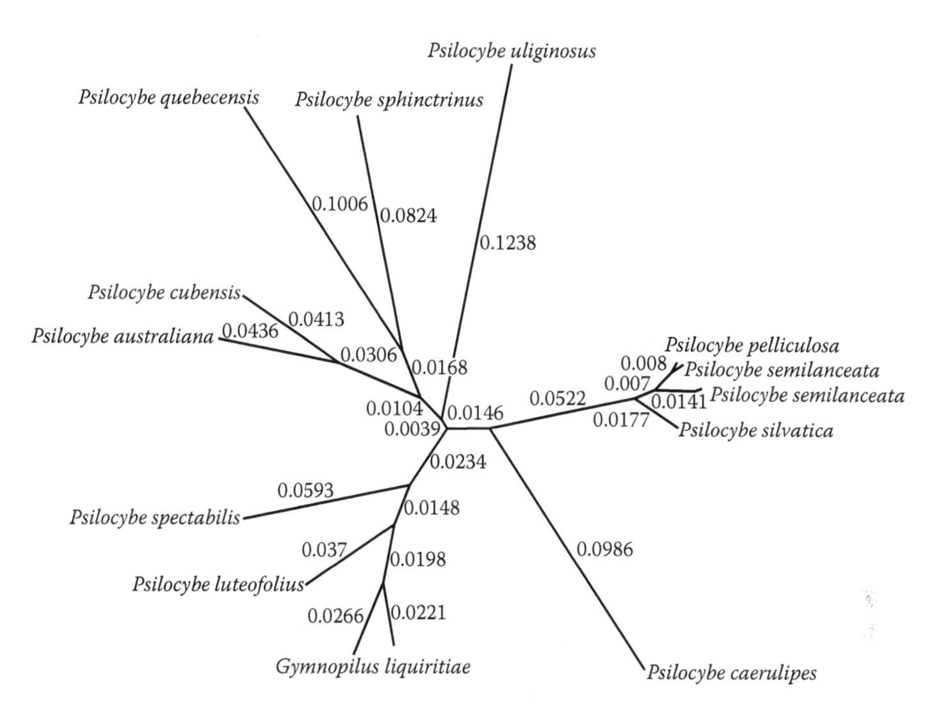

FIGURE 3.4 Phylogenetic similarity of hallucinogenic mushrooms within the ITS1 sequence (Nugent et al. 2004).

mushroom (*Amanita verna*), funeral bell (*Galerina marginata*), deadly fibrecap (*Inocybe rubescens*), false morel (*Gyromitra esculenta*), fool's webcap (*Cortinarius orellanus*), naked brimcap (*Paxillus involutus*), common ink cap (*Coprinopsis atramentaria*), fly agaric (*Amanita muscaria*), false blusher (*Amanita pantherina*), false death cap (*Amanita citrina*), sickener (*Russula emetica*), and Satan's Bolete (*Boletus satanas*).

The current taxonomy of hallucinogenic mushrooms is not completely clear. As shown in Figure 3.4, the species *Psilocybe semilacenta* and *Psilocybe pelliculosa* are ambiguously classified in spite of a high DNA-differentiating potential within the ITS1 region. Perhaps this is a misclassification of the species carried out on the basis of morphological features.

3.5 DETECTION METHODS FOR HALLUCINOGENIC AND POISONOUS MUSHROOMS

3.5.1 Isolation of Pure DNA Samples

An increasingly thorough understanding of the genomes of mushrooms brings many benefits. It may help physicians in coming up with a rapid diagnosis and contribute to the improvement of treatment. In addition, new genetic tests can help detect crimes related to narcotic mushrooms. Identification of mushroom species can be carried out with the analysis of DNA, RNA, and morphological characteristics of mushrooms. The most common molecular targets are ITS1 and ITS2 sequences

(Internal Transcribed Spacers) between the DNA sequences encoding subunits 18S, 5,8S, and 28S of the ribosomal RNA (White et al. 1990) and the sequence of the gene fragment coding for *gpd* - glyceraldehyde 3-phosphate dehydrogenase (Kotłowski et al. 2000). In the correct identification of species of mushrooms, based on samples collected for taxonomic purposes or clinical samples which require quick identification, it is important to use efficient methods of isolation of the purest DNA for PCR amplification and sequencing. One such universal method of DNA isolation has been described by Wołoszyn (2015). It may be used for samples of both fresh and processed mushrooms. In the first step, the sample is ground and then heated in TE buffer (10 mM Tris, 1 mM EDTA) to denature the proteins. The next step is fungal cell lysis with chloroform and sodium dodecyl sulfate (SDS). The stage of freezing the samples is to intensify the process of lysis of the fungal cells by creating sharp ice crystals. In a further step, the addition of guanidine hydrochloride is intended to liquidate the sample via the denaturation of proteins bound to nucleic acids. This step allows the efficient isolation of nucleic acids in the sample flow through a bed of silica. The nucleic acids are selectively bound to the silica bed and the remainder of the sample with the proteins and other components flows through the bed. Rinsing with ethanol allows to purify the nucleic acids bound to the silica bed, and then their elution from the bed with the TE buffer (10 mM Tris, 1 mM EDTA) makes it possible to obtain DNA with a high degree of purity suitable for PCR amplification.

It is best to perform species diagnostics of nucleic acids isolated from poisonous and hallucinogenic mushrooms with the participation of primer sequences complementary to the variable regions ITS1 and ITS2 located within the *rrn* operon. Due to the presence of several copies of the *rrn* operon in the genome of mushrooms, this method has a higher sensitivity than assays of molecular targets that occur only once. However, the sequence analysis of ITS1 and ITS2 shows that very closely related species of mushroom *Amanita muscaria* and *Amanita pantherina* have almost identical sequences, making it difficult to identify species in PCR assay, which detects the presence or absence of a particular species of fungus. Moreover, the death cap specimen and its white varieties have a high homology within the ITS sequence, which complicates the design of species-specific probes for the detection of individual species. For these purposes, better suited are *gpd* gene intron sequences, with a greater volatility than the sequences of the *rrn* operon.

3.5.2 Detection of the Genes Coding for Toxins by PCR

Amatoxins and phallotoxins in comparison to other known cyclic peptides present in mushrooms are biosynthesized on ribosomes and therefore classified as ribosomally synthesized and post-translationally modified peptides (RiPPs) (Hallen et al. 2007). The currently known sequences of genes encoding amatoxins and phallotoxins for eight different mushroom species made it possible to design PCR-primers specific to toxins regardless of mushroom species. For example detection of alpha and beta amanitins can be conducted by using primers AMAF 5´- GCDACBCGTCTTCCCATCTGGGG and AMAR 5´–GCYTCGCCACGAGTGAGGA, and for detections of phallotoxins using primers FALF 5´—GCBACBCGTCTTCCYGCYTGGCT, and FALR 5´—CTCGCCACGAGTGAGGAGRCGGT (Wołoszyn 2015).

3.6 CONCLUDING REMARKS

In recent years, mushrooms have been demonstrated to contain many beneficial compounds. They can be a rich source of antioxidant, antibacterial, and antiviral compounds. Mushrooms also help in the treatment of cardiovascular diseases and even cancer. Furthermore, as saprophytes, they intake nutrients from dead organisms and organic substrates, releasing elements which can then be included again in biochemical cycles. All in all, mushrooms play an important role in the ecosystem. Collecting and eating wild mushrooms is a popular pastime in many countries, representing an important element in the national food culture. However, the lack of basic knowledge about the morphological characteristics of edible and poisonous mushrooms is a frequent cause of poisonings in individuals and sometimes entire families. Such unfortunate events are especially frequent in autumn and summer. Less experienced mushroom pickers often apply totally inadequate criteria to recognize poisonous mushrooms. They tend to ascribe only a few minor characteristics to poisonous mushrooms, such as a bitter taste, blackening of silver spoons, redness, or yellowing of the mushroom flesh after salting. There are many other common techniques applied to distinguish poisonous mushrooms, but usually they are fundamentally wrong, and their common acceptance is a major cause of the constantly large number of poisonings. Other factors contributing to the occurrence of mushroom poisonings are mushroom collection by children; picking the juvenile forms with undeveloped morphological features; the habit of clipping the picked mushrooms just below the cap; and mushrooming in woods with abundant undergrowth or with scant natural light. An additional problem is the high similarity of many species: there exist many toxic look-alikes of edible mushrooms. Mushroom poisonings are usually characterized by severe clinical symptoms, often requiring liver transplantation and sometimes resulting in death. Recent years have also seen an increased interest in hallucinogenic mushrooms. According to the law, possession and trade of mushrooms containing narcotics is a crime. Therefore, accurate identification of species of mushrooms that contain toxic substances, also those illegal, is very important for the purposes of legal and medical proceedings. The statistics show the necessity of improving the treatment of poisonings caused by mushrooms. In many countries, we still have an insufficient number of qualified individuals to ensure implementation of the most modern treatment techniques, among others, by albumin dialysis or transplantation of the liver. In order to reduce such serious effects of poisoning, as well as their frequency, it is important to raise public awareness in this regard as well as the preparation of medical services to function properly at every stage of the treatment process. What is very important here is efficient and accurate diagnosis.

REFERENCES

Bushnell, D.A., P. Cramer, and R.D. Kornberg. 2002. Structural basis of transcription: α-Amanitin–RNA polymerase II cocrystal at 2.8 Å resolution. *Proc Natl Acad Sci USA* 99(3): 1218–1222.

Chilton, W.S. and J. Ott. 1976. Toxic metabolites of Amanita pantherina, A. cothurnata, A. muscaria and other Amanita species. *Lloydia* 39(2–3): 150–157.

Enjalbert, F., G. Cassanas, S. Rapior, C. Renault, and J.P. Chaumont. 2004. Amatoxins in wood-rotting Galerina marginata. *Mycologia* 96(4): 720–729.

Grzymala, S. and R. Fiksinski. 1960. Use of micro-electrofiltration in the precipitation of thermal decomposition products of orellanine in the volatile phase. *Postepy Hig Med Dosw.* 14: 699–702. [in Polish].

Hallen, H.E., H. Luo, J.S. Scott-Craig, and J.D. Walton. 2007. Gene family encoding the major toxins of lethal Amanita mushrooms. *Proc Natl Acad Sci USA* 104(48): 19097–19101.

Kretz, O.H., E.E. Creppy, and G. Dirheimer. 1991. Characterization of bolesatine and toxic proteins from the mushroom Boletus satanas Lenz and its effects on kidney cells. *Toxicology* 66(2): 213–24.

Kotłowski R., P. Myjak, and J. Kur. 2000. Specific detection of Amanita phalloides mycelium and spores by PCR amplification of the gpd (glyceraldehyde-3-phosphate dehydrogenase) gene fragment. *J Food Biochem* 24: 201–212.

List, P.H. and P. Luft. 1968. Gyromitrin, the poison of Gyromitra esculenta. 16. On the fungi contents. *Arch Pharm Ber Dtsch Pharm Ges* 301(4): 294–305. [in German].

Luo, H., S.Y. Hong, R.M. Sgambelluri, E. Angelos, X. Li, and J.D. Walton. 2014. Peptide macrocyclization catalyzed by a prolyl oligopeptidase involved in α-amanitin biosynthesis. *Chem Biol* 21(12): 1610–1617.

Nugent, K.G. and B.J. Saville. 2004. Forensic analysis of hallucinogenic mushrooms: A DNA-based approach. *Forensic Sci Int* 140: 147–157.

Sgambelluri, R.M., S. Epis, D. Sassera, H. Luo, E.R. Angelos, and J.D. Walton. 2014. Profiling of amatoxins and phallotoxins in the genus Lepiota by liquid chromatography combined with UV absorbance and mass spectrometry. *Toxins (Basel)* 6(8): 2336–2347.

White, T.J., T. Bruns, S. Lee, and J.W. Taylor. 1990. Amplification and direct sequencing of fungal ribosomal RNA genes for phylogenetics. Pp. 315–322 In: PCR Protocols: A Guide to Methods and Applications, eds. Innis, MA, Gelfand DH, JJ Sninský, and TJ White. Academic Press, New York.

Wołoszyn, A. 2015. Master's Thesis entitled: Discovering of new gpd gene fragment sequences of poisonous mushrooms Amanita pantherina and Tricholoma equestre and development of new detection method for amanitin and phallotoxin independently from mushroom species. Gdansk University of Technology, Department of Molecular Biotechnology and Microbiology. Gdansk, Poland.

4 Marine Phycotoxins and Seafood Safety

Gustaaf M. Hallegraeff

CONTENTS

4.1 INTRODUCTION

Microscopic marine unicellular algae form an important component of the plankton diet of shellfish such as mussels, oysters, scallops as well as larval crustaceans and fish. Under favorable environmental conditions of light, temperature, salinity, water column stability, and nutrients, algal populations of only a few cells can quickly multiply into dense blooms containing millions of cells per dm^3, which sometimes can discolor the seawater. Most algal blooms appear to be harmless events, but under exceptional conditions, they can become so densely concentrated that they deplete the oxygen in the water. This can cause indiscriminate kills of fish and invertebrates in sheltered bays. Other algal species can kill fish by damaging the sensitive fish gill membranes either mechanically or through the release of ichthyotoxins that usually are harmless to humans.

An essentially different phenomenon is the production by certain species of dinoflagellates, diatoms, and cyanobacteria of potent neurological toxins, which can find their way through fish and shellfish to humans. When humans eat seafood contaminated by these microalgae, they may suffer a variety of gastrointestinal and neurological illnesses. These poisoning syndromes include Paralytic Shellfish Poisoning (PSP), which in extreme cases can lead to death through respiratory paralysis; Diarrhetic Shellfish Poisoning (DSP), which causes severe gastrointestinal problems and may promote stomach tumors; Neurotoxic Shellfish Poisoning (NSP), which also can cause respiratory distress via aerosol toxins; and Amnesic Shellfish Poisoning (ASP), which can lead to permanent brain damage (short-term memory loss) (Table 4.1). Problems caused by cyanobacterial toxins include liver damage from hepatotoxic peptides or PSP from neurotoxic alkaloids. Toxic cyanobacterial blooms are primarily confined to fresh water and brackish water environments, but increasingly can discharge into coastal environments and also contaminate seafood. Ciguatera is essentially a tropical fish food-poisoning syndrome well known from coral reef areas. Humans consuming contaminated fish can suffer from gastrointestinal and neurological illnesses, and in extreme cases, can die from respiratory failure.

Although toxic algal blooms, in a strict sense, are completely natural phenomena that have occurred throughout recorded history, in the past four decades, the public health and economic impacts of such events appear to have increased in frequency, intensity, and geographic distribution (Hallegraeff 1993).

Global climate change is adding a new level of uncertainty to many seafood safety monitoring programs (Hallegraeff 2010), as are range extensions of harmful algal bloom species by ship ballast water transport and increased sea surface temperatures. The greatest problems for human society will be caused by being unprepared for significant range extensions or the increase of algal biotoxin problems in currently poorly monitored areas. Increased vigilance in seafood biotoxin monitoring programs is, therefore, recommended.

4.2 PARALYTIC SHELLFISH TOXINS

4.2.1 Symptoms and Causative Organisms

One of the first recorded fatal cases of human PSP after eating shellfish contaminated with dinoflagellate toxins was in 1793, when Captain George Vancouver and his crew landed in British Columbia in an area now known as Poison Cove. He noted that for local Indian tribes, it was taboo to eat shellfish when the sea water became bioluminescent due to dinoflagellate blooms (Dale and Yentsch 1978).

TABLE 4.1
Clinical Symptoms of Various Types of Fish and Shellfish Poisoning

Paralytic Shellfish Poisoning (PSP)	Diarrhetic Shellfish Poisoning (DSP)	Amnesic Shellfish Poisoning (ASP)	Neurotoxic Shellfish Poisoning (NSP)	Azaspiracid Shellfish Poisoning (AZP)	Ciguatera Fish Poisoning (CFP)
Causative Toxin					
Saxitoxins, gonyautoxins, sulfocarbomoyl saxitoxins	Okadaic acid, Dinophysis toxins	Domoic acid and isomers	Brevetoxin	Azaspiracid	Ciguatoxin
Symptoms					
Mild Case					
Within 30 min: tingling sensation or numbness around lips, gradually spreading to face and neck; prickly sensation in fingertips and toes; headache, dizziness, nausea, vomiting, diarrhea	After 30 min to a few hours (seldom more than 12 h): diarrhea, nausea, vomiting, abdominal pain	After 3–5 h: nausea, vomiting, diarrhea, abdominal cramps	After 3–6 h: chills, headache, diarrhea; muscle weakness, muscle and joint pain; nausea and vomiting	Similar to DSP. Nausea, vomiting, severe diarrhea, stomach cramps	Symptoms develop within 12–24 h of eating fish. Gastrointestinal symptoms: diarrhea, abdominal pain, nausea, vomiting

(Continued)

TABLE 4.1 (*Continued*)
Clinical Symptoms of Various Types of Fish and Shellfish Poisoning

Paralytic Shellfish Poisoning (PSP)	Diarrhetic Shellfish Poisoning (DSP)	Amnesic Shellfish Poisoning (ASP)	Neurotoxic Shellfish Poisoning (NSP)	Azaspiracid Shellfish Poisoning (AZP)	Ciguatera Fish Poisoning (CFP)
Extreme Case					
Muscular paralysis; pronounced respiratory difficulty; choking sensation; death through respiratory paralysis may occur within 2–24 h after ingestion	Chronic exposure may promote tumor formation in the digestive system	Decreased reaction to deep pain; dizziness, hallucinations, confusion; short-term memory loss; seizures	Paraesthesia; altered perception of hot and cold; difficulty in breathing, double vision, trouble in talking and swallowing		Neurological symptoms: numbness and tingling of hands and feet; cold objects feel hot to touch; difficulty in balance; low heart rate and blood pressure; rashes. In extreme cases, death through respiratory failure
Treatment					
Patient has stomach pumped and is given artificial respiration. No lasting effects	Recovery after three days, irrespective of medical treatment				No antitoxin or specific treatment is available. Neurological symptoms may last for months or years. Calcium and mannitol may help to relieve symptoms

The causative dinoflagellate (*Alexandrium tamarense/catenella* species complex, initially classified as *Gonyaulax, Protogonyaulax* or *Gessnerium*) was first identified in the 1930s in California, but until the 1970s, it was known only from the temperate waters of Europe, North America, and Japan. The causative alkaloid toxins (saxitoxins) were first chemically characterized in the 1960s, but by the 1990s, PSP was well documented from throughout the Southern Hemisphere. Other species of the dinoflagellate genus *Alexandrium*, such as *A. minutum*, as well as the phylogenetically unrelated dinoflagellates *Gymnodinium catenatum* and tropical *Pyrodinium bahamense* are now also widely implicated. Globally, this is the most widespread shellfish toxin. Paralytic Shellfish Toxins (PSTs) block the sodium channels of excitable membranes of the nervous system and associated muscles, inhibiting action potentials and nerve transmission impulses. In vertebrates, the peripheral nervous system is particularly affected. Typical symptoms of poisoning include tingling and numbness of the extremities, progressing to muscular incoordination, respiratory distress, and muscular paralysis, leading in extreme cases to death by asphyxiation.

4.2.2 Toxin Chemistry and Action Levels

The first PST to be chemically characterized was named saxitoxin after the butter clam *Saxidomus* from which it was isolated. Since then, at least 20 other toxin fractions have been identified from plankton and shellfish. These toxins all resemble the parent molecule saxitoxin but differ in the type and localization of derivation (Figure 4.1a). PST can be grouped conveniently into carbamate toxins (saxitoxin STX, neosaxitoxin NEOSTX, gonyautoxins GTX 1–4), sulfamate toxins (gonyautoxins 5, 6; fractions C_1–C_4), and decarbamoyl gonyautoxins. Australian shellfish contaminated with *G. catenatum* contained predominantly fractions C_1–C_4 (Oshima et al. 1987), but when contaminated with *A. tamarense,* contained STX, GTX2,3, NEOSTX, GTX1,4) and when contaminated by *A. minutum,* contained gonyautoxins 1–4 (Oshima et al. 1989a). Low PST concentrations have also been found in the digestive system of Tasmanian abalone and rock lobsters (Dowsett et al. 2011). These different PST fractions exhibit widely different toxic potencies when injected intraperitoneally into mice, ranging from 2,045 MU (mouse units)/μmole (saxitoxin) to 16 MU/μmole (C_1), in which 1 MU (mouse unit) is the amount of toxin required to kill a mouse weighing 20 g in 15 min upon intraperitoneal injection. Now mouse bioassays are increasingly being phased out, the applicability of Toxicity Equivalence Factors (TEFs) based on mouse intraperitoneal potency is increasingly being questioned and expected to be replaced in future with mouse oral potency factors (Munday et al. 2013). This approach would significantly increase the potency of, for example, neosaxitoxin.

The ultimate toxicity of shellfish to humans depends not only on the abundance and toxic potency of the dinoflagellates being filtered but also on the chemical transformations of the various toxins, either by the shellfish themselves or during food storage, food processing, and food digestion by human consumers. In humans, 120–180 μg PSP can produce moderate symptoms, 400–1,060 μg PSP can cause death, but 2,000–10,000 μg is more likely to constitute a fatal dose, with the body weight of the patient being an important variable. While the predominance

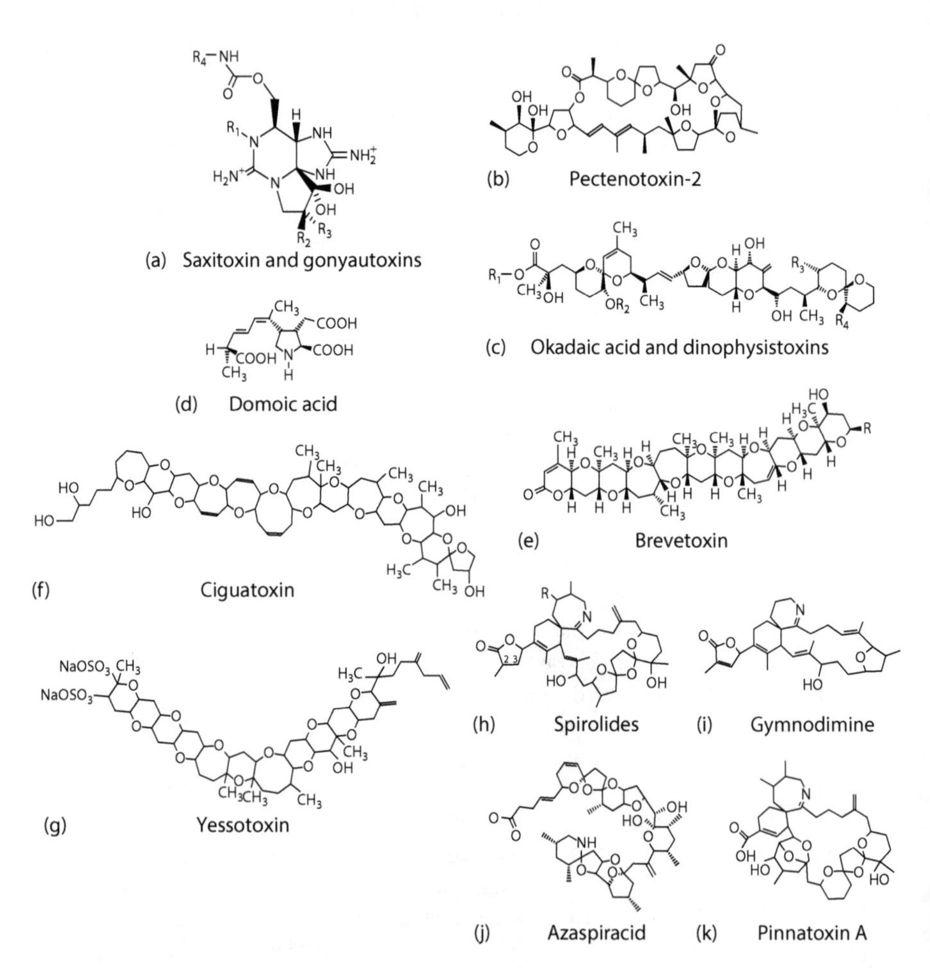

FIGURE 4.1 Chemical structures of key seafood algal toxins. (Modified after Cembella, A.D., *Phycologia*, 42, 420–447, 2003.)

of sulfamate toxins in Tasmanian shellfish contaminated with *G. catenatum* thus suggests a low health risk to humans, these sulfamate fractions can easily be transformed under mild acidic conditions to the corresponding carbamate toxins. Fraction C_1 thus transforms into GTX_2, C_2 into GTX_3, C_3 into GTX_1, and C_4 into GTX_4, with a concomitant 10 to 100-fold increase in toxicity. For this reason, the C_{1-4} toxins are often referred to as cryptic PST. While these conversions are easily accomplished *in vitro* in the laboratory, we still do not know under what conditions these conversions may also occur *in vivo* in the human stomach. Until the precise fate of these toxins can be determined, the most conservative toxin regulatory level (0.8 mg STX equivalent per kg shellfish meat) has been internationally adopted. This is based on an observed lethal level in human adults at 10,000 μg, with moderate symptoms appearing at 1,000 μg (which can be the result of eating, for example, 12 clams weighing 100 g at toxin levels of 0.8 mg/kg). This US Food and Drug Administration quarantine level has been internationally adopted.

When seafood products reach this level, the affected area should be closed to both recreational and commercial shellfish harvesting and not reopened until levels decline. In the Philippines alone, *Pyrodinium* has now been responsible for more than 2,000 human illnesses and 100 deaths resulting from the consumption of contaminated shellfish as well as sardines and anchovies (Hallegraeff and MacLean 1989). Because of its higher toxic potential, a lower alert level of 40 μg PSP/100 g shellfish is employed in some SE Asian countries.

4.2.3 Detection of PST

Historically, the AOAC mouse bioassay (AOAC 1990) was the only internationally, legally accepted method for PST toxins. In this bioassay, 100 g of shellfish meat is macerated in a blender, gently boiled for 5 min with 100 cm^3 0.1 N HCl, and 1 cm^3 of the clarified extract (pH adjusted to 2.0–4.0) injected intraperitoneally into a 20 g test mouse. The toxicity of the solution is established by measuring the time from injection to the mouse's last gasping breath, using a table of dose/death time relationships and correcting for the precise weight of the test animal. Substantial errors can result in estimating dose at long or short death times, and sample extracts, therefore, need to be diluted by trial and error to achieve death times in the range of 5–7 min. Test results can be calibrated against pure saxitoxin and expressed as mg STX equivalents per kg of shellfish meat. The method is relatively easy to perform and requires no special equipment. The major disadvantage is its poor precision (±20%) and insensitivity (detection limit is 0.5 mg saxitoxin /kg).

In the past decades, stricter ethical standards for animal experiments in most countries and drawbacks inherent in the mouse bioassay have led to the development of alternative chemical assays. The most successful methods involve the alkaline oxidation of PSP toxins to fluorescent derivatives using periodic acid in sodium phosphate buffer, their separation by high-performance liquid chromatography (HPLC), and detection by fluorometry. The early HPLC methods developed by Sullivan et al. (1985) and Oshima et al. (1989b) found widespread following. The first method uses a polymer PRP column and gradient elution to separate the 10 most common PST in a single 20-min run. The second method uses a C8 bonded silica gel column and isocratic elution to separate all known 20 or so PST fractions in three separate chromatographic runs for sulfamate toxins, gonyautoxins, and saxitoxins, respectively. Shellfish with simple toxin profiles (e.g., *A. minutum*) can be adequately analyzed with the Sullivan method, whereas complex toxin profiles (e.g., *G. catenatum*) can be resolved only with the Oshima method. HPLC methods offer increased sensitivity (0.1–0.2 mg/kg) and increased precision (5–10%) compared with mouse bioassays and can operate continuously with automated injection systems. An important further refinement of the HPLC method using a precolumn oxidation step was introduced by Lawrence et al. (2005). In this case, the oxidation occurs immediately after sample extraction and prior to HPLC analysis, so that the HPLC separation is of the reaction products as opposed to the STXs themselves as done in the postcolumn method. Modification of the HPLC/FLD (fluorescence detection)/MS (mass spectrometric detection) method by adding a combination of strong anion- and cation-exchangers-enabled ion chromatographic separation of all PST toxins within a single chromatographic run (Jaime et al. 2001). Another recent improvement is the application of hydrophilic interaction liquid chromatography (HILIC) HPLC-MS/MS analysis of PST (Boundy et al. 2015). These chemical methods still require international validation before results can become legally accepted. Jellett Biotek Ltd (now renamed Scotia) developed a rapid semiquantitative immuno test kit for PST toxins (Jellett et al. 2002), with further improvements marketed by Abraxis™, Neogen™, and Europroxima™. The varying mixtures and cross-reactivities of the antibodies used in these test kits provide varying results against different STX profiles (De Grasse et al. 2014; Jawaid et al. 2015; Turner et al. 2015). Radioreceptor binding assays for PST (Doucette et al. 1991) and a method based on the saxitoxin-binding protein saxiphilin (Negri and Llewellyn 1998) have also been developed. The ability to reliably determine whether the total of PST toxins are present below or above the regulatory level of 0.8 mg/kg is the ultimate criterion for choice of a particular analytical method.

4.3 DIARRHETIC SHELLFISH TOXINS

4.3.1 Symptoms and Causative Organisms

Severe vomiting, nausea, and diarrhea symptoms in human shellfish consumers were first recorded in the Netherlands in the 1960s (Kat 1985), but the term DSP was first coined in 1976 from Japan, where it caused problems for the scallop fishery (Yasumoto et al. 1980). The first dinoflagellate implicated was *Dinophysis fortii* (in Japan), followed by *D. acuminata* (in Europe), *D. acuta, D. norvegica* (in Scandinavia), and the benthic dinoflagellate *Prorocentrum lima*. Between 1976 and 1982, some 1,300 DSP cases were reported in Japan, in 1981 more than 5,000 cases in Spain, and in 1983 some 3,300 cases in France. In 1984 in Sweden, DSP problems caused a shutdown of the mussel industry for almost a year. Increasing problems of contamination of seafood with pectenotoxins (not regulated) have also been noted (Burgess and Shaw 2001). The known global distribution of DSP now includes Japan, Europe, Chile, Thailand, Canada, Australia, New Zealand, and most recently the USA. The clinical symptoms of DSP often may have been mistaken for those of bacterial gastric infections and the problem may be much more widespread than currently thought. Unlike in PSP, no human fatalities have been reported and patients usually recover within 3 days. However, some of the toxins involved could act as stomach tumor promotors and thus produce chronic problems in shellfish consumers (Suganuma et al. 1988).

4.3.2 Toxin Chemistry and Action Levels

The causative DST toxins are fat-soluble polyether compounds (Figure 4.1h,i). The first toxin to be characterized chemically was okadaic acid (OA), originally isolated from the sponge *Halichondria okadai* but now thought to have been derived from associated benthic dinoflagellate *P. lima*. Subsequent research revealed the presence in shellfish of okadaic acid derivatives, termed Dinophysis toxins (DTX), pectenotoxins

(PTX, after the scallop genus *Pecten*) (Lee et al. 1989), DTX2, and an isomer from Irish mussels, pectenotoxin 2 from *D. fortii* in the Adriatic Sea, and numerous other analogues. Diarrheagenic effects have only been proven for OA, DTX1, and DTX3, whereas PTX1 - 4 causes liver necrosis. Some diarrheagenic toxins (OA and DTX1) are potent inhibitors of protein phosphatases, and this mode of action may be linked to the observed diarrhea, degenerative changes in absorptive epithelium of the small intestine, and to tumor promotion.

As a result of the diversity of toxins involved, compared with other shellfish toxins such as PST and AST, the action level for DST toxins set by regulatory authorities varies considerably from country to country. Japan uses 0.05 MU/g = 50 MU/kg edible tissue (1 MU = 4 μg OA), taking into consideration the weight that the digestive gland represents of total shellfish tissue, while Canada uses 1 μg OA equivalent per g digestive gland, but this does not take into consideration the variation in percentage of the weight of the digestive gland. At present, satisfactory regulatory levels are known only for the OA series (including OA, DTX1,2, and the DTX3 complex), which are all phosphatase inhibitors and diarrhetic in action. In the European Union, OA/DTX analogues are regulated with the quarantine level for the sum of both toxin groups in bivalves set at 0.16 mg/kg, while 0.2 mg OA equivalent/kg is the action level currently adopted by the Food Standards Australia New Zealand.

4.3.3 Detection of DST

An intraperitoneal mouse bioassay procedure developed by the Japanese Ministry of Health and Welfare (1981) proved to be susceptible to producing false positive results due to the presence of contaminating free fatty acids in shellfish digestive glands (DGs) at certain times of the year. This method has now been generally abandoned and also in Japan since 2015 has been replaced by LC-MS. A feeding method with white rats was used successfully in the Netherlands (Kat 1985) but has since been discontinued. While the intraperitoneal mouse bioassay estimates total toxicity due to a range of lipophilic compounds, the oral dosage rat bioassay evaluates the diarrhetic effect of only certain DST toxins. With the decision in the European Union to cease the use of mouse and rat bioassays for lipophilic toxins, reliable chemical analytical methods are increasingly applied. An HPLC method first developed for separating DST toxins by Lee et al. (1987) greatly advanced this field of research. Shellfish DGs are homogenized and extracted with 80% methanol in water, the DSP toxins esterified to fluorescent esters with 9-anthryldiazomethane (ADAM), and the toxins then separated by HPLC and monitored by fluorometry. Problems with the implementation of this method resulted from the poor stability of the ADAM reagent and the presence of coextractives in shellfish tissues, necessitating a silica column cleanup following the derivatization step (Quilliam 1995). Semiquantitative immunoassay test kits for quick detection of OA and/or DTX1 are available (e.g., Abraxis, UBE Industries, and Tokyo DSP Check™ kit). While these chemical and immunological techniques represent an important step forward, they are still not sufficiently reliable as a routine method to accurately detect the full range of toxins involved. OA and DTX1 have been identified as inhibitors of protein phosphatases, and this property has been explored in radioactive and colorimetric assays for their detection (Tubaro et al. 1996). The primary toxins produced by the dinoflagellates are water-soluble DTX4 or derivatives, which cannot be detected by ADAM LC procedures but probably do not contribute significantly to DST shellfish contamination. Furthermore, the discovery of an esterase in the outer wall of dinoflagellates led to the recognition that hydrolysis during handling and extraction of shellfish and plankton can lead to erratic results (Quilliam 1998). Liquid chromatography–mass spectrometry (LC-MS) is currently the only efficient and comprehensive option for analysis of lipophilic DST toxins. The ability to reliably determine whether the OA series of DST toxins are present below or above the regulatory level of 0.2 mg OA equivalent/kg is the ultimate criterion for choice of a particular analytical method.

4.4 AMNESIC SHELLFISH POISONS

4.4.1 Symptoms and Causative Organisms

ASP was first recognized in 1987 on Prince Edward Island, Canada, where it caused 3 deaths and 105 cases of acute human poisoning following the consumption of blue mussels (Bates et al. 1989). The memory loss associated with extreme cases of human intoxication led to the description of the syndrome as ASP. This problem was eventually shown (Bates et al. 1989; Wright et al. 1989) to have derived from the chain-forming diatom *Pseudo-nitzschia multiseries.* Until this discovery, diatoms were not regarded as sources of toxins. Since then, other *Pseudo-nitzschia* species shown to be toxic include *P. australis*, *P. brasiliana*, *P. calliantha*, *P. cuspidata*, *P. delicatissima*, *P. fraudulenta*, *P. galaxiae*, *P. granii*, *P. multistriata*, *P. pseudodelicatissima*, *P. pungens*, *P. seriata*, and *P. turgidula* (Trainer et al. 2012). To date, reports of domoic acid in seafood products have been mainly confined to North America and Canada, while only insignificant concentrations have been detected in other parts of the world such as Europe, Australia, Japan, and New Zealand. Of further concern is domoic acid production by the unrelated diatoms *Nitzschia navis-varingica* from tropical shrimp aquaculture ponds and *N. bizertensis* from Tunesia (Lundholm and Moestrup 2000; Smida et al. 2014).

4.4.2 Toxin Chemistry and Action Levels

The causative compound domoic acid (Figure 1b) is an excitatory amino acid acting as a glutamate antagonist on the kainate receptors of the central nervous system. Humans affected in Canada had consumed mussels containing 300–1,200 mg/kg of domoic acid. Seabird mortalities have been related to consumption of domoic-acid-contaminated fish in California and Mexico. In addition to bivalve shellfish, razor clams as well as the hepatopancreas and viscera of dungeness crab (USA) have also been found to be contaminated. The proposed regulatory level in Canada of 20 mg/kg tissue (AOAC 1991) has been adopted by other countries screening for the toxin. This is based on the observation of an effect on certain consumers at an estimated domoic acid concentration of 200 g/kg wet weight, with a factor of 0.1 applied for safety reasons. It is recognized that isomers of domoic acid also exist and possibly can contribute to toxicity.

4.4.3 Detection of AST

During the early days of the Canadian crisis, domoic acid was extracted from shellfish using the standardized extraction procedure for mouse bioassay of PST toxins (Lawrence et al. 1989) but with longer observation times (up to 4 hrs). At toxin levels >40 mg/kg domoic acid, mice exhibit characteristic scratching symptoms, but this bioassay method is now generally considered not sensitive enough to accurately estimate the proposed quarantine level in Canada of 20 mg/kg tissue (AOAC 1991). HPLC is now the preferred analytical technique for the determination of domoic acid in shellfish. A very sensitive procedure, based on reaction with 9-fluorenylmethylchloroformate to form the fluorenylmethoxycarbonyl derivative and HPLC analysis with fluorescence detection, has been developed for monitoring of domoic acid in marine matrices such as seawater and phytoplankton (Pocklington et al. 1990). The detection limit is as low as 15 pg/ cm^3 for domoic acid in seawater. This procedure has been adapted to shellfish tissue extracts (Quilliam et al. 1989, 1995). Domoic acid is extracted from shellfish tissues by homogenization with methanol-water (1:1, v/v). The concentration of domoic acid is determined by HPLC with ultraviolet absorbance detection. Sample extracts are injected following dilution and filtration of the crude extract or after cleanup on strong anion-exchange solid-phase extraction cartridges. The latter provides selective isolation of domoic acid and related compounds from interfering substances such as tryptophan, as well as preconcentration, to facilitate analysis of trace levels. A photodiode array detector can be used to examine UV spectra in order to confirm domoic acid, but this option may not always be available. The detection limit is 20–30 ng/g. A neuroreceptor binding assay for AST has been developed based on binding to the kainate-glutamate receptor in rat brain synaptosomes, using 3H-kainic acid as a standard (Van Dolah et al. 1994). Immunological test kits for ASP are also available (e.g., Biosense Laboratories, Abraxis, and Neogen).

4.5 NEUROTOXIC SHELLFISH POISONS

4.5.1 Symptoms

Until 1993, NSP, caused by polyether brevetoxins produced by the unarmored dinoflagellate *Karenia brevis*, was considered endemic to the Gulf of Mexico and the east coast of Florida, where "red tides" had been reported as early as 1844. An unusual feature of this organism is the formation by wave action of toxic aerosols that can lead to respiratory asthma-like symptoms in humans. Unexpectedly, in early 1993, more than 180 human shellfish poisonings were reported from New Zealand, putatively caused by a mixed bloom of *K. mikimotoi* and related species (Haywood et al. 2004). Earlier claims that *raphidophyte* blooms of *Chattonella*, and possibly the related genera *Fibrocapsa* and Heterosigma, can produce brevetoxin-like compounds have been rejected (McNabb et al. 2006). In humans, the symptoms of NSP include respiratory distress, as well as eye and nasal membrane irritation, caused principally by exposure to sea-spray aerosols and by direct contact with toxic algal blooms while swimming. No human fatalities from brevetoxin poisoning have ever been reported. The toxins implicated in neurological shellfish poisoning are considered to be primarily ichthyotoxins (fish killing toxins), but they are also known to accumulate in shellfish.

4.5.2 Toxin Chemistry and Action Levels

Brevetoxins are polyether ladder toxins. Many of these lipid-soluble cyclic polyether compounds have been characterized, but due to the chemical lability of the brevetoxins, analysis of these compounds continues to be problematic (Yasumoto et al. 1989). The New Zealand shellfish toxins (tentatively coded TX1, TX2, and TX3; Satake et al. 1996) differ from well-characterized Florida *K. brevis* dinoflagellate toxins (PbTx1-8) in either the side chain, the cyclic ether skeleton, or both (Figure 4.1c). Brevetoxins and their derivatives exert their toxic effect by specific binding to site-5 of voltage-sensitive sodium channels. In Florida and North Carolina, shellfish harvesting is suspended when cell concentrations of *K. brevis* exceed 5,000 cells/dm^3 or seafood toxins exceed 200 MU/kg. This latter regulatory level has also been adopted by New Zealand. Respiratory problems in humans occur at about 10^5–10^6 cells/dm^3, while fish kills only happen at $>10^6$ cells/dm^3. Levels of NST during the 1993 New Zealand shellfish poisoning outbreak reached 5920 MU/kg (Trusewich et al. 1996).

4.5.3 Detection of NST

The currently accepted method for the determination of NST is the American Public Health Association (APHA 1985) procedure based on diethyl-ether extraction of shellfish tissue followed by mouse bioassay. The APHA protocol is widely used in the USA, where the problem of NSP is most acute. After the detection of NST in New Zealand in 1993, the Ministry of Agriculture and Fisheries Regulatory Authority improved the sample preparation method by utilizing acetone extraction of lipophilic components, followed by partitioning into dichloromethane (Hannah et al. 1985). Sample extracts are prepared for mouse injection, and the bioassay results are calculated in mouse units. The Hannah procedure is very effective in extracting unknown lipid-soluble toxins from shellfish containing NSP toxins, and the method presents certain advantages compared with the APHA protocol. However, the subsequent discovery of a novel bioactive compound (gymnodimine; Figure 4.1f; MacKenzie et al. 1996; Seki et al. 1996), produced by the dinoflagellate *K. selliformis*, a common species in New Zealand waters during neurotoxic events, has forced the local health authorities to return to the APHA diethyl—ether extraction procedure. Gymnodimine is not extractable by diethyl—ether, but it causes very rapid mouse deaths when the dichloromethane procedure is used, while this compound is not considered to present a risk to human health. A sensitive radioreceptor assay for brevetoxin is based on binding to site-5 on the voltage-dependent sodium channel in rat brain synaptosomes, using ^3H-$PbTx_3$ for quantification (Trainer et al. 1995). HPLC-MS is currently the method of choice (McNabb et al. 2006).

4.6 CIGUATERA FISH POISONING

4.6.1 Symptoms and Causative Organisms

Ciguatera Fish Poisoning (CFP) is a debilitating human illness caused by eating tropical seafood contaminated by ciguatoxins (CTX). Ciguatera has long been reported throughout the Caribbean ["cigua" is Spanish for "one poisoned from snails"], the Hawaiian Islands, French Polynesia, tropical and subtropical Australia (Kohli et al. 2014), Southeast Asia, and Indian Ocean. More recently, reports are appearing in previously ciguatera-naïve locations such as the Canary Islands, Mediterranean, Gulf of Mexico, Atlantic Ocean off North Carolina, USA (34.7°N), Angola and Cameroon (Africa), and Pakistan. Ciguatera is now spreading by the causative organism and toxin production appearing in new regions as well as by globalised seafood trade exporting ciguatera risk between nations. Ciguatera causes fish markets to ban product sales based on species, size, and geographic location such as entire estuaries (e.g., Platypus Bay, Australia). Humans consuming contaminated fish such as red bass, chinaman fish, moray eel, and paddle tail can suffer from gastrointestinal and neurological illnesses, and in extreme cases can die from respiratory failure. Ciguatera is rarely lethal for human consumers of tropical coral reef fish, but can inflict significant health impacts through persistent human neurological problems caused by the fact that the toxins accumulate in the human body. The most common fish associated with CFP are groupers, barracudas, hogfish, snappers, carang, old wife, kingfish, parrotfish, and small surgeon fish. Eating of these target fish species from known ciguatoxic areas is discouraged or sometimes forbidden, and the taking of small fish is recommended because large fish may have accumulated too much toxin. Tracking down the origin of ciguatoxic fish in the market place poses a major challenge due to the mobility of fish. Regional differences in ciguatera toxin profiles in the Pacific, Caribbean, and Indian Oceans may explain variations in clinical symptoms. Gastrointestinal symptoms are stronger in the Caribbean, while neurological symptoms dominate in the Pacific. Similarly, mannitol treatment has clinical utility in the Pacific, but is regarded ineffective in the Caribbean. There is no immunity; toxins are cumulative and persistent, and the debilitating symptoms often recur. The disease often goes unreported by victims or misdiagnosed by medical or paramedical personnel. In some instances, victims of ciguatera have sought financial compensation through legal action (e.g., Sydney fish market, Australia) adding significantly to the economic costs of any ciguatera event and extending the length of time that an event may impact upon a community as court processes may be slow to resolve.

The causative organisms are benthic *Gambierdiscus* dinoflagellates that live in epiphytic association with bushy red, brown, and green seaweeds (up to 200,000 cells/100 g of algae) and also occur free in sediments and coral rubble. These dinoflagellates produce the potent neurotoxins gambiertoxin and maitotoxin, which accumulate through the food chain, from small fish grazing on the coral reefs into the organs of bigger fish that feed on them (the principal toxin fraction in fish is ciguatoxin). While in a strict sense, this is a completely natural phenomenon, from being a rare disease two centuries ago, ciguatera now has reached epidemic proportions in French Polynesia. In the period 1960–1984, more than 24,000 patients were reported from this area, which is more than six times the average for the Pacific as a whole (Skinner et al. 2011). Evidence is accumulating that reef disturbance by hurricanes, military, and tourist developments, as well as coral bleaching (linked to global warming) and perhaps in future increasing coral damage due to ocean acidification, are increasing the risk of ciguatera. A recent game changer has been the elucidation via molecular tools that what was once thought to be a single causative dinoflagellate is now considered a species complex of 11 different morphospecies (Litaker et al. 2009). At least four *Gambierdiscus* species (*G. belizeanus*, *G. caribaeus*, *G. carolinianus* and *G. carpenteri*), are distributed globally, with the other seven found only in the Pacific (*G. australes*, *G. pacificus*, *G. polynesiensis*, *G. toxicus*, *G. yasumotoi*), Indian (*G.toxicus*), or the Atlantic Oceans (*G. ruetzleri*, *G. excentricus*). This finding sheds new light on the previously recognised >100-fold variation in toxicity, but also suggests a much broader range of environmental tolerances. Of the described species, *G. polynesiensis*, *G. australes*, *G. belizeanus*, *G. pacificus*, and *G. excentricus* are currently known to be ciguatoxic.

4.6.2 Toxin Chemistry

CTX are lipid-soluble polyether compounds consisting of 13 to 14 rings fused by ether linkages into a most rigid ladder-like structure (Figure 4.1e). They are relatively heat-stable molecules that remain toxic after cooking and exposure to mild acidic and basic conditions. CTX are readily transferred through the food web from dinoflagellates, to herbivorous fish, to carnivorous fish, and ultimately to humans. On current evidence CTX in fish is the result of both accumulation of CTXs and biotransformation of gambiertoxins (GTXs), while bioaccumulation of water-soluble maitotoxin (MTX) remains unresolved. CTX are the most potent sodium channel toxins known, causing toxicity at extremely low concentrations and which (together with matrix effects) challenges detection levels by existing analytical methods.

4.6.3 Detection of CTX

Ciguatoxin (CXT) in carnivorous fish poses a health risk at extremely low levels of 0.1 μg/g, which together with the requirement for chemical clean-up procedures from fish flesh, poses significant analytical challenges. Antibody-based assays and sodium-channel binding assays hold the most promise as cost-effective screens to detect ciguateric fish prior to consumption, but until high-affinity antibodies to CTX become available, the intraperitoneal mouse bioassay still remains the principal method of detection for many laboratories. Alternative animal assays using chicken, cat, mongoose, brine shrimp, mosquito, and fly larvae have also been explored. CTXs do not possess a distinctive UV chromophore for monitoring via liquid chromatography, but can readily be detected as sodium or ammonium adducts via mass spectrometry. Pacific (P-CTX-1) and Caribbean (C-CTX-1) CTX exhibit slight structural differences (Lewis et al. 1998). No publicly available analytical CTX standards exist, and the only available screening test Cigua-Check™ is no longer available because of unacceptable rates of false negative and false positive results.

4.7 CYANOBACTERIAL TOXINS

4.7.1 Symptoms and Causative Organisms

Cyanobacterial toxins can kill domestic and wild animals that drink from the shores of eutrophic ponds, lakes, and reservoirs, and contaminate human drinking water with teratogens and tumor promotors, but they can also accumulate in the digestive system of freshwater (Negri and Jones 1995) and brackish water shellfish (Falconer 1993, 2013; Falconer et al. 1992). Nodularin has also been detected in fish and prawns from the Gippsland Lakes. Several species of fresh water and brackish water cyanobacteria (blue-green algae) can produce liver-damaging hepatotoxic peptides (*Nodularia spumigena, Microcystis aeruginosa*), hepatotoxic alkaloids (*Cylindrospermopsis raciborskii*), and neurotoxic alkaloids (*Anabaena circinalis*). The brackish water species *N. spumigena* produces recurrent toxic blooms in the Baltic Sea. The freshwater species *A. circinalis* produced a bloom stretching 1,000 km in the Darling River, Australia, in November–December 1991. The increasing frequency, intensity, and geographic distribution of toxic cyanobacterial blooms pose an increasing threat to established shellfish industries in the estuaries in which these river systems discharge.

4.7.2 Action Levels

Adequate regulatory levels for cyanobacterial toxins in seafood have yet to be agreed on, but guideline values of 83 μg microcystin/kg shellfish, 39 μg microcystin/kg prawns, and 39 μg microcystin/kg finfish have been suggested (Falconer 2013). By comparison, safe concentrations for peptide toxins in drinking water as adopted by WHO are <1 $\mu g/dm^3$ (Falconer 1993). New groups of toxins from freshwater cyanobacteria await discovery.

4.8 OTHER PHYCOTOXINS

Increasing social awareness of seafood safety and increased monitoring by ever more sophisticated analytical methods are continuously bringing to light new compounds of potential public health significance, such as fast-acting, lipophilic toxins. These include spirolides from the dinoflagellate *A. ostenfeldii*, prorocentrolide from the dinoflagellate *P. maculosum*, gymnodimine from the dinoflagellate *K. selliformis*, and pinnatoxin from the dinoflagellate *Vulcanodinium rugosum*. While these toxins cause rapid death in mice upon intraperitoneal injection with lipophilic extracts, a link with human poisonings has not been established. Azaspiracids are another recently identified group of shellfish toxins, produced by the dinoflagellate *Azadinium* and responsible for azaspiracid poisoning (AZP) and which is now regulated (Satake et al. 1998).

The syndrome Azaspiracid Shellfish Poisoning was first coined in 1998 in association with human DSP-like poisonings after consumption in the Netherlands of Irish mussels, but the causative dinoflagellate *Azadinium spinosum* was not identified until 2009 (Tillmann et al. 2009). This taxon and four related nontoxic species *A. obesum*,

A. poporum, *Amphidoma caudatum*, and *A. languida* are now known from the North Atlantic, Mediterranean, Black Sea, Mexico, Argentina, Indian Ocean, Korea, and China. The causative azaspiracids (AZA) have unique spiro-ring assemblies (Figure 4.1j; Satake et al. 1998) and a cyclic amine instead of a cyclic imine as found with dinoflagellate toxins such as spirolides, pinnatoxin, gymnodimine, and prorocentrolides. Unlike DST polyether toxins, AZP toxins can be distributed throughout shellfish tissues and hence the conventional DSP mouse assay that utilizes only the hepatopancreas for testing can seriously underestimate. Only LC-MS and LC-MS-MS methods can unambiguously detect AZP toxin. The European Union has now established a regulatory limit of 0.16 mg AZA/kg whole shellfish flesh, but no limit has yet been agreed on by Food Standards Australia New Zealand.

A new class of fast-acting, lipophilic toxins that has been receiving increasing attention includes spirolides (Figure 4.1g) from the dinoflagellate *A. ostenfeldii*, yessotoxin and analogues (YTX, Figure 4.1d; named after the scallop *Patinopecten yessoensis*) from the gonyaulacoid dinoflagellates *Lingulodinium polyedrum*, *Protoceratium reticulatum*, and some strains of *Gonyaulax spinifera* have high intraperitoneal toxicity, but its oral potency is very low. Pinnatoxins produced by the dinoflagellate *V. rugosum* are novel amphoteric polyether macrocycles, known from Chinese razor clams (*Pinna*), and South Australian and New Zealand oysters (Rhodes et al. 2011). These cyclic imines all exhibit high intraperitoneal as well as oral potency to mice, but human oral potency has not yet been convincingly demonstrated and these compounds are not regulated (EFSA 2010).

It is perplexing that the human society is still confronted with new HAB phenomena. The benthic dinoflagellate *Ostreopsis ovata*, known from the Mediterranean for more than two decades, came into prominence in 2005 along Italy's Genoan coastline (Ciminiello et al. 2006). Over 200 people were hospitalised with skin irritation and respiratory problems; however, paradoxically, no evidence of palytoxin or its congeners known to be produced by this species has yet been found in tested aerosols. Palytoxin can be sequestered in fish and crabs (considered responsible for clupeotoxicity), but bioaccumulation in shellfish has not yet been demonstrated.

4.9 REGULATORY APPROACHES

If precautions are not taken, public health problems and economic damage through reduced local consumption and reduced exports of seafood products can be considerable. Poisonous seafood neither looks nor tastes different from uncontaminated seafood, and cooking and other treatments of shellfish do not destroy the toxins. Seafood industries potentially contaminated by toxic algal species therefore need to run costly monitoring programmes to check for toxic algae in the water and, whenever these are present, regular tests for toxins in associated seafood products need to be carried out. While some toxic algal species (e.g., *G. catenatum* and *P. bahamense*) can readily be microscopically recognized from phytoplankton net tows even at low magnification, many others (e.g., *Alexandrium*, *Azadinium*, and *Pseudo-nitzschia*) require expert light and/or electron microscopy or the application of sophisticated molecular probes. Many shellfish industries employ phytoplankton surveys as an early warning system and a trigger to commence more expensive testing for toxins in seafood products. Broad toxin screening methods often use mouse bioassays, which are now increasingly phased out in many countries due to stricter ethical standards for animal experiments. Once the seafood toxin risks of a local shellfish industry are well defined, rapid toxin screen test kits can be used to reliably determine whether toxins are present at or below the regulatory level. Only in the latter case, decisive and often expensive chemical methods such as LC-MS (Hess 2008) are then applied upon which to base seafood closures. Increasing emphasis is placed on testing for algal toxins out in the field (DeGrasse et al. 2014), for example, in scallops on board ship, thus avoiding the costly risk that a catch needs to be confiscated and destroyed upon arrival at the docks. The justification for scrutiny of fisheries products for phycotoxins is to prevent significant health effects, economic hardships, and trade disadvantages. Although this can result from a genuine toxic threat, it can also result from the so-called "halo effect" whereby bad publicity affects the sale of all seafood products, including those that are toxin free. The use of inappropriate testing methodologies (producing false positive or false negative results) or the choice of inappropriate toxin action levels can seriously confound the public image of seafood safety.

The competency of regulatory authorities also plays a critical role. Internationally, either health or fisheries departments tend to assume control of seafood safety issues. Examples of the first are the US Food and Drug Administration or the Japanese Ministry of Health, while an example of the latter is the New Zealand Ministry of Agriculture and Fisheries (MAF). A combined approach occurs in Canada by the Department of Fisheries and Oceans, and the Department of Health and Welfare. Internationally accepted regulatory limits (also called "quarantine levels" or "action levels" or "alert levels") have almost invariably been established by health authorities. For example, the PST regulatory limit was created by the US Food and Drug Administration, the AST regulatory limit by Health and Welfare, Canada, and the DST regulatory limit by the Japanese Ministry of Health and Welfare. In general, the most appropriate control of seafood toxins would be by fisheries departments (which apply the same regulatory limits) before seafood products reach consumers.

REFERENCES

American Public Health Association (APHA). 1985. Method for *Ptychodiscus brevis* toxins. In: *Laboratory Procedures for the Examination of Seawater and Shellfish*, 5th edition, American Public Health Association, Washington, DC, pp. 64–80.

Association of Official Analytical Chemists (AOAC). 1990. Paralytic shellfish poison. Biological method. Final action. sec 959.08. In: K. Hellrich (ed), *Official Methods of Analysis*, 15th edition. Association of Official Analytical Chemists, Arlington, VA, pp. 881–882.

Association of Official Analytical Chemists (AOAC). 1991. Domoic acid in mussels, liquid chromatographic method, first action 1991. Official Methods of Analysis. Association of Official Analytical Chemists, secs 991.26, Arlington, VA.

Bates, S.S., C.J. Bird, A.S.W. de Freitas, R. Foxall, M. Gilgan, L.A. Hanic et al. 1989. Pennate diatom *Nitzschia pungens* as the primary source of domoic acid, a toxin in shellfish from Eastern Prince Edward Island, Canada. *Can. J. Fish Aquatic Sci.* 46(7): 1203–1215.

Burgess, V. and G. Shaw. 2001. Pectenotoxins–An issue for public health. A review of their comparative toxicology and metabolism. *Environ. Int.* 27: 275–283.

Boundy, M.J., A.I. Selwood, D.T. Harwood, P.S. McNabb, and A.D. Turner. 2015. Development of a sensitive liquid chromatography-mass spectrometry method for high throughput analysis of paralytic shellfish toxins using graphitised carbon solid phase extraction. *J. Chromatogr. A* 1387: 1–12.

Cembella, A.D. 2003. Chemical ecology of eukaryotic microalgae in marine ecosystems. *Phycologia* 42(4): 420–447.

Ciminiello, P., C. Dell'Aversano, E. Fattorusso, M. Forino, G.S. Magno, L. Tartaglione et al. 2006. The Genoa 2005 outbreak, determination of putative palytoxin in Mediterranean *Ostreopsis ovata* by new liquid chromatography tandem mass spectrometry method. *Anal. Chem.* 78: 6153–6159.

Dale, B. and C.M. Yentsch. 1978. Red tide and paralytic shellfish poisoning. *Oceanus* 21(3): 41–49.

De Grasse, S., S. Conrad, P. DiStefano, C. Vanegas, D. Wallace, P. Jensen et al. 2014. Onboard screening dockside testing as a new means of managing paralytic shellfish poisoning risks in federally closed waters. *Deep Sea Res. Part II Top Stud. Oceanogr.* 103: 288–300.

Dowsett, N., G. Hallegraeff, P. van Ruth, R. van Ginkel, P. McNabb, B. Hay et al. 2011. Uptake, distribution and depuration of Paralytic Shellfish Toxins from *Alexandrium minutum* in Australian greenlip abalone, *Haliotis laevigata*. *Toxicon* 58: 101–111.

Doucette, G.J., M.M. Logan, J.S. Ramsdell, and F.M. van Dolah. 1991. Development and preliminary validation of a microtiter plate-based receptor binding assay for paralytic shellfish poisoning toxins. *Toxicon* 35: 625–636.

EFSA. 2010. Scientific opinion on marine biotoxins in shellfish-Cyclic imines (spirolides, gymnodimines, pinnatoxins and pteriatoxins). *EFSA J.* 8(6): 1626.

Falconer, I.R. (ed). 1993. *Algal Toxins in Seafood and Drinking Water*. Academic Press, New York, 211 pp.

Falconer, I.R. 2013. Cyanobacterial toxin accumulation in shellfish, finfish and crustaceans: Guidelines for consumer safety. In: C. McLeod et al. (eds), *Proceedings of the 9th International Conference on Molluscan Shellfish Safety*, March 17–22, 2013. Sydney, Australia, pp. 122–125.

Falconer, I.R., A. Choice, and W. Hosja. 1992. Toxicity of edible mussels (*Mytilus edulis*) growing naturally in an estuary during a water bloom of the blue-green alga *Nodularia spumigena*. *Environ. Toxicol. Water Qual.* 7: 119–123.

Hallegraeff, G.M. 1993. A review of harmful algal blooms and their apparent global increase. *Phycologia* 32: 79–99.

Hallegraeff, G.M. 2010. Ocean climate change, phytoplankton community responses and harmful algal blooms: A formidable predictive challenge. *Journal of Phycology* 46: 220–235.

Hallegraeff, G.M. and J.L Maclean. (eds). 1989. Biology, Epidemiology and Management of *Pyrodinium* Red Tides. ICLARM Conference Proceedings 21, Manilla, Phillipines, 286 p.

Hannah, D.J., D.G. Till, T. Deverall, P.D. Jones, and M. Fry. 1995. Extraction of lipid-soluble marine biotoxins. *J. AOAC Int.* 78: 480–483.

Hess, P. 2008. What's new in toxins? In: Ø. Moestrup et al. (eds), *Proceedings of the 12th International Conference on Harmful Algae*, IOC-UNESCO, Copenhagen, pp. 360–370.

Haywood, A.J., K.A. Steidinger, E.W. Truby, P.R. Bergquist, J. Adamson, and L. Mackenzie. 2004. Comparative morphology and molecular phylogenetic analysis of three new species of the genus *Karenia* (Dinophyceae) from New Zealand. *J. Phycol.* 40: 165–179.

Jaime, E., C. Hummert, P. Hess, and B. Luckas. 2001. Determination of paralytic shellfish poisoning toxins by high-performance ion-exchange chromatography. *J. Chromatogr.* A929(1–2): 43–49.

Jawaid, W., K. Campbell, K. Melville, S.J. Holmes, J. Rice, and C.T. Elliott. 2015. Development and validation of a novel lateral flow immunoassay (LFIA) for the rapid screening of paralytic shellfish toxins (PSTs) from shellfish extracts. *Anal. Chem.* 87: 5324–5332.

Japanese Ministry of Health and Welfare. 1981. Method of testing for diarrhetic shellfish toxin. *Food Sanitation Res.* 7: 60–65.

Jellett, J.F., R.L. Roberts, M.V. Laycock, M.A. Quilliam, and R.E. Barrett. 2002. Detection of paralytic shellfish poisoning (PSP) toxins in shellfish tissue using MIST Alert, a new rapid test, in parallel with the regulatory AOAC mouse bioassay. *Toxicon* 40: 1407–1425.

Kat, M. 1985. *Dinophysis acuminata* blooms, the distinct cause of Dutch mussel poisoning. In: D.M. Anderson, A.W. White, and D.G. Baden (eds), *Toxic Dinoflagellates*, Elsevier, Amsterdam, the Netherlands, pp. 73–77.

Kohli, G.S., S.A. Murray, B.A. Neilan, L.L. Rhodes, T. Harwood, K.F. Smith et al. 2014. High abundance of the potentially maitotoxic dinoflagellate *Gambierdiscus carpenteri* in temperate waters of New South Wales, Australia. *Harmful Algae* 39: 134–145.

Lawrence, J.F., C.F. Charbonneau, C. Menard, M.A. Quilliam, and P.G. Sim. 1989. Liquid chromatographic determination of domoic acid in shellfish products using the paralytic shellfish poison extraction procedure of the association of official analytical chemists. *J. Chromatogr.* 462: 349–356.

Lawrence, J.F., B. Niedzwiadek, and C. Menard. 2005. Quantitative determination of paralytic shellfish poisoning toxins in shellfish using prechromatographic oxidation and liquid chromatography with fluorescence detection: Collaborative study. *J. AOAC Int.* 88(6): 1714–1732.

Lee, J.S., T. Yanagi, R. Kenma, and T. Yasumoto. 1987. Fluorometric determination of diarrhetic shellfish toxins by high-performance liquid chromatography. *Agric. Biol. Chem.* 51(3): 877–881.

Lee, J.S., M. Murata, and T. Yasumoto. 1989. Analytical methods for determination of diarrhetic shellfish toxins. In: S. Natori, K. Hashimoto, and Y. Ueno (eds), *Mycotoxins and Phycotoxins*, Elsevier, Amsterdam, the Netherlands, pp. 327–334.

Lewis, R.J., J.P. Vernoux, and I.M. Brereton. 1998. Structure of Caribbean ciguatoxin isolated from *Caranx latus*. *J. Am. Chem. Soc.* 120: 5914–5920.

Litaker, R.W., M.W. Vandersea, M.A. Faust, S.R. Kibler, M. Chinain, M.J. Holmes et al. 2009. Taxonomy of *Gambierdiscus* including four new species, *Gambierdiscus caribaeus*, *Gambierdiscus carolinianus*, *Gambierdiscus carpenteri* and *Gambierdiscus ruetzleri* (Gonyaulacales, Dinophyceae). *Phycologia* 48(5): 344–390.

Lundholm, N. and Ø.J. Moestrup. 2000. Morphology of the marine diatom *Nitzschia navis-varingica,* sp. nov. (Bacillariophyceae), another producer of the neurotoxin domoic acid. *J. Phycol.* 36(6): 1162–1174.

MacKenzie, L., A. Haywood, J. Adamson, P. Truman, D. Till, T. Seki et al. 1996. Gymnodimine contamination of shellfish in New Zealand. In: T. Yasumoto, Y. Oshima, and Y. Fukuyo (ed). *Harmful and Toxic Algal Blooms*, Intergovernmental Oceanographic Commission of UNESCO, Paris, France, pp. 97–100.

McNabb, P., L. Rhodes, J. Adamson, and P. Holland. 2006. Brevetoxin—An elusive toxin in New Zealand waters. *Afr. J. Marine Sci.* 28: 375–377.

Munday, R., K. Thomas, R. Gibbs, C. Murphy, and M.A. Quilliam. 2013. Acute toxicities of saxitoxin, neosaxitoxin, decarbamoyl saxitoxin and gonyautoxins 1&4 and 2&3 to mice by various routes of administration. *Toxicon* 76: 77–83.

Negri, A. and L. Llewellyn. 1998. Comparative analyses by HPLC and the sodium channel and saxiphilin ^{3}H-saxitoxin receptor assays for paralytic shellfish toxins in crustaceans and molluscs from tropical North West Australia. *Toxicon* 36: 283–298.

Negri, A.P. and G.J. Jones. 1995. Bioaccumulation of paralytic shellfish poisoning (PSP) toxins from the cyanobacterium *Anabaena circinalis* by the freshwater mussel *Alathyria condola*. *Toxicon* 33: 667–678.

Oshima, Y., K. Hasegawa, T. Yasumoto, G.M. Hallegraeff, and S.I. Blackburn. 1987. Dinoflagellate *Gymnodinium catenatum* as the source of paralytic shellfish toxins in Tasmanian shellfish. *Toxicon* 25: 1105–1111.

Oshima, Y., M. Hirota, T. Yasumoto, G.M. Hallegraeff, S.I. Blackburn, and D.A. Steffensen. 1989a. Production of paralytic shellfish toxins by the dinoflagellate *Alexandrium minutum* Halim from Australia. *Bull. Jap. Soc. Sc. Fish.* 55: 925.

Oshima, Y., K. Sugino, and T. Yasumoto. 1989b. Latest advances in HPLC analysis of paralytic shellfish toxins. In: S. Natori, K. Hashimoto, and Y. Ueno (eds), *Mycotoxins and Phycotoxins'88*, Elsevier, Amsterdam, the Netherlands, pp. 319–326.

Pocklington, R., J.E. Milley, S.S. Bates, C.J. Bird, A.S.W. Frejtas, and M.A. Quilliam. 1990. Trace determination of domoic acid in seawater and phytoplankton by high-performance liquid chromatography of the fluorenylmethoxycarbonyl (FMOC) derivative. *Int. J. Environ. Anal. Chem.* 38(3): 351–368.

Quilliam, M.A. 1995. Analysis of diarrhetic shellfish poisoning toxins in shellfish tissue by liquid chromatography with fluorometric and mass spectrometric detection. *J. AOAC Int.* 78: 555–570.

Quilliam, M.A. 1998. AOAC General Referee Report 1997, Committee on Natural Toxins: Phycotoxins. *J. AOAC Int.* 82: 773–781.

Quilliam, M.A., P.G. Sim, A.W. McCulloch, and A.G. McInnes. 1989. High performance liquid chromatography of domoic acid, a marine neurotoxin, with application to shellfish and plankton. *Int. J. Environ. Anal. Chem.* 36: 139–154.

Quilliam, M.A., M. Xie, and W.R. Hardstaff. 1995. A rapid extraction and cleanup procedure for the liquid chromatographic determination of domoic acid in unsalted seafood. *J. AOAC Int.* 78(2): 543–554.

Rhodes, L., K. Smith, A. Selwood, P. McNabb, R. Munday, S. Suda et al. 2011. Dinoflagellate *Vulcanodinium rugosum* identified as the causative organism of pinnatoxins in Australia, New Zealand and Japan. *Phycologia* 50: 624–628.

Satake, M., A. Morohashi, K. Murata, H.F. Kaspar, and Y. Yasumoto. 1996. Chemical studies on the NSP toxins in the green shell mussels from New Zealand. In: T. Yasumoto, Y. Oshima, and Y. Fukuyo (eds), *Harmful and Toxic Algal Blooms, The Proceedings of the Seventh International Conference on Toxic Phytoplankton*, July 12–16, 1995, Sendai, Japan. International Oceanographic Commission of UNESCO, Paris, France, pp. 487–490.

Satake, M., K. Ofuji, H. Naoki, K.J. James, A. Furey, T. McMahon et al. 1998. Azaspiracid, a new marine toxin having unique spiro ring assemblies, isolated from Irish mussels, *Mytilus edulis*. *J. Am. Chem. Soc.* 120: 9967–9968.

Seki, T., M. Satake, L. MacKenzie, H.F. Kaspar, and T. Yasumoto. 1996. Gymnodimine, a novel toxic imine isolated from the oveaux strait oysters and *Gymnodinium* sp. In: T. Yasumoto, Y. Oshima, and Y. Fukuyo (eds), Harmful and Toxic Algal Blooms. Intergovernmental Oceanographic Commission of UNESCO, Paris, France, pp. 495–498.

Skinner, M.P., T.D. Brewer, R. Johnstone, L.E. Fleming, and R.J. Lewis. 2011. Ciguatera fish poisoning in the Pacific Islands (1998 to 2008). *PLOS Negl. Trop. Dis.* 5(12): 1–7.

Smida, D.B., N. Lundholm, W.H.C.F. Kooistra, I. Sahraoui, M.V. Ruggiero, Y. Kotaki et al. 2014. Morphology and molecular phylogeny of *Nitzschia bizertensis* sp.nov.-a new domoic acid producer. *Harmful Algae* 32: 49–63.

Suganuma, M., H. Fujiki, H., Suguri, S. Yoshizawa, M. Hirota, M. Nakayasu et al. 1988. Okadaic acid: An additional non- phorbol-12-tetradecanoate 13-acetate-type tumor promoter. *Proc. Nat. Acad. Sci. USA* 85: 1768–1771.

Sullivan, J.J., J. Jonas-Davies, and L.L. Kentala. 1985. The determination of PSP toxins by HPLC and autoanalyzer. In: D.M. Anderson, A. White, and D.G. Baden (eds), *Toxic Dinoflagellates*. Elsevier, London, pp. 275–280.

Tillmann, U., M. Elbrächter, B. Krock, U. John, and A. Cembella. 2009. *Azadinium spinosum* gen. et sp.nov. (Dinophyceae) identified as a primary producer of azaspiracid toxins. *Europ. J. Phycol.* 44: 63–79.

Trainer, V.L., D.G. Baden, and W.A. Catterall. 1995. Detection of marine toxins using reconstituted sodium channels. *J. AOAC Int.* 78: 570–573.

Trainer, V.L., S.S. Bates, N. Lundholm, A.E. Thessen, W.P. Cochlan, N.G. Adams et al. 2012. *Pseudo-nitzschia* physiological ecology, phylogeny, toxicity, monitoring and impacts on ecosystem health. *Harmful Algae* 14: 271–300.

Trusewich, B., J. Sim, P. Busby, and C. Hughes. 1996. Management of marine biotoxins in New Zealand. In: T. Yasumoto, Y. Oshima, and Y. Fukuyo (eds), *Harmful and Toxic Algal Blooms, Proceedings of the VII International Conference on Toxic Phytoplankton*, July 1995, Sendai, Japan. IOC/UNESCO, pp. 27–30.

Tubaro, A., C. Florio, E. Luxich, S. Sosa, R.D. Loggia, and T. Yasumoto. 1996. A protein phosphatase 2A inhibition assay for a fast and sensitive assessment of okadaic acid contamination in mussels. *Toxicon* 34: 743–752.

Turner, A.D., S. Tarnovius, S. Johnson, W.A. Higman, and M. Algoet. 2015. Testing and application of a refined rapid detection method for paralytic shellfish poisoning toxins in UK shellfish. *Toxicon* 100: 32–41.

Van Dolah, F.M., E.L. Finley, B.L. Haynes, G.J. Doucette, P.D. Moeller, and Dr J.S. Ramsdell. 1994. Development of rapid and sensitive high throughput pharmacological assays for marine phycotoxins. *Natural Toxins* 2: 189–196.

Wright, J.L.C., R.K. Boyd, A.S.W. Defreitas, M. Falk, R.A. Foxall, W.D. Jamieson et al. 1989. Identification of domoic acid, a neuroexcitatory amino acid, in toxic mussels from eastern P.E.I. *Can. J. Chem.* 67: 481–490.

Yasumoto, T., Y. Oshima, W. Sugawara, Y. Fukuyo, H. Oguri, T. Igarashi et al. 1980. Identification of *Dinophysis fortii* as the causitive organism of diarrhetic shellfish poisoning. *Bull. Jpn. Soc. Sci. Fish.* 46: 1405–1411.

Yasumoto, T., M. Murata, J.S. Lee, and K. Torigoe. 1989. Polyether toxins produced by dinoflagellates. In: S. Natori, K. Hashimoto, and Y. Ueno (eds), *Mycotoxins and Phycotoxins '88, Bioactive Molecules*, vol. 10, Elsevier, Amsterdam, the Netherlands, pp. 375–382.

5 Biogenic Amines

Sevim Köse

CONTENTS

5.1 INTRODUCTION

Biogenic amines (BAs) are defined as low-molecular-weight basic nitrogenous compounds that possess biological activity. These are organic bases that can be divided into several groups according to their chemical structure—aliphatic (e.g., cadaverine, putrescine, spermine, and spermidine), aromatic (e.g., phenylethylamine and tyramine) and heterocyclic (e.g., histamine and tryptamine), or in relation to the number of amino groups into monoamines (phenylethylamine and tyramine) and diamines (histamine, cadaverine, and putrescine). Several authors had also classified cadaverine, putrescine, spermine, and spermidine among polyamines. BAs can also be grouped as volatile such as phenylethylamine and nonvolatile (e.g., histamine, cadaverine, putrescine, spermine, agmatine, and tryptamine). Figure 5.1 shows the chemical structures of the most important amines in terms of food safety and quality.

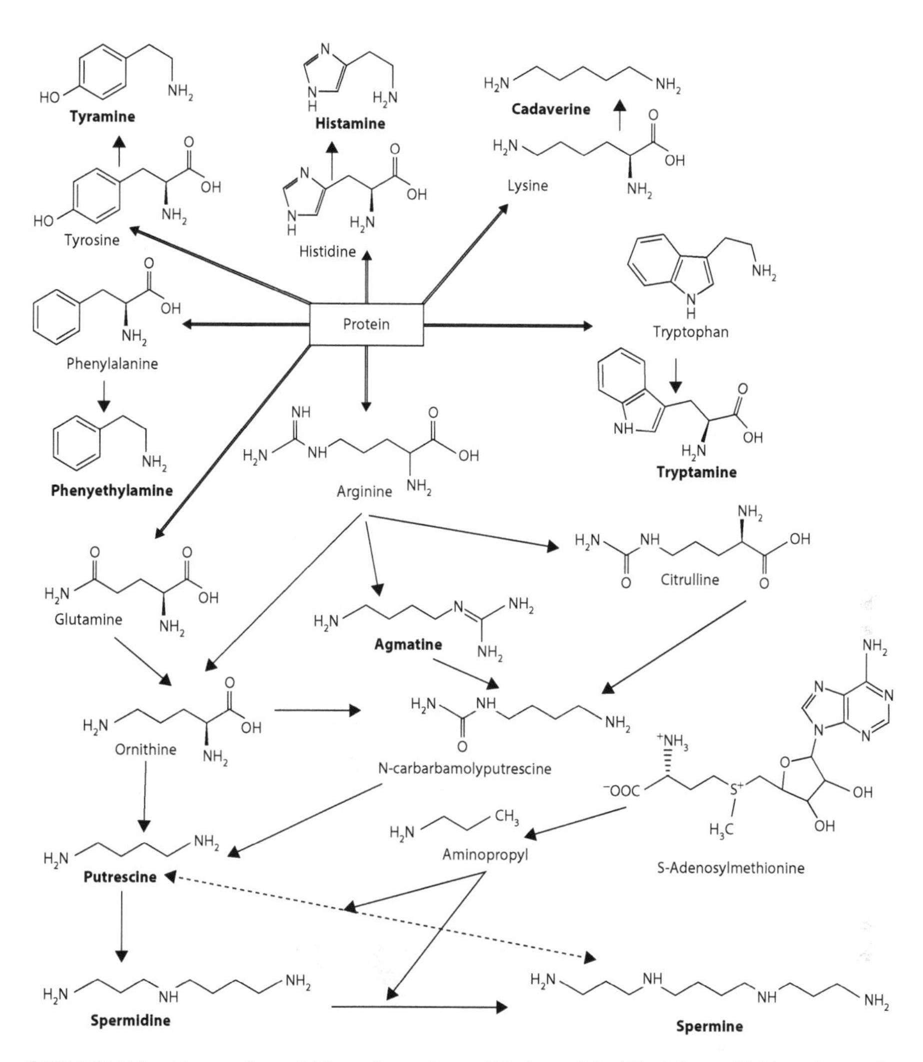

FIGURE 5.1 Generation of biogenic amines. (Updated/Modified from Halász, A. et al., *Trends Food Sci. Technol.*, 5, 42–49, 1994; Restuccia, D. et al., Accumulation of biogenic amines in foods: Hazard identification and control options, in *Microbial Food Safety and Preservation Techniques*, eds. R.R. Rai and J.A. Bai, Chapter 4, CRC Press, 2014, pp. 53–74.)

Various BAs such as serotonin, histamine, and tyramine are reported to play important roles in many human and animal physiological functions as well as in plants. They are sources of nitrogen and precursors for the synthesis of hormones, alkaloids, nucleic acids, and proteins. They can also influence various physiological processes in the organism such as the regulation of body temperature, intake of nutrition, and increase or decrease of blood pressure. For example, in plants, putrescine, spermidine, and spermine take role in cell division, flowering, fruit development, response to stress, and senescence, whereas polyamines are important for the growth, renovation, and metabolism of every organ of animal and human body and essential for maintaining the high metabolic activity of the normal functioning and immunological system of gut. Among the beneficial contribution of BAs, some are reported to contribute to the flavor and taste of food. Although BAs have essential roles in the benefit of living organisms, the amounts necessary for physiological body functions are limited; therefore, excess concentrations usually taken via ingestion of food are reported to cause toxicological effect to the organisms. Toxicological effects of BAs can be examined in two categories, namely, food poisoning and cancer.

The most common health effect of BAs is known as food poisoning implicated with various foods, particularly fish. Histamine is the main causative BA to cause food poisoning covering the majority of reported food poisoning cases (Hungerford 2010), whereas some of the other BAs have been claimed to potentiate histamine food poisoning (HFP) (Karovičová and Kohajdová 2005). Moreover, certain BAs formed due to decomposition of foods (e.g., putrescine and cadaverine) or during processing (e.g., tyramine) are reported to have the potential to cause illness, even in the absence of histamine.

The second type of toxicological effects of BAs is linked to their role in the formation of carcinogenic *N*-nitroso compounds. Among the BAs, agmatine, putrescine, spermine, and spermidine are reported to be potential precursors for the formation of carcinogenic *N*-nitroso compounds in the presence of nitrite (NO_2^-). The importance of putrescine, spermidine, and spermine in tumor growth is also widely recognized, and the inhibition of polyamine biosynthesis in tumor-bearing individuals is reported to be one of the major targets of cancer therapy research (Karovičová and Kohajdová 2005). BAs are also a concern for food quality due to their formation during decomposition of foods, particularly fish. Therefore, different studies have been reported to estimate their roles in food spoilage as well as food safety. Although some useful BA indexes are reported, however, so far, none has been found useful application for the estimation of food spoilage and the risk of food safety (Koral and Köse 2012).

Numerous review articles summarized the studies carried on the formation, preventive measures, and presence of these amines in variety of food types, analytical methods as well as toxicological effects to humans and animals, and epidemiology of food poisoning cases associated with BAs. Studies on these amines, particularly histamine, are still in concern to food safety authorities as well as food scientists and analytical chemists due to their involvement in number of recent food poisoning cases/outbreaks despite the strict control measures applied throughout the world. Therefore, recent studies usually concentrated on preventive measures of BAs in various foods. These studies can be categorized into four main groups as:

1. Innovation studies relating to preventive measures on BAs that investigate the formation of BAs in various foods including new products under different processing and storage conditions to highlight on preventive measures
2. Investigating the degradation of BAs previously formed in foods
3. Fast and/or accurate measurement of BAs in foods leading to development of various new analytical methods
4. Epidemiological studies

Therefore, the aim of this chapter is to cover recent developments on controlling health risk of BAs in foods including epidemiology, methodology, and preventive measures in various foods.

5.2 FORMATION OF BAs

5.2.1 Introduction

BAs in foods are formed mainly by decarboxylation of amino acids or by amination and transamination of aldehydes and ketones. Removal of the α-carboxyl group from a proteinous amino acid leads to the corresponding BA. These amines are generated in course of microbial, vegetable, and animal metabolisms. Decarboxylation of BAs in food and beverages occurs either as the result of endogenous amino acid decarboxylase activity in raw food materials, or by the growth of decarboxylase-positive microorganisms under conditions favorable to enzyme activity. However, it has been found that some of the aliphatic amines can be formed *in vivo* by amination from corresponding aldehydes (Silla Santos 1996). Amine production has been associated with the protective mechanisms of microorganisms against an acidic environment to supply alternative metabolic energy when bacterial cells are exposed to suboptimal substrate conditions (Anli and Bayram 2008). It was claimed that the presence of BAs might serve as a useful indicator of food spoilage due to the possibility of the increased production of decarboxylases during the microbial spoilage of food (Halász et al. 1994).

The precursors of the main BAs involved in food poisoning, and their metabolic pathways can be seen in Figure 5.1. Putrescine, a catabolic product of ornithine or arginine pathways, can be converted into spermidine, which can form spermine. During storage and processing of foods, prerequisites for the formation of BAs are reported as (i) the availability of free amino acids (FAAs); (ii) the existence of decarboxylase-positive microorganisms; and (iii) the presence of suitable preconditions allowing the growth, decarboxylase synthesis, and activity of these bacteria. In the set of metabolic pathways that break down amino acids into smaller units, several reactions are also reported as decarboxylation, transamination, deamination, and desulfurization (Anli and Bayram 2008; Restuccia et al. 2014). The factors that have impact on the production of the FAAs, the decarboxylating enzyme, and also their level of activity affects the type and the amount of BAs present in foods. Factors associated with the raw material (food composition, pH, handling conditions such as the substrate source and reaction medium) directly affect the availability of FAAs, whereas the presence of enzyme is closely connected to microbiological aspects (bacterial species and strain, bacterial growth). These factors are obviously interdependent and are further influenced by the technological processes associated with the types of food derivative and storage conditions. The combined action of these factors is what chiefly determines the final concentrations of BAs, because it determines either directly or indirectly the presence and the activity of the substrate and enzyme.

5.2.2 Availability of FAAs

The FAAs play a fundamental role in the formation of BAs in foods, in that they are the precursors of amines and, moreover, constitute a substrate for microbial growth. They either occur as such in foods, or may be liberated through proteolysis. Microbial strains with high proteolytic enzyme activity also help to increase the availability of these amino acids.

Although precursor amino acids of BAs usually are found in many protein-rich foods, such as cheese and fish, some fish species have low histidine contents. Therefore, they are not associated with HFP. As HFP is often reported with fish and fish products, presence of histamine in these products is strictly regulated by the government authorities. Therefore, studies on histamine and histidine in foods have been mainly focused on these products. Free histidine is generally found in large amounts in the muscle of fatty, red-meat, active, and migratory species compared to that in the white meat of slower species. Therefore, formation of histamine primarily relates to marine fish species and is not a potential hazard when freshwater fishes are used as raw material. Table 5.1 shows the list of fish species that present a potential health hazard for HFP (FAO-WHO 2013).

Some food processing methods, particularly fermentation, are important in terms of their role to increase FAAs in food matrix that further lead to formation of BAs. This is often the case for fish and cheese. During the ripening processes of fermentation, proteolytic enzymes can break protein in foods down to FAAs, which are the precursors of BAs. Therefore, high contents of BAs in various fermented fish and cheeses are often reported.

Many compounds contributing to the flavor of cheeses derive from amino acids. During the cheese ripening, the action of proteases liberates peptides that are further catabolized by amino peptidases producing FAAs or small peptides that can be metabolized by bacteria. However, some amino acids can be used by decarboxylating bacteria to produce undesirable BAs that present health risk to human. Relatively high amounts of histamine are reported in fermented foods, particularly fish and cheese (Restuccia et al. 2014). After fish, cheese is the next most commonly implicated food item associated with food poisoning; the first reported case occurred in 1967 in the Netherlands and involved Gouda cheese (Silla Santos 1996).

5.2.3 Presence of Decarboxylase-Positive Microorganisms

Many microorganisms possessing decarboxylase enzymes are able to produce amines. Therefore, the amount and type of amine formed in a food not only depends on the nature of the commodity but also on the microorganisms present. Many bacteria species are reported to be capable of decarboxylating one or more amino acids. These bacteria belong to various genera such as *Bacillus*, *Citrobacter*, *Clostridium*, *Escherichia*, *Klebsiella*, *Proteus*, *Pseudomonas*, *Photobacterium*, *Shigella*, and the lactic acid bacteria (LAB) such as *Lactobacillus*, *Pediococcus*, and *Streptococcus* (Silla Santos 1996). Studies on the decarboxylate activity of microorganisms in

TABLE 5.1
Fish Species Commonly Reported for Histamine Food Poisoning and/or Presenting Histamine Health Risk Due to High Levels of Histamine

Family	Common English Names	Genera and/or Species[a]	Histidine Levels mg/kg
Ammodytidae	Lesser eel	*Ammodytes tobianus* (Sandeel)	
Arripidae	Kahawai	*Arripis* spp., *A. trutta* (Kahawai)	12420
Belonidae	Garfish	*Belone belone*	6084–6685
Carangidae	Yellowtail, Amberjack	*Seriola* spp., *Seriola lalandi* (Amberjack or Kingfish)	7320, 5500–15800
		S. quinqueradiata (Japanese)	2470–11600
		S. dumerili (Rudder Fish)	2860
	Mackerel, Jack Jack	*Caranx* spp., *Oligoplites saurus, Selene* spp., *S. rivoliana* (Yellowtail, longfin), *Urapsis secunda, Carangoides bartholomaei, C. crysos* (Blue Runner), *Nematistius pectoralis* (Roosterfish), *Alectis indica* (Crevalle), *Trachurus* spp., *T. capensis* (Cape H.), *T. truchurus* (Atlantic H.), *T. murphyi* (Chilean)	
		Caranx georgianus	1800–6300
		Elagatis bipinnulata (Rainbow Runner)	7090
		T. novaezelandiae	2720
		T. japanicus (Mackerel, Horse)	172–3680
	Kohera	*Decapterus koheru* (Yellowtail)	2300–2700
	Queenfish, Talang	*Scomberoides* spp., *S. commersonnianush*	
Chanidae	Milkfish	*Chanos chanos*	4410–5340, 25070
Clupeidae	Herring, Shad	*Alosa* spp., *Dorosoma* spp. (Gizzard S.), *Ethmalosa fimbriata* (Bonga), *Nematalosa vlaminghi* (Western/ Australian gizzard), *Tenualosa ilisha* (Hilsa S.), *A. pseudoharengus, Etrumeus teres, Ilisha* spp., *Opisthopterus tardoore* (Pacific Thread), *Pellona ditchela, Clupea* spp. (Sild & roe), *Opisthonema* spp. (Thread), *C. bentincki* (Araucanian), *C. pallasii pallasii* (Pacific), *Harengula* spp., *H. thrissina* (Pacific), *Spratelloides gracilis* (Silver-stripe)	
		Clupea harengus (Atlantic)	1230–2950

(*Continued*)

TABLE 5.1 (*Continued*)
Fish Species Commonly Reported for Histamine Food Poisoning and/or Presenting Histamine Health Risk Due to High Levels of Histamine

Family	Common English Names	Genera and/or Species[a]	Histidine Levels mg/kg
Clupeidae	Menhaden	*Brevoortia* spp., *B. patronus (Gulf), Ethmidium maculatum (Pacific)*	
		B. tyrannus (Atlantic)	1860–2790
	Pilchard or Sardine	*Sardinella* spp., *Amblygaster sirm (Spotted S.), S. aurita (Round S.), S. longiceps (Sardine, Indian Oil), S. gibbosa (Goldstripe), S. maderensis (Madeiran)*	
		Sardina pilchardus (European)	2888
		Sardinops sagax (Pilchard Japanese)	1227–7626
	Sprat, Bristling	*Sprattus* spp., *Sprattus antipodum*	3900
Coryphaenidae	Mahi-Mahi	*Coryphaena hippurus* (Dolphinfish)	1829–9370
Engraulidae	Anchovy	*Anchoa* spp., *Anchoviella* spp., *Cetengraulis mysticetus* (Anchoveta, Pacific), *Engraulis ringens* (Peruvian), *E. capensis* (S. African), *Stolephorus* spp.	
		Engraulis encrasicolus (European A.)	6200
		Engraulis japonicus (Japanese A.)	4810
Hexagrammidae	Mackerel, Atka	*Pleurogrammus monopterygius* (Okhotsk Atka), *P. azonus*	2500
Hemiramphidae	Piper	*Hyporhamphus* spp.	3200
Istiophoridae	Spearfish, Sailfish, Marlin	*Tetrapturus* spp., *Istiophorus albicans, I. platypterus, Makaira* spp.	
		Makaira mazara (Black M.)	7630
		M. mitsukurii (Striped M.)	8310–13200
Lutjanidae	Jobfish Snapper	*Aphareus* spp., *Aprion virescens, Pristipomoides* spp.	
Mugilidae	Mullet	*Mugil cephalus*	2060–7600
		Mugil curema	1333[b]
Pomatomidae	Bluefish	*Pomatomus saltatrix*	
Pristigasteridae	Indian pellona	*Ilisha* spp., *Pellona ditchela*	
		Salmo salar (Atlantic S.)	130–300
		Oncorhynchus tshawytscha (Chincook S.)	70–288
		O. keta (Chum S.)	70–670
		O. kisutch (Coho S.)	219–970
		O. macrostomus (Amago S.)	188–441
		O. masou (Cherry S.)	387–2362
		O. nerka (Sockeye S.)	240–590
		O. gorbuscha (Pink S.)	408–1557

(*Continued*)

TABLE 5.1 (*Continued*)
Fish Species Commonly Reported for Histamine Food Poisoning and/or Presenting Histamine Health Risk Due to High Levels of Histamine

Family	Common English Names	Genera and/or Species[a]	Histidine Levels mg/kg
Scombridae	Tuna	*Thunnus* spp., *Allothunnus fallai (Slender), Auxis* spp., *Euthynnus* spp., *Katsuwonus pelamis, T. thynnus* (A. Bluefin), *T. atlanticus* (Blackfin)	
		E. affinis (Kawakawa)	10900
		Katsuwonus pelamis (Skipjack T.)	13400–20000
		Thunnus tonggol (Longtail T.)	11540
		Thunnus alalunga (Albacore),	4600–6790
		T. albacares (Yellowfin)	2123–12200
		T. maccoyii (Southern Bluefin)	6670
		T. obesus (Bigeye Tuna)	7450
		T. orientalis (Pacific Bluefin T.)	6850–7110
	Bonito	*Cybiosarda elegans (Leaping), Sarda* spp., *Sarda sarda* (Atlantic Bonito)	
		Auxis thazard,	4330–10100
		Gymnosarda unicolor (Dogtooth Tuna),	669
		Orcynopsis unicolor (Plain T.)	759
		Sarda spp.	62215
	Mackerel	*Gasterochisma melampus* (Butterfly Kingfish), *Grammatorcynus* spp., *Rastrelliger brachysoma* (Mackerel Short), *R. kanagurta* (Indian M.), Scomberomorus spp. (Spanish M.), *S. commerson* (Narrow-Barred Spanish), *S.cavalla* (Spanish, King M.)	
		Auxis tapeinocephalus (Mackerel Frigatate)	14600
		Pneumatophorus diego	5193–5999
		Scomber scombrus (Atlantic Mackerel)	2000–4500
		S. japonicus (Chub Mackerel)	1063–8020
		S. australasicus (Blue Mackerel)	2600
		S. niphonius (Japanese/Spanish)	1990–2180
	Wahoo	*Acanthocybium solandri*	
Scomberesocidae	Saury	*Cololabis saira, Scomberesox saurus saurus*	16100
Xiphiidae	Swordfish	*Xiphias gladius*	

Source: FDA, Fish and fishery products hazards and controls guidance. 4th edn. 2011; Köse, S., *Turkish J. Fish. Aquatic Sci.*, 10, 139–160, 2010; FAO-WHO. Joint FAO/WHO Expert Meeting on the Public Health Risks of Histamine and Other Biogenic Amines from Fish and Fishery Products, 2013.

[a] Parenthesis represent specific common name of the species.

[b] Millán et al. *Revista Científica*. 13, 339–346, 2003.

terms of BA formation in different food products usually rely on the combination of three different approaches. These are the following:

1. Presumptive determination of BA forming microorganisms isolated from foods either containing high BA values and/or implicated with poisoning incidents caused by BAs. The oldest method for determining the role of microorganisms on the BA formation was based on the presumptive estimation of growth performance of microorganisms in the presence of precursor amines. This method applied to quantitative determination of histamine forming bacteria (HFB) using a differential plating medium containing L-histidine (Niven et al. 1981) and a pH indicator. Later, this method was modified and applied to various food products. The presumptive results for specific microorganisms isolated from the selective media are further verified using amino acid decarboxylase broths as confirmatory media containing precursor amino acids. Determination of BAs in the culture media is also included in some studies
2. Later, studies included testing BA decarboxylating activity of selected microorganisms, usually bacteria for precursor amino acids of specific BAs. Culture broths containing these amino acids are used for the growth of specific bacteria, and then determination of BAs in the culture was carried out. The findings in these studies are usually further confirmed on real foods or food media for BA forming ability
3. Recent studies have focused on identification of decarboxylating gene of the specific bacteria strains, and then they are further confirmed for their ability on the formation of BAs using both culture broth and real food media

Although numerous bacteria have been reported to possess amino acid decarboxylase activity, only certain species found in foods have been implicated in the formation of significant levels of BAs enough to pose toxicological effect. Wide variations in histamine formation have been observed even among strains of the same species (Halász et al. 1994). For example, Gardini et al. (2012) demonstrated that *Streptococcus thermophilus* PRI60 can produce high histamine levels in cheese while the strain PRI40 of the same species is recorded as nonhistamine producer. Moreover, Kučerová et al. (2009) reported that most strains of *Enterococcus faecium* isolated from different cheese and milk samples showed tyrosine decarboxylase positive activity while both positive and negative activities were observed for histidine. The variation in the decarboxylating activity might be attributed to the conditions in foods affecting bacterial growth. *Morganella morganii*, *Klebsiella pneumoniae*, *Proteus vulgaris*, and *Hafnia alvei* are known to originate from fish-implicated incidents of HFP.

Most of the amino acid decarboxylases require pyridoxal 5 - 1-phosphate (pyridoxal-P or PLP) as an essential coenzyme. Biodegradative decarboxylases do not show strict specificity toward the substrates, and when the primary amino acid substrate is absent, structurally similar amino acids may be decarboxylated to form other BAs to provide pH homeostasis. In the pathway of amino acid catabolism, generally, the combined action of decarboxylases and a functional substrate/product transmembrane exchanger results in a proton motive force, which generates alkalinization of the cytoplasm (Restuccia et al. 2014). A decarboxylase with a given amino acid specificity is adjacent to an exchanger with an equally strict amino acid/BA specificity, as was reported for histidine/histamine, tyrosine/tyramine, aspartate/alanine, ornithine/putrescine, and glutamate/g-aminobutyrate decarboxylation systems (Restuccia et al. 2014). The arginine deiminase pathway is the other type in which arginine is converted into ornithine (Figure 5.1). A very similar pathway consists of one transport step, and the sequential activities of three enzymes have been described for agmatine, the decarboxylation product of arginine, which yields putrescine (Halász et al. 1994; Restuccia et al. 2014). In this pathway, the transporter is responsible for the combined uptake and excretion of substrate and product, respectively, that is, arginine/ornithine and agmatine/putrescine exchange (Restuccia et al. 2014).

Table 5.2 shows microorganisms commonly associated with the formation of BAs in various food products. Both gram-positive and gram-negative bacteria, and some yeasts are confirmed for their ability to form BAs and also isolated from various foods containing high levels of various BAs. Extensive studies showed that the ability of microorganisms to form BAs *in vitro* does not reflect the actual production in food, as environmental parameters (temperature, water activity, pH, precursor availability), microbiological factors (flora competition or presence of BA degraders), and optimal decarboxylase enzyme activity can all influence the amine production (Restuccia et al. 2014). High levels of certain BAs in foods, such as putrescine, spermidine, spermine, and cadaverine, are reported to be an indicative of undesired microbial activity (Shalaby 1996; Restuccia et al. 2014). However, the capability of microorganism to form BAs is generally considered a strain-specific characteristic rather than a species property. Therefore, it is usually difficult to find precise correlations between BA contents and microbial counts as also reported by various researches in literature for different foods (Halász et al. 1994; Restuccia et al. 2014).

Microorganisms with the amino acid decarboxylase positive activity are either naturally present in food products or may be introduced by contamination before, during, or after food processing and even during storage. In fish, BA producing bacteria are most likely to be present on the gills or skin, or in the gastrointestinal tract. Transfer of these bacteria to the flesh of the fish, where FAAs may be present, leads to development of BAs. Transfer can occur from the gastrointestinal tract after harvesting, through migration, or via rupture or spillage of gastric contents during gutting. Microorganisms may also be transferred from the skin or gills during filleting or skinning. In the case of fermented foods and beverages, the applied starter cultures may also affect the production of BAs (Halász et al. 1994). In fermented foods, LAB can contribute to BA formation as they are present in raw materials, are part of the starter culture, or contaminate the product during processing. To this regard, a number of authors have suggested the ability to produce BAs to be a negative trait when selecting a starter, secondary, or adjunct culture to be used for making fermented products. Various strains LAB (Table 5.2) are capable of decarboxylating amino acids in several foods like cheese, fermented meat, vegetables, and beverages (Russo et al. 2010; Restuccia et al. 2014). Some *Enterobacteriaceae* are usually associated with the production of high amounts of putrescine, cadaverine, and histamine in spoiled foods such as fish and meat products (Table 5.2). Recent studies indicated the ability of certain LAB strains (*L. brevis* from wine and *L. curvatus* and *E. faecalis* isolated from cheese) to produce putrescine by agmatine deamination instead of the ornithine decarboxylation pathway, although putrescine synthesis was initially associated with gram-negative bacteria, particularly the members of *Enterobacteriaceae*.

TABLE 5.2
Commonly Reported Biogenic Amine Forming Microorganisms Isolated from Various Food and Food Products

Food	Biogenic Amines	Microorganisms with Decarboxylase Activity	
Fish	Histamine	*Enterobacteriaceae, Morganella morganii, M. psychrotolerans, Klebsiella pneumoniae, Hafnia alvei, Proteus* spp. (*P. mirabilis, P. vulgaris*), *Enterobacter* spp. (*E. clocae, E. aerogenes*), *Serratia* spp. (*S. fonticola, S. liquefaciens*), *Citrobacter freundii, Clostridium* spp., *Pseudomonas* spp. (*P. fluorescens, P. putida*), *Aeromonas* spp., *Plesiomonas shigelloides, Photobacterium* spp. (*P. phosphoreum*)	Emborg et al. (2005), Dalgaard et al. (2008), Ladero et al. (2010), Restuccia et al. (2014)
	Putrescine	*Enterobacteriaceae, Pseudomonaceae*	
	Cadaverine	*Enterobacteriaceae, Pseudomonaceae, Lactobacillus, Enterococcus, and Staphylococcus*	
	Tyramine	*Lactobacillus* spp. (*L. brevis, L. hilgardii, L. plantarum*), *Enterococcus* spp. (*E. faecium*)	
Cheese	Histamine	*Lactobacillus* spp. (*L. buchneri, L. curvatus*), *Enterococcus* spp. (*E. faecium*), *Enterobacteriaceae, Streptococcus thermophilus PRI60*	Kučerová et al. (2009), Gardini et al. (2012), Ladero et al. (2010), Restuccia et al. (2014)
	Putrescine	*Enterobacteriaceae* (*Enterobacter, Serratia, Escherichia, Salmonella, Hafnia, Citrobacter, Klebsiella*) *Lactobacillus* spp. (*L. brevis, L. hilgardii, L. buchneri, L. plantarum, L. zeae*), *Enterococcus* spp. (*E. faecium, E. faecalis*), *Leuconostoc mesenteroides, Oenococcus oeni*	
	Tyramine	*Enterococcus* spp. (*E. faecalis, E. faecium, E. durans, E. hirae*), *Lactobacillus* spp. (*L. brevis, L. lactis, L. curvatus, L. hilgardii, L. plantarum*), *Leuconostoc* spp. (*L. mesenteroides*), *Carnobacterium* spp., *Staphylococcus* spp.	
Wine	Histamine	*Lactobacillus* (*L. hilgardii, L. parabuchneri, L. rossiae*), *Oenococcus oeni, Pediococcus* spp. (*P. cerevisiae, P. parvulus*), *Leuconostoc mesenteroides*	Ladero et al. (2010), Restuccia et al. (2014)
	Putrescine	*Lactobacillus* spp. (*L. buchneri, L. hilgardii, L. brevis, L. plantarum*), *Leuconostoc mesenteroides, Oenococcus oeni*	
	Cadaverine	*Enterobacteriaceae, Bacillus, Clostridium, Listeria, Staphylococcus*	
	Tyramine	*Lactobacillus* spp. (*L. hilgardii, L. brevis, L. plantarum*), *Leuconostoc* spp. (*L. mesenteroides*), *Enterococcus faecium*	
	Phenylethylamine	*Lactobacillus* spp. (*L. hilgardii, L. brevis*)	

(*Continued*)

TABLE 5.2 (*Continued*)
Commonly Reported Biogenic Amine Forming Microorganisms Isolated from Various Food and Food Products

Food	Biogenic Amines	Microorganisms with Decarboxylase Activity	
Beer	Histamine	*L. buchneri*	Kalač et al. (2002)
Meat	Histamine	*Enterobacteriaceae, Staphylococcus capitis*	Ladero et al. (2010), Restuccia et al. (2014)
	Tyramine	*Staphylococcus* spp. (*S. carnosus, S. xylosus, S. epidermidis, S. saprophyticus*), *Lactobacillus* spp. (*L. brevis, L. bavaricus, L. curvatus, L. plantarum, L. sakei*), *Carnobacterium* spp. (*Carnobacterium divergens, C. piscicola*)	Ercan et al. (2013), Ladero et al. (2010), Restuccia et al. (2014), Karovičová and Kohajdová (2005)
	Putrescine	*Enterobacteriaceae, Enterococcus* spp., *Enterobacter cloacae, Morganella morganii, Pseudomonas, Serratia liquefaciens, Pseudomonas* spp.	
	Cadaverine	*Enterobacteriaceae, Pseudomonas* spp.	
	Putrescine	*Leuconostoc mesenteroides, Lactobacillus* spp.	
	Tyramine	*Lactobacillus* spp.	

Source: Updated from Restuccia, D., U.G. Spizzirri, F. Puoci, I.O. Parisi, M. Curcio, and N. Picci. 2014. Accumulation of biogenic amines in foods: Hazard identification and Ccontrol options. In: R.R. Rai and J.A. Bai (eds) *Microbial Food Safety and Preservation Techniques*. Boca Raton, FL: CRC Press, pp. 53–74, Chapter 4.

In fact, LAB are reported to be the main bacteria responsible for putrescine production in wine. Similarly, some LAB strains were recently reported to produce histamine in wine despite the main responsible bacteria for this process as *Oenococcus oeni*. Decarboxylase activity was also observed in some species belonging to the genera *Micrococcus* and *Staphylococcus* in fermented sausages (Restuccia et al. 2014).

5.2.4 Conditions for BA Formation

Conditions for the formation of BAs are mostly related to the factors affecting to the growth of microorganisms that have decarboxylating activity and to the ability of decarboxylating reactions of enzymes. These are mainly described as pH, oxygen content, temperature, and salt and sugar contents of foods.

5.2.4.1 pH

It has been reported that amino acid decarboxylase activity is stronger in an acidic environment. In earlier studies, the optimum pH for decarboxylating activity was suggested in a range of 2.5–6.5 (Halász et al. 1994), but later it was limited to 4.0–5.5 (Marcobal et al. 2006). Two main mechanisms are reported acting simultaneously in relation to pH effect on BA formation. One of which affects the microbial growth by acidity inhibiting the growth of microorganisms while other influencing the production and activity of the enzyme. In low-pH environments, bacteria are more stimulated to produce decarboxylase as a part of their defense mechanisms against acidity. The pH contents of foods vary according to the changes during processing and storage. Since fish muscles contain relatively low amount of glycogen compared with mammalian muscles, the final postmortem pH is consequently higher making fish meat more susceptible to microbial attack. However, the level of pH at this stage is not as low as to accelerate the decarboxylate activity of bacterial enzymes as mentioned above. Therefore, other factors, such as temperature, influence the bacterial growth increasing BA formation in fresh fish.

Acidic conditions of marinades make the tissue cathepsins more active resulting in the degradation of some muscle proteins into peptides and amino acids which are the precursors of BAs. The influence of glucono δ-lactone (GDL) on the reduction of pH in dry sausages was reported by Karovičová and Kohajdová (2005). Low pH in sausages can lead to increase decarboxylase activity of bacteria.

5.2.4.2 Oxygen (O_2)

Oxygen supply also appears to have a significant effect on the biosynthesis of BAs. It has been reported that *E. cloacae* produces about half the quantity of putrescine in anaerobic compared with aerobic conditions, and *K. pneumoniae* synthesizes significantly less cadaverine but acquires the ability to produce putrescine under anaerobic conditions (Halász et al. 1994; Restuccia et al. 2014). There are different processing and packaging methods that provide anaerobic conditions in foods to prolong the shelf life by preventing or delaying oxidation and microbial spoilage. In such environments, the growth of some microorganism strains that have decarboxylase activity can be affected. However, it has been reported that the success of inhibition largely depends on the type of microflora, its environmental conditions, such as temperature, and also the gas mix used in case of modified atmosphere packaging (MAP); it may also be product specific (Naila et al. 2010). The redox potential of the medium is also known to influence the BA production. Conditions resulting in a reduced redox potential stimulate histamine production, and histidine decarboxylase activity seems to be inactivated or destroyed in the presence of oxygen (Restuccia et al. 2014).

5.2.4.3 Temperature

The quantitative production of BAs is often reported to be time/temperature (TT) dependent. The amine production rate usually increases with the increasing temperature up to certain level while the production is minimum at low temperatures due to the inhibition of microbial growth and the reduction of enzyme activity. The optimum temperature for the formation of BAs by mesophilic bacteria has been reported to be between 20°C and 37°C, whereas the production of BA decreases below 5°C or above 40°C (Restuccia et al. 2014). Influence on the amine formation by bacteria is commonly reported for different amines, for example, *E. cloacae* produced 2 mg/mL putrescine after 24 hours' incubation at 20°C but was unable to synthesize amine at 10°C, although *K. pneumoniae* was not as sensitive to temperature but did show less extensive cadaverine production at 10°C than at 20°C (Halász et al. 1994). Table 5.3 shows temperature effect on the formation of BAs in various food products.

TABLE 5.3
Development of Important Biogenic Amines in Various Fish and Food Products at Certain Temperatures

		(mg/kg for Solid Foods, mg/L for Liquids)				
Food Type	**Temp/Time**	**HIS**	**PUT**	**CAD**	**TYR**	**References**
Sardine (*Sardina pilchardus*)	4°C/15 days	203	114	100	16.0	Özogul and Özogul (2006)
	22°C/12 h	577	420	<d.l	16.0	Prester et al. (2009)
	24°C/24 h	620				Visciano et al. (2007)
Anchovy (*E. encrasicolus*)	0°C/5 days	0.46	3.09	5.26	2.8	Pons-Sánchez-Cascado et al. (2006)
	10°C/24 h	11.0				Rossano et al. (2006)
	20°C/24 h	750				Rossano et al. (2006)
Mackerel (*S. scombrus*)	22°C/12 h	40	56	<d.l	47.0	Prester et al. (2009)
Indian mackerel (*Rastrelliger kanagurda*)	3 ± 1°C/6 days	26.2	18.1	14.9		Zare et al. (2013)
	10°C/3 days	422.3	56.8	93.8		
Chub mackerel (*S. japonicus*)	20–23°C/24 h	1500	80	200		Mendes (1999)
Mahi-mahi (*C. hippurus*)	32°C/24 h	2500				Baranowski et al. (1990)
Skipjack tuna (*K. pelamis*)	21°C/2 days	1533	65	649		Rossi et al. (2002)
Yellowfin tuna (*T. albacares*)	4°C/5 days	25.6	1.7	<d.l		Due et al. (2002)
	25°C/10 h	7.1	1.9	7.2		Staruszkiewicz et al. (2004)
	31°C/10.5 h	131	6.7	19		Staruszkiewicz et al. (2004)
Herring (*C. harengus*)	10°C/2 days	236	10	147	17.0	Mackie et al. (1997)
Whole bonito (*S. sarda*)	4°C/7 days	113.8	24.6	101.3	33.6	Koral and Köse (2012)
Fish sauce	20°C, 30 days	2800				Kuda et al. (2012)
Pork meat	5°C/8 days	4.0	16.9	38.6		Halász et al. (1994)
	5°C/15 days	9.9	18.9	43.0		
	−20°C/8 days	0.5	4.4	27.5		
	−20°C/15 days	0.5	11.2	41.2		
Cheese	−18°C/180 days	27.8	31.7	43.7	157.2	Andiç et al. (2009)
	4°C/180 days	219.6	525.2	1166.9	643.3	
Beer	21°C/4 days	1.2	5.1	1.4	6.0	Kalač et al. (2002)
	21°C/8 days	2.0	5.8	1.5	16.6	

Source: Updated from Prester, L., *Food Addit. Contamm. Part A.* 28, 1547–1560, 2011.
d.l.: detection limit; HIS: *histamine*; PUT: *putrescine*; CAD: *cadaverine*; TYR: *tyramine.*

Histamine is formed more commonly as a result of high temperature spoilage than that of long term, relatively low temperature spoilage. However, there are a number of opportunities for histamine to be formed under more moderate abuse temperature conditions. HFP can also be caused by psychrotolerant bacteria (*M. psychrotolerans* and *Photobacterium phosphoreum*) due to their ability of producing toxic concentrations of histamine at temperatures as low as 2°C (Emborg et al. 2005). Dalgaard et al. (2008) also pointed out that both bacteria can produce histamine in toxic levels at 0°C–5°C. Therefore, histamine formation during extended storage of fish at low temperature must not be disregarded (Köse 2010).

5.2.4.4 Sodium Chloride (NaCl) and Sugars

Sodium chloride and sugar are added to foods as either preservative additives or to improve taste. These additives are often used together for fermented foods and also important factors in the formation of BAs during this process. Their effect appears to depend on several factors (concentration, processing conditions, and others). In particular, NaCl plays an important role in microbial growth and, therefore, influences the activity of the amino acid decarboxylase. Many studies demonstrated marked decrease in BA formation in the increase of NaCl concentration. It was reported that NaCl concentration in a range from 3.5% to 5.5% could inhibit histamine formation (Suzzi and Gardini 2003). For example, the ability of *L. buchneri* to form histamine is partly inhibited at the 3.5% salt content, and its formation is stopped at 5.0%. The influence of the salt can be attributed to the reduced cell yield obtained in the presence of high NaCl concentration and to a progressive disturbance of the membrane located in microbial decarboxylase enzymes (Restuccia et al. 2014). However, the presence of NaCl activates tyrosine decarboxylase activity and inhibits histidine decarboxylase activity (Silla Santos 1996). Hence, it can be assumed that the effect of NaCl in inhibiting and stimulating BA production is strain specific.

The presence of fermentable carbohydrate such as glucose can increase both growth and amino acid decarboxylase of bacteria. It has been demonstrated that the acidification produced by sugars in the fermentation process influences the formation of BAs. The optimum glucose concentration for the formation of decarboxylase enzymes is 0.5%–2.0%, while levels in excess of 3.0 % inhibit enzyme formation. This is related to the effect of reduced pH on microorganism growth and the activity of enzymatic systems (Restuccia et al. 2014).

5.3 TOXICITY OF BAs

5.3.1 Introduction

Low concentrations of BAs are usually tolerated by the human body, and they are very rapidly metabolized to physiologically less active degradation products by specific enzymes in intestinal tract of healthy persons. However, these amines can have adverse effects when present at high concentrations and pose a health risk for sensitive individuals (Prester 2011). Therefore, BAs do not usually represent any health hazard to individuals unless large amounts are ingested, or the natural mechanism for the catabolism of the amines is inhibited or genetically deficient (Halász et al. 1994).

Specific enzymes in the intestinal tract of mammals have detoxifying role in the metabolizing normal dietary intake of BAs. Oxidation is the main route of BA detoxification following ingestion by amine oxidases at the gut level (Hungerford 2010). Dietary polyamines such as putrescine, spermidine, and spermine are catabolized by several enzymes: polyamine oxidase (PAO EC 1.5.3.11), diamine oxidases (DAO, EC 1.4.3.6), spermidine/spermine acetyltransferase, and possible other oxidases present in intestine and liver such as histamine *N*-methyltransferase (HNMT) (Prester 2011). Monoamine oxidase (MAO)-A predominates in the stomach, intestine, and placenta and has polar aromatic amines as preferred substrates. MAO-B predominates in the brain and selectively deaminates nonpolar aromatic amines. Tyramine is a substrate for either form of MAO (EC 1.4.3.4); MAO-A is responsible for the intestinal metabolism of tyramine, thereby preventing its systemic absorption. In humans, DAO is the main responsible enzyme for catabolizing histamine. Moreover, detoxification was also reported for tyramine, histamine, and phenylethylamine by *N*-methyltransferases or acetylation (Hungerford 2010; Prester 2011).

However, upon intake of high loads of BAs with foods, this detoxification system is unable to eliminate BAs sufficiently resulting in poisoning. Moreover, in case of insufficient DAO-activity, caused by various factors, such as genetic predisposition, gastrointestinal diseases, or inhibition of DAO-activity due to secondary effects of medicines or alcohol, already low amounts of BAs cannot be metabolized efficiently (Anli and Bayram 2008; Prester 2011). People with gastrointestinal problems (gastritis, irritable bowel syndrome, Crohn's disease, stomach, and colonic ulcers) are at risk because the activity of oxidases in their intestines is usually lower than that in healthy individuals. In women, there is premenstrual decrease in the activity of B-type MAO. Patients, who are taking medicines with inhibiting effect to MAO and DAO such as antihistamines, antimalarial agents, psychopharmaceutics, might have a changed metabolism of BA, which can lead to inhibit or decrease the detoxification activity. Also, injuries of intestinal mucosa can reduce the function of BA detoxification enzymes (Karovičová and Kohajdová 2005).

In the case of histamine toxicity, the potentiating effect of other BAs present in foods such as tyramine, putrescine, and cadaverine was reported due to their competition with histamine-metabolizing enzymes (Halász et al. 1994; Shalaby 1996; Prester 2011). For this reason, even low dietary intake of histamine can cause clinical signs of food intolerance (Hungerford 2010; Prester 2011). Therefore, the presence of other BAs in foods is important to estimate the toxicity of dietary histamine in foods. Halász et al. (1994) reported that the determination of the exact toxicity threshold of BAs in individuals is extremely difficult since the toxic dose is strongly dependent on the efficiency of the detoxilication mechanisms of different individuals. Aminoguanidine, anserine, carnosine, agmatine, and tyramine inhibit DAO, and phenylethylamine, tryptamine, octopamine possess inhibiting effect on *N*-methyltransferase (Karovičová and Kohajdová 2005).

Varying levels of BAs are reported for causing toxicity to humans and animals (Halász et al. 1994; Shalaby 1996; Prester 2011). An intake of 5–10 mg of histamine can be considered as defecting to some sensitive people, 10 mg is considered as tolerable limit, 100 mg induce a medium toxicity, and 1000 mg is highly toxic. About 100–800 mg/kg tyramine and 30 mg/kg phenylethylamine have been reported to be toxic doses in foods (Halász et al. 1994). The consumption of foods containing high amount of BAs is reported to cause some adverse effects such as headaches, hypo- or hypertension, nausea, cardiac palpitation, renal intoxication (Table 5.4) and in severe cases intracerebral hemorrhage or even death (Anli and Bayram 2008). The most common symptoms were rash, diarrhea, flushing, and headache (Halász et al. 1994). Some food migraines are related to BAs, particularly tyramine and phenylethylamine (EFSA 2011).

The clinical signs of BA poisoning normally appear between 30 minutes to a few hours following BA ingestion and disappear within 24 hours. The severity of clinical symptoms depends on the type and the amount of BAs ingested, and the correct functioning of the detoxification system that could be influenced by various factors. Therefore, the dose–response anomalies can be expected in the toxicity of BAs. With regard to human susceptibility, it is clearly evidenced that certain physiological/pathological status can modify the sensitivity against BAs. For example, during pregnancy, there is a physiological increase of DAO production (up to 500-fold), which would explain the remissions of food intolerance while individuals affected by gastritis, irritable bowel syndrome, Crohn's disease, etc., are more sensible due to lower oxidase activity. In addition, several studies reported inhibition of enzymes involved in the detoxification process by various drugs such as antidepressant drugs, which can inhibit MAO activity resulting in an increase on tyramine sensitivity up to 13-fold depending on the drugs used. Therefore, individuals taking nonselective MAO inhibitor (MAOI) drugs are recommended to avoid the consumption of tyramine-rich foodstuffs (fermented fish, cheese, salami, sausage, soy sauce, etc.) (Restuccia et al. 2014).

Some studies also showed evidence that smoking tobacco reduces MAO levels by up to 40% together with other components present in cigarettes (Restuccia et al. 2014). One other important risk factor is the quantity of BA-rich food in a meal, which makes the prediction of the phenomenon of BA accumulation difficult. Moreover, foods rich in BAs like cheese are frequently consumed with alcoholic fermented beverages such as beer or wine, which increases the permeability of intestinal epithelial cells to BAs, enhancing the toxic effect (Silla Santos 1996). This phenomenon is referred to as the BA synergistic effect and may explain the reason that aged cheese is more toxic than an equivalent of histamine administration in aqueous solution (Restuccia et al. 2014).

5.3.2 Toxicity of Histamine

Toxicity of histamine was first implicated with Scombroid fish such as tuna, bonito, and mackerel. Therefore, originally it is known "Scombroid fish poisoning." Later, it was associated with other foods, so it is called as "histamine food poisoning" (Köse 2010). HFP is frequently misdiagnosed due to its typical symptoms that mimic those of allergy (Köse 1993; Restuccia et al. 2014). Histamine poisoning is characterized by the symptoms mainly, headaches, vertigo, nausea and vomiting, enhanced secretion of gastric mucosa, gastrointestinal cramps, stomach ache, diarrhea, hypotension, tachycardia, extrasystoles, and itching (Table 5.4; Restuccia et al. 2014).

TABLE 5.4
Toxicological Effects of Biogenic Amines

Biogenic Amines	Levels	Pharmaceutical Effects	Symptoms	
			Mild/Moderate Poisoning	Severe Poisoning
Histamine	5–10 mg toxic to some sensitive people, 10 mg tolerable limit, 100 mg induce a medium toxicity 1000 mg is highly toxic	Liberates adrenaline and noradrenaline, excites the smooth muscles of the uterus, the intestine, and the respiratory tract, stimulates both sensory and motor neurons, controls gastric acid secretion	In skin: itching, swelling, flushing, rash, urticaria Neurological: headache, dizziness, tremor Gastrointestinal: nausea, abdominal cramps, diarrhea, vomiting Other: rhinitis oral burning sensation/tingling, metallic, bitter, or peppery taste, swelling of tongue, dry mouth, dyspnea	Bronchospasm, respiratory distress, hypotension or hypertension, tachycardia Rarely wheezing or loss of consciousness due to hypotension Acute pulmonary edema, exacerbation of asthma Myocardial infarction and even refractory myocardial dysfunction requiring biventricular assist devices
Tyramine	100–800 mg/kg	Peripheral vasoconstriction, increases the cardiac output, causes lacrimation and salivation, increases respiration, increases blood sugar level, releases noradrenaline from the sympathetic nervous system	Causes migraine, headache, neurological disorders, nausea, vomiting, respiratory disorders, hypertension dizziness, and discomfort	
Putrescine and cadaverine		Increased cardiac output, Potentiate the toxicity of other amines	Hypotension, bradycardia, paresis of the extremities, tachycardia, carcinogenic effects Hypotension	
Phenylethylamine	30 mg/kg	Increases the blood pressure Releases noradrenaline from the sympathetic nervous system	Causes migraine	
Tryptamine		Increases the blood pressure		

Source: Updated from Anli, R.E., and M. Bayram, *Food Rev. Int.*, 25, 86–102, 2008.

Histamine is present in mast cells and basophils, and its biological effects are usually seen only when it is released in large amounts in the course of allergic and other reactions. Histamine exerts its toxic effects by interacting with four types of receptors (H_1, H_2, H_3, H_4) on cellular membranes of humans and other species (Silla Santos 1996; Restuccia et al. 2014). It causes dilatation of peripheral blood vessels, capillaries, and arteries, thus resulting in hypotension, flushing, and headache (EFSA 2011). H_1 receptors are responsible for the histamine-induced contraction of intestinal smooth muscle causing abdominal cramps, diarrhea, and vomiting, whereas H_2 receptors located on the parietal cells and take role in gastric acid secretion. It was also claimed that pain and itching associated with the urticarial lesions may be due to sensory and motor neuron stimulation through H_1 receptors (Karovičová and Kohajdová 2005). The role of H_4 receptor is less known, but it is also reported to involve in histamine toxicity (Hungerford 2010; EFSA 2011).

Due to the variability in dose–response anomaly in histamine toxicity in humans, earlier researchers suggested that other compounds such as "a mast cell degranulator" such as cis urocanic acid may be responsible in histamine toxicity (Hungerford 2010). Later, toxicity associated with dietary histamine has been confirmed by various clinical studies (Prester 2011; Feng et al. 2016).

Treatment of histamine toxic effect is possible with antihistaminic drugs (Karovičová and Kohajdová 2005; EFSA 2011; FAO-WHO 2013). H_1-receptor antagonists have been used for the treatment of allergic conditions, whereas H_2-receptor antagonists have been available for the treatment of gastric ulcers. H_3-receptor was used for the treatment of central nervous system disorders. The role of H_3 receptors in learning and memory indicates that H_3-receptor antagonists could have a role in the treatment of memory disorders such as Alzheimer's disease (Karovičová and Kohajdová 2005; EFSA 2011). Histamine is also converted into inactive acetylhistamine in the intestine, presumably by bacterial enzymes. The human kidney has a considerable capacity for removing histamine from blood. When healthy individuals were infused intravenously with histamine, a large proportion was methylated by the kidney and excreted in the urine and a smaller proportion was excreted unchanged in the urine (Karovičová and Kohajdová 2005; EFSA 2011).

5.3.3 Tyramine Toxicity

Tyramine, tryptamine, and β-phenylethylamine have been reported as vasoactive amines. The toxicology of tyramine was reported as supporting the efflux of catecholamines from the sympathetic nervous system and the adrenal medulla and may cause an increase of the mean arterial blood pressure and heart rate by peripheral vasoconstriction, resulting in hypertensive crisis. Tyramine also dilates the pupils and the palpebral tissue, causes lacrimation and salivation, accelerates respiration, and increases the blood sugar content (Russo et al. 2010).

Toxicity of tyramine is often reported as "the cheese reaction" due to common association with cheese. It is a pathological condition commonly associated to adverse interaction between MAOIs, a class of antidepressant drugs, and high amounts of dietary tyramine (Russo et al. 2010). An adverse side MAOIs (which are used to disturb the catabolic pathway of serotonin to relieve the depressive crisis of patients) effect is reported as their concurrent failure to inactivate the strong vasopressor tyramine. The resulting hypertensive reactions in more severe cases can lead to shock and death by brain hemorrhage (Karovičová and Kohajdová 2005; Kantaria and Gokani 2011). As in the histamine poisoning cases, dose–response situation varies in the toxicity of dietary tyramine, although ingestion of 125 mg/kg tyramine has been reported to be necessary for the occurrence of this condition (Restuccia et al. 2014). It has been reported that the presence of 6 mg in one or two usual servings is thought to be sufficient to cause a mild adverse event while 10–25 mg will produce a severe adverse event in those using MAOI drugs. For unmedicated adults, 200–800 mg of dietary tyramine is needed to induce a mild rise in blood pressure. Although polyamines such as pustrescine and cadaverine are considered not hazardous for human health, they are known to contribute a dangerous synergistic effect on histamine or tyramine toxicity by inhibiting MAO, DAO, and hydroxymethyl transferase (Kantaria and Gokani 2011; Karovičová and Kohajdová 2005; Restuccia et al. 2014).

The first case of tyramine associated with cheese was reported by a neurologist who noticed that his wife, who was receiving MAOI treatment, had severe headaches (caused by cerebral vasoconstriction followed by dilation) and migraines when eating cheese. Rarely, the increase in blood pressure results in a hypertensive crisis in some individuals. This situation can cause end-organ damage to the heart or central nervous system. Raised levels of tyramine in the brain have been associated with neurological disorders such as schizophrenia, Parkinson's disease, depression, and Reyes' syndrome (Kantaria and Gokani 2011).

The main dietary intake of tyramine and other vasoactive amines comes from cheese and some fermented foods. As in the case of fish, BAs are often distributed unevenly within the cheese depending on several production conditions. Proteolysis is a crucial factor, because it allows high formation of FAAs that provide a rich substrate for BA formation. It was reported that conditions of accelerated or enhanced proteolysis resulted in a dramatic increase of BA during cheese ripening. Higher levels of BA are reported for hard cheeses than unripened cheeses (Novella-Rodríguez et al. 2002). Another critical issue is the occurrence of microflora able to transform the FAAs into the correspondent BA. In cheese, the main microorganisms with decarboxylase activity belong to the genera *Enterococcus* and *Lactobacillus*. In particular, *Enterococcus faecalis*, *E. faecium*, and *E. durans* strains are considered very strong tyramine producers. Therefore, although tyramine is the most frequent BA found in cheese, reaching levels higher than 1000 mg/kg, it is difficult to correlate BA concentration with microorganism content (Russo et al. 2010).

5.3.4 BAs Relating to Cancer

Prester (2011) reported that polyamines are involved in neoplastic cell growth. Therefore, various studies have been carried out on polyamine-reduced diet, and such diet was proposed as a part of nutritional therapy to prostate cancer patients. However, the potential therapeutic tool of a diet free of polyamine in neoplastic growth is still subject to further investigations. Due to the importance of dietary polyamines in cancer therapy, it is of interest to examine the contents of individual polyamines in food. Past studies reported that decomposed foods such as fermented fish contain higher polyamine levels than fresh foods indicating the importance of avoiding spoiled or ripened foods for cancer patients (Prester 2011; Restuccia et al. 2014).

The accumulation of BAs in certain foods, particularly fermented fish and meat, is also linked to formation of carcinogenous nitrosamines (NAs). These are *N*-nitroso compounds generally formed by the reaction of a nitrosating agent derived from either nitrite salts or nitrogen oxide with a substance having an amine group. The effect of crude (impure) salt and heating was also reported as to enhance NA formation in food products (Silla Santos 1996; Al Bulushi et al. 2009; Prester 2011). These compounds can also form endogenously in human body, especially intragastrically. Figure 5.2 shows the nitrosation of amines (Prester 2011).

In 1978, the International Agency for Research on Cancer (IARC) classified various NAs with respect to cancer risk for humans. The IARC considers *N*-nitrosodimethylamine (NDMA) and *N*-nitrosodiethylamine into a group of probably carcinogenic to human, and *N*-nitrosodibutylamine (NDBA), *N*-nitrosopiperidine (NPIP), and *N*-nitrosopyrrolidine (NPYR) into the group of possibly carcinogenic to human. Among these NAs, NDMA is the most commonly encountered volatile NA in food samples (Yurchenko and Mölder 2006). The United States has set 10 μg/kg NPYR as the maximum allowable limit in bacon (Al Bulushi et al. 2009) while not many countries including the European Union (EU) Commission set regulations for NAs originated from food. Estonian government has maximum permitted concentration of the sum of two NAs (NDMA and NDEA) in fresh and smoked fish, which is 3 μg/kg (Yurchenko and Mölder 2006). The EU regulations (EU 1993) relate to the release of the *N*-nitrosamines and *N*-nitrosatable substances from elastomer or rubber teats and soothers (Köse 2010).

Although various causes have been implicated with the formation of NAs in foods, the mechanisms of NA formation in food products and factors influencing their formation have not been clearly elucidated (Köse 2010). The nitrosable secondary amines such as dimethylamine (DMA), agmatine, spermine, spermidine, and so on can form NAs by reaction with nitrite (NO_2^-), whereas tertiary amines produce a range of labile *N*-nitroso products (Karovičová and Kohajdová 2005). Various factors

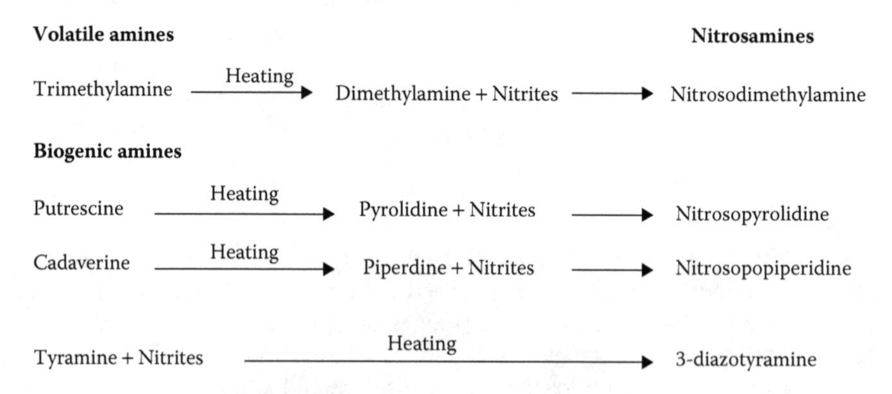

FIGURE 5.2 Nitrosation of fish amines. (Redrawn from Prester, L., *Food Addit. Contamm. Part A.*, 28, 1547–1560, 2011.)

have been reported to affect NA formation in food products. Nitrite in foods is the main precursing agent in the formation of NAs along with other amines (Figure 5.2).

Nitrite is commonly used as sodium nitrite ($NaNO_2$) for food coloring, flavoring, and preservation (Prester 2011). $NaNO_2$ is added to meat and seafood products as preservative agents and also to develop and fix the typical bright pink color associated with cured and smoked meats. Nitrite can also be formed by nitrifying bacteria in the presence of high nitrate (NO_3^-) in foods. In fact, sodium nitrate ($NaNO_3$) is used primarily in the curing of food such as fermented sausages and dry-cured meats that require long production times. In these food items, $NaNO_3$ serves as a reservoir for the production of $NaNO_2$, through the bacterial reduction of $NaNO_3$. Nitrite inhibits the growth of pathogens, including *Clostridium botulinum* and some meat-spoilage bacteria (Epley et al. 1992). The antimicrobial activity of $NaNO_2$ has also been demonstrated for of other foodborne pathogens, including *Listeria monocytogenes*, and its activity is enhanced in conjunction with NaCl, pH, temperature, and a_w (Nyachuba et al. 2007).

The DMA is known as the most abundant nitrosatable precursors in nitrite-cured fish meat (Yurchenko and Mölder 2006). This amine is formed from trimethylamine (TMA), which is a spoilage compound of marine fishes. However, BAs subjected to heat may also form nitrosatable amines. Putrescine and cadaverine, which are commonly found in decomposed fish and shellfish, may generate NAs such as NPYR and NPIP (Figure 5.2; Yurchenko and Mölder 2006; Al Bulushi et al. 2009). Furthermore, it was reported that dietary tyramine is converted to a mutagen compound, 3-diazotyramine (3-DT) (after treatment with nitrite under acidic conditions) that induced carcinoma of the oral cavity in rats (Ochiai et al. 1984; Prester 2011).

Studies on NAs in foods mainly concentrate on the factors in the formation of these amines and accumulation in different food products. Few studies also reported method developments in detecting NAs in foods, which is important to correct estimation of their levels. Many variables influence NA levels: amount of nitrite added during processing, concentrations of amines in meat, type and amounts of other ingredients used in processing, actual processing conditions, length of storage, storage temperatures, and method of cooking (Epley et al. 1992). Low amount of NAs were detected in fresh fish, whereas the levels of these compounds in fish products and fried fish were reported considerably high and even may exceed the tolerance limit of 3 μg/kg (Yurchenko and Mölder 2006; Al Bulushi et al. 2009). Past studies reported relatively high concentrations of NAs in traditionally fermented fish products (FFPs) (Ahn et al. 2003).

Ingestion of nitrite is also known to cause health risk. The ingestion of 8–15 g of nitrite can cause severe gastroenteritis with abdominal pain, blood in stool and urine, weakness, and collapse. Chronic ingestion of smaller doses can cause dyspepsia, mental depression, and headache. Due to health risk also arise from consumption of nitrite and its reported association in the formation of NAs, the amount to be added to the foods is also regulated by most authorities. The addition of $NaNO_3$ and $NaNO_2$ to meats is regulated by the US Department of Agriculture/Food Safety and Inspection Service (USDA/FSIS) and allowed between 100 and 200 mg/kg $NaNO_2$ and $\leq$500 mg/kg $NaNO_3$ in cured meats (Nyachuba et al. 2007). The use of these agents is also permitted in some types of smoked fish (e.g., smoked salmon).

However, the use of $NaNO_3$ and $NaNO_2$ in smoked fish is regulated by U.S. Food and Drug Administration (FDA) (Nyachuba et al. 2007). Brazilian cheesemakers are allowed to add 20 g of nitrate/400 L of milk during manufacturing of certain types of cheeses, whereas Dutch and Canadian cheesemakers are also permitted to add 15 and 20 g nitrate/100 L of milk, in the production of certain cheeses (Oliveira et al. 1995).

Varying studies have been carried out on the effects of different factors on the formation of NAs. Pensabene et al. (1974) studied the influence of high heat on the cooking bacon. They reported that frying bacon at 176.6°C for 6 minutes, 204.4°C for 4 and 10 minutes, the levels of NPYR were obtained as 10, 17, and 19 μg/kg. Thus, they concluded that well-done or burned bacon probably is potentially more hazardous than less well-done bacon. They also pointed out that bacon cooked by microwave has less NAs than fried bacon. Therefore, they advised consumers to cook bacon properly (Epley et al. 1992). Huang et al. (1981) also studied the effect of heat on the formation of NAs in salted fish. They detected NDMA in all samples whether cooked or uncooked, whereas NDEA was determined in more batches of the steamed fish than of the uncooked or fried fish. They reported that NDPA was detected in both steamed and fried samples and NDBA in only the fried samples. Neither was detected in the uncooked samples. However, *N*-nitrosomorpholine (NMOR) occurred in the uncooked samples. Therefore, they concluded that only certain NAs are formed from precursors during cooking. It was also reported that NPYR can be formed from putrescine or spermidine in fatty foods at high temperature and in the presence of water (Karovičová and Kohajdová 2005).

5.3.5 Histamine, Gizzerosine, and Gizzard Erosion in Poultry

The toxicity effect of BAs, particularly histamine to chickens, is called gizzard erosion (GE) mainly characterized by decreases in feed efficiency and enlargement of the proventriculus resulting in decreased weight gain and feed consumption and chicken' mortality at severe cases. GE is also known as "black vomiting" due to the presence of black vomit in gizzards of affected chickens (Harry et al. 1975). The toxicity of histamine to chickens implicated with feeds containing high levels of BAs, particularly histamine, has been reported since 1970s. The other amines such as putrescine and cadaverine, which are elevated along with histamine in abused fish meal, were also known to induce clinical changes in gastric morphology of chickens and may potentiate the effects of histamine *in vivo* by inhibiting intestinal histamine-catabolizing enzymes (Köse 1993; Fairgrieve et al. 1994). Other factors including mycotoxins, adenovirus, feed starvation, and sulfur amino acid deficiency have been reported to cause GE chickens. In 1993, Japanese scientists isolated another GE-causing substance named as gizzerosine, which is 2-amino-9-(4-imidazolyl)-7-azanonanoic acid (Figure 5.3) that was formed by the reaction of histamine or histidine and lysine during overheating of brown fish meal (Köse 1993).

Although the role of BAs in GE has been questioned by some authors, several researchers proved that BAs, specifically histamine can cause GE in broiler chickens. Barnes et al. (2001) conducted two studies to determine the effects of histamine and cadaverine on broilers growth and the incidence of pathologies associated with

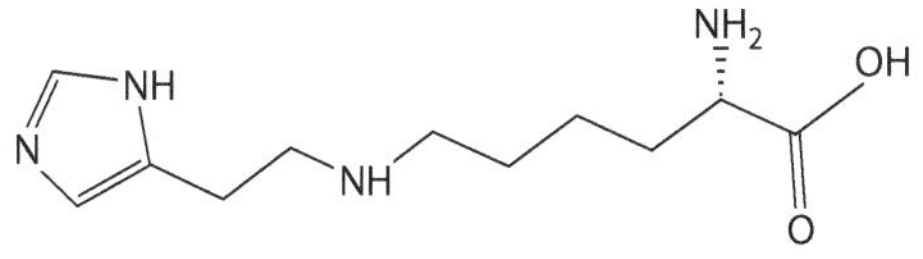

FIGURE 5.3 The structure of gizzerosine.

proventriculus. They observed that histamine at 1 and 2 g/kg or the combination of histamine and cadaverine (1 g/kg each) reduced body weight and feed conversion at 21 days of age. They also found that histamine and cadaverine increased the total number of incidence and severity of GE and proventriculus ulcers.

Limited studies exist on the toxicity effects of fish meals containing gizzerosine, histamine, or other BAs on other animals. Few studies reported inconclusive results of feeding trials on fish and shrimps (Fairgrieve et al. 1994; Opstvedt et al. 2000; Tapia-Salazar et al. 2001). Fairgrieve et al. (1994) carried out a feeding trial on rainbow trout with the supplementation of histamine (2 g/kg) and combination of putrescine and cadaverine (0.5 g/kg each). They reported no depressing effect on the feed intake, growth, or feed conversion and no signs of acute toxicity or mortality occurred in 16 weeks of study, although they observed stomach distension syndrome.

FAO-WHO (2013) reported that the toxicological responses of animals to histamine depend on the method of administration, and the toxicological effects differ among species. Oral administration of histamine, alone or together with spoiled tuna, produced emesis in pigs while an emetic response was also reported in dogs by Blonz and Olcott (1978). Intraduodenal injection of histamine produced only transient hypotension in dogs and cats, whereas a histamine-containing yeast extract produced a wider variety of effects in cats, including increased volume and acidity of stomach acid, increased hematocrit and limb volume, and enhanced electromyographic activity (FAO-WHO 2013). Feeding trials to test the toxicological effects of BAs and gizzerosine have long been forgotten since the late 2000s and the research on the GE of broilers usually directed to other causes (Opstvedt et al. 2000; Tapia-Salazar et al. 2001).

5.4 EPIDEMIOLOGY OF POISONING CAUSED BY BAs

Although food poisoning cases/outbreaks resulted by BAs occur worldwide, there is still a lack of complete reporting on this aspect. In some countries, this illness is not even notifiable yet because affected individuals do not always seek a medical attention and physicians can easily misdiagnose the cases. Many countries do not take enough effort to collect and disseminate information on incidents of this illness. Therefore, the true statistics on this disease are unknown.

The reported cases/outbreaks have been mainly done for HFP, previously known as "scombroid fish poisoning" due to its association with *Scombroid* fish species. HFP is common and occurs worldwide. Dalgaard et al. (2008) reported that HFP accounted for 32% of all seafood-borne incidents of human disease in England and

Wales during the 1990s and 38% of all seafood associated outbreaks in the United States. Only rare cases are reported for other BAs, such as tyramine in cheese. Epidemiological studies are usually carried out at developed countries, such as Japan, United States, and Britain. The disease was first described in 1799 in Britain and reemerged in the medical literature in the 1950s when outbreaks were reported in Japan. In the United States, the first cases were documented in 1968. Since then, cases have been described in a number of different settings, including restaurants, cafeterias, schools, army barracks, and medical conferences (Feng et al. 2016). The largest outbreak ever reported, involving 2656 people, was recorded in Japan in 1973 (Feng et al. 2016). In the United States, between 1988 and 1997, HFP was officially reported in 145 outbreaks involving 811 people from at least 20 states. Between 1998 and 2008, there were official reports of 333 outbreaks involving 1383 people, resulting in 59 hospitalizations (Feng et al. 2016). However, HFP cases are still known as underreported due to misdiagnosis and the inherent barriers in reporting cases to public health organizations. Recent data reported by CDC (2014) showed that 40 outbreaks occurred between 2009 and 2012, involving 136 people, resulting in one hospitalization (Feng et al. 2016). Other than United States, HFP is most frequently reported in Japan, New Zealand, and the Britain. From 1998 to 2008, 89 histamine fish poisoning incidents affecting 1577 individuals (with no deaths) were reported in Japan, giving an average of around 8 incidents with 150 patients every year. Among these incidents, the leftover food samples were analyzed for histamine and the concentrations were varied from below the detection limit to 1267 mg/100 g in samples, with 8% containing <100 mg/kg, and 12% <200 mg/kg (FAO-WHO 2013). Fletcher (2010) revised HFP data from 2000 to 2009 and reported 31 outbreaks mostly involving smoked fish, particularly smoked kahawai. Therefore, during this period there have been two major recalls for hot-smoked kahawai produced by the same company. Cases have also been documented in various other countries. Only one death has been recorded worldwide (Feng et al. 2016).

Diagnosing HFP is sometimes difficult since certain types of symptoms of this illness are also known to be characteristic of other foodborne diseases. Only the cutaneous symptoms, such as rash and urticaria, which do not occur in all cases, can be used to distinguish HFP from other foodborne intoxications. It is claimed that many doctors are unaware of the possible alternative diagnosis of HFP, which are often misidentified as food allergy (Köse 1993). Therefore, three possible ways to distinguished HFP from other food allergy incidents have been suggested as:

1. The lack of a previous history of allergic reactions to the incriminated food
2. The high attack rate in group outbreaks
3. The detection of high levels of histamine in the incriminated food

Suspected HFP cases must be confirmed by the authorities using effective surveillance methods that involve fast histamine analysis in the incriminated food. Most countries are lack of effective methods to confirm and report HFP cases. Table 5.5 shows some HFP incidents implicated with fish products reported for various countries since 2000.

TABLE 5.5
Type of Fish Involved in Histamine Fish Poisoning in Various Countries Since 2000

Species	Scientific Name	Country	Year	Number of Cases	Histamine Level (mg/kg)	References
Tuna		Senegal	2010	71	4900	FAO-WHO (2013)
Tuna		Scotland	2009	4		James et al. (2013)
Kingfish		New Zealand	2009	3		Fletcher (2010)
Fish cube	*Tetrapturus angustirostris*	Taiwan	2007	347	>400	Chen et al. (2010)
Fried fermented tuna		Thailand	2007	91	4460	FAO-WHO (2013)
Tuna		Israel	2005–2007	46		Lavon et al. (2008)
Tuna		USA	2006	11	>500	CDC (2007)
Dried milkfish	*Chanos chanos*	Taiwan	2006	3	616	Tsai et al. (2007b)
Tuna dumbling		Taiwan, China	2006	7	1608	Chen et al. (2008)
Marlin		Japan	2006	32		FAO-WHO (2013)
Smoked kahawai		New Zealand	2004	11		Fletcher (2010)
Yellowtail	*Seriola lalandi*	South Africa	2004	19		Auerswald et al. (2006)
Fried billfish	*Makaira nigricans*	Taiwan	2004	59	>1500	Tsai et al. (2007a)
Swordfish	*Xiphias gladius*	Taiwan	2004	43	859–2937	Chang et al. (2008)
Smoked kahawai		New Zealand	2003	25		Fletcher (2010)
Saury		Japan	2003	8	320	Miki et al. (2005)
Yellowfin Tuna	*Thunnus albacares*	Australia	2003	6	470–490	Hall (2003)
Escolar fish		USA	2003	42	2000–3800	Feldman et al. (2005)
Tuna		Scotland	2002	3		James et al. (2013)
Smoked kahawai		New Zealand	2002	20		Fletcher (2010)
Dried sardine		Japan	2002	1	1700	Kanki et al. (2004)
Tuna & Tuna steak		Scotland	2001	14		James et al. (2013)
Canned mackerel		Taiwan	2001	3	500–1539	Tsai et al. (2005)
Garfish	*Belone belone*	Denmark	2001	13	1000–2000	Dalgaard et al. (2006)

Source: Updated from Prester, L., *Food Addit. Contamm. Part A.* 28, 1547–1560, 2011.

The best surveillance programs and guidelines were reported for developed countries such as United States, United Kingdom, Japan, and New Zealand. Therefore, incidences are most commonly reported from these countries. The reports from such countries are usually confirmed through their efficient surveillance programs. The countries such as author's country lacking suitable reporting program for this purpose, usually rely on the affected victims' calling "Disease Report Centers" or reports by doctors who treated affected individuals. Therefore, such reports are unconfirmed results. Reports from scientists from different countries have also been published over the years. In such reports, histamine contents of incriminated products are commonly analyzed (Tsai et al. 2005; 2007a, 2007b). Centers for Disease Control and Prevention of United States gave a useful guideline on confirmation of foodborne-disease outbreaks including histamine poisoning (URL-1). According to the guideline, patients diagnosed with histamine fish poisoning have symptoms starting with 1 minute–3 hours; usually 1 hour with flushing, dizziness, burning of mouth and throat, headache, gastrointestinal symptoms, urticaria, and generalized pruritus. The pharmacological effects and common symptoms of food poisoning caused by different BAs are shown in Table.5.4.

5.5 REGULATORY ISSUES

A hazardous level of histamine for human health has been suggested as 500 mg/kg, although low levels as 50 mg/kg have been reported in histamine poisoning (Köse 2010; FDA 2011). Based on the reported cases, Shalaby (1996) suggested guideline levels for histamine content of fish as regard to health hazard as follows: (i) <50 mg/kg (safe for consumption), (ii) 50–200 mg/kg (possibly toxic), (iii) 200–1000 mg/kg (probably toxic), (iv) >1000 mg/kg (toxic and unsafe for human consumption). However, in most cases, histamine levels with implicated fish have been above 200 mg/kg, often above 500 mg/kg (Lehane and Olley 2000; Hungerford 2010). The reasons of the variability in dose–response for histamine toxicity are explained in above sections. Except for tyramine, currently no recommendations about the levels of other BAs in humans have been suggested. For adults, values of 100–800 mg/kg for dietary tyramine and 30 mg/kg for dietary phenylethylamine have been reported as toxic doses in foods. However, in individuals using MAOI drugs, the ingestion of 60 mg/kg of dietary tyramine can cause migraine, whereas 100–250 mg/kg will produce a hypertensive crisis (Silla Santos 1996).

In early reports, upper limits of 100 mg histamine/kg in foods, 2 mg histamine/L in alcoholic beverages, and 100–800 mg/kg tyramine and 30 mg/kg β-phenylethylamine in foods have been suggested (Halász et al. 1994). Currently, regulation of BAs is usually set for histamine in fish and fish products and rarely in other foods. The contents of tyramine in cheese and beverages and NAs in foods are also regulated in various countries.

The European Union Directive (EC 2007: Directive No: 1441/2007) regulated histamine in fish belonging to the following families: *Scombridae*, *Clupeidae*, *Engraulidae*, *Coryfenidae* (Coryphaenidae), and *Pomatomidae*, *Scombresosidae*. According to the regulation, nine samples must be taken from each batch of fish species, and these must fulfill the following requirements:

- The mean value must not exceed 100 mg/kg
- Two samples may have a value of more than 100 mg/kg but less than 200 mg/kg
- No sample may have a value exceeding 200 mg/kg

However, the EU regulations stipulated higher critical levels of histamine or "the fishery products which have undergone enzyme maturation treatment in brine and manufactured from fish species associated with a high amount of histidine" (EC 2007). According to the regulation,

- Two samples may have a value of more than 20 mg/100 g but less than 40 mg/100 g
- No sample may have a value exceeding 40 mg/100 g

Histamine is generally not uniformly distributed in decomposed solid foods such as fish, meat, and cheeses. For this reason, FDA (2011) claims that if 50 mg/kg is found in one section of fish, it means that it is possible for other sections to exceed 500 mg/kg, which is considered as the toxic level to human. Therefore, FDA set the stricter acceptable histamine value for fish species (specified under FDA guidelines) based on data collected from numerous outbreaks. The upper allowable limit for histamine is stated as 50 mg/kg for fish and fish products (FDA 2011). Nutritional Codex of the Slovak Republic determined the maximal tolerable limit for histamine in beer and fish as 20 and 200 mg/kg, respectively, and for tyramine in cheese as 200 mg/kg. The Netherlands Institute of Dairy Research and the Czech Republic recommended the upper limit for histamine as 100–200 mg/kg in meat products (Karovičová and Kohajdová 2005).

The legislation of certain countries allows the rejections of wines with histamine content higher than legal limits. The upper limits for histamine in wine in some European countries are 2 mg/L histamine for Germany, 3 mg/L for Holland, 5 mg/L for Finland, 5–6 mg/L for Belgium, 8 mg/L for France, and 10 mg/L for Switzerland and Austria (Russo et al. 2010). Codex standards for fish sauce requires below 400 mg histamine/kg of fish sauce in any sample unit tested (FAO-WHO 2013). The Canadian Fish Inspection Agency set up the maximum limit for histamine in fish sauce at 200 mg/L, whereas the FDA set it at 500 mg/L (Brillantes and Samosorn 2001).

Since histamine and tyramine intolerance has become an increasing problem over the last few decades, the food industry has investigated producing foods with histamine and tyramine levels as low as possible (Bodmer et al. 1999). Due to high toxicity effect of these compounds to the susceptible people such as ones taking medical treatment, it would be of great interest to certify some fish such as hake as histamine free or low histamine (Baixas-Nogueras et al. 2001).

Although no regulations were set for histamine in fish meal for animal consumption, fish meal containing low histamine below 500 mg/kg is accepted as high-quality product by the traders and is paid over 25% per ton than the common low-quality products containing histamine over 1000 mg/kg (Pers. Comm. with fish meal producers in Turkish Black Sea Region).

Using nitrite or nitrate is usually reported for meat rather than fish products. Therefore, health risk usually expected for meat products. The United States has set 10 μg/kg NPYR as the maximum allowable limit in bacon (Al Bulushi et al. 2009) while not many countries including the EU regulations set regulations for NAs originated from food (Köse 2010). Estonian government has maximum permitted concentration of the sum of two NAs (NDMA and NDEA) in fresh and smoked fish as 3 μg/kg (Yurchenko and Mölder 2006). The EU regulations relate to the release of the *N*-nitrosamines and *N*-nitrosatable substances from elastomer or rubber teats and soothers (EU 1993). However, as nitrite is necessary in the chemical pathway of NA formation, the regulating bodies are more concerned in controlling the amount of nitrite added to food during processing. For example, the US government allows 100–200 mg/kg nitrite for vacuum-packed (VP) cold smoked fish while EU does not allow nitrite in food products (FDA 2011).

5.6 BA CONTENTS OF FOODS

5.6.1 Raw Fish

5.6.1.1 Introduction

In nonfermented foods, the presence of BAs above a certain level is considered as indicative of undesired microbial activity. Therefore, the amine level could be used as an indicator of microbial spoilage. However, as stated by Silla Santos (1996), the presence of BAs in food does not necessarily correlate with the growth of spoilage organisms because they are not all decarboxylase positive. Levels of histamine, putrescine, and cadaverine usually increase during spoilage of fish and meat, whereas levels of spermine and spermidine decrease during this process.

In this section, the term "raw fish" was used as "fresh fish" to avoid misunderstanding of the word "fresh" for unprocessed food and "fresh" for quality (i.e., recently harvested and/in good quality). Therefore, we preferred the term "raw fish" meaning it is marketing without processing or raw material prior to processing.

Formation of BAs in raw fish kept at chilled or frozen conditions is limited since these conditions retard bacterial growth and enzymatic activity. Therefore, most past studies recorded very low levels for very fresh fish, whereas high contents of BAs detected for spoiled fish (Prester 2011; FAO-WHO 2013). In fact, the history of histamine poisoning outbreaks/cases is often linked to fish kept at TT abused conditions (Hungerford 2010; Köse 2010). Studies with different fish species containing high-precursor amino acids further demonstrated that fish kept at warm temperatures at long period of time would result in high contents of BAs (Table 5.4).

5.6.1.2 Histidine-Rich Fish

Histidine decarboxylating bacteria can be part of the natural microflora in the skin, gills, and gut of a freshly caught fish (FAO-WHO 2013). The bacterial action could start after harvesting fish usually at its postmortem stage. These bacteria can multiply rapidly at the suitable temperature conditions and form histamine even before postmortem proteolysis occurs. Therefore, histamine can reach high levels before the formation of organoleptic spoilage indicators. Once bacterial multiplication has occurred and histidine decarboxylases are produced, enzyme activity can continue slowly at refrigeration temperatures, even after bacterial growth has ceased. Histamine formation at chilled conditions is also expected at longer storage period, although cold storage is one of the preventive measures for controlling BA formation in foods.

About 20 fish families covering over 100 fish species are reported to present health risk for HFP (Table 5.1). These fish species contain high levels of free histidine ranging from 2600 to 25070 mg/kg. Some species were included in this group not on the basis of free histidine content but rather on reported illnesses of histamine intoxication. The free histidine levels of *Salmonidae* family have been reported as in the range from 70 to 2362 mg/kg. However, species only under six families were regulated by the EU and Codex, namely, *Scombridae*, *Clupeidae*, *Engraulidae*, *Coryphaenidae*, *Pomatomidae*, and *Scomberesocidae*. Other fish and marine/freshwater species may allow the formation of other unsafe BAs such as cadaverine and putrescine (FAO-WHO 2013).

The contents of BAs in fisheries raw material are of concern due to health hazard described above and monitoring the levels, particularly histamine is necessary to be included in hazard analysis and critical control points (HACCP) plan of any seafood processing plant. Low histamine levels usually are targeted at the raw material stage before processing and/or during fresh storage because the amount is likely to increase to unsafe levels with time. Hundreds of studies reported different levels of BAs for many types of freshwater and marine fish and other seafood, particularly for the species listed as unsafe species for histamine health risk since 1980s (FAO-WHO 2013). It was identified that the percentage of histamine over safety risk of 100 mg/kg is low for fresh fish while high percentage falls into levels even over 500 mg/kg for fermented or spoiled fish samples (FAO-WHO 2013).

Prester (2011) reported that most studies with histidine-rich fishes followed similar trend of histamine accumulation during storage (Table 5.3). Some of the work carried out at author's laboratory also supported these findings (Koral and Köse 2012, 2015). It was reported that after 12 hours at 22°C, histamine contents in sardines and mackerel reached a level of 50 mg/kg, thus they were considered unfit for humans (Prester 2011). According to author's experience, marine captured fishes usually reached to market within 1 to 12 hours depending on the different factors such as distance from the market and loading capacity, etc. Therefore, controlling BA formation, particularly at chilled storage, is very important. Histamine health risk is often reported due to fish kept at abused temperatures. The toxic histamine levels (>500 mg/kg) were reported for anchovy, sardines and mackerel stored at 20°C–25°C, and for mahi-mahi at 32°C within 24 hours (Baranowski et al. 1990; Rossano et al. 2006; Prester et al. 2009; Prester 2011).

The most common BAs reported in raw seafood are histamine, putrescine, cadaverine, tyramine, spermine, and spermidine. These amines are commonly reported for fish species such as anchovy, bonito, mackerel, herring, tuna, sardines. The formation of other BAs in decomposed histidine-rich species has been reported as considerably lower than histamine value at similar conditions (Prester 2011). Therefore, quantification of several other BAs correlated with fish decomposition is recommended (Prester 2011). For this reason, several studies tried to link different BA levels with the spoilage of fish species (Mietz and Karmas 1977; Veciana-Nogués et al. 1997; Özogul and Özogul 2006). Two different BA indexes were reported as Quality Index (QI) and the Biogenic Amine Index (BAI) with the following formulae:

$$QI = (\text{histamine} + \text{putrescine} + \text{cadaverine})/(1 + \text{spermidine} + \text{spermine})$$

$$BAI = (\text{histamine} + \text{putrescine} + \text{cadaverine} + \text{tyramine})$$

It was reported that BAI correlates well with the organoleptic quality of tuna and sardines (Veciana-Nogués et al. 1997; Özogul and Özogul 2006). However, different studies suggested different levels of BAI for different fishes at certain conditions (Veciana-Nogués et al. 1997; Özogul and Özogul 2006; Koral and Köse 2012, 2015). Moreover, past studies also proved that the levels of amines used in the formulae can vary in great extend depending on several factors (Köse 2010; Prester 2011). Therefore, usefulness of these indexes in terms of estimating fish spoilage is rather questionable. The type and amount of bacteria with decarboxylating amine activity present in different batches of fish with the same species potentially lead to different amount of amines at varying levels. However, certain storage conditions that suppress bacterial activity may help to stabilize or limit the unfavor of amine formation. Recent studies carried out at the author's laboratory demonstrated that anchovy, Atlantic bonito, and shad with unsafe histamine levels that were stored at different chilling conditions were already scored unfit for human consumption by the sensory panelists (Koral and Köse 2012, 2015). The values of other BAs in these samples were detected as lower than 100 mg/kg with some exceptions (Koral and Köse 2012, 2015). Although these findings might suggest that sensory evaluation of chilled fish might help to avoid BAs in these fish species, more studies at the same conditions with different batches are needed to draw a conclusion. Interestingly, Koral and Köse (2012) reported about 163 mg/kg spermidine in fresh bonito but decreased during the chilled storage.

5.6.1.3 Histidine-Poor Fish

Several studies demonstrated that histamine formation in white-muscle fish was far below the legal limits set for fish species by FDA and EU. In fact, so far no report exists for histamine poisoning implicated with the consumption of histidine-poor fish (Baixas-Nogueras et al. 2005; Prester 2011). Putrescine and cadaverine were the main amines formed in histidine-poor fish such as hake and trout. Therefore, these amines were mainly used as an indicator of quality of histidine-poor fish (Prester 2011).

Low levels of histamine formation were usually reported for cephalopods, crustaceans, and shellfish. However, high values of other BAs such as putrescine, cadaverine, and tyramine were reported for these species. Hu et al. (2012) demonstrated that putrescine, cadaverine, and tyramine levels increase during storage both at ambient and refrigerated storage although low amounts in the fresh samples. Agmatine has been proposed as a freshness indicator for cuttlefish (*Sepia officinalis*) and for some other squid species stored in ice (Zhao et al. 2007; Prester 2011). Although the possible role of agmatine in intoxication caused by BAs is uncertain, it is reported that it may act as a potentiator in toxicity of other BAs such as histamine and tyramine (Halász et al. 1994). There are few data about BA level in other cephalopods (Prester 2011). The presence of other BAs such as cadaverine and putrescine in *Crustacea* also was reported as their use to identify their decomposition. Among these amines, putrescine was suggested as the best indicator of decomposition for penaeid shrimp and Norway lobster (*Nephrops norvegicus*) stored at a wide range of temperatures while cadaverine production followed a pattern similar to that of putrescine in several species of *Crustacea* (Zhao et al. 2007; Prester 2011). Prester (2011) reported that histamine and tyramine contents have not been detected at any stage of Norway lobster storage. Therefore, the species of *Crustacea* have been suggested as a suitable food for people requiring for histamine-restricted diet. Various studies also reported lower amounts of histamine and tyramine in bivalves than fish species (Prester 2011). However, overall polyamine levels in some bivalve molluscs have been reported as relatively high (4300 mg/kg), which is important due to their role in health and diseases. A large variation was observed in the amine levels of various bivalve species as 150 mg/kg for putrescine and 65 mg/kg for spermidine and 80 mg/kg for cadaverine (Prester 2011).

5.6.2 Fruits and Vegetables

Halász et al. (1994) reported different factors associated with the accumulation of some BAs in plants. Agmatine and putrescine formation in plants are linked to the conditions of potassium and magnesium deficiency and high ammonium concentrations. Considerable variations in estimated amine content is also known to associate with different degrees of maturity of plants, so very different amine concentrations have been published for the same type of fruits. High amine levels have been reported for orange juice (noradrenaline, tryptamine), tomato fruit (tyramine, tryptamine and histamine), banana fruit (tyramine, noradrenaline, tryptamine, and serotonin), plum fruit (tyramine, noradrenaline), and spinach leaves (histamine) (Halász et al. 1994). It is reported that phenethylamine in chocolate is derived from the roasted cocoa bean, and its concentration in the final product varies considerably. High levels of phenylethylamine have also been reported for certain species of mushrooms. Histamine and cadaverine have been detected in carrageenan from algae (Silla Santos 1996). Reports on the hygienic status of leafy vegetables indicate the association of high microbial numbers and the presence of BA, both with the fresh and packed products. Number of the dominant groups was recorded as *Pseudomonadaceae* and *Enterobacteriaceae* (Halász et al. 1994).

5.6.3 Fresh Meat

Fresh and processed pork meat contains high levels of adrenaline, spermidine, and spermine but low levels of noradrenaline, putrescine, histamine, cadaverine, and tyramine. In cooked and uncooked ground beef and in pork meat, various BAs have been identified. Large amounts of cadaverine present in beef have been associated with heavy contamination by *Enterobacteriaceae* (Halász et al. 1994; Karovičová and Kohajdová 2005).

The most prevalent BAs in meat and meat products are tyramine, cadaverine, putrescine, and also histamine. The only amines present at significant levels in fresh meat are spermidine and spermine. High spermine contents, usually between 20 and 60 mg/kg, are usual in meat and meat products of warm-blooded animals. Spermidine levels in meat rarely exceed 10 mg/kg (Ruiz-Capillas and Jiménez-Colmenero 2004). Therefore, an opposite relation between spermidine and spermine contents is typical for foods of animal origin as compared with plant products. Some amines such as tyramine, putrescine, and cadaverine can be formed during storage of meat. As tyramine concentrations in stored beef were found the highest on the meat surface, it can be reduced effectively by washing (Stadnik and Dolatowski 2010). Prolong storage even at chilled conditions increased some amine levels, particularly spermidine and tyramine and cadaverine for products in VPs (Ruiz-Capillas and Jiménez-Colmenero 2004; Stadnik and Dolatowski 2010).

5.6.4 Processed Foods

5.6.4.1 Introduction

Some HFB are reported to be halotolerant or halophilic. However, efficient dry salting processes for various food products such as salted fish are unlikely to allow such bacteria to grow due to low a_w values (Köse 2010). The a_w and salt contents of most dry salted commercial, home-made, and laboratory made dry salted fish products have been reported as under 0.77% and 15% water phase salt (WPS), respectively, at both ambient and refrigerated conditions (Koral et al. 2013). Such conditions are effective enough to prevent BA formation and bacteria growth at both room and cold temperatures during maturation and subsequent storage conditions (Köse 2010). It is reported that some HFB can still be isolated from both salted and brined fish products (Köse 2010). Therefore, care should be taken after desalting. Veciana-Nogues et al. (1997) pointed out that formation of BAs can sharply increase in salted products during desalting period and packing in oil as applied in Spain. High levels of BAs can be obtained in commercial dry salted or brined fish products. The main reason is closely linked to previously formed BAs and/or decarboxylating enzymes in the poor quality raw material. According to author's observations, it is a common habit that retail processors usually process their fish using dry salting or brining if they cannot sell their fresh fish within the same day although currently some started to freeze fish for the retail display at the following days. The past studies at author's laboratory also demonstrated that maturing brined fish products at room temperature present health risk for histamine and/or other BAs such as cadaverine, putrescine, and tyramine if brining is carried out at <25% salt concentrations (Koral et al. 2013; Köse et al. 2015). High levels of histamine and other BAs are reported for brined fish products kept at elevated temperatures. Therefore, unless heavily salted brine (25%<) is used, cold storage conditions are advised for maturing and storage (Köse 2010). Although cold storage and brine (salt) together have been reported to be very effective for controlling histamine formation in fish products, such prevention is only effective until certain period of time. Usually, products are safe within the sensory shelf life especially for small-sized fish such as anchovies (Köse et al. 2015).

The studies with other salted food types also proved the effect of salt concentration on the BA formation, and low levels usually obtained with products salted in high concentrations (Chong et al. 2011). *Enterobacteriaceae* is often reported as responsible for the histidine decarboxylase activity to produce histamine (Bover-Cid et al. 2009). In salt-fermented soybean paste, higher salt content (12%) had the lower BA levels compared to lower salt condition (6% and 8% salt) (Kim et al. 2005). Various studies also found the high salt content can control the BA formation in different salted foods such as Feta cheese (Bover-Cid et al. 2009; Chong et al. 2011).

5.6.4.2 Marinated Products

Previous studies reported low levels of histamine and other BAs in different types of commercial marinated fish products kept at cold storage conditions (0°C–4°C) with some exceptions (Köse et al. 2012). However, high levels of BAs, particularly histamine, have been detected in marinated fish products matured and stored at ambient temperatures (Gökoğlu 2003). It is advised to use lightly salted raw material to obtain a good quality product in the case of marinades prepared from presalted raw material. In such conditions, elevated temperatures can allow histamine formation during long maturation and/or storage period (Köse 2010). Gökoğlu (2003) demonstrated that BAs, particularly histamine levels in two different marinated sardine reached to unsafe levels within a day during maturation at ambient temperature (25 ± 2°C).

5.6.4.3 Smoked and Dried Products

Past literature reported high contents of histamine in various smoked fish products that exceeds either the FDA or EU-permitted levels (Lehane and Olley 2000; Köse et al. 2012; Koral et al. 2013). However, hot smoking is a safe method in prevention of BA formation due to high heat practically sterilizes the product and denatures enzymes, imparting some degree of preservation but does not destroy histamine already formed (Lehane and Olley 2000). Therefore, high BA levels in smoked fish are usually associated with poor handling and TT abuse of raw material. Since hot smoked fish products are known to contain lower amount of salt than cold smoked fish and other salted fish products, recontamination with bacteria and storage at elevated temperature conditions may allow BA formation. Emborg et al. (2005) reported high histamine concentration of >7000 mg in VP tuna, which caused histamine fish poisoning, and they linked high concentration with the growth of psychrotolerant *M. morganii*-like bacteria or with *Photobacterium phosphoreum* in VP fish. A number of the HFB are facultative anaerobes that can grow in reduced oxygen environments (Tsai et al. 2007b; Mah and Hwang 2009).

Some drying methods also include salting prior to drying. As in the salting method, decreasing a_w is the same preserving factor for dried fish products as well as for other dried foods. Since low a_w values directly affect bacterial activities, these products present low health risk for BAs. However, previously formed histamine or other BAs in raw material may lead to high amounts in the dried portions that explain the involvement of HFP with dried fish products reported by earlier publications with high histamine values found in the meals of affected people (Table 5.5; Tsai et al. 2007b).

5.6.4.4 Canned Fish Products

High heat process in canning kills bacteria and destroys the enzymes but not able to destroy high levels of histamine, which is a heat-resistant compound (Köse 1993). Moreover, canned products properly sealed do not allow bacterial contamination unless defects occur in sealing such as impacts during transportation. Therefore, low levels of BAs are expected in canned fish products or other foods providing that BAs in raw materials were also low amount prior to packing and processing. Recent studies also supported this fact that low amount of BAs was reported for good quality canned fish products (Prester 2011). However, high levels of histamine up to 520 mg/kg were detected in many canned fish samples in Korea, Mexico, and Brazil, indicating the bad handling and storage of raw materials used in canning. In Taiwan, the percentage of unacceptable canned fish samples was 4.2% (Tsai et al. 2005; Prester 2011). It was also pointed out that histamine accumulation often occurs after frozen histidine-rich fish are thawed and kept for long periods at room temperature before further processing (Tsai et al. 2005; Prester 2011). Karovičová and Kohajdová (2005) pointed out that the quantification of histamine in canned products indicates the thermostability of the molecule. Odors that normally signal decomposition to the organoleptic analyst may be modified, reduced, or eliminated by thermal processing; therefore, histamine is a useful indicator of decomposition in some canned fish products.

5.6.4.5 BAs in Packed Seafood

The inclusion of carbon dioxide (CO_2) may inhibit the growth and increase the lag phase of microorganism with amino acid decarboxylase. Various studies reporting the successful inhibition of BAs using MAP in fish and chicken meat and found better inhibitory effect compared to VP (Chong et al. 2011). Emborg et al. (2005) reported that histamine achieved toxic level in chilled VP tuna steaks at 2°C but MAP with 40% CO_2/60% O_2 was reported to inhibit the histamine formation. The effect of MAP on retarding the production of BAs was studied with MAP for different fresh fish, such as sardine, herring, garfish, and hake. Gallas et al. (2010) also showed that the higher oxygen (75% O_2, 25% CO_2) had significant lower BA concentration in chicken meat compared to MAP of 75% N_2 and 25% CO_2. Recently, chitosan film packaging was found to have the best histamine inhibitory effect in Atlantic bonito fillet followed by MAP, VP, and cling film packaging (Alak et al. 2011).

5.6.5 BA Contents in Fermented Foods

5.6.5.1 Introduction

Using various microbial strains, fermentation conditions, such as different microorganisms, substrates, temperature, time of fermentation and chemical engineering achievements, enable us to manufacture hundreds of types of dairy/cheeses, fermented milk products), vegetables (sauerkraut, pickles, olives), meat and fish products (e.g., fermented sausages and fish sauce), alcoholic beverages (wine, beer, cider), bread, and vinegar and other food acids. Despite the wide variety of these products, tastes, and textures, in the majority of the cases, only two types of fermentations are used: lactic acid and ethanolic fermentation. The function of both is to change conditions, so unwanted spoiling or pathogenic microorganisms would not grow and alter the food. The main reason for higher amount of BAs in fermented foods was explained as the presence of nonprotein nitrogen fraction FAAs, the main precursors of BAs, which increases during fermentation. The FAA concentration in fermented products depends on the activity of endogenous enzymes, which is in turn favored by the denaturation of proteins as a consequence of acidity increase, dehydration, and action of NaCl (Suzzi and Gardini 2003). Temperature is one of the other factors significantly affect BA formation. Ercan et al. (2013) reported that fermentation processes usually between 7°C and 28°C generally increase BA formation. In addition, the microorganisms responsible for the fermentation process may contribute to the accumulation of BAs (Stadnik and Dolatowski 2010; Latorre-Moratalla et al. 2014). However, the concentration of BAs may vary in fermented products with comparable microbial flora, indicating that the complex interaction of factors is involved in their production. Moreover, the differences in the amount of the precursor amino acids in the foods can lead to the variation for the concentrations and types of BAs in fermented products. Processing method is also an important factor in such variation in the amine levels since certain processing conditions such as drying, cooking, and application of salt and/or other additives can either suppress or favor microbial and enzyme activity in the fermentation or ripening process of these products. Therefore, BA contents of fermented food products are discussed under different food types considering the similar effects on BA formation.

5.6.5.2 BA Contents of Fermented Meat Products

Staphylococci are strongly related to proteolytic processes during meat fermentation, although most LAB, mainly lactobacilli, have also shown a proteolytic or amino peptidase activity on meat proteins to obtain essential FAAs. In fact, species of lactobacilli prevalent in dry fermented sausages, such as *Lactobacillus sakei* or *L. curvatus*, have been implicated in the hydrolysis of meat proteins and the generation of FAAs. At the same time, some of these microorganisms use the FAAs as substrates for further metabolic reactions (deamination, dehydrogenation, and transamination), many of which are related to the development of aromas and flavors characterizing fermented and ripened meat products. However, unlike the above reactions, microbial decarboxylation of certain FAA results in the undesired formation of BAs. Aminogenesis in dry fermented sausages is a strain-dependent enzymatic activity of technological fermentative microbiota but also undesired contaminant microorganisms. Therefore, dry fermented sausages gather all requirements for BA accumulation, the presence of microorganisms, availability of FFA precursors, and the favorable environmental conditions for bacterial growth and decarboxylase activity (Latorre-Moratalla et al. 2014).

The most prevalent BAs in meat and meat products are reported as tyramine, cadaverine, putrescine, and histamine (Jairath et al. 2015). The contents of these amines tend to vary depending on the different product types, but Fermented Meat Products (FMPs) constitute considerably higher amount of BAs (Ruiz-Capillas and Jiménez-Colmenero 2004; Stadnik and Dolatowski 2010). Low levels of BAs were also reported by various authors for different FMPs, such as 17 mg/kg tryptamine in salami and 2.6, 0.9, 9.6 mg/kg putrescine, tyramine, and spermine in fermented pepperoni sausages (Kim et al. 2005). However, very high levels up to 1000 mg/kg were detected in many commercial FMPs around the world (Ruiz-Capillas and Jiménez-Colmenero 2004). Recently, Papavergou et al. (2012) surveyed BA levels of FMPs in Greek retail market and found that the concentration of tyramine, putrescine, histamine, and cadaverine was in the range of 0–510, 0–505, 0–515, and 0–690 mg/kg, respectively. Eerola et al. (1998) reported histamine, tyramine, putrescine, and cadaverine levels up to 200, 320, 580, 790 mg/kg in Finnish dry sausages. Therefore, these amines were commonly used as the estimation of meat quality, and various BAI formulae were suggested by various researchers. Cadaverine and putrescine were the most commonly used in these indexes for various FMPs. Histamine and tyramine were also included in some of the formulae applied to different products such as hamburger and dry sausages (Ruiz-Capillas and Jiménez-Colmenero 2004).

Amine content and profiles in FMPs may vary depending on various extrinsic and intrinsic factors during the manufacturing process, such as pH, redox potential, temperature, NaCl. The hygienic quality of raw materials is known as one of the extrinsic factors affecting BA concentration. However, the same raw material can lead to very different amine levels in final products depending on the presence of decarboxylating microorganisms, either derived from environmental contamination or from starter cultures, and the conditions supporting their growth and activity. Among the extrinsic factors, storage conditions were commonly studied for amine formation in FMPs, and past research concluded that amine levels in meat products were affected by the storage conditions and while cooking did not affect the concentrations with the exception of spermine, spermine levels decreased during heat treatment. The possible bacterial sources of putrescine and cadaverine in chill-stored VP beef were studied. The studies showed that putrescine and cadaverine contents increased during storage, whereas spermidine and spermine contents decreased (Halász et al. 1994). This phenomenon was attributed to the differences in the reaction rates of amine synthesis and amine deamination. Putrescine, cadaverine, spermidine, and spermine levels changed less during storage at −20°C than at 5°C. Several trials have been conducted in an attempt to determine whether levels of particular amines in certain foods can be correlated with bacterial counts (Halász et al. 1994). Some studies reported decarboxylating activity of LAB in various fermented foods including meat products. *Carnobacterium divergens* was found responsible for tyramine formation in VP meat, the formation of putrescine and cadaverine was caused by *Enterobacteriaceae* or strains of *Pseudomonas* spp. (Halász et al. 1994).

The contents of some BAs were used for the estimation of bacterial quality of different foods such as meat, cheese, and wine. For ground beef, putrescine was suggested as a potential for use as a bacterial index. Certain correlation levels were also linked BAs to bacteria counts, such as putrescine with the total aerobic counts, cadaverine with coliform counts. *Pseudomonas* strains that are known to be the dominant microorganisms in chilled meats mainly produce putrescine, whereas strains of *Enterobacteriaceae* preferentially form cadaverine (Halász et al. 1994). It was reported that the occurrence of BAs in fermented sausages may originate from contaminated raw material or from the fermentation process itself.

5.6.5.3 BA Contents of Fermented Fish

Numerous FFPs exist in the world, and the most commonly used types originate from SE Asia. Traditionally, the term "fermented fish" covers both enzyme-hydrolyzed and microbial FFPs; however, a clear distinction has not been made between these products (Köse 2010). Most FFPs also involve salting and occasionally smoking, marinating, and drying. FFPs can be grouped under three categories:

1. Products usually prepared from whole fish with the addition of salt to reduce a_w to prevent microbial spoilage (e.g., fish paste and fish sauce). The enzymes for the fermentation process come partly from the fish digestive system and partly from the bacteria that are naturally present in the fish and salt.
2. Products prepared with different forms of fish with the addition of carbohydrates as substrate and salt. Fermentation is carried out by naturally occurring microorganisms.
3. Products similar to second type except that starter cultures are added for fermentation.

It was reported that the fermentation process of fish may fulfill the conditions required for abundant formation of BAs, such as availability of FAAs, presence of decarboxylase-positive microorganisms, and the conditions allowing bacterial growth, which are decarboxylase synthesis and decarboxylase activity (Köse 2010). Very high histamine levels have been reported for FFPs, particularly Asian origin. The highest amounts were recorded for fish sauces of different varieties, such as 200–600 mg/L in Thai fish sauce, 430 mg/L in *nampla*, 1380 mg/L in Korean anchovy sauce (Brillantes and Samosorn 2001). Recent studies also identified high levels of histamine in fish sauce. In Japan, Kuda et al. (2012) reported very high values of histamine for fish sauce *nukazuke* from sardine as 383–1172 mg/L histamine, from mackerel as 408 mg/L, although low values were also determined for the same type of products from different companies indicating high variation in the factors influencing BA formation in this type of products. Fish paste is another type of FFPs, although it is sometimes included in other salted fish product group by different publications. High levels of histamine and other BAs were also observed for this product by different studies. Ten fish paste products originated from Turkey and EU countries were analyzed at the author's laboratory for BAs (Köse et al. 2012). Only three samples contained unacceptable levels of histamine, the highest amount accounted as 1544 mg/kg for the anchovy fish paste sample originated from Greece, whereas 166 and 192 mg/kg histamine were found for samples from Turkey made from anchovy and sardine. Low values for other fish paste products were below 5 mg/kg, with the exception of one sample from Italy. Due to the EU restrictions, such products are usually produced and stored at cold storage conditions in the EU countries.

Although few food poisoning outbreaks have been attributed to FFPs, high levels of histamine and other BAs have been detected by several researchers suggesting that cases were left unreported (Köse 2010). Other possible reason may be that some of these products, especially fish sauce, are consumed in small amounts as an ingredient with/or side dish along with other dishes that is likely to reduce the risk. Therefore, the permitted level for FFPs is higher for various authorities compared to nonfermented fish (EC 2005).

Different bacteria species were isolated from FFPs such as LAB, yeasts, and *Enterobacteriaceae*. Some of the bacteria are identified as fermentative bacteria often used as starter cultures. Therefore, this situation creates a major problem in preventing BA formation in these products. The other important factor is the temperature used for fermentation. Many processing techniques used in FFPs involve ambient conditions. Due to difficulty in preventing histamine formation in most SE Asian FFPs, especially in fish sauce, several studies concentrated on decreasing histamine levels using inhibition effect of additives or using other degradative compounds such as enzymes (Tapingkae et al. 2010; Köse 2010).

5.6.5.4 BA Contents of Cheese

Cheese is a traditional fermented food product and different varieties are known around the world, many are specific to a certain region due to traditional processing methods and specific strains of microorganisms involving in the ripening period. Montel et al. (2014) reported that more than 400 microorganisms including LAB, yeasts, and molds have been detected in raw milk. This biodiversity decreases in cheese cores, where a small number of LAB species become dominant and persists on the cheese surfaces. Diversity between cheeses is due to particularly to wide variations in the dynamics of the same microbial species in different cheeses.

Although fresh milk normally contains very low levels of histamine (<0.3 mg/kg), commercially available pasteurized or ultra high temperature (UHT) treated milk already shows slightly higher histamine content. Upon fermentation of milk, a considerable increase of histamine content often occurs, leading to contents of up to 7 mg/kg histamine in sour cream and even slightly higher levels in yogurt. Finally, in cheese production a rather drastic increase of histamine content often occurs, leading to maximum histamine levels up to 2500 mg/kg in aged cheese (Bodmer et al. 1999). However, although high levels of BAs, particularly histamine and tyramine, were reported for different types of cheeses, low values were also recorded. Large amounts of BAs in cheese could indicate a failure, from a hygienic point of view, in the milk used for cheese products or during the cheese making (Karovičová and Kohajdová 2005; Spizzirri et al. 2013).

Halász et al. (1994) reported that increases in the BA contents of cheeses may be due to the decarboxylating activity of various microorganisms found among starter LAB species, nonstarter LAB, and/or other spontaneous microflora. However, it is difficult to find a straight correlation between microbial counts and BA content in cheese, because amine-producing abilities of different strains of various bacteria differ widely (Spizzirri et al. 2013). Moreover, several extrinsic processing factors may also play an important role in BA formation. These are pasteurization of milk, pH, salt-in-moisture levels (WPS), and ripening temperature. The pH of cheese is reported between 5.0 and 6.5, which is optimum for the activity of most decarboxylases. Moreover, formation of BAs is further accelerated by high temperatures during production cheese and by the prolonged ripening (Gardini et al. 2012; Spizzirri et al. 2013).

5.6.5.5 BA Contents of Alcoholic and Nonalcoholic Beverages

Since alcohol is an inhibitor of MAOs, the control of BAs in fermented beverages is considerably important for consumer's health. BAs in wine could also cause commercial import and export difficulties. Karovičová and Kohajdová (2005) reported three possible origins for BAs in wines. They can be present in the must, can be formed by yeasts during malolactic fermentation, or result from the action of bacteria involved in malolactic fermentation. The maceration of grape skins during vinification promotes extraction of grape components such as phenolic compounds, protein, amino acids, and polysaccharides. Grape skin maceration practices commonly applied during red wine production include cold maceration. Pectolytic enzymes are often added to grape must to increase the yield of juice, clarify the must, extract compounds from the grape skins, and facilitate pressing and filtration. Carbonic maceration and thermovinification are less conventional grape skin extraction methods that can be applied during winemaking (Smit et al. 2013).

Many different BAs in various amounts and compositions have been identified in beer and wine. The most detected BAs in wine have been reported as histamine, tyramine, putrescine, isopentylamine, and phenylethylamine (Bodmer et al. 1999). Putrescine, cadaverine, and tyramine are the most representative BAs in beer. Although histamine contents of fresh and good quality grape juice have a very low, almost neglectable histamine content, wine derived from this grape juice can have a considerable, unacceptable histamine levels. Alcohol is known to impair DAO-activity; therefore, extremely low levels of histamine and other BAs in alcoholic beverages are of crucial importance and of special interest to the consumer (Bodmer et al. 1999). For this reason, some wine producers have developed new methods for productions of high-quality wine and sparkling wines with the application of efficient HACCP plans. Later, studies with wine products obtained from European markets showed that sparkling and Cherry wines processed with conventional method contained higher histamine values than wine originated from modified methods (Bodmer et al. 1999). Legislation of certain countries allows the rejections of wines with histamine content higher than legal limits. The upper limits for histamine in wine in some countries vary between 2 and 10 mg/L histamine.

5.6.6 BA Contents of Other Food Types

Karovičová and Kohajdová (2005) reported that the manufacturing of sauerkraut coursed in three steps characterized by active microorganisms, which produced BAs are *Leuconostoc mesenteroides*, producing putrescine in content about 250 mg/kg, *Lactobacillus* spp., producing putrescine and tyramine, and *Pediococcus cerevisiae*, producing histamine in content about 200 mg/kg. BAs, especially putrescine, accumulate in sauerkraut brine. They also reported that cadaverine, histamine, putrescine, spermidine, and tyramine were often found in the lactic acid fermented vegetables such as carrot and red beet in content ranging from 1 to 15 mg/kg.

5.7 METHODOLOGY FOR BAs

5.7.1 Introduction

Detection of BAs in foods has an important role on the preventive measures for food safety. Analytical methods are generally used on the investigation of potential food poisoning incidents, for verification of food production processes (including HACCP) as well as a measure of quality (freshness) of both raw materials and finished products (EFSA 2011; Restuccia et al. 2014). Analysis of most compounds can be carried out at the varying levels of accuracy. The factors that can influence the choice of method used are the actual need for accuracy, time consideration, technical skills involved, the expense, and the availability of reagents or equipment used (Köse 1993). The earliest methods used for detecting histamine were bioassays, which were qualitative methods depended on the guinea pig ileum contraction assay or using biological systems (Köse 1993). Since then high numbers of test methods have been developed for the determination of BAs in food and food products including both qualitative and quantitative methods with a varying accuracy. Since histamine is the main amine regulated for fish and fish products over the years, the most developments on the methodology on this aspect were usually applied on histamine analysis in fish. However, soon after the incidents of HFP associated with other food types and the recognition of the role of other BAs in food intoxication and quality, analytical techniques have also been modified or developed for different food product types for analysis of all BAs.

5.7.2 Method Selection

The choice of methodology is limited by three main target uses, namely, (i) analysis of BAs in processing plants, mainly at the defined critical control points (CCPs), and verification of HACCP and quality management (QM) plans for food safety and quality issues; (ii) controlling BAs by the government authorities for monitoring and risk assessment purposes; and (iii) research work on food safety and quality issues.

Histamine detection is usually included in HACCP plan of the food processors and government control program due to existing regulation for histamine in foods. Therefore, some methods specifically target histamine analysis, particularly in fish and fish products. Analytical methods specific to histamine analysis include well-accepted fluorometric method by the Association of Official Analytical Chemists (AOAC 977.13) (Hungerford 2010), the spectrofluorometric method, the colorimetric enzyme test and enzyme immunoassay (EIA), and/or enzymatic methods (Hungerford 2010; FAO-WHO 2013). Developing chromatographic methods with a variety of different approaches enabled us to determine all BAs including histamine in food products. These methods range from simple and inexpensive thin layer chromatography (TLC) procedures to more powerful liquid chromatography–mass spectrometry (LC-MS) methods (Hungerford 2010). These techniques are reviewed and discussed by various authors over the years (Lehane and Olley 2000; Dalgaard et al. 2008; Hungerford 2010; Erim 2013).

Each method has strengths and limitations, and they vary in terms of related cost, operator expertise, analytical time per sample, portability, etc. It is difficult to find a simple, fast, inexpensive yet highly accurate method for BA analysis. Qualitative methods used mainly for histamine analysis. They are usually simple, inexpensive, and fast methods but not very sensitive; therefore, they are preferred for the purpose as fast screening of histamine at CCPs in the HACCP application at food plants and may be for a quick result at official control points during marketing. These methods are usually produced into commercial test kits for portable use. The test kits are often set to 50 ppm, which is the upper limit defined by FDA, and if positive results are obtained, further analysis are carried out using a suitable quantitative method for confirmation. Codex standards propose the use of the fluorometric method (AOAC 997.13) or other scientifically equivalent validated methods for this purpose (FAO-WHO 2013). However, high-performance liquid chromatography (HPLC) is the most extensively used techniques in determining BAs in different kinds of foods. EC (2005) also requires using HPLC method since 2005 for histamine analysis in fisheries products. The suggested method is based on the method used by Eerola et al. (1993) with minor differences. Modification of this procedure was later published by different authors (Köse et al. 2011).

5.7.3 Extraction Procedures

In an analytical method for foods, one has to first consider the suitable extraction procedure. Very similar procedures for the extraction of the amines from different food matrixes were applied before chromatographic analysis. In the HPLC procedures, solid samples are extracted with various acids (e.g., trichloroacetic acid, hydrochloric, perchloric, thiodipropionic, or methanesulfonic acids), solvents (mainly petroleum ether, chloroform, and methanol), and filtration (Erim 2013; Restuccia et al. 2014). Three types of solvents have mainly been used for the extraction of BAs with a range of concentration of 0.6 M for perchloric acid, 5%–10% for trichloroacetic acid, and 0.1 M for HCl (Karovičova and Kohajdová 2005). Acid treatment is also reported that it deproteinizes the extracts. Wine samples are used directly or after a simple polyvinylpolypyrrolidone (PVPP) treatment and then filtration to remove phenolic compounds (Erim 2013). Methanol was suggested for a suitable solvent for milk product for the extraction of BAs at the increased temperature (60°C) (Karovičova and Kohajdová 2005). Some authors suggest extraction with butanol or butanol-chloroform at basic pH for the clean-up of samples. It is reported that some parameters significantly influence the extraction and recovery of BAs (e.g., pH) (Karovičova and Kohajdová 2005; Erim 2013). The author of this chapter also experienced filtering problems with formic acid with fish in oil. The relative extraction efficiencies of these solvents depend on the type and nature of the BAs and the food from which they are being extracted. The solid-phase extraction (SPE) has provided a more efficient choice than classical liquid extraction by virtue of the wide availability of sorbent materials and of the fact that the need to dispose of organic solvents is avoided (Karovičova and Kohajdová 2005).

5.7.4 Separation Techniques for Removing Interfering Compounds

Two main problems need to be overcome for the analytical procedures designed for analysis of histamine detection only, and for all BAs. One is the necessity of the separation of BAs and removal of other interfering compounds in the food matrix such as histidine. For the procedures applied to histamine detection only, removal of other existing BAs is also required. Second, since many amines show neither natural UV absorption nor fluorescence, most liquid chromatographic methods require that amines should be derivatized before detection (Spizzirri et al. 2013). Therefore, the large majority of assays employ fluorometric and UV detection with precolumn or postcolumn derivatization techniques (Erim 2013; FAO-WHO 2013).

Different types of derivatization reagents have been applied in methods using derivatization step as ninhydrin and o-phthalaldehyde, as a postcolumn derivatization reagent, dansyl and dabsyl chloride, benzoyl chloride, fluorescein, 9-fluorenylmethyl chloroformate with precolumn derivatization (Köse 1993; Erim 2013). The advantages and disadvantages of using different derivatization reagents and different methodology have been discussed in detail by Erim (2013) and also experienced by the author. Paleologos et al. (2003) pointed out that in almost all approaches, the derivatized amines have to undergo extraction in a suitable organic solvent, evaporation to dryness, and redissolution before injection in the HPLC system. Thus, the risk of sample loss and contamination is introduced along with extensive analysis time. Furthermore, the chromatographic conditions result either in insufficient separation or prolonged analysis, which may require longer than an hour. Therefore, more rapid and simple quantitative analytical methods without derivatization steps are needed for quantitative analysis, particularly for regulatory purposes for fishery products.

Most of the separation methods applied to BAs in foods and food products use reversed-phase HPCL with detection schemes based on precolumn or postcolumn derivatization to produce fluorescent products or strong chromophores (Hungerford 2010; Erim 2013). It has also been reported that traditional HPLC methods suffer from various drawbacks such as cumbersome sample preparation, problems of derivatization stability, by-products interference, complex instrumentation, skilled operator, and/or long time of analysis. Other popular separation-based methods have been reported as ion chromatography (IC) developed by Cinquina et al. (2004), capillary electrophoresis reported by Sato et al. (2006), and gas chromatography–MS (GC-MS) (Hungerford 2010). Some novel LC methods coupled with mass spectrometric detection (LC-MS) with novel precolumn derivatization approaches have been reported (Hungerford 2010; Sagratini et al. 2012; Erim 2013).

5.7.5 Quantitative Methods with Direct Detection of BAs

The LC or GC methods that do not require derivatization also exist in literature, such as solid-phase microextraction GC-MS (Erim 2013), HPLC tandem MS (HPLC-MS/MS) (Sagratini et al. 2012), HPLC-MS/MS using polar hydrophilic interaction liquid chromatography (HILIC) stationary phase (Gosetti et al. 2007), matric solid-phase dispersion with HPLC-MS/MS (Gianotti et al. 2008) and HPLC method with evaporative light scattering detection (ELSD) (Restuccia et al. 2011). However, it was reported that high polarity of BAs is known as a drawback for conventional HPLC in terms of analyte separation that often leads to coelution of BAs (Sirocchi et al. 2014). Therefore, IC is being a more suitable approach allowing a rather straightforward separation since at low pH all analytes exist in the ionized form, whereas in HPLC careful control of pH is necessary to achieve a good separation. It was also reported that impurities in conventional HPLC eluents (acetonitrile, methanol) may also have a negative effect on MS detection (Song et al. 2004). In contrast to HPLC, in IC, neutral impurities elute in the void volume thus enabling us to completely remove them from the system that is often not possible in HPLC. Replacing HPLC with IC separation overcomes the mentioned problems, since IC columns designed specifically for separation of BAs and they are readily available on the market (Pompe 2016, Pers. Comm.). Table 5.6 summarizes some of the most recent BA analytical techniques applied to various food products using MS detection without a derivatization step.

To avoid derivatization steps, LC methods were coupled with pulsed amperometric detection (PAD) or integrated PAD (IPAD) using noble-metal electrodes in alkaline media (Saccani et al. 2005). However, disadvantages of these methods were reported as their requirement of a postcolumn addition of a pH modifier. However, techniques using suppressed conductivity or MS detection do not need any precolumn or postcolumn modification. A suppressed conductivity method was proposed by Cinquina et al. (2004) for the determination of histamine in tuna. This method only was tested for four BAs. Later, Saccani et al. (2005) compared IC-MS/MS to suppressed conductivity methods for analyzing several BAs in meat and meat products. Although they observed similar separation with six BAs (namely, histamine, cadaverine, putrescine, agmatine, phenylethylamine, and spermine), tyramine could not be detected by MS if suppressed conductivity detection was used because tyramine is removed by the suppressor. This might be a problem especially when dealing with cheese samples, where tyramine is one of the main occurring BAs. It was pointed out that tyramine could be detected by MS only when the separator column is directly connected to the mass detector. However, they also stressed that methanesulfonic acid eluent is not compatible with mass spectrometric detector. Saccani et al. (2005) reported that they carried out a test with an MS compatible acid such as formic acid that enabled tyramine detection; however, this eluent did not allow them a full separation of all the other amines. They indicated that the relatively high concentration of formic acid is necessary for the tyramine elution.

Restuccia et al. (2011) have developed a new LC method with evaporative light scattering detector and validated it for BA determination in cheese. ELSD is known more affordable than mass spectrometry and is also compatible with a broad range of solvents and gradient elution. Although this method had the advantage of the elimination of the derivatization procedure drawbacks, a severe matrix effect in cheese has been reported (Spizzirri et al. 2013).

5.7.6 Commercial Test Kits for Histamine Analysis

An interest in "portable" procedures for field analysis capable of rapid screening particularly fishery products at dockside has led to the development of commercial

TABLE 5.6
Recent Advanced Methods for Detecting Biogenic Amines in Foods with Nonderivatization Approach

Food Sample	Analytes	Sample Treatment	Separation Method	Detection	LOD & LOQ	References
Fish	PUT, CAD, HIS, PHE, SPM, TYR, TRP	5%TCA, SPE	HPLC, C18 column, (250 × 4.0 mm, 5 µm) A: ammonium formate, formic acid, water, pH3.3, B: methanol	MS/MS	LOD: 0.02–0.25 mg/kg LOQ: 0.07–0.75 mg/kg	Sagratini et al. (2012)
Fish	PUT, CAD, HIS, TYR, 3 volatile amines	0.6M $HClO_4$	UHPLC, BEHC18column, 1002.1 mm, 1.7 µm A: methanol, B: formic acid solution	MS/MS	LOQ: 25 µg/kg for all, 60 µg/kg for trimethylamine	Romero-Gonzáles et al. (2012)
Fish & fish products	AGM, CAD, PHE, HIS, PUT, TYR, TRP, URO	Matrix solid-phase dispersion CN-silica sorbent/ammonium formate, acetonitrile eluent	UHPLC-HILIC, BEH-HILIC column, (150 × 2.1 mm,1.7 µm) A: ammonium formate buffer B: acetonitrile	Orbitrap mass spectrometry	LOD: 0.0237–2.58 ppm LOQ: 0.0791–8.61 ppm	Self et al. (2011)
Cheese	HIS, SPM, SPMD, TYR, PUT, PHE	0.1M HCl, SPE	HPLC, RP cation exchange column, 5 µm A: acetonitrile/water, trifluoro acetic acid (0.05%) B: acetonitrile/water, trifluoroacetic acid (0.35%)	Evaporative light scattering detection	LOD: 1.4–3.6 mg/L LOQ: 3.6–9.3 mg/L	Restuccia et al. (2011)
Cheese	HIS, SPD, SPE, TYR, PUT, CAD, AGM, PHE	0.1M HCl, SPE	LC, RP cation exchange column, A: acetonitrile/water 5 / 95 (v/v) containing trifluoroacetic acid (0.06%, v/v); B: acetonitrile/water 5 / 95 (v/v) containing trifluoroacetic acid (0.45%, v/v)	Evaporative light scattering detection	LOD: 1.0–3.2 mg/L (0.8–2.6 mg/kg)	Spizzirri et al. (2013)
Beer, herb tea, dairy, beverage, vinegar	SPM, SPMD, PHE, HIS, AGM, TRY, TRP, CAD, PUT, OCT, SER, DOP, CAM, ALA		Ion-pair LC, silica-phenyl-hexyl column,(150 × 2 mm, 3 µm) perfluorocarboxylic acids as ion pair reagents A: nonafluoropentanoic acid (NFPA) in water, B: NFPA in methanol	Chemiluminescent nitrogen detector	LOD: 0.1–0.4 µg/mL	Sun et al. (2011)

(Continued)

TABLE 5.6 (*Continued*)
Recent Advanced Methods for Detecting Biogenic Amines in Foods with Nonderivatization Approach

Food Sample	Analytes	Sample Treatment	Separation Method	Detection	LOD & LOQ	References
Beer	Ethanolamine, TRY, tryptophan		Microchip capillary electrophoresis, glass microchannel chips, effective length: 75 mm 20 mM phosphate buffer (pH 2.5)	Amperometric detection Ruthenium coated glassy carbon electrodes	LOD: 1.4–6.8 mg/L	Dossi et al. (2011)
Wine	HIS, PHE, TRY		CITP-CZE, ITP column 140 mm, 800 μm, CZE column: 160 mm, 300 μm, ITP: Leading electrolyte: Potassium, pH: 6; Terminating electrolyte: e-amino caproic acid pH: 4.3; CZE: Background electrolyte: e-aminobutyric acid (GABA), HEC; pH: 4.1	UV-280n	LOD: 0.33–0.37 mg/L LOQ: 0.49–0.55 mg/L	Ginterová et al. (2012)
Meat (beef, chicken, lamb, rabbit)	HIS, PUT, CAD, PHE, SER, SPM, SPMD, TRP, TRY, AGM	5%TCA, SPE STRATA cartridges	RP-80A analytical column (250 × 4.6 mm I.D., particle size 4 μm) ammonium formate 5 mM and formic acid in water pH: 3.3 and methanol.	MS/MS	LOD: 0.002–0.1 mg/L LOQ: 0.008–0.5 mg/	Sirocchi et al. (2014)

Source: Updated from Erim, F.B., *Trends Anal. Chem.*, 52, 239–247, 2013.
Biogenic amines: HIS: histamine; TRY: tyramine; TRP: tryptamine; SPMD: spermidine; SPM: spermine; PUT: putrescine; CAD: cadaverine; PHE: phenylethylamine; AGM: agmatine; OCT: octopamine, SER: serotonin, DOP: dopamine, CAM: caminobutyric acid, ALA: b-alanine. MS/MS: tandem quadrupole mass spectrometer; Q-TOFMS: quadrupole time-of-flight mass spectrometer; LOD: limit of detection; LOQ: limit of quantification; UHPLC: ultra-high- performance liquid chromatography; HPLC: high-performance liquid chromatography; SPE: solid-phase extraction; LC: liquid chromatography; RP: reversed-phase; TCA: trichloroacetic acid; HEC: Hydroxyethylcellulose; URO: urocanic acid; ITP: Isotachophoresis; CITP-CZE: Capillary Zone Electrophoresis with isotachophoresis.

test kits proposed for HACCP plan applications (Rogers and Staruszkiewicz 2000). Several types of commercial test kits available in the market based on their quantitative properties as semiquantitative (or qualitative) and quantitative methods (Köse et al. 2011). Commercial test kits mainly based on immunoassay methods for histamine analyses have become popular because of their user friendliness and reduced time requirements compared to those of traditional analytical techniques. However, they are easily affected by the sample matrix and other application conditions. Therefore, evaluating the compatibility of test kits against approved quantitative methods are of interest for both test kit producing companies and scientists. Moreover, on a regular base, some companies such as Labour Diagnostica Nord, Germany (LND), participate at external quality assessment schemes such as CHEK, Netherland and Food Analysis Performance Assessment Scheme to prove reliability of their methods for marketing policy. They claim that their results usually are successful (URL-2), and they use this information to modify the existing methods (LDN, 2011, Pers. Comm.). So far, two test kits are approved by AOAC using Performance Testing. The first approved commercial immunoassay test method by AOAC is Veratox by Neogen Cooperations with an approval number AOAC-RI 070703. It is a competitive direct ELISA intended for the quantitative analysis of histamine in fish, such as tuna, bluefish, and mahi-mahi, and in fish meal. The second method that was more recently approved is HistaSure ELISA Fast Track by LDN with an approval number AOAC-021402. It is also a competitive ELISA techniques intended for the quantitative determination of histamine in fresh/frozen yellowfin tuna, canned tuna-chunk light in water, fresh/frozen mahi-mahi, canned sardines in oil and fish meal. LDN Company also produced other histamine test kits and commercialized for many years. These are HistaSure™ ELISA High Sensitive (a quantitative ELISA) designed for any kind of food types, HistaSure™ Dipstick assay (immunogold) for all fish samples for screening purposes, HisQuick™ (a colorimetric assay) for quantitative determination of histamine in fish meal only. Other commercial test kits based on immunoassays and other types are revised by various publications (Hungerford 2010; Köse et al. 2011). The most commonly reported ones are ALERT Histamine by Neogen, United States; HISTAMARINE by Immunotech, France; EIA for Histamine in fish extract, K1-HTM and K3-HTM in raw and canned fish by Immuno-Tech., United States; HistaMeter by Biomedix, United States, and Transia Tube Histamine as semiqualitative and quantitative methods by Diffchamb, Sweden. Some test kits are named differently by the partner company of LDN Company as RIDASCREEN, although they are the same kits as stated by the owner of LDN (Manz B. 2008, Germany; Pers. Comm.) as a marketing policy.

Several studies have been carried out on the evaluation of different types of test kits compared to well-accepted quantitative methods mainly HPLC. These studies are reviewed and discussed by Rogers and Staruszkiewicz (2000), Köse et al. (2011), Hungerford and Wu (2012). Among these studies, HPLC is mainly applied for the evaluation of test kits for fish and fish products due to the requirement of EU for regulatory purposes (EC 2005). However, fluorometric method is officially required for the analysis of histamine in fishery products by FDA, and therefore, evaluation of commercial test kits was also compared for this method (Rogers and Staruszkiewicz 2000). The results of previous studies indicated that performance of test kits can vary according to type of product used as well as the method that is used for evaluation (Köse et al.

2011). Most existing test kit methods have also been evaluated at the author's laboratory and found that Histamine Food EIA and HistaSure kits by LDN and Veratox by Neogen proved to be well correlated with HPLC method (Köse et al. 2011). The main advantage of HistaSure kit is that although this method is set for 50 ppm histamine value (which is the FDA permitted level), it can be set to different cut-off levels starting with 5–200 ppm by adjusting the extraction volume. Total assay time including sample preparation is also very short takes between 20 and 30 minutes. However, most test kits use water for extraction of histamine from food, so this might be a disadvantage in accurate quantitative determination. Future studies will probably focus on this aspect including other drawbacks. HistaSure Fast Track which is also a modified version of HistaSure gives promise to wide application of use in food industry.

In recent years, novelty approaches for determination of BAs in different foods have emerged. Some of these are biosensors, voltammetric measurements and ion mobility spectrometry (IMS). These techniques are well discussed in Erim (2013). It was pointed out that although they enable relatively low detection limits and sufficient repeatability, they are somewhat complex and do not allow for determination of all of the BAs considered important in the field of food safety. The development of novel sensors for BA analysis appears to provide alternative methods to separation techniques. The advantages of sensors are their low cost, short analytical time, and the possibility of their use on site (Erim 2013). However, they are not selective to all individual amines. Generally, total BA contents are obtained via sensors. Due to lack of selectivity, they are sensitive to the food matrix, and the accuracy of the results requires to be checked with a reliable method before using a sensor on a new food sample (Erim 2013).

Tao et al. (2012) revised the methodology used for the determination of gizzerosine. They pointed out the difficulties in using simple and reliable methods. Therefore, they established a simple, rapid method for gizzerosine analysis in fish meal called paper electrophoresis. They reported the linearity of gizzerosine estimation using this method was within the range 30–1000 ng. They claimed that gizzerosine was satisfactorily detected and completely separated from histamine and other interfering compounds. The advantage of this method over existing methods is that this method does not require expensive instruments or tedious pretreatment to eliminate interfering compounds such as histamine or histidine. Compared to HPLC method, it also uses fewer reagents. The authors claimed that it is suitable for monitoring gizzerosine in fish meal containing as low as 10 ppm gizzerosine.

5.8 CONTROL MEASURES FOR BAs

5.8.1 Introduction

There are two main approaches to control the presence of BAs in foods. These are the following:

1. Controlling accumulation of BAs in foods during transporting, storage, and processing. This is well achieved by applying an efficient HACCP plan by the processors including necessary good manufacturing and hygienic plans

(GMP, GHP), and similar approach by the fresh food distributors using mainly GHP and TT control
2. Degradation of previously formed BAs in foods, particularly applied to fermented foods

The current control options to minimize BA occurrence in foods are mainly focused on the food processing level that also includes raw material handling and storage (Restuccia et al. 2014). Therefore, implementation of an efficient HACCP plan by the experts would easily overcome this problem. Maintenance of hygienic quality of raw materials and through production processes, and implementation of specific conditions to inhibit (or eliminate) growth and activity of BA decarboxylating microorganisms are the target of many control approaches stated in the literature (Restuccia et al. 2014). This is mainly done by GHP. However, once the decarboxylating enzymes are formed, these enzymes can continue to decarboxylate the precursor FAAs to BAs unless their activities are also inhibited or retarded. Moreover, physical and chemical spoilage of foods promotes the bacterial attack and increase the activity. The other important aspect often overlooked is the contribution of endogenous enzymes in BA formation. The available precursor FAA concentrations in food products are closely depend on the activity of endogenous enzymes (e.g., digestive enzymes in fish guts or cathepsins in meat) which is in turn favored by the denaturation of proteins into small peptides or amino acids that can be metabolized by decarboxylating bacteria. Therefore, control strategies must also include preventing chemical and physical degradation of foods prior to processing or marketing. Restuccia et al. (2014) summarized the most commonly applied preventive approaches to prevent BA formation in various foods. FDA (2011) usually provides good guidelines for handling and storage of fishery products in terms of avoiding food health hazards including histamine.

After harvesting, foods follow two ways to reach consumers, namely, (i) through direct marketing that high possibly involves storage at certain stages due to marketing necessities and (ii) reach to processing plants and then processed before marketing to consumers. This route also involves storage at certain stages of marketing. Other than their contribution to sensory and nutritional attributes, the majority of the processing techniques target prevention or delaying the bacterial and enzymatic activities in foods (i.e., they are designed for preserving foods and maintaining food safety). For this reason, controlling BA formation in foods is of importance at the raw material stage and fresh marketing. Therefore, controlling strategies of BAs in food and food products are examined under two groups as preventive approaches at raw material stage including fresh marketing and the prevention at processing stage. In both stages, varying methods are applied to limit bacterial growth and inhibit bacterial and enzymatic activities in foods.

5.8.2 Preventing BA Formation at Raw Material Stage Including Fresh Food Marketing

5.8.2.1 Introduction

At this stage, the factors affecting the BA formation are (i) the natural microbial flora of foods, harvesting techniques; (ii) natural properties of the foods such as nutrient contents; (iii) handling conditions during harvesting, transport, and storage that allow physical damage and bacterial contamination; and (iv) storage conditions, particularly TT issues relating to bacterial and enzymatic activity. All these factors can be controlled mainly by four effective ways as using safe harvesting methods, eliminating microorganisms, TT control, and applying proper handling methods. These are explained below.

5.8.2.2 Hygienic Conditions

Hygienic conditions must start at the stage of harvesting of foods, through handling, and storage to avoid further contamination. Each food originates from different environment with a varying microbial load and species. Although safe agriculturing and harvesting techniques exist, foods with low number of bacteria cannot always possible. In the HACCP plan, it is stated that food from polluted waters should not be accepted at the raw material receiving step. However, this is usually the case for enteric bacteria which is an indicator of pathogenic bacteria. So products are often checked for the presence of either *E. coli* or coliform. A wide range of bacteria are confirmed for BA decarboxylate activity. Routine testing of total number and specific type of bacteria in foods to take control action is not a practical way to avoid unsafe conditions. Therefore, it is advised to treat all the products with the assumption that they are likely to contain high numbers of amine forming bacteria.

The presence of BAs in raw materials is usually associated with spoilage, suggesting poor hygienic practices, and may also indicate other food safety issues. Therefore, decarboxylating activity of the microorganisms should be prevented in fresh commodities by improving food-handling standards through a preventative strategy from harvest/slaughtering to the consumer, implying that food quality and safety management relying on HACCP should be regarded as the primary approach (Hungerford 2010; Restuccia et al. 2014). At the same time, GHP along with proper cleaning and disinfection procedures should be carefully implemented starting from primary production. Microorganisms originating from animals (i.e., intestines, skin, fish gills) can be spreaded to other sites, surfaces, and equipment during handling of fresh raw materials (e.g., during degutting and filleting of fish, slaughtering, cutting, and mincing of meat), and consequently promote the accumulation of BAs during further processing and/or storage (Restuccia et al. 2014). Although evisceration and removal of the gills of fish in a sanitary manner may reduce microorganisms and enzymes in the guts, under unsanitary conditions, these steps may accelerate the process of histamine development in the edible portions of the fish by spreading the bacteria to the fish flesh (FDA 2011).

Food safety authorities already implemented effective GHP over the years including all food types. Legislations set by various authorities such as EU and good guidelines on GMP and even animal health are given by various organizations. Different methods are carried out to decrease or destroy the existing microorganisms in freshly harvested food products. Washing is the traditional method often applied to fresh foods, and it lowers microbial load to a certain point but not effective enough to avoid the risk unless it is combined with other supporting techniques such as using ozonized water and high-pressure washing. However, not all food types allow all types of washing methods and some foods may not be washable at all. Therefore, other method such as application of UHT such as for milk is necessary. High hydrostatic pressure (HHP) is also gained a wide application to sterilize raw foods for fresh marketing. Restuccia et al. (2014) reported that intervention strategies to improve the hygiene of raw materials should include, whenever possible, thermal treatments. Boiling milk after milking has been a traditional attitude even at household productions for long years to avoid food safety and to provide safe storage for fresh use or further processing into yogurt, butter, and cheese. In particular, pasteurization is the most common milk treatment used during cheesemaking to reduce the number of pathogenic and spoilage microorganisms. Many authors found that pasteurization is able to reduce the concentration of BAs in milk and dairy products. In fact, many decarboxylating bacteria such as *Enterobacteriaceae* and *Enterococcus* spp. do not survive thermal treatment, this being the main explanation for the lower BA contents generally found in cheeses from pasteurized milk in comparison with those obtained from raw milk. Therefore, deficient hygienic conditions can promote contamination with BA-producing microorganisms during the manufacture of dairy products after the thermal treatment has been accomplished. To this regard, the accumulation of elevated concentrations of BAs has been reported in cheeses derived from pasteurized milk (Restuccia et al. 2014).

5.8.2.3 TT Control

TT binomial is the most important risk factor for the formation of histamine and other BAs during the handling and storage of fresh commodities (e.g., meat and seafood products). For this reason, a strict adherence to the cold chain should be accomplished and low temperatures should be applied during storage to inhibit proteolytic and decarboxylase activity of bacteria. Apart from mesophilic aminogenic organisms, which can be controlled by preventing TT abuse, psychrotolerant bacteria are also relevant in relation to BA production in fish stored at chill temperature. Freezing and temperatures near 0°C inhibit growth and activity of decarboxylating microorganisms and therefore constitute the most effective way to prevent BA accumulation in fresh products, and thus also in raw materials. However, once the BA decarboxylase enzymes have been formed, they can continue to produce BAs in the foods even if the bacteria are not active. The enzymes can be active at or near refrigeration temperatures. The enzymes are also likely to remain stable while in the frozen state and may be reactivated very rapidly after thawing (FDA 2011; Köse 2010). After thawing, frozen meat and fish are less susceptible to BA accumulation than unfrozen counterparts, probably because the microbiota is reduced to some extent as a result of the freezing process (EFSA 2011). However, thawed foods, particularly fish, are more susceptible to spoilage due to possible damage to the muscle cells due to freezing may potentiate the chemical and bacterial spoilage.

FDA (2011) recommended that rapid chilling of fish immediately after death is the most important element in any strategy for preventing the formation of histamine, especially for fish exposed to warmer waters or air. The time required to lower the internal temperature of fish after capture will be dependent upon a number of factors including (Köse 2010):

1. *The harvest method*: Delays in removing fish from a long line may significantly limit the amount of time left for chilling and may allow some fish to

heat up after death. The quantity of fish landed in a purse seine or on a long line may exceed a vessel's ability to rapidly chill the product

2. *The size of the fish*: Bigger fish will be chilled down slower than small sized fish
3. *The chilling method*: As a consequence of reduced contact area and heat transfer, ice alone takes longer to chill fish than ice slurry or recirculated refrigerated sea water or brine does. The quantity of ice or ice slurry and the capacity of refrigerated sea water or brine systems must be suitable for the quantity of catch

Although FDA (2011) gave a valuable guide on how long fish should be kept at/or exposed to certain temperatures for a safe shelf life in relation to histamine formation, such guidance is more suitable or much easier to be used for fresh/frozen fish marketing for developed countries where seafood safety regulations are effectively in use. There are several factors that can affect such guidances. Moreover, environmental conditions may differ around the world at different regions. Therefore, the following guidelines are advised for better TT control strategies (Köse 2010). To monitor total exposure time of implicated fish before processing can be carried out depending on processors' choices, if they can trace fish harvesters (fishermen or farmers) through their recordings or not. If the answer is "YES," then they can set up their critical limit as decided TT depending on the experimental histamine test results for such delivery conditions as well as the type of processing to be applied. If the answer is "NO," then processors should apply several critical limits to monitor histamine formation. These are (i) checking the temperature of fish and water at arrival, (ii) checking sensory quality of fish (set up the freshest quality parameters as given in several guidances), (iii) testing histamine levels at the arrival for suspected lot using rapid test kits and set up critical histamine levels according to the type of processing method, and (iv) if fish arrived as frozen, then the processors can perform histamine testing for a specified critical limit according to type of processing method, then continue TT monitoring during storage and thawing.

5.8.2.4 Sensory Evaluation of Foods

FDA (2011) pointed out that although sensory evaluation is generally used to screen fish for spoilage odors, such examination alone is ineffective control for histamine. Moreover, toxic histamine levels can also be observed in fish despite their acceptable sensory quality (Köse 2010). Federal Register (1995) reported that the best quality fish has histamine values less than 10 ppm, while histamine values between 10 and 30 ppm are accepted as middle quality and 30–50 ppm histamine value is critical since it is close to the level of FDA regulation (50 ppm). Therefore, histamine testing is an effective way of monitoring its formation at raw material stage before processing. However, approved histamine testing procedures are time consuming and require technical skills that are mostly lacking at processing companies. Practical test kits are suggested to be used during monitoring histamine hazard in the HACCP plan (Köse 2010).

Recent studies carried out at the author's laboratory demonstrated the storage quality of certain fresh fish species (anchovy and Atlantic bonito) was well correlated with the safe histamine levels at various chilled conditions (Koral and Köse 2012, 2015). Although these findings might suggest that sensory evaluation of chilled fish might help to avoid these fish species, more studies at the same conditions with different batches are needed to draw a conclusion. Some studies with BAs were also proved a good correlation with the quality of certain foods such as fish and cheese. Therefore, they used the BA levels to estimate the quality of foods, and several indexes were suggested as given at the earlier sections of this chapter. Sensory quality of foods is easier to estimate, so the author suggests that scientists should focus on finding sensory schemes or formulae with sensory scores to estimate the risk of BAs.

5.8.2.5 Handling and Harvesting Conditions

The handling and harvesting conditions relating to microbial contamination and spoilage have been mentioned above. Good handling and harvesting conditions would help to decrease activity of the existing enzymes and microorganisms. Normally, meat and fish flesh is safe from microorganisms, but the animals contain high load of microorganisms. Physical damage during harvesting and transport can lead to spreading bacteria from surface of the food through internal parts. Catching methods of fish and slaughthering methods can also affect their shelf life that leads to unfavor bacteria attack. For example, fish caught by gillnet (which gives more stress and damage to fish) goes into rigor and post rigor stage faster fish caught by a hook or rod with less stressed conditions. It is reported that bacterial spoilage starts after the post rigor stage.

5.8.3 Control at Processing Steps

5.8.3.1 Introduction

At this stage, HACCP is the primary control approach, which also includes GHP and GMP. GHP is reported the presequisitive program of the HACCP plan applied to a food processing (Köse 2010). Most processing methods are usually designed for preventing health hazards including microbiological and chemical hazards. CCPs set for pathogenic bacteria can easily eliminate the decarboxylate bacteria activity in foods during processing and storage of processed foods. The main parameters to be monitored as critical limits to control bacteria growth and toxin formation including BAs are suggested as pH, salt content, temperature, time, and water activity. Some processing techniques may require screening tests for histamine and bacteria analysis using test kits. These are also known as the main parameters affect BA formation in foods.

5.8.3.2 Thermal Treatments and Freezing

Providing good quality raw material with the proper control measures taken prior to processing, pressured cooking, and pasteurization (canning) is the best method followed by freezing in controlling BA formation in foods. Canning or pasteurization is known to kill microorganisms in foods and also destroy the enzymes. Although freezing also inhibits bacterial growth, some enzymes previously formed in raw material may still continue to be active.

5.8.3.3 Fermented Foods

There are three main factors that promote BA formation in fermented foods or during fermentation. First one is pointed out by Restuccia et al. (2014) as proteolysis that cannot be inhibited for these foods such as cheeses or fermented sausage manufacture because it is an essential process for coagulation and ripening. Second is warm production temperature used for some fermentation procedures, which can promote the growth of BA forming bacteria. Third, some starter cultures used in fermentation procedures, which may also have amino acid decarboxylating activity. Therefore, additional care must be taken for such foods including (i) minimizing any additional source of decarboxylating microorganisms (by avoiding recontamination and choosing safe starter cultures), (ii) assuring an optimal water quality and brine for salting, and (iii) using preservatives such as spices and ingredients during manufacturing (Restuccia et al. 2014). Some control measures are given below.

5.8.3.3.1 Application of GHP

The hygienic quality of raw materials and ingredients should also be assured to facilitate the dominance of starter bacteria from the early stages of fermentation (Restuccia et al. 2014). To this regard, a useful example is represented by the so-called low histamine technology (Bodmer et al. 1999) based on both the preventive approach (through GHP, GMP, and HACCP) and the implementation of specific technological measures for the manufacture of traditional alcoholic beverages (Bodmer et al. 1999). Similarly, some publications reported low levels of BAs from cheese products that are certified as "Protected Designation of Origin (PDO)" meaning that cheese be produced in a defined area under a specific standard of identity (Spizzirri et al. 2013).

5.8.3.3.2 Starter Culture Selection

BA formation in fermented foods has often been attributed to the activity of the nonstarter microflora. However, an indirect role of the starter LAB has been hypothesized as the peptidases released by the lysis of starter LAB could be essential in providing precursor amino acids (Restuccia et al. 2014). Therefore, it was suggested that the selection of starter cultures is important. They should be chosen from strains that are negative for BA decarboxylating activity but able to grow well at the temperature intended for fermentation while suppressing the growth of wild amine-producing microflora (Restuccia et al. 2014). For this reason, selection must be carried out with the consideration of varying factors such as product formulation (salt, sugar, preservatives, spices) and processing parameters (temperature, relative humidity, time, etc.). In this respect, the European Food Safety Authority (EFSA) has introduced a system for a premarket safety assessment of selected taxonomic groups of microorganisms, leading to a Qualified Presumption of Safety (QPS), which is European equivalent of the Generally Recognized as Safe (GRAS) status (EFSA 2007).

Some bacteria species used in fermentation have been reported to delay the formation of BAs as degradating activity. Moreover, a rapid and sharp decrease in pH is recognized as a key factor to reduce the growth of contaminated microorganisms, this pH level can also stimulate decarboxylation reactions in surviving microbiota as a response against unfavorable acidic environments (Restuccia et al. 2014).

The protective performance of starter cultures to prevent BA accumulation will also be strongly conditioned by the adaptation of strains to the particular fermentation ecology, which can be better if strains are isolated from the same product or type of product. Standardized commercial preparations can be less effective than indigenous starters, although the influence is strain dependent. For example, in fermented sausages, *L. sakei* and *L. curvatus* are well adapted to the meat (Latorre-Moratalla et al. 2014; Restuccia et al. 2014).

Fermentation environment provides optimum conditions for starter cultures enabling them highly competitive to outgrow spontaneous fermenting flora and can efficiently inhibit gram-negative contaminating bacteria. In fact, it was confirmed that starter cultures including decarboxylase-negative strains of *L. sakei* are the most protective as they reduce the overall amine accumulation by up to 95% in comparison with 30%–40% achieved with other commercial starters consisting of *L. plantarum* and *Pediococcus* spp. Mixed starter cultures, not only of LAB, but with other species involved in meat fermentation will contribute to control a wider variety of microorganisms with decarboxylase activity (Restuccia et al. 2014).

5.8.3.3.3 Fermentation Parameters

Optimization of the technological conditions will favor proper implantation and development of the starter culture for fermentation. Different technological variables have been reported as appropriate measures to prevent the accumulation of BAs during processing and prolonged storage. These are (i) temperature and relative humidity of the ripening conditions, (ii) the modification of the type or concentration of fermentable sugar, and/or (iii) the addition of nontherapeutic antimicrobials (sulfite, etc.) and additives (Restuccia et al. 2014). Among these parameters, the temperature at which fermentation takes place influences the formation of BAs. In fact, controlling fermentation temperature has been advised as a very useful parameter for preventing tyramine formation in dry sausage, chiefly by assuring conditions favorable to starter growth. The reason was explained as higher fermentation temperature allows the starter culture to outgrow nonstarter LAB (Restuccia et al. 2014).

Various publications exist in literature demonstrated the effects of additives and preservatives on the reduction of BA formation by inhibiting bacterial growth and decarboxylase activity. Among these, sodium sorbate, potassium sorbate, sodium hexametaphosphate at 2%, citric acid, succinic acid, d-sorbitol, and malic acid have commonly applied to delay the formation of BAs in seafood and meat products. Naturally occurring specific inhibitory substances in spices and additives (curcumin, capsaicin, and piperine) as well as ginger, garlic, green onion, red pepper, clove, and cinnamon have also been shown to limit BA formation (Köse 2010; Restuccia et al. 2014). Mah and Hwang (2009) reported successful reduction of histamine in salted and fermented fish with the addition of glycine in culture with a reduction of 32.6%, 78.4%, 93.2%, 100.0%, and 100.0% for putrescine, cadaverine, histamine, tyramine, and spermidine, respectively (Mah and Hwang 2009). They also observed that, during the ripening of *Myeolchijeot*, overall BAs were reduced by down to 63.0% and 73.4%, in samples prepared with 0% and 20% NaCl, respectively. However, few studies also reported negative effect of additives and preservatives on amine accumulation and claimed that they can increase BA formation in fermented foods such as sausages (Komprda et al. 2004). A putrefactive odor was observed within 2 days at chill storage reports when sodium sorbate and sodium hexametaphosphate were applied to sardines (Restuccia et al. 2014). Good fermentation practices have also demonstrated low levels of BAs in alcoholic beverages such as wine (Bodmer et al. 1999; Smit et al. 2013).

5.8.3.4 Other Traditional Foods

Other processing methods applying heat such as hot smoking, ready to eat products (cooked) also have similar action on the destruction of decarboxylating bacteria and inactivating enzymes. However, recontamination with bacteria is often reported for these foods. Therefore, effective monitoring strategies are necessary in the HACCP plans. Drying is another processing method that inhibits bacterial growth and enzymatic activity due to very low a_w, which is usually targeted to below 0.83. Addition of salt, sugar, or other preserving ingredients increases their long stability. However, packaging used for dried foods is the main CCP after drying step during processing (Köse 2010). These food products can easily absorb moisture, so humidity control in storage rooms or VP is often applied. Although formation of BAs at marinated products are expected due to their suitable pH levels, low temperatures can eliminate bacteria growth and their activity. There are different salting types but mainly divided into two groups by processing techniques as brining and dry salting. Depending on salt concentrations, these methods can also be safe in preventing BA formation due to low a_w levels and high salt content can inhibit bacteria growth and enzyme activity. However, foods salted at low concentrations, such as lower than 25% for brining fish, must present health risk, and therefore, maturation at low temperatures are required (Koral et al. 2013; Köse et al. 2015).

Recently, an EU funded integrated project under sixth Frame programme for RTD called Traditional United Europe Food (TRUEFOOD) (No: FOOD -CT-2006 - 016264) has worked on traditional food products in terms of food safety and nutritional quality. The project demonstrated and published various safe handling and risk assessment approaches to prevent health risks including BAs in traditional food products of European countries including Turkey. Some of the useful guidelines and results are open to public at the following webpage, which will particularly help to brewers, cheesemakers, and fish processors to avoid BA health risk. *http://www.truefood.eu/public_deliverable.asp*.

5.8.4 Degrading Methods

In the literature, attempts to destroy BAs once they are formed in the final product have also been described. In particular, irradiation may be an effective method acting by direct radiolysis of BAs and by reducing the number of bacteria responsible for BA production (Kim et al. 2005) considering that the ionizing radiation inactivates the microorganisms by damaging the nucleic acid of cells (Farkas 2006). However, although irradiation can be appropriate in eliminating BAs in foods once formed, it may pose some adverse effects on the aspects of food nutrition and organoleptic properties. High temperature treatments have also been shown to be unsuitable to destroy formed BAs, because these compounds are reported to be heat stable.

Therefore, cooking or prolonged exposure to heat will not eliminate the toxin (Shalaby 1996; Restuccia et al. 2014).

Some bacteria are known as amine oxidizers since they can oxidize BAs into aldehyde, hydrogen peroxide, and ammonia. These bacteria are proposed to decrease BAs levels in fish sauce, sausage, or wine fermentation. The equilibrium between amines formed and degraded finally determines the BA level in food (Restuccia et al. 2014). Tapingkae et al. (2010) have reported a histamine dehydrogenase enzyme purified from *Natrinema gari* BCC 24369 have an effect on degrading histamine in Thai fish sauce by 70%. Other methods include the use of microorganisms with BA decarboxylate activity and enzymes such as DAO. BA-degrading bacteria could be introduced into a food-processing step to degrade the BAs in the food, or the bacteria could be used as a starter for fermented foods. These strategies are potential control measures where it is difficult to control BA levels through the traditional means of refrigeration and to eliminate already formed BAs in food. However, these methods are not according to the general principles of food hygiene that rely on prevention rather than elimination of problems after they appear. Moreover, they have not been proven as effective and feasible (Restuccia et al. 2014).

Although some studies reported that if HHP is applied to raw material, a reduction in the number of bacteria may inhibit BA formation. Although reduction of BA concentrations has been shown in studies dealing with fish and meat, other papers reported an increase in BA concentration after HHP. Therefore, the effect of HHP is still unclear and need more investigation (Restuccia et al. 2014). Some safety organizations such as EFSA has great concern on amine toxicity, particularly in fermented foods. It has been underlined by the Question No. EFSA-Q-2009-00829, adopted on September 21, 2011, and by the technical reports drafted by the Rapid Alert System for Food and Feed (RASFF) (Leuschner et al. 2013). Following the annual meeting in 2009, EFSA issued a self-tasking mandates to the Panel on Biological Hazards on risk based control of BA formation in fermented foods (EFSA-Q-2009-00829). In this context, EFSA sent requests to the MRA Network to assist in the collation of data on BAs and on microbial contamination of fresh produce in the context of Regulation (URL-3).

5.8.5 Control of NAs in Foods

Many factors have been reported to influence NA formation or degradation in food (Yurchenko and Mölder 2006; Al Bulushi et al. 2009; Köse 2010). These are summarized as follows:

1. The level of nitrate and nitrite in food or water that is used to process food
2. The type of bacteria present in the product or contaminated via water (because some of them may accelerate nitrosating reaction and increase NA amount, e.g., bacteria can convert nitrate to nitrite)
3. The purity of salt has been shown to have inhibitory action on the formation of NAs, whereas impure salt, particularly with high nitrite content, can accelerate its formation

4. The pH of the product (low pH enhances NA formation in fish products, and the optimum pH for the formation of the highest levels of NAs has been found to be 3.8)
5. Species of the fish and the food type
6. The temperature (although *in vitro* formation of NPYR and NPIP has been found to occur at high temperature, such as 160°C for 2 hours, the reaction between nitrite and putrescine was found to occur at low temperature such as 22°C over 6 days)
7. The quality of food prior to processing (some fish can contain high amount of BAs that can affect NA formation)
8. The type of processing methods (e.g., the United States allows addition of $NaNO_2$ in smoked fish to prevent *C. botulinum*, but the EU does not allow it)

All these factors are studied *in vitro*; however, little is known about the effect of these factors *in vivo* (Al Bulushi et al. 2009). Thus, one expects that formation of NAs in food products produced from food containing high levels of BAs may be significant. Although NDMA and NPIP increase significantly in meat products treated with nitrite during storage, little is known about the impact of storage conditions on the formation of these compounds in fish products (Al Bulushi et al. 2009).

Ahn et al. (2003) reported that gamma irradiation has a possibility to reduce *N*-nitrosamines in salted and fermented anchovy sauce. They reported that NDMA and NPYR levels were decreased by radiation at 5 kGy or above after storage. Considering the possible effects on NA formation in fish products, it is advisable to use good quality fish and water, limited amount of nitrite, pure salt and apply GHP (Köse 2010). Nitrite level in foods is often regulated by the food authorities and products often recall due to failure of applying to the standards. Just recently, USDA (2015) has recalled approximately 12,566 pounds of beef, pork, and poultry products. Using $NaNO_3$ not declared on the product label was given among the reasons of rejection. Such amount of rejected products not only indicates the risk on food safety but also shows the high economical loss.

5.8.6 Control of BAs and Gizzerosine in Fish Meal

Histamine is usually found as the main amine which concerns food industry since its association with toxic effect with poultry, and therefore, low histamine levels leaded higher value for the products. It is reported that standard fish meal should contain lower histamine and gizzerosine contents reflecting to fresher raw material and the type of processing method. Maximum level in a standard fish meal for histamine is reported as 1000 mg/kg histamine. For standard/fair average quality products amine limits are generally not needed and therefore not normally specified (IFFO 2013). Pet feed producers also use fish meal and oil in their products. They prefer fish meal containing stickwater meal due to high gel binding ability; however, they also prefer low histamine value (Çağatay Yem 2011, Pers. Comm.). However, it is difficult to obtain low histamine value with fish meal containing solids from recovered stickwater by evaporators and dryers since it was demonstrated that most histamine in fish meal is accumulated in stickwater during cooking and high concentrations were observed (Köse 1993; Köse et al. 2003). It is known that the quality of fish meal and its price relate to its histamine content. Prime quality fish meal with less than 500 mg/kg of fish meal, will cost an average of 25% more per ton than common fish meal. Since histamine is heat stable, therefore, the best control must be at raw material stage. According to author's experience, although most fish meal plants have established in high capacity, in heavy fishing season, long storage period of raw materials at room temperature is often observed. Most fish meal processing companies do not apply chilled storage; however, better hygienic conditions are applied during transportation and storage prior to processing at many countries including Turkey. Due to recent attempts to produce fish oil by human consumption, GHP is also applied at these plants. It is reported that GE could be prevented by avoiding overheating of fish meal, using cimetidine in the diet and addition of antioxidants (e.g., ethoxyquin and butylated hydroxytoluene) for fish meal with a high fat content (Köse 1993).

5.9 CONCLUDING REMARKS

This chapter demonstrates us how foods rich in essential amino acids necessary for human healthy diet can also become a threat to our health if not treated in suitable conditions. Although food poisoning associated with BAs are not as deadly as other food intoxication incidents, HFP is listed among the top causes for seafood poisoning cases and many left unreported. Due to difficulties in tracking the affected patients, an efficient surveillance program to establish the true epidemiology of food poisoning caused by BAs is necessary. Most countries have the policy of "no report, no problem" and tracing usually relies on voluntary reports. Since 1970s, hundreds of publications and many official databases from various countries reported very high BA contents, particularly histamine above toxic levels for numerous food samples from different varieties state the high health risk from these amines. However, similar reports with low levels with the same food types indicate the prevention measures are often possible. An efficient HACCP plan covering all the stages of food line easily can prevent this health risk. Difficulties in preventing BA formation in fermented foods usually relate to microbiological issues and the temperature used in traditional products. Knowing the current developments in genetic engineering and advanced methodology in food microbiology, such as polymerase chain reaction (PCR) techniques, it is not difficult to obtain safe cultures for fermented food industry. Although prevention is usually done at manufacturer's step, the control is driven by government authorities. Both quantitative and qualitative reliable analytical methods exist for the use of each party. However, fast and reliable test methods usually designed for histamine analysis for regulatory purposes. It is advised that future studies should focus on "improvements in the surveillance programs covering all BA health risk," clarification on the decarboxylating activity of different strains of microorganisms, formation of gizzerosine in different foods, and the effect of different processing techniques on the formation and degradation, developing quick test methods for other BAs such as tyramine.

ACKNOWLEDGMENTS

The author appreciates the help of Dr. Nuran Kahriman for drawing chemical compounds.

REFERENCES

Ahn, H.J., J.H. Kim, C. Jo, H.S. Yook, H.J. Lee, and M.W. Byun. 2003. N-nitrosamine reduction in salted and fermented anchovy sauce by ionizing irradiation. *Food Cont.* 14: 553–557.

Alak, G., S.A. Hisar, O. Hisar, and H. Genççelep. 2011. Biogenic amines formation in Atlantic bonito (*Sarda sarda*) fillets packaged with modified atmosphere and vacuum, wrapped in chitosan and cling film at 4°C. *Eur. Food Res. Technol.* 232(1): 23–28.

Al Bulushi, I., S. Poole, H.C. Deeth, and G.A. Dykes. 2009. Biogenic amines in fish: Roles in intoxication, spoilage, and nitrosamine formation-A review. *Crit. Rev. Food Sci. Nutr.* 49(4): 369–377.

Andiç, S., H. Gençcelep, Y. Tunçtürk, and Ş. Köse. 2009. The effect of storage temperatures and packaging methods on properties of Motal cheese. *J. Dairy Sci.* 93: 849–859.

Anli, R.E., and M. Bayram. 2008. Biogenic amines in wines. *Food Rev. Int.* 25: 86–102.

Auerswald, L., Morren, C. and A.L. Lopata. 2006. Histamine levels in seventeen species of fresh and processed South African seafood. *Food Chem.* 98: 231–239.

Baixas-Nogueras, S., S. Bover-Cid, M.T. Veciana-Nogués, A. Mariné-Font, and M.C. Vidal-Carou. 2005. Biogenic amine index for freshness evaluation in iced Mediterranean hake (*Merluccius merluccius*). *J. Food Prot.* 68(11): 2433–2438.

Baranowski, J.D., H.A. Frank, P.A. Brust, M. Chongsiriwatana, and R.J. Premaratne. 1990. Decomposition and histamine content in mahi-mahi (*Coryphaena hippurus*). *J. Food Protect.* 53: 217–222.

Barnes, D.M., Y.K. Kirby, and K.G. Oliver. 2001. Effects of biogenic amines on the growth and the incidence of proventricular lesions in broiler chickens. *Poult. Sci.* 80(7): 906–911.

Blonz, E.R., and H.S. Olcott. 1978. Effects of orally ingested histamine and/or commercially canned spoiled skipjack tuna on pigs, cats, dogs and rabbits. *Comp. Biochem. Physiol. C.* 61(1): 161–163.

Bodmer, S., C. Imark, and M. Kneubühl. 1999. Biogenic amines in foods: Histamine and food processing. *Inflamm. Res.* 48(6): 296–300.

Bover-Cid, S., S. Torriani, V. Gatto, R. Tofalo, G. Suzzi, and N. Belletti. 2009. Relationships between microbial population dynamics and putrescine and cadaverine accumulation during dry fermented sausage ripening. *J. Appl. Microbiol.* 106(4): 1397–1407.

Brillantes, S., and W. Samosorn. 2001. Determination of histamine in fish sauce from Thailand using a solid phase extraction and high-performance liquid chromatography. *Fish. Sci.* 67: 1163–1168.

CDC. 2007. http://www.cdc.gov/mmwr/preview/mmwrhtml/mm5632a2.htm.

CDC. 2014. http://www.cdc.gov/foodborneoutbreaks/default.aspx

Chen, H.C., H.F. Kung, W.C. Chen, W.F. Lin, D.F. Hwang, Y.C. Lee, and Y.H. Tsai. 2008. Determination of histamine and histamine-forming bacteria in tuna dumpling implicated in a food-borne poisoning. *Food Chem.* 106: 612–618.

Chen, H.C., Y.R. Huang, H.H. Hsu, C.S. Lin, W.C. Chen, C.M. Lin, and Y.H. Tsai. 2010. Determination of histamine and biogenic amines in fish cubes (*Tetrapturus angustirostris*) implicated in a food-borne poisoning. *Food Cont.* 21: 13–18.

Chong, C.Y., F. Abu Bakar, A.R. Russly, B. Jamilah, and N.A Mahyudin. 2011. The effects of food processing on biogenic amines formation. *Int. Food Res. J.* 18(3): 867–876.

Cinquina, A.L, A. Calì, F. Longo, L. De Santis, A. Severoni, and F. Abballe. 2004. Determination of biogenic amines in fish tissues by ion-exchange chromatography with conductivity detection. *J. Chromatogr. A.* 1032: 73–77.

Dalgaard, P., J. Emborg, A. Kjølby, N.D. Sørensen, and N.Z. Ballin. 2008. Histamine and biogenic amines formation and importance in seafood. In: T. Børresen (ed) *Improving Seafood Products for the Consumer*, Cambridge, UK: Woodhead Publishing, pp. 292–324.

Dalgaard, P., H.L. Madsen, N. Samieian, and J. Emborg. 2006. Biogenic amine formation and microbial spoilage in chilled garfish (Belone belone belone) – effect of modified atmosphere packaging and previous frozen storage. *J. Appl. Microbiol.*, 101: 80–95.

Dossi, N., R. Toniola, A. Pizzariello, S. Susmel, and G. Bontempelli. 2011. A modified electrode for the electrochemical detection of biogenic amines and their amino precursors separated by microchip capillary electrophoresis. *Electrophoresis* 32: 906–912.

Du, W. X., C.M. Lin, A.T. Phu, J. Cornell, M. Marshall, and C.I. Wei. 2002. Development of biogenic amines in yellowfin tuna (Thunnus albacares): effect of storage and correlation with decarboxylase-positive bacterial flora. *J Food Sci.* 67: 292–301.

EC. 2005. Commission Regulation (EC) No 2073/2005No. 2073/2005. of 15 November 2005 on microbiological criteria for foodstuffs. (Text with EEA relevance). OJ L 338, 22.12.2005.

EC. 2007. Commission Regulation (EC) No 1441/2007 of 5 December 2007. Amending Regulation (EC) No 2073/2005 on microbiological criteria for foodstuffs. L 322/12-29. https://www.fsai.ie/uploadedFiles/Reg1441_2007(1).pdf.

Eerola, S., R. Hinkkanen, E. Lindfors, and T. Hirvi. 1993. Liquid chromatographic determination of biogenic amines in dry sausages. *J. AOAC Int.* 76(3): 575–577.

Eerola, H.S., Saugués, A.X.R. and T.K. Hirvi. 1998. Biogenic amines in Finnish dry sausages. *J. Food Safety.* 18:127–138.

EFSA. 2007. Opinion of the Scientific Committee on a request from EFSA on the introduction of a Qualified Presumption of Safety (QPS) approach for assessment of selected microorganisms referred to EFSA. *EFSA J.* 587: 1–16.

EFSA. 2011. Scientific opinion on risk based control of biogenic amine formation in fermented foods. *EFSA J.* 9(10): 2393.

Emborg, J., B.G. Laursen, and P. Dalgaard. 2005. Significant histamine formation in tuna (*Thunnus albacares*) at 2°C—effect of vacuum—and modified atmosphere-packaging on psychrotolerant bacteria. *Int. J. Food Microbiol.* 101: 263–279.

Epley, R.J., P.B. Addis, and J.J. Warthesen. 1992. Nitrite in meat. Available from University of Minnesota. Extension Service (http://www.extension.umn.edu/distribution/ nutrition/DJ0974.html). Posted February 5, 2007. (accessed April 5, 2016).

Ercan, S.Ş., H. Bozkurt, and Ç. Soysal. 2013. Significance of biogenic amines in foods and their reduction methods. *J. Food Sci. Engineer.* 3: 395–410.

EU. 1993. (93 / 11/EEC). Concerning the release of the N-nitrosamines and N-nitrosable substances from elastomer or rubber teats and soothers. *Off. J. Eur. Com.* No L 93/37. http://eur-lex.europa.eu/legal-content/HU/TXT/?uri=URISERV:l21088

Erim, F.B. 2013. Recent analytical approaches to the analysis of biogenic amines in food samples. *Trends Anal. Chem.* 52: 239–247.

Fairgrieve, W.T., M.S. Myers, R.W. Hardy, and F.M. Dong. 1994. Gastric abnormalities in rainbow trout (*Oncorhynchus mykiss*) fed amine-supplemented diets or chicken gizzard erosion-positive fish meal. *Aquaculture.* 127: 219–231.

FAO-WHO. 2013. Joint FAO/WHO Expert Meeting on the Public Health Risks of Histamine and Other Biogenic Amines from Fish and Fishery Products, July 23–27, 2012. Rome, Italy: FAO.

FDA. 2011. U.S. Department of Health and Human Services Food and Drug Administration, Center for Food Safety and Applied Nutrition. Fish and fishery products hazards and controls guidance. 4th edn. Available at http://www.fda.gov/FoodGuidances (accessed February 2, 2016).

Farkas, J. 2006. Irradiation for better foods. *Trends Food Sci. Technol.* 17: 148–152.

Federal Register. 1995. Decomposition and histamine raw, frozen tuna and mahi-mahi; canned tuna; and related species. *CPG 540.525.* 60(149): 39754–30956.

Feng, C., S. Teuber, and M.E. Gershwin. 2016. Histamine (Scombroid) fish poisoning: A Comprehensive review. *Clinic. Rev. Allerg. Immunol.* 50: 64–69.

Feldman, K.A., S.B. Werner, S. Cronan et al. 2005. A large outbreak of scombroid fish poisoning associated with eating escolar fish (Lepidocybium flavobrunneum). *Epid. Infect.* 133: 29–33.

Fletcher, G.C. (ed). 2010. Research of relevance to histamine poisoning in New Zealand. A review. *MAF Technical Paper No: 2011/70.* New Zealand: Ministry of Agriculture.

Gallas, L., E. Standarová, I. Steinhauserová, L. Steinhauser, and L. Vorlová. 2010. Formation of biogenic amines in chicken meat stored under modified atmosphere. *Acta Vet. Brno.* 79: S107–S116.

Gardini, F., F. Rossi, L. Rizzotti, S. Torriani, L. Grazia, C. Chiavari, F. Coloretti, and G. Tabanelli. 2012. Role of *Streptococcus thermophilus* PRI60 in histamine accumulation in cheese. *Int. Dairy J.* 27: 71–76.

Gianotti, V., U. Chiuminatto, E. Mazzucco, F. Gosetti, M. Bottaro, P. Frascarolo, and M. Gennaro. 2008. A new hydrophilic interaction liquid chromatography tandem mass spectrometry method for the simultaneous determination of seven biogenic amines in cheese. *J. Chromatogr. A.* 1185: 296–300.

Ginterová, P., J. Marák, A. Staňová, V. Maier, J. Ševčík, and D. Kaniansky. 2012. Determination of selected biogenic amines in red wines by automated online combination of capillary isotachophoresis-capillary zone electrophoresis. *J. Chromatogr. B.* 904: 135–139.

Gosetti, F., E. Mazzucco, V. Gianotti, S. Polati, and M.C. Gennaro. 2007. High performance liquid chromatography/tandem mass spectrometry determination of biogenic amines in typical Piedmont cheeses. *J. Chromatogr. A.* 1149: 151–157.

Gökoğlu, N. 2003. Changes in biogenic amines during maturation of sardine (*Sardina pilchardus*) marinade. *Fish Sci.* 69: 823–829.

Halász, A., A. Baràth, L. Simon-Sarkadi, and W. Holzapfel. 1994. Biogenic amines and their production by microorganisms in food. *Trends Food Sci. Technol.* 5: 42–49.

Hall, M. 2003. Something fishy: Six patients with an unusual cause of food poisoning. *Emerg. Med. (Fremantle)* 15(3): 293–295.

Harry, E.C., J.F. Tucker, and A.P. Lauresen. 1975. The role of histamine and fish meal in the incidence of gizzard erosion and pro-ventricular abnormalities in the fowl. *Br. Poult. Sci.* 16: 69–78.

Huang, D.P., J.H.C. Ho, K.S. Webb, B.J. Wood, and T.A. Gough. 1981. Volatile nitrosamines in salt-preserved fish before and after cooking. *Food Cosmet. Toxicol.* 19: 167–171.

Hu, Y., Z. Huang, J. Li, and H. Yang. 2012. Concentrations of biogenic amines in fish, squid and octopus and their changes during storage. *Food Chem.* 135: 2604–2611.

Hungerford, J.M. 2010. Scombroid poisoning: A review. *Toxicon.* 56: 231–243.

Hungerford, J.M., and W.H. Wu. 2012. Comparison study of three rapid test kits for histamine in fish: BiooScientific MaxSignal enzymatic assay, Neogen Veratox ELISA, and the Neogen Reveal Histamine Screening test. *Food Cont.* 25. 448–457.

IFFO. 2013. http://www.iffo.net (accessed April 23, 2013).

Jairath, G., P.K. Singh, R.S. Dabur, M. Rani, and M. Chaudhari. 2015. Biogenic amines in meat and meat products and its public health significance: A review. *J. Food Sci. Technol.* 52(11): 6835–6846.

James, C., S. Derrick, G. Purnell, and S.J. James. 2013. Review of the risk management practices employed throughout the fish processing chain in relation to controlling histamine formation in at-risk fish species. FSAS Project. Grimsby, UK: Grimsby Institute.

Kalač, P., J. Šavel, M. Kržek, T. Pelikánová, and M. Prokopová. 2002. Biogenic amine formation in bottled beer. *Food Chem.* 79: 431–434.

Kanki, M., T. Yoda, M. Ishibashi, and T. Tsukamoto. 2004. Photobacterium phosphoreum caused a histamine fish poisoning incident. *Int J Food Microbiol.* 92: 79–87.

Kantaria, U.D., and R.H. Gokani. 2011. Quality and safety of biogenic amines. Int. J. Res. Pharm. *Biomedic. Sci.* 2(4): 1461–1468.

Karovičová, J. and Z. Kohajdová. 2005. Biogenic Amines in Food. *Chem. Pap.* 59(1): 70–79.

Kim, J.H., D.H. Kim, H.J. Ahn, H.J. Park, and M.W. Byun. 2005. Reduction of the biogenic amine contents in low salt-fermented soybean paste by gamma irradiation. *Food Cont.* 16(1): 43–49.

Koral, S., and S. Köse. 2012. The effect of filleting and ice application on the quality and safety of Atlantic bonito (*Sarda sarda*) at refrigerated storage. *Int. J. Food Sci. Technol.* 47: 210–220.

Koral, S., and S. Köse. 2015. Evaluation of biogenic amine development of anchovy (*Engraulis encrasicolus*) muscle compared to its quality changes at different chilling conditions. *J. Food Health Sci.* 1(3): 150–165.

Koral, S., B. Tufan, A. Ščavničar, D. Kočar, M. Pompe, and S. Köse. 2013. Investigation of the contents of biogenic amines and some food safety parameters of various commercially salted fish products. *Food Cont.* 32: 597–606.

Köse, S. 1993. Investigation into toxins and pathogens in fish meal production. PhD Thesis Loughborough, UK: Loughborough University Tech.

Köse, S. 2010. Evaluation of seafood safety health hazards for traditional fish products: Preventive measures and monitoring issues. *Turkish J. Fish. Aquatic Sci.* 10: 139–160.

Köse, S., B. Tufan, and S. Koral. 2015. Determining the quality changes of salted anchovies produced from previously frozen raw material for a year. *World Seafood Congress 2015*. September 5-10, Grimsby, UK. http://www.seafish.org/about-seafish/news-and-events/events/world-seafood-congress-september-2015.

Köse, S., N. Kaklıkkaya, S. Koral, B. Tufan, K.C. Buruk, and F. Aydın. 2011. Commercial test kits and the determination of histamine in traditional (ethnic) fish products-evaluation against an EU accepted HPLC method. *Food Chem.* 125: 1490–1497.

Köse, S., P. Quantick, and G. Hall. 2003. Changes in the levels of histamine during processing and storage of fish meal. *Anim. Feed Sci. Technol.* 107: 161–172.

Köse, S., S. Koral, B. Tufan, M. Pompe, A. Ščavničar, and D. Kočar. 2012. Biogenic amine contents of commercially processed traditional fish products originating from European countries and Turkey. *Eur. Food Res. Technol.* 235: 669–683.

Komprda, T., D. Smela, P. Pechova, L. Kalhotka, J. Stencl, and B. Klejdus. 2004. Effect of starter culture, spice mix and storage time and temperature on biogenic amine content of dry fermented sausages. *Meat Sci.* 67: 607–616.

Kučerová, K., H. Svobodová, S. Tuma, I. Ondráčková, and M. Plockvá. 2009. Production of biogenic amines by *Enterococci*. *Czech J. Food Sci.* 27(2): S50–S55.

Kuda, T., Y. Izawa, S. Ishii, H. Takahashi, Y. Torido, and B. Kimura. 2012. Suppressive effect of *Tetragenococcus halophilus,* isolated from fish-nukazuke, on histamine accumulation in salted and fermented fish. *Food Chem.* 130: 569–574.

Latorre-Moratalla, M.L., S. Bover-Cid, J. Bosch-Fusté, M.T. Veciana-Nogués, and M.C. Vidal-Carou. 2014. Amino acid availability as an influential factor on the biogenic amine formation in dry fermented sausages. *Food Cont.* 36: 76–81.

Lavon, O., Y. Lurie, and Y. Bentur. 2008. Scombroid fish poisoning in Israel, 2005–2007. *Israel Med. Assoc. J.* 10: 789–792.

Lehane, L., and J. Olley. 2000. Histamine fish poisoning revisited. *Int J. Food Microbiol.* 58(1–2): 1–37.
Leuschner, R.G.K., H. Aglika, T. Robinson, and M. Hugas. 2013. The Rapid Alert System for Food and Feed (RASFF) database in support of risk analysis of biogenic amines in food. *J. Food Comp. Anal.* 29: 37–42.
Mah, J.H., and H.J. Hwang. 2009. Effects of food additives on biogenic amine formation in *Myeolchi-jeot*, a salted and fermented anchovy (*Engraulis japonicus*). *Food Chem.* 114: 168–173.
Mackie, I.M., L. Pirie, A.H. Ritchie, and H. Yamanka. 1997. The formation of non-volatile amines in relation to concentrations of free basic amino acids during postmortem storage of the muscle of scallop (Pecten maximus), herring (Clupea harengus) and mackerel (Scomber scombrus). *Food Chem.* 60: 291–295.
Marcobal, A., B. de las Rivas, M.V. Moreno-Arribas, and R. Muñoz. 2006. Evidence for horizontal gene transfer as origin of putrescine production in *Oenococcus oeni* RM83. *App. Environ. Microbiol.* 72: 7954–7958.
Mendes, R. 1999. Changes in biogenic amines of major Portuguese bluefish species during storage at different temperatures. *J Food Biochem.* 23: 33–43.
Mietz, J.L., and E. Karmas. 1977. Chemical index of canned tuna determined by high-pressure liquid chromatography. *J. Food Sci.* 42: 155–158.
Miki, M., Ishikawa, T. and H. Okayama. 2005. An outbreak of histamine poisoning after ingestion of the ground saury paste in eight patients taking isoniazid in tuberculous ward. *Intern. Med.* 44: 1133–1136.
Millán, R., Izquierdo, P., Allara, M., Torres, G., García, A. and Y. Barboza. 2003. Effect of temperature and storage time on microbial quality and histamine production in Lisa (Mugil curema). *Revista Científica.* 13(5): 339–346.
Montel, M.C., S. Buchin, A. Mallet, C. Delbes-Paus, D.A. Vuitton, N. Desmasures, and F. Berthier. 2014. Traditional cheeses: Rich and diverse microbiota with associated benefits. *Int. J. Food Microbiol.* 177: 136–154.
Naila, A., S. Flint, G. Fletcher, P. Bremer, and G. Meerdink. 2010. Control of biogenic amines in food – Existing and emerging approaches. *J Food Sci.* 75(7): R139–R150.
Niven, C.F., M.B. Jeffrey, and D.A. Corlett. 1981. Differential plating medium for quantitative detection of histamine-producing bacteria. *Appl. Env. Microbiol.* 41(1): 321–322.
Novella-Rodríguez, S., M.T. Veciana-Nogués, A. Trujillo-Mesa, and M.C. Vidal-Carou. 2002. Profile of biogenic amines in goat cheese made from pasteurized and pressurized milks. *J. Food Sci.* 67: 2940–2944.
Nyachuba, D.G., C.W. Donnelly, and A.B. Howard. 2007. Impact of nitrite on detection of *Listeria monocytogenes* in selected ready-to-eat (RTE) meat and seafood products. *J. Food Sci.* 72(7): M267–M275.
Ochiai, M., K. Wakabayashi, M. Nagao, and T. Sugimura. 1984. Tyramine is a major mutagen precursor in soya sauce, being convertible to a mutagen by nitrite. *Gann* 75(1): 1–3.
Oliveira, C.P., M.B.A. Glória, J.F. Barbour, and R.A. Scanlan. 1995. Nitrate, nitrite, and volatile nitrosamines in whey-containing food products. *J. Agric. Food Chem.* 43: 967–969.
Opstvedt, J., H. Mundheim, E. Nygard, H. Aase, and I.H. Pike. 2000. Reduced growth and feed consumption of Atlantic salmon (*Salmo salar* L.) fed fish meal made from stale fish is not due to increased content of biogenic amines. *Aquaculture* 188: 323–337.
Özogul, F., and Y. Özogul 2006. Biogenic amine content and biogenic amine quality indices of sardines (*Sardina pilchardus*) stored in modified atmosphere packing and vacuum packing. *Food Chem.* 99: 574–578.
Paleologos, E.K., S.D. Chytiri, I.N. Savvaidis, and M.G. Kontominas. 2003. Determination of biogenic amines as their benzoyl derivatives after cloud point extraction with micellar liquid chromatographic separation. *J. Chromatogr. A.* 1010: 217–224.
Papavergou, E.J., I.N. Savvaidis, and I.A. Ambrosiadis. 2012 Levels of biogenic amines in retail market fermented meat products. *Food Chem.* 135: 2750–2755.

Pensabene, J.W., W. Fiddler, R.A. Gates, J.C. Fagan, and A.E. Wasserman. 1974. Effect of frying and other cooking conditions on nitrosopyrrolidine formation in bacon. *J. Food Sci.* 39(2): 314–316.

Pons-Sánchez-Cascado, S., M.T. Veciana-Nogués, S. Bover-Cid, A. Mariné-Font, and M.C. Vidal-Carou. 2006. Use of volatile and non-volatile amines to evaluate the freshness of anchovies stored in ice. *J. Sci. Food Agri.* 86: 699–705.

Prester, L. 2011. Biogenic amines in fish, fish products and shellfish: A review. *Food Add. Contam. Part A.* 28(11): 1547–1560.

Prester, L.J., J. Macan, V.M. Varnai, T. Orct, J. Vukušič, and D. Kipčic. 2009. Endotoxin and biogenic amine levels in Atlantic mackerel (*Scomber scombrus*), sardine (*Sardina pilchardus*) and Mediterranean hake (*Merluccius merluccius*) stored at 22°C. *Food Add. Contam.* 26: 355–362.

Restuccia, D., U.G. Spizzirri, F. Puoci, G. Cirillo, M. Curcio, O.I. Parisi, F. Iemma, and N.A. Picci. 2011. A new method for the determination of biogenic amines in cheese by LC with evaporative light scattering detector. *Talanta* 85: 363–369.

Restuccia, D., U.G. Spizzirri, F. Puoci, I.O. Parisi, M. Curcio, and N. Picci. 2014. Accumulation of biogenic amines in foods: Hazard identification and control options. In: R.R. Rai and J.A. Bai (eds) *Microbial Food Safety and Preservation Techniques.* Boca Raton, FL: CRC Press, pp. 53–74, Chapter 4.

Romero-González, R., M.I. Alarcón-Flores, J.L.M. Vidal, and A.G. Frenich. 2012. Simultaneous determination of four biogenic and three volatile amines in anchovy by ultra-high-performance liquid chromatography coupled to tandem mass spectrometry. *J. Agric. Food Chem.* 60: 5324–5329.

Rogers, P.L., and W.F. Staruszkiewicz. 2000. Histamine test kit comparison. *J. Aquatic Food Product Technol.* 9(2): 5–17.

Rossano, R., L. Mastrangelo, N. Ungaro, and P. Riccio. 2006. Influence of storage temperature and freezing time on histamine level in the European anchovy *Engraulis encrasicolus* (L., 1758): A study by capillary electrophoresis. *J. Chromatogr. B.* 830: 161–164.

Rossi, S, C. Lee, P.C. Ellis, and L.F. Pivarnik. 2002. Biogenic amines formation in bigeye tuna steaks and whole skipjack tuna. *J. Food Sci.* 67(6): 2056–2060.

Ruiz-Capillas, C., and F. Jiménez-Colmenero. 2004. Biogenic amines in meat and meat products. *Crit. Rev. Food Sci.* 44: 489–499.

Russo, P., G. Spano, M.P. Arena, V. Capozzi, F. Grieco, and L. Beneduece. 2010. Are consumers aware of the risks related to biogenic amines in food? *Current Res. Technol. Education Top. App. Microbiol. Micr. Biotechnol.* 2: 1087–1095.

Saccani, G., E. Tanzi, P. Pastore, S. Cavalli, and M. Rey. 2005. Determination of biogenic amines in fresh and processed meat by suppressed ion chromatography-mass spectrometry using a cation-exchange column. *J. Chromatogr. A.* 1082: 43–50.

Sagratini, G., M. Fernández-Franzón, F. De Berardinis, G. Font, S. Vittori, and J. Mañes. 2012. Simultaneous determination of eight underivatised biogenic amines in fish by solid phase extraction and liquid chromatography-tandem mass spectrometry. *Food Chem.* 132: 537–543.

Sato, M., Z.H. Tao, K. Shiozaki, T. Nakano, T. Yamaguchi, T. Yokoyama, N. Kan-No, and E. Nagahisa. 2006. A simple and rapid method for the analysis of fish histamine by paper electrophoresis. *Fish. Sci.* 72: 889–892.

Self, R.L., W.H. Wu, and H.S. Marks. 2011. Simultaneous quantification of eight biogenic amine compounds in tuna by matrix solid-phase dispersion followed by HPLC orbitrap mass spectrometry. *J. Agr. Food Chem.* 59: 5906–5913.

Shalaby, A.R. 1996. Significance of biogenic amines in food safety and human health. *Food Res. Int.* 29: 675–690.

Silla Santos, M.H. 1996. Biogenic amines: Their importance in food. *Int. J. Food Mic.* 29: 213–231.

Sirocchi, V., G. Caprioli, M. Ricciutelli, S. Vittori, and G. Sagratini. 2014. Simultaneous determination of ten underivatized biogenic amines in meat by liquid chromatography-tandem mass spectrometry (HPLC-MS/MS). *J. Mass Spectrom.* 49: 819–825.

Smit, A.Y., W.J. du Toit, M. Stander, and M. du Toit. 2013. Evaluating the influence of maceration practices on biogenic amine formation in wine. *LWT-Food Sci. Technol.* 53: 297–307.

Song, Y., Z. Quan, J.L. Evens, E.A. Byrd, and Y.M. Liu. 2004. Enhancing capillary liquid chromatography/tandem mass spectrometry of biogenic amines by pre-column derivatization with 7-fluoro-4-nitrobenzoxadiazole. *Rapid Commun. Mass Spectrom.* 18: 989–994.

Spizzirri, U.G., D. Restuccia, M. Curcio, O.I. Parisi, F. Iemma, and N. Picci. 2013. Determination of biogenic amines in different cheese samples by LC with evaporative light scattering detector. *J. Food Comp. Anal.* 29: 43–51.

Stadnik, J., and Z.J. Dolatowski. 2010. Biogenic amines in meat and fermented meat products. *Acta Sci. Pol. Technol. Aliment.* 9(3): 251–263.

Staruszkiewicz, W.F., J.D. Barnett, P.L. Rogers, R.A. Jr. Benner, L.L. Wong, and J. Cook. 2004. Effects of on-board and dockside handling on the formation of biogenic amines in mahi-mahi (*Coryphaena hippurus*), skipjack tuna (*Katsuwonus pelamis*), and yellowfin tuna (*Thunnus albacares*). *J. Food Prot.* 67(1): 134–141.

Sun, J., H.X. Guo, D. Semin, and J. Cheetham. 2011. Direct separation and detection of biogenic amines by ion-pair liquid chromatography with chemiluminescent nitrogen detector. *J. Chromatogr. A.* 1218: 4689–4697.

Suzzi, G., and F. Gardini. 2003. Biogenic amines in dry fermented sausages: A review. *Int. J. Food Microbiol.* 88: 41–54.

Tao, Z., M. Sato, K. Wu, H. Kiyota, T. Yamaguchi, and T. Nakano. 2012. A simple, rapid method for gizzerosine analysis in fish meal by paper electrophoresis. *Fish Sci.* 78: 923–926.

Tapia-Salazar, M., T.K. Smith, A. Harris, D. Ricque-Marie, and L.E. Cruz-Suarez. 2001. Effect of dietary histamine supplementation on growth and tissue amine concentrations in blue shrimp *Litopenaeus stylirostris*. *Aquaculture* 193: 281–289.

Tapingkae, W., S. Tanasupawat, K.L. Parkin, S. Benjakul, and W. Visessanguan. 2010. Degradation of histamine by extremely halophilic archaea isolated from high salt-fermented fishery products. *Enzyme Microb. Technol.* 46(2): 92–99.

Tsai, Y.H., H.F. Kung, T.M. Lee, Y.C. Lee, H.F. Kung, C.H. Wu, H.M. Hsu, H.C. Chen, T.C. Huang, and Y.H. Tsai. 2005. Determination of histamine in canned mackerel implicated in a foodborne poisoning. *Food Cont.* 16(7): 579–585.

Tsai, Y.H., H.F. Kung, H.C. Chen, S.C. Chang, H.H. Hsu, and C.I. Wei. 2007b. Determination of histamine and histamine-forming bacteria in dried milkfish (*Chanos chanos*) implicated in a food-borne poisoning. *Food Chem.* 105: 1289–1296.

Tsai, Y.H., H.S. Hsieh, H.C. Chen, S.H. Cheng, T. Chai, and D.F. Hwang. 2007a. Histamine level and species identification of billfish meats implicated in two food-borne poisoning. *Food Chem.* 104: 1366–1371.

URL-1.http://www.cdc.gov/foodsafety/outbreaks/investigating-outbreaks/confirming_diagnosis.html

URL-2. http://www.ldn.de/

URL-3. EC 2073 / 2005. http://www.efsa.europa.eu/en/supporting/pub/89e

USDA. 2015. http://www.fsis.usda.gov/wps/portal/fsis/topics/recalls-and-public-health-alerts/current-recalls-and-alerts (accessed on November 2015).

Veciana-Nogués, M.T., A. Marineé-Font, and M.C. Vidal-Carou. 1997. Biogenic amines as hygienic quality indicators of tuna. Relationships with microbial counts, ATP-related compounds, volatile amines and organoleptic changes. *J. Agr. Food Chem.* 45: 2036–2041.

Visciano, P G. Campana, L. Annunziata, A. Vergara, and A. Ianieri. 2007. Effect of storage temperature on histamine formation in *Sardina Pilchardus* and *Engraulis Encrasicolus* after catch. *J. Food Biochem.* 31: 577–588.

Yurchenko, S., and U. Molder. 2006. Volatile N-Nitrosamines in various fish products. *Food Chem.* 96: 325–333.

Zare, D., K. Muhammad, M.H. Bejo, and H.M. Ghazali. 2013. Changes in uracanic acid, histamine, putrescine and cadaverine levels in Indian mackerel (Rastrelliger kanagurta) during storage at different temperatures. *Food Chem.* 139: 320–325.

Zhao, Q.X., J. Xu, C.H. Xue, W.J. Sheng, R.C. Gao, Y. Xue, and Z.J. Li. 2007. Determination of biogenic amines in squid and white prawn by high-performance liquid chromatography with postcolumn derivatization. *J Agric Food Chem.* 55: 3083–3088.

6 Mycotoxins

Sui-Sheng T. Hua, Perng-Kuang Chang, and Jeffrey Palumbo

CONTENTS

6.1 INTRODUCTION

Mycotoxins are naturally occurring toxins produced by filamentous fungi that affect many agricultural crops. Over 300 mycotoxins have been identified, of which about 20 have been shown to occur naturally in food at sufficient levels posing food safety concerns (Bennet and Klich 2003; Wild and Gong 2009; Wu et al. 2014). The majority of these toxins are produced by fungi in the genera, *Aspergillus*, *Penicillium*, and *Fusarium*. The most commonly occurring mycotoxins are aflatoxins (B_1, B_2, G_1, G_2, and M_1), ochratoxin A (OTA), patulin, citrinin, sterigmatocystin, fumonisins (B_1, B_2, and B_3), zearalenone, T-2 and HT-2 toxins, nivalenol, and deoxynivalenol (DON). Among them, aflatoxin B_1 (AFB_1), which is hepatocarcinogenic, poses greatest threat to human health, especially in individuals with hepatitis B (Henry et al. 1999, 2002). Others also present a health threat. For instance, OTA has been shown to cause cancer of the kidneys in animals. Exposure to high levels of fumonisins (B_1, B_2, and B_3) has also been reported to cause liver and kidney damages in experimental animals (Peraica et al. 1999; Wild and Gong, 2009; Wu et al. 2014). The mycotoxins discussed in this chapter are aflatoxins, ochratoxins, ochratoxins A, fumonisins, patunin, and citrinin.

Mycotoxin content in food is monitored and regulated in many countries around the world. Currently, more than 100 countries have regulations regarding mycotoxin levels in the food and feed (van Egmond et al. 2007). In the United States, the Food and Drug Administration (FDA) has set the maximum total aflatoxins limit for tree nuts that are intended for human consumption at 20 ng g^{-1} (Food and Drug Administration 1996). The European Union (EU), a major importer of California tree nuts and dry fruits, has in the past applied tolerance levels as low as 2 ng g^{-1} for AFB_1 and 4 ng g^{-1} for total aflatoxins (European Commission 2005, 2006). These limits have recently been somewhat relaxed, with current allowable limits of 8 ng g^{-1} for AFB_1 and 10 ng g^{-1} for total aflatoxins (Commission Regulation (EU) No 165/2010). The European Commission's Scientific Committee for Food has set a limit at 5 ng g^{-1} OTA in dried fruit intended for direct consumption. EU regulatory limits for fumonisins in maize range from 0.2 to 2 ng g^{-1} and US FDA recommended limits are 2–4 ng g^{-1}.

Undoubtedly, mycotoxin is a unique challenge to food safety worldwide. According to FAO, at least 25% of the world's food crops are contaminated with mycotoxins, at a time when the production of agricultural commodities is barely sustaining the increasing population (Boutrif and Canet 1998). The global volume of such agricultural products as maize, groundnuts, copra, palm nuts, and oilseed cake, which are high-risk commodities, is about 100–200 million tonnes of which come from the developing countries (FAO 1997). The disposal of contaminated products or their diversion to nonhuman uses is not always practical and could seriously compromise the world food supply. Efforts to reduce and eliminate mycotoxins in human foods and animal feedstuffs are based on two major concerns: (1) the adverse effects of mycotoxin-contaminated crops or feeds on human or animal health and productivity and (2) potential residues of mycotoxins or toxic metabolites in edible animal food products.

Reducing mycotoxin levels in food is a high-priority research. Preharvest interventions include production of genetically enhanced resistant crops, development of appropriate agronomic practices, determination of optimal stage for harvesting crops, and investigation of novel biocontrol and chemical control methods. Postharvest contamination by mycotoxigenic fungi usually occurs during storage and transportation and is normally a consequence of improper drying or exposure of the product to condensation or rain. Potential postharvest control measures include optimizing storage and transportation conditions, sorting to remove contaminated product, and applying chemical methods to prevent fungal growth. The development of biological control methods based on ecological and environmental parameters will be reviewed in this chapter.

6.2 AFLATOXIN: SOURCES, AFFECTED FOODS, AND BIOSYNTHESIS

Aflatoxins are a family of fungal secondary metabolites exclusively produced by species in the genus of *Aspergillus*. The commonly recognized species that produce aflatoxins are *A. flavus*, *A. parasiticus*, *A. nomius*, *A. tamarii*, *A. pseudotamarii*, *A. bombycis*, *A. ochraceoroseus*, *A. parvisclerotigenus*, *A. minisclerotigenes*, and *A. arachidicola* (Cary et al. 2005; Pildain et al. 2008; Varga et al. 2010).

Aflatoxin contamination of agricultural commodities mainly corn, peanuts, tree nuts often arises from field conditions conducive to fungal growth such as insect damages and environmental stresses, for example, high heat and drought to the host plants before harvest. Aflatoxins are believed to be primarily produced by the two species of *A. flavus* and *A. parasiticus*. The former makes only aflatoxins B_1 and B_2, whereas the latter makes four major aflatoxins, B_1, B_2, G_1 and G_2. The B-type aflatoxins show blue fluorescence under long-wave ultra violet light and are different from the green fluorescent G-type aflatoxins. Recently, *A. nomius*, which produces both B- and G-type aflatoxins, has been reported to be the most common species found in Brazil nuts (Calderari et al. 2013). Contamination of crops by aflatoxins is a global concern because of associated economical losses that result from inferior crop quality, reduced animal productivity, and impacts on international trade and public health.

To minimize human exposure to aflatoxins, 48 countries have specific regulations limiting total aflatoxins in foodstuffs and 21 countries have regulations for aflatoxins in feedstuffs (FAO 1995). In the United States, FDA has established regulatory guidelines to prevent the sale of commodities if contamination by aflatoxins exceeds allowed levels. The FDA has set limits of 20 ng g^{-1} total aflatoxins for interstate commerce of food and feedstuff and 0.5 ng g^{-1} aflatoxin M_1 in milk. The European Commission has set the limits on groundnuts to be further processed at 15 ng g^{-1} for total aflatoxins and 8 ng g^{-1} for AFB_1 and for nuts and dried fruits subject to further processing at 10 ng g^{-1} for total aflatoxins and 5 ng g^{-1} for AFB_1. The aflatoxin standards for cereals, dried fruits, and nuts intended for direct human consumption are even more stringent, and the limit for total aflatoxins is 4 and 2 ng g^{-1} for AFB_1 (Otsuki et al. 2001; Molyneux et al. 2007; Trucksess and Scott 2008). The detection of high levels of aflatoxins in Brazil nuts has been widely reported by several importing countries. Codex Alimentarius Commission thus has recommended limits for aflatoxins in Brazil nuts for further processing to be set at 15 ng g^{-1} and for direct consumption at 10 ng g^{-1} (Calderari et al. 2013, IJFM).

A. flavus has a broad ecological niche and can reproduce abundantly (Hedayati et al. 2007). Genetic diversity of *A. flavus* populations has been demonstrated by vegetative compatibility grouping (VCG) and DNA fingerprinting (Horn and Green 1995; McAlpin et al. 2005; Hua et al. 2006, 2012). The spores of *A. flavus* can infect wounded plant tissues (Diener et al. 1987; Horn et al. 2005). Infection of corn, peanuts, cotton seeds, almonds, or pistachios by *A. flavus* creates the potential for production of aflatoxins. Although in many cases the sources of infections are unknown. The fungal spores can be found in the soil or in the air. Contamination may spread from previously infested almonds (mummy nuts) or other pests. Spores can be transferred by the navel orangeworm (NOW) and grow on nut meats. Aflatoxin contamination is aggravated by factors such as insect damage, drought, and high temperatures.

Technology advancement in DNA sequencing has provided a powerful tool to study genes and genetics of aflatoxin biosynthesis at the genome scale. The aflatoxin gene cluster is located on chromosome III near a subtelomeric region (Yu et al. 2004; Payne et al. 2008). The genome sequence data have been deposited in the National Center for Biotechnology Information (NCBI) GenBank database (http://www.ncbi.nlm.nih.gov) under accession AAIH02000000. The data are also available through the *A. flavus* website (http://www.aspergillusflavus.org). The *A. parasiticus* strain SU-1 genome has recently been sequenced (Linz et al. 2014). Like *A. flavus*, *A. parasiticus* also contains eight chromosomes. In *A. flavus* and *A. parasiticus*, a complete aflatoxin pathway gene cluster consisting of 30 genes has been confirmed within an 80 kb DNA sequence. More than 25 genes are involved in the biosynthesis of aflatoxins via the polyketide pathway.

A regulatory gene, *aflR*, and a coregulatory gene, *aflJ* (*aflS*) are required for the expression of several identified genes in the pathway (Amaike and Keller 2011). At least 16 enzyme-catalyzed steps are required to complete the synthesis of AFB_1 from norsolorinic acid, the first stable intermediate. Other advanced techniques such as DNA microarrays and RNA sequencing (RNA-Seq) have been developed to study genome-wide gene expression. These approaches have proved a wealth of information with regard to how biotic factor such as major regulators of LaeA (Georgianna et al. 2010), VeA (Cary et al. 2015) and NsdC (Gilbert et al. 2016), and abiotic factor, for example, volatiles (Chang et al. 2014, 2015; Hua et al. 2014), inhibitor (Lin et al. 2013), and water activity (Zhang et al. 2014) influence expression of aflatoxin biosynthesis genes.

6.3 OCHRATOXINS: SOURCES AND AFFECTED FOODS

Ochratoxins are pentaketide mycotoxins composed of dihydroisocoumarin covalently linked to β-phenylalanine. The form that most commonly occurs in food is OTA, which is also the most toxic. At least 29 species of *Aspergillus* and *Penicillium* are known to produce OTA. The OTA-producing *Aspergillus* species belong to subgenus *Circumdati*, among sections *Circumdati, Nigri*, and *Flavi*. Members of section *Circumdati* that have been shown to produce OTA include *A. ochraceus*, *A. steynii*, *A. westerdijkiae*, *A. affinis*, *A. cretensis*, *A. flocculosus*, *A. fresenii* (formerly *A. sulphureus*), *A. muricatus*, *A. pseudoelegans*, *A. roseoglobosus*, *A. occultus*, and *A. pulvericola*. Other species that are weak or inconsistent producers under laboratory conditions include *A. ostianus, A. melleus, A. persii, A. salwaensis*, *A. sclerotiorum*, *A. subramanianii*, and *A. westlandensis* (Frisvad et al. 2004; Visagie et al. 2014). In section *Nigri*, the species identified as OTA producers are *A. carbonarius*, *A. niger*, *A. welwitschiae*, *A. lacticoffeatus*, and *A. sclerotioniger* (Samson et al. 2004; Nielsen et al. 2009). *A. tubingensis* has variously been reported as OTA-producing and OTA-nonproducing, but there is evidence that extrolytes from *A. tubingensis* with similar high-performance liquid chromatography (HPLC) retention patterns likely were misidentified as OTA (Storari et al. 2012). *A. alliaceus* and synonymous or closely related species *A. albertensis* and *A. lanosus* are OTA-producing members of section *Flavi* (Bayman et al. 2002; McAlpin and Wicklow 2005). The only *Penicillium* species confirmed to produce OTA are *P. verrucosum* and *P. nordicum* (Cabañes et al. 2010).

Several food products have the potential to be contaminated with OTA. Cereals, such as barley, oats, wheat, and rice, are at risk for OTA contamination. The most likely source for OTA contamination in grains grown in temperate and cool climates is *P. verrucosum* (Duarte et al. 2010). Because many food processing steps do not remove or destroy OTA, products derived from those grains, including beer and breakfast cereals, also are at risk for OTA contamination (Mateo et al. 2007; Lee and Ryu 2015). In warmer, subtropical and tropical climates, coffee, cocoa, dried fruits, and nuts are at risk for OTA contamination, in which *A. ochraceus*, *A. westerdijkiae*, and *A. steynii* are the most frequent producers (Logrieco et al. 2003). *A. carbonarius* and to a lesser extent *A. niger* are the most likely sources of OTA contamination in grapes and grape products including wine and raisins (Mateo et al. 2007; Palumbo et al. 2015).

6.4 *FUSARIUM* MYCOTOXINS: SOURCES AND AFFECTED FOODS

Fusarium species and other fungi produce several classes of mycotoxins, including fumonisins, trichothecenes, and zearalenone. *Fusarium verticillioides* (formerly *F. moniliforme*) and *F. proliferatum* are the major sources of fumonisins (FB_1, FB_2, and FB_3) due to their widespread occurrence on corn (Rheeder et al. 2002). More recently, *A. niger* and *A. welwitschiae* were discovered to produce fumonisins (FB_2 and FB_4), which may then become contaminants in grapes and wine (Frisvad et al. 2007; Logrieco et al. 2009; Mogensen et al. 2010; Knudsen et al. 2011; Palumbo et al. 2011).

Trichothecene mycotoxins, such as T-2 toxin, DON and nivalenol, and zearalenone are major classes of mycotoxins produced by *Fusarium* species, including *F. sporotrichioides*, *F. graminearum*, and *F. culmorum*. While there is evidence suggesting human toxicity, the importance of these mycotoxins in agriculture is considered largely to be with regard to their presence in animal feeds. This group of toxins has been reviewed elsewhere (e.g., Yazar and Omurtag 2008) and will not be discussed in this chapter.

6.5 PATULIN AND CITRININ: SOURCES AND AFFECTED FOODS

Patulin is a polyketide lactone mycotoxin produced by approximately 60 species of fungi in 30 genera. The primary patulin producers of importance to food production are *Penicillium expansum*, as well as other *Penicillium*, *Aspergillus*, and *Byssochlamys* species. Patulin is most predominantly found in apples infected with *P. expansum* and apple products (juices, purees, and ciders) made from infected apples. There have also been reports of patulin contamination appearing in tomatoes, cheeses, and shellfish.

Citrinin is a polyketide mycotoxin produced by several fungal species, most predominantly *Aspergillus* and *Penicillium* species, as well as species of *Monascus*. Citrinin adds to total mycotoxin contamination in grains, where it may cooccur with OTA, as well as in apples, where it may cooccur with patulin. *Monascus* species are traditionally used for fermented products, such as red yeast rice, which are therefore at risk for citrinin contamination unless steps are taken to ensure that citrinin-nonproducing *Monascus* strains are used for the fermentations (Bennet and Klich 2003).

6.6 TOXICITY AND MODE OF ACTION OF MYCOTOXINS

The outbreak of Turkey "X" disease in 1960 resulted in the death of more than 10,000 turkeys after being fed with aflatoxin-contaminated peanut meal (Blount 1961). Since then, many studies have established the mutagenic, tetratogenic, and hepatocarcinogenic properties of aflatoxins. Among the four aflatoxins, B_1 is the most carcinogenic, and the toxicity of the group is in the order of $B_1 > G_1 > B_2 > G_2$. AFB_1 contains a double bond in the terminal furan ring. This bond is commonly oxidized by hepatic enzymes into an epoxide that can intercalate into DNA. The liver is the primary target of aflatoxins. The activation of AFB_1 by microsomal cytochrome P-450 is required for its carcinogenic effect (Eaton and Gallagher 1994).

The liver P-450 enzyme is able to convert AFB_1 to metabolites of increased polarity including AFB_1-8, 9-epoxide. It is this carcinogen that ultimately binds covalently to the N7 position of guanine in DNA in the codon 249 of the p53 tumor suppressor gene (Denissenko et al. 1999). This results in defective repair of DNA damages in cells and leads to guanine (G) to thymine (T) transversion. The presence of DNA-aflatoxin adducts in urine is an indication of the G to T mutation in the specific site of p53. This mutation hot spot in p53 is frequently associated with human hepatocarcinoma. The International Agency for Research on Cancer (IARC) has designated aflatoxin as a human liver carcinogen (Wogan 2000). Children are particularly affected by aflatoxin exposure, which leads to stunted growth, delayed development, liver damage, and liver cancer (Wu et al. 2014). Adults have a higher tolerance to exposure, but they are also at risk. No animal species is immune. Aflatoxins are among the most carcinogenic substances known. After entering the body, aflatoxins may be metabolized by the liver to a reactive epoxide intermediate or hydroxylated to become the less harmful M_1.

The toxic effect of aflatoxins on animal and human health is referred to as aflatoxicosis. In animal models, aflatoxicosis often results in proliferation of the bile duct, centrilobular necrosis in and fatty infiltration of the liver, and other hepatic lesions. Although acute aflatoxicosis in humans is rare, several lethal outbreaks have been reported. In 2004, an aflatoxicosis outbreak in rural Kenya resulted in 317 cases and 125 deaths. Contaminated maize was responsible for the outbreak, and officials found AFB_1 levels as high as 4.4 parts per million (ppm), 220 times the Kenyan regulatory threshold (Azziz-Baumgartner et al. 2005; Lewis et al. 2005; Montville and Matthews 2008). In addition, *A. flavus* is the second leading cause of invasive aspergillosis and is the most common cause of superficial infection. Disease associated with *A. flavus* includes chronic granulomatous sinusitis, keratitis, cutaneous aspergillosis, wound infections, and osteomyelitis (Hedayati et al. 2007). *A. flavus* is second only to *A. fumigatus* as the cause of human invasive aspergillosis by exposing to fungal spores.

Ochratoxins are secondary metabolites produced by *Aspergillus* and *Penicillium* strains, which can be found on cereals, coffee, and grape as well as on all kinds of food commodities of animal origin in many countries. The most frequent is OTA, which is nephrotoxic and immunosuppressive. Owing to its limited solubility in water, OTA absorbed from the gastrointestinal tract binds strongly to plasma proteins. This results in reabsorption of OTA in the kidney and enterohepatic recirculation. Therefore, biotransformation or renal clearance of OTA is delayed significantly in the body, resulting in a relatively long half-life of approximately 35 days (Pfohl-Leszkowicz and Manderville 2007; Sorrenti et al. 2013). OTA is produced most commonly by the fungi *P. verrucosum*, *A. carbonarius*, and *Aspergillus ochraceus*, which can produce OTA across a wide range of temperatures (0°C–37°C) in multiple agricultural commodities. Hence, OTA can contaminate a wide variety of foods and can also bioaccumulate in the blood and milk of animals exposed to OTA.

The risks of fumonisin B_1 have been evaluated by The World Health Organization's International Programme on Chemical Safety (IPCS) and the Scientific Committee on Food (SCF) of the European Commission. They determined a tolerable daily intake (TDI) for FB_1–FB_3, alone or in combination of 2 μg kg^{-1} body weight. FB_1 bears a clear structural similarity to the cellular sphingolipids, and this similarity has been shown to disturb the metabolism of sphingolipids by inhibiting the enzyme ceramide synthase leading to accumulation of sphinganine in cells and tissues. FB_1 is neurotoxic, hepatotoxic, and nephrotoxic in animals, and it has been classified as a possible carcinogen to humans (Riley et al. 2001; Stockmann-Juvalla and Savolainen 2008) because FB_1 disrupts sphingolipid metabolism; this could affect folate uptake and cause neural tube defect (NTD). In 1990 and 1991, a sudden outbreak of NTDs occurred along the Texas–Mexico border. It is believed that this outbreak might have been due to high levels of FB_1 that were detected in corn during previous years. Coincidentally, regions in China and South Africa with high corn consumption show a high prevalence of NTD (Marasas 2001; Blom et al. 2006). Other studies show that higher levels of concentrations of FB_1, FB_2 and *F. verticillioides* are present in corn growing in regions with a high percentage of esophageal cancer. This is in contrast with regions with low levels of *F. verticillioides*, FB_1, and FB_2 in corn. In addition, people with a high corn intake are at higher risk to develop esophageal cancer than people with low corn intake. This correlation is observed for people in regions of Italy, Iran, Kenya, Zimbabwe, Brazil, and United States with high incidence of esophageal cancer (Lozano et al. 2012; Zhang et al. 2012).

Patulin is a mycotoxin produced by a variety of molds, in particular, *Aspergillus* and *Penicillium*, most commonly found in rotting apples. In general, the amount of patulin in apple products is viewed as a measure of the quality of the apples used in production. In addition, patulin has been found in other foods such as grains, fruits, and vegetables. Although not considered a particularly potent toxin, a number of studies have shown patulin to be genotoxic (Bennet and Klich 2003; Puel et al. 2010). Several countries have instituted patulin restrictions in apple products. The World Health Organization (WHO) recommends a maximum concentration of 50 μg L^{-1} in apple juice. In the EU, the limit is set to 50 μg kg^{-1} in both apple juice and cider and to half of that concentration, 25 μg kg^{-1}, in solid apple products, and 10 μg kg^{-1} in products for infants and young children. Citrinin acts as a nephrotoxin in all species in which it has been tested, but its acute toxicity varies. The toxin has been implicated as a cause of Balkan nephropathy and a form of cardiac beriberi (Bennet and Klich 2003).

6.7 PREHARVEST MYCOTOXIN CONTROL METHODS

Current preharvest intervention strategies include enhancing crops resistance via genetic engineering, developing of appropriate agronomic practices, determining optimal stage for harvesting crops, and implementing novel biocontrol and chemical methods for mycotoxin control.

The use of chemical fungicides has resulted in development of pest resistance and resurgence. In addition, use of fungicides in certain agricultural systems is impractical due to the expense, risk of environmental pollution, and negative effects to human health (Ferron and Deguine 2005). Biological control of insect pests, plant pathogens, and weeds is the only major alternative to the use of pesticides in agriculture and forestry. Accordingly, microorganisms naturally present in agricultural ecosystems are being studied as environmentally compatible alternatives to traditional chemical methods for controlling plant diseases and fungi associated with mycotoxin production. Biological control can reduce the harmful effect of phytopathogenic or mycotoxigenic fungi while having a minimal impact on the environment (Janisiewicz and Korsten 2002; Fravel 2005; Castoria et al. 2008; Droby et al. 2009; Tsitsigiannis et al. 2012; Chulze et al. 2015).

Numerous studies have been undertaken in search of bacterial antagonists of mycotoxigenic fungi that control fungal growth and/or inhibit mycotoxin production. A review by Palumbo et al. (2008) describes interactions between aflatoxin-, fumonisin-, trichothecene-, and ochratoxin-producing fungi and species of several bacterial genera, including *Pseudomonas*, *Bacillus*, *Streptomyces*, *Microbacterium*, *Enterobacter*, *Burkholderia*, and others. Another review by Chulze et al. (2015) summarizes several studies demonstrating antagonistic activities of *Bacillus*, *Pseudomonas*, *Streptomyces*, *Microbacterium*, and other genera against *F. graminearum* and DON in wheat, *F. verticillioides* and fumonisin in maize, and *Aspergillus* species and aflatoxin and ochratoxin in peanuts and grapes.

More recently, rhizosphere bacteria have been isolated from peanut and maize that have been used for seed treatments to reduce *A. flavus* rhizosphere populations in those crops (Aiyaza et al. 2015; Navya et al. 2015). The bacterial isolates with the most promising antifungal activity are *Pseudomonas* and *Bacillus* species. Although these studies showed activity against *A. flavus*, field studies using the same bacterial seed treatments in maize showed no reduction of *F. verticillioides* or fumonisins, suggesting that multiple application strategies might be necessary for effective control of both fungi in maize. In contrast, Lizárraga-Sánchez et al. (2015) conducted a field study using seed and foliar inoculation of maize with *Bacillus cereus,* which resulted in reduced *F. verticillioides* disease incidence as well as reduced total fumonisin levels in maize kernels. Similarly, seed treatments using *B. amyloliquefaciens* reduced *F. verticillioides* infection and fumonisin contamination in field-grown maize (Pereira et al. 2010). Strains of other *Bacillus* species, such as *B. subtilis* and *B. mojavensis*, produce surfactins that inhibit *A. flavus* and *F. verticillioides* growth (Mohammadipour et al. 2009; Bacon et al. 2012). The diversity of bacteria with antimycotoxigenic activity includes lactic acid bacteria such as *Pediococcus pentosaceus*, which inhibits fumonisin production in *F. verticillioides* (Dalié et al. 2012) and ds *rhamnosus* and *L. plantarum*, which show reduction of zearalenone production by *F. graminearum* (Dogi et al. 2013). Bacterial inhibition of mycotoxigenesis has also been described in *Streptomyces* species (Verheecke et al. 2015) and in *Stenotrophomonas rhizophila*, which produces the cyclic dipeptides, cyclo (L-ala-L-pro) and cyclo (L-val-L-pro) that inhibit transcription of aflatoxin biosynthetic pathway genes in *A. parasiticus* (Jermnak et al. 2013).

Preharvest control of aflatoxin contamination of field crops has been a main goal of current research to mitigate the adverse effects aflatoxins on agricultural commodities. One of the strategies being used is to introduce nonaflatoxigenic *A. flavus* isolates into agricultural fields at a large scale to displace native aflatoxigenic strains. To date, the biocontrol method has shown a great promise for controlling aflatoxin contamination in cotton-, maize-, and peanut-growing regions in the southern United States (Dorner 2009; Jaime-Garcia and Cotty 2010). In the United States, two nonaflatoxigenic *A. flavus* strains, AF36 and NRRL21882, are registered with Environmental Protection Agency (EPA) as biopesticides for prevention of aflatoxin contamination. AF36 has been applied on cotton in Arizona and on corn in Texas for years with great efficacy; it was also tested on pistachio in California (Robens 2008). The vegetative compatibility group, YV36, to which AF36 belongs is also endemic to corn-growing regions in Mexico (Ortega-Beltran et al. 2016). This raises the possibility of using AF36 by Mexico in their aflatoxin prevention programs. NRRL21882 is the active ingredient of a commercialized biopesticide for controlling aflatoxin contamination in peanuts. Pilot field tests in Georgia and Alabama showed that it reduced aflatoxin in farmers' stock peanuts by 85%–98% (Dorner 2009). The technology later patented has been licensed and is currently marketed by Syngenta under the trade name, Afla-Guard®. This biopesticide is currently also registered for use in Brazil. A similar biocontrol management strategy is being pursued in Nigeria (Donner et al. 2010) and in Kenya where aflatoxin poisoning outbreaks have occurred in recent years (Probst et al. 2007). This technology was also tested in China (Yin et al. 2009). *A. flavus* AF051 (Jiang et al. 2009), the strain used in China, is highly competitive against natural aflatoxin-producing strains. Application of AF051 to soil of peanut fields displaced natural *Aspergillus* populations by up to 99%.

Yeast species are promising biocontrol agents because they do not produce allergenic spores and they are usually nonpathogenic. Saprophytic yeasts have been studied as potential biological control agents for the control of various fungal pathogens, including *Botrytis cinerea, Penicillium spp.* Biological control by yeasts has been mainly used to manage postharvest losses due to these fungal infections in apples, grapes, pears × peach, sweet cherries, and citrus. A number of commercial yeast products have been developed in recent years. The yeast *Metschnikowia fructicola* is the active ingredient in the commercial biocontrol product Shermer, which is marketed for the control of postharvest diseases of fruits and vegetables. *Candida oleophila* and *C. sake* are active ingredients of commercial products of BioNext and Candifruit, respectively. Furthermore, the selected yeast strains can be applied in combination with suitable fungicides to maximize the efficacy of biocontrol while reducing the amount of fungicides on food products. Yeast species can develop quickly in leaf, fruit, and flower surfaces, excluding the other microorganism growth by means of competition for space and nutrient. The use of yeasts in postharvest biocontrol formulations apparently presents advantages over other organisms. Yeasts are easy to cultivate, fast growing, and are present in a variety of environmental niches (Janisiewicz and Korsten 2002; Fravel 2005; Bleve et al. 2006; Pal and Gardener 2006; De Felice et al. 2008; Droby et al. 2009; Hua 2013).

Aspergillus flavus Papa 827, a *nor* mutant played an important role in a visual screening for yeast biocontrol agents to inhibit aflatoxin biosynthesis (Papa 1984; Hua et al. 1999). The *nor* mutant has a mutation in the gene coding for norsolorinic acid reductase, thus aflatoxin biosynthesis is blocked at this step. The accumulated norsolorinic acid, a bright red-orange pigment can be easily visualized. The rationale for using the *nor* mutant as an indicator strain is that accumulation of the red-orange pigment during growth implies that the aflatoxin biosynthetic pathway is operating up to the formation of norsolorinic acid. If no such pigment is produced, it implies that aflatoxin biosynthesis is inhibited at an earlier step in the pathway and that this inhibition also may occur in field strains of aflatoxigenic *A. flavus*.

Two hundred strains of yeasts were initially screened for their ability to prevent the growth of *A. flavus* by this visual bioassay. A few species of yeasts have been identified to inhibit both the growth of *A. flavus* and aflatoxin production to various extents (Hua et al. 1998, 1999). One isolate in particular, WRL-076 is greatly effective in inhibiting both the growth and aflatoxin production of *A. flavus*. The yeast strain was identified to be *Pichia anomala* by the Central Bureau for Fungal Culture (CBS), Baarn, the Netherlands. The species has recently been renamed as *Wickerhamomyces anomalus* (Kurtzman et al. 2008). Throughout this review the yeast will be referred to as *P. anomala*, rather than *W. anomalus*, mainly because it was the nomenclature used in many previous publications. Several strains from this species have been demonstrated to control fungal pathogens of stored wheat and fruits (Petersson and Schnurer 1998; Petersson et al. 1998; Jijakli 2011).

The biocontrol efficacy of a strain of yeast, *P. anomala* WRL-076, has been evaluated further on pistachio flowers, leaves, nut-fruits and almond leaves, and corn. Spore production of *A. flavus* was reduced by about 80% in pistachio flowers sprayed with the yeast. Wounded pistachio nut fruits inoculated with yeast decrease spore production of *A. flavus*. Almond nuts sprayed with the yeast showed much less fungal growth (Hua 2002, 2004, 2006, 2013). Field experiments conducted in Texas (Isakeit et al. 2007) indicated that *P. anomala* significantly reduced the level of preharvest aflatoxin in corn as much as 70%. The report also demonstrated that there was a trend of reduced aflatoxin levels with *P. anomala* treatments, but two applications of *P. anomala* at silk stage of corn resulted significant reduction in aflatoxin with a p value of 0.05 ($p = 0.05$).

An important requirement for the commercialization of biocontrol agents is the ability to economically produce large quantities of the microorganisms, and the development of formulations for good shelf life is also critical. Live *P. anomala* yeast cells are required for its broad application in food and agriculture industries. A stable liquid formulation is highly desirable for *P. anomala* WRL-076 because of easy dispersion in water and delivery to crops. The biocontrol yeast grows well in nutrient broth to a high concentration of 10^9 cells mL^{-1}. One of the liquid formulations developed for *P. anomala* WRL-076 preserved cell viability up to 83% even after cold storage for 12 months. In that formulation, intracellular sorbitol and trehalose synergistically enhanced yeast viability (Hua et al. 2015). *P. anomala* WRL-076 has been commercially licensed for developing biocontrol products.

REFERENCES

Aiyaza, M., S.T. Divakara, S.C. Nayaka, P. Hariprasad, and S.R. Niranjana. 2015. Application of beneficial rhizospheric microbes for the mitigation of seed-borne mycotoxigenic fungal infection and mycotoxins in maize. *Biocontrol Sci. Tech.* 25: 1105–1119.

Amaike, S., and N.P. Keller. 2011. *Aspergillus flavus*. *Ann. Rev. Phytopath.* 49: 107–133.

Azziz-Baumgartner, E., K. Lindblade, K. Gieseker, H.S. Rogers, S. Kieszak, H. Njapau, R. Schleicher, L.F. McCoy, A. Misore, and K. DeCock. 2005. Case-control study of an acute aflatoxicosis outbreak, Kenya, 2004. *Environ. Health Perspec.* 113: 1779–1783.

Bacon, C.W., D.M. Hinton, T.R. Mitchell, M.E. Snook, and B. Olubajo. 2012. Characterization of endophytic strains of *Bacillus mojavensis* and their production of surfactin isomers. *Biol. Control.* 62: 1–9.

Bayman, P., J.L. Baker, M.A. Doster, T.J. Michailides, and N.E. Mahoney. 2002. Ochratoxin production by the *Aspergillus ochraceus* group and *Aspergillus alliaceus*. *Appl. Environ. Microbiol.* 68: 2326–2329.

Bennett, J.W., and M. Klich. 2003. Mycotoxins. *Clin. Microbiol. Rev.* 16: 497–516.

Bleve, G., F. Grieco, G. Cozzi, A. Logrieco, and A. Visconti. 2006. Isolation of epiphytic yeasts with potential for biocontrol of *Aspergillus carbonarius* and *A. niger* on grape. *Int. J. Food Microbiol.* 108: 204–209.

Blom, H. J., G. M. Shaw GM, M. den Heijer, and R. H. Finnel. 2006. Neural tube defects and folate: Case far from closed. *Nat. Rev. Neurosci.* 7: 724–731.

Blount, W.P. 1961. Turkey "X" disease. *Turkeys* 9: 55–58.

Boutrif, E., and C. Canet. 1998. Mycotoxin prevention and control: FAO programmes. *Revue de Médecine Vétérinaire* 149: 681–694.

Cabañes, F.J., M.R. Bragulat, and G. Castellá. 2010. Ochratoxin A producing species in the genus *Penicillium*. *Toxins* 2: 1111–1120.

Calderari, T.O., B.T. Iamanaka, J.C. Frisvad, J.I. Pitt, D. Sartori, J.L. Pereira, M.H. Fungaro, and M.H. Taniwaki. 2013. The biodiversity of *Aspergillus* section *Flavi* in Brazil nuts: From rainforest to consumer. *Int. J. Food Microbiol.* 160: 267–272.

Cary, J.W., M.A. Klich, and S.B. Beltz. 2005. Characterization of aflatoxin-producing fungi outside of *Aspergillus* section *Flavi*. *Mycologia* 97: 425–432.

Cary, J.W., Z. Han, Y. Yin, J.M. Lohmar, S. Shantappa, P.Y. Harris-Coward, B. Mack et al. 2015. Transcriptome analysis of *Aspergillus flavus* reveals *veA*-dependent regulation of secondary metabolite gene clusters, including the novel aflavarin cluster. *Eukaryotic Cell* 14: 983–997.

Castoria R., S.A.I. Wright, and S. Droby. 2008. Biological control of mycotoxigenic fungi in fruits. In: R. Barkai-Golan, and N. Paster (ed), *Mycotoxins in Fruits and Vegetables*, Academic Press, pp. 311–333.

Chang, P.K., L.L. Scharfenstein, B. Mack, J. Yu, and K.C. Ehrlich. 2014. Transcriptomic profiles of *Aspergillus flavus* CA42, a strain that produces small sclerotia, by decanal treatment and after recovery. *Fungal Genet. Biol.* 68: 39–47.

Chang, P.K., S.S. Hua, S.B. Sarreal, and R.W. Li. 2015. Suppression of aflatoxin biosynthesis in *Aspergillus flavus* by 2-phenylethanol is associated with stimulated growth and decreased degradation of branched-chain amino acids. *Toxins (Basel)* 7: 3887–3902.

Chulze, S.N., J.M. Palazzini, A.M. Torres, G. Barros, M.L. Ponsone, R. Geisen, M. Schmidt-Heydt, and J. Köhl. 2015. Biological control as a strategy to reduce the impact of mycotoxins in peanuts, grapes and cereals in Argentina. *Food Addit. Contam.* 32: 471–479.

Dalié, D., L. Pinson-Gadais, V. Atanasova-Penichon, G. Marchegay, C. Barreau, A. Deschamps, and F. Richard-Forget. 2012. Impact of *Pediococcus pentosaceus* strain L006 and its metabolites on fumonisin biosynthesis by *Fusarium verticillioides*. *Food Contr.* 23: 405–411.

De Felice, D.V., M. Solfrizzo, F. De Curtis, G. Lima, A. Visconti, and R. Castoria. 2008. Strains of *Aureobasidium pullulans* can lower ochratoxin A contamination in wine grapes. *Phytopathol.* 98: 1261–1270.

Denissenko, M.F., J. Cahill, T.B. Koudriakova, N. Gerber, and G.P. Pfeifer. 1999. Quantitation and mapping of aflatoxin B_1-induced DNA damage in genomic DNA using aflatoxin B_1-8,9-epoxide and microsomal activation systems. *Mutation Res.* 425: 205–211.

Diener, U.L., R.J. Cole, T.H. Sanders, G.A. Payne, L.S. Lee, and M.A. Klich. 1987. Epidemiology of aflatoxin formation by *Aspergillus flavus*. *Annu. Rev. Phytopathol.* 25: 249–270.

Dogi, C.A., A. Fochesato, R. Armando, B. Pribull, M.M.S. de Souza, I. da Silva Coelho, D. Araújo de Melo, A. Dalcero, and L. Cavaglieri. 2013. Selection of lactic acid bacteria to promote an efficient silage fermentation capable of inhibiting the activity of *Aspergillus parasiticus* and *Fusarium graminearum* and mycotoxin production. *J. Appl. Microbiol.* 114: 1650–1660.

Donner, M., J. Atehnkeng, R.A. Sikora, R. Bandyopadhyay, and P.J. Cotty. 2010. Molecular characterization of atoxigenic strains for biological control of aflatoxins in Nigeria. *Food Addit. Contam.* 27: 576–590.

Dorner, J.W. 2009. Development of biocontrol technology to manage aflatoxin contamination in peanuts. *Peanut Sci.* 36: 60–67.

Droby, S., M. Wisniewski, D. Macarisin, and C. Wilson. 2009. Twenty years of postharvest biocontrol research: Is it time for a new paradigm? *Postharvest Biol. Tech.* 52: 137–145.

Duarte, S.C., A. Pena, and C.M. Lino. 2010. A review on ochratoxin A occurrence and effects of processing of cereal and cereal derived food products. *Food Microbiol.* 27: 187–198.

Eaton, D.L., and E.P. Gallagher. 1994. Mechanisms of aflatoxin carcinogenesis. *Annu. Rev. Pharmacol. Toxicol.* 34: 135–172.

European Commission. 2005. Rapid Alert System for Food and Feed (RASFF)—2005 Weekly Overview.

European Commission. 2006. The Rapid Alert System for Food and Feed (RASFF) Annual Report 2005.

FAO. 1997. Worldwide Regulations for Mycotoxins 1995. A Compendium. Rome, Italy: *FAO Food and Nutrition Paper 64*.

Ferron, P., and J-P. Deguine. 2005. Crop protection, biological control, habitat management and integrated farming. *A Review. Agron. Sustain. Dev*. 25: 17–24.

Food and Drug Administration. 1996. Compliance Policy Guides Manual. Sec.555.400, 268; Sec. 570.500, 299.

Frisvad, J.C., J.M. Frank, J.A.M.P. Houbraken, A.F.A. Kuijpers, and R.A. Samson. 2004. New ochratoxin A producing species of *Aspergillus* section *Circumdati*. *Stud. Mycol.* 50: 23–43.

Frisvad, J.C., J. Smedsgaard, R.A. Samson, T.O. Larsen, and U. Thrane. 2007. Fumonisin B_2 production by *Aspergillus niger. J. Agric. Food Chem.* 55: 9727–9732.

Fravel, D.R. 2005. Commercialization and implementation of biocontrol. *Annu. Rev. Phytopathol.* 43:337–359.

Georgianna, D.R., N.D. Fedorova, J.L. Burroughs, A.L. Dolezal, J.W. Bok, S. Horowitz-Brown, C.P. Woloshuk, J. Yu, N.P. Keller, and G.A. Payne. 2010. Beyond aflatoxin: Four distinct expression patterns and functional roles associated with *Aspergillus flavus* secondary metabolism gene clusters. *Mol. Plant Pathol.* 11: 213–226.

Gilbert, M.K., B.M. Mack, Q. Wei, J.M. Bland, D. Bhatnagar, and J.W. Cary. 2016. RNA sequencing of an *nsdC* mutant reveals global regulation of secondary metabolic gene clusters in *Aspergillus flavus*. *Microbiol. Res.*182: 150–161.

Hedayati, M. T., A. C. Pasqualotto, P. A.Warn, P. Bower, and D. W. Denning. 2007. *Aspergillus flavus*: Human pathogen, allergen and mycotoxin producer. *Microbiol.* 153: 1677–1692.

Henry, S.H., F.X. Bosch, and J.C. Bowers. 2002. Aflatoxin, hepatitis and worldwide liver cancer risks. *Adv. Exp. Med. Biol.* 504: 229–233.

Henry, S.H., F.X. Bosch, T.C. Troxell, and P.M. Bolger. 1999. Public health-reducing liver cancer-global control of aflatoxin. *Science* 286: 2453–2454.

Horn, B.W., and R.L. Green. 1995. Vegetative compatibility within populations of *Aspergillus flavus*, *A. parasiticus*, and *A. tamari* from a peanut field. *Mycologia.* 87: 324–332.

Hua, S.S.T. 2002. Potential use of saprophytic yeast to reduce populations of *Aspergillus flavus* in almond and pistachio orchards. In: I. Battle, I. Hormaza, and M. T. Espiau (eds), *Proceedings of the Third International Symposium of Pistachio and Almond. Acta Horticulture*, International Society for Horticultural Science (ISHS) in Belgium 591: 527–530.

Hua, S.S.T. 2004. Application of a yeast, *Pichia anomala* strain WRL-076 to control *Aspergillus flavus* for reducing aflatoxin in pistachio and almond. *IOBC Bullet.* 27: 291–294.

Hua, S.S.T. 2006. Progress in prevention of aflatoxin contamination in food by preharvest application of *Pichia anomala* WRL-076. In: A. Mendez-Vilas (ed), *Recent Advances in multidisciplinary Applied Microbiology*. Weinheim, Germany: Wiley-VCH Verlag GmbH&Co. KGaA, pp. 322–326.

Hua, S.S.T. 2007. Environmental Adaptation of *Pichia anomala* WRL-076 as an effective biocontrol agent for pre-harvest application. *IOBC Bullet.* 30: 241–244.

Hua, S.S.T. 2013. Biocontrol of *Aspergillus flavus* by *Pichia anomala*. In: A. Mendez-Vilas (ed), *Microbial Pathogens and Strategies for Combating Them: Science Technology and Education*, vol. 2. Spain: Formatex Research Center, pp. 1067–1072.

Hua, S.S.T., C.E. McAplin, P.K. Chang, S.B.L. Sarreal. 2012. Characterization of aflatoxigenic and non-aflatoxigenic *Aspergillus flavus* isolates from pistachio. *Mycotoxin Res* 28: 67–75.

Hua, S.S.T., C.E. McAlpin, and S.B. Ly. 2006. Population of *Aspergillus flavus* on pistachio buds and flowers. In: A. Mendez-Vilas (ed.). Recent Advances in multidisciplinary Applied Microbiology, Wiley-VCH Verlag GmbH&Co. KGaA, Weinheim, Germany, pp. 440–445.

Hua, S.S.T., A.S. Taurin, S.N. Pandey, L. Chang, P.K. Chang. 2007. Characterization of *AFLAV*, a *Tfl/Sushi* retrotransposon from *Aspergillus flavus*. *Mycopathologia* 163: 97–104.

Hua, S.S., B.J. Hernlem, W. Yokoyama, and S.B. Sarreal. 2015. Intracellular trehalose and sorbitol synergistically promoting cell viability of a biocontrol yeast, *Pichia anomala*, for aflatoxin reduction. *World J. Microbiol. Biotechnol.* 31: 729–734.

Hua, S.S.T., C.E. McAplin, P.K. Chang, and S.B.L. Sarreal. 2012. Characterization of aflatoxigenic and non-aflatoxigenic *Aspergillus flavus* isolates from pistachio. *Mycotoxin Res.* 28: 67–75.

Hua, S.S.T., J.L. Baker, and M. Flores-Espiritu. 1999. Interactions of saprophytic yeasts with a *nor* mutant of *Aspergillus flavus*. *Appl. Environ. Microbiol.* 65: 2738–2740.

Hua, S.S.T., J.L. Baker, and O.K. Grosjean. 1998. Improvement of the quality and value of pistachios and almonds through preharvest biocontrol of *Aspergillus flavus*. In: L. Ferguson, and D. Kester (eds), *Proceedings of the Second International Symposium of Pistachios and Almonds, Acta Horticulturae No. 470*. Leuven, Belgium: International Society for Horticultural Science.

Hua, S.S.T., J.J. Beck, S.B.L. Sarreal, and W. Gee. 2014. The major volatile compound 2-phenylethanol from the biocontrol yeast, *Pichia anomala*, inhibits growth and expression of aflatoxin biosynthetic genes of *Aspergillus flavus*. *Mycotoxin Res.* 30: 71–78.

Isakeit, T., F.J. Betran, G. Odvody, and S.S.T. Hua. 2007. Efficacy of *Pichia anomala* WRL-076 to control aflatoxin on corn in Texas, 2005. *Plant Dis. Manag. Reports.* 1: FC021.

Jaime-Garcia, R., and P.J. Cotty. 2010. Influence of crop rotation on persistence of the atoxigenic strain *Aspergillus flavus* AF36 in Arizona. *Phytopathol.* 100: S55.

Janisiewicz, W., and L. Korsten. 2002. Biological control of postharvest diseases of fruits. *Annu. Rev. Phytopathol.* 40: 411–441.

Jermnak, U., A. Chinaphuti, A. Poapolathep, R. Kawai, H. Nagasawa, and S. Sakuda. 2013. Prevention of aflatoxin contamination by a soil bacterium of *Stenotrophomonas* sp. that produces aflatoxin production inhibitors. *Microbiology* 159: 902–912.

Jiang, J., L. Yan, and Z. Ma. 2009. Molecular characterization of an atoxigenic *Aspergillus flavus* strain AF051. *Appl. Microbiol. Biotechnol.* 83: 501–505.

Jijakli, M.H. 2011. *Pichia anomala* in biocontrol for apples: 20 years of fundamental research and practical applications. *Antonie Leeuwenhoek* 99: 93–105.

Knudsen, P.B., J.M. Mogensen, T.O. Larsen, and K.F. Nielsen. 2011. Occurrence of fumonisins B_2 and B_4 in retail raisins. *J. Agric. Food Chem.* 59:772–776.

Kurtzman, C.P., C.J. Robnet, and E. Basehoar-Powers. 2008. Relationships among species of *Pichia*, *Issatchenkia* and *Williopsis* determined from multigene phylogenetic analysis and the proposal of *Barnettozyma* gen. *nov.*, *Lindnera* gen. *nov.* and *Wickerhamomyces* gen. *nov. FEMS Yeast Res.* 8: 939–954.

Lee, H.J., and D. Ryu. 2015. Significance of ochratoxin A in breakfast cereals from the United States. J. *Agric. Food. Chem.* 63: 9404–9409.

Lewis, L., M. Onsongo, H. Njapau, H. Schurz-Rogers, G. Luber, S. Kieszak, J. Nyamongo et al. 2005. Aflatoxin contamination of commercial maize products during an outbreak of acute aflatoxicosis in eastern and central Kenya. *Environ. Health Perspec.* 113: 1763–1767.

Lin, J.Q., X.X. Zhao, Q.Q. Zhi, M. Zhao, and Z.M. He. 2013. Transcriptomic profiling of *Aspergillus flavus* in response to 5-azacytidine. *Fungal Genet. Biol.* 56: 78–86.

Linz, J.E., J. Wee, and L.V. Roze. 2014. *Aspergillus parasiticus* SU-1 genome sequence, predicted chromosome structure, and comparative gene expression under aflatoxin-inducing conditions: Evidence that differential expression contributes to species phenotype. Eukaryot Cell. 13: 1113–1123.

Lizárraga-Sánchez, G.J., K.Y. Leyva-Madrigal, P. Sánchez-Peña, F.R. Quiroz-Figueroa, and I.E. Maldonado-Mendoza. 2015. *Bacillus cereus sensu lato* strain B25 controls maize stalk and ear rot in Sinaloa, Mexico. *Field Crops Res.* 176: 11–21.

Logrieco, A., A. Bottalico, G. Mulé, A. Moretti, and G. Perrone. 2003. Epidemiology of toxigenic fungi and their associated mycotoxins for some Mediterranean crops. *Eur. J. Plant Pathol.* 109: 645–667.

Logrieco, A., R. Ferracane, M. Haidukowsky, G. Cozzi, A. Visconti, and A. Ritieni. 2009. Fumonisin B_2 production by *Aspergillus niger* from grapes and natural occurrence in must. *Food Addit. Contam.* 26: 1495–1500.

Lozano, R, M. Naghavi, K. Foreman, S. Lim, K. Shibuya, V. Aboyans, J. Abraham, T. Adair et al. 2012. Global and regional mortality from 235 causes of death for 20 age groups in 1990 and 2010: A systematic analysis for the Global Burden of Disease Study 2010. *Lancet* 380: 2095–2128.

Marasas, W.F. 2001. Discovery and occurrence of the fumonisins: A historical perspective. *Environ. Health Perspect.* 109 (S2): 239–243.

Mateo, R., A. Medina, E.M. Mateo, F. Mateo, and M. Jimenez. 2007. An overview of ochratoxin A in beer and wine. *Int. J. Food Microbiol.* 119: 79–83.

McAlpin, C.E., D.T. Wicklow, and B.W. Horn. 2002. DNA fingerprinting analysis of vegetative compatibility groups in *Aspergillus flavus* from a peanut field in Georgia. *Plant Dis.* 86:254–258.

McAlpin, C.E., D.T. Wicklow, and C. Platis. 1998. Genotypic diversity of *Aspergillus parasiticus* in an Illinois corn field. *Plant Dis.* 82: 1132–1135.

Mogensen, J.M., T.O. Larsen, and K.F. Nielsen. 2010. Widespread occurrence of the mycotoxin fumonisin B_2 in wine. *J. Agric. Food Chem.* 58: 4853–4857.

Mohammadipour, M., M. Mousivand, G.S. Jouzani, and S. Abbasalizadeh. 2009. Molecular and biochemical characterization of Iranian surfactin-producing *Bacillus subtilis* isolates and evaluation of their biocontrol potential against *Aspergillus flavus* and *Colletotrichum gloeosporioides*. *Can. J. Microbiol.* 55: 395–404.

Molyneux, R.J., N. Mahoney, J.H. Kim, and B.C. Campbell. 2007. Mycotoxins in edible tree nuts. *Internat. J. Food Microbiol.* 119: 72–78.

Montville, T. J., K.R. Matthews. 2008. Food Microbiology, An Introduction. Washington: ASM Press, p. 428.

Navya, H.M., J. Naveen, P. Hariprasad, and S.R. Niranjana. 2015. Beneficial rhizospheric microorganisms mediated plant growth promotion and suppression of aflatoxigenic fungal and aflatoxin contamination in groundnut seeds. *Ann. Appl. Biol.* 167: 225–235.

Nielsen, K.F., J.M. Mogensen, M. Johansen, T.O. Larsen, and J.C. Frisvad. 2009. Review of secondary metabolites and mycotoxins from the *Aspergillus niger* group. *Anal. Bioanal. Chem.* 395: 1225–1242.

Ortega-Beltran, A., L.C. Grubisha, K.A. Callicott, and P.J. Cotty. 2016. The vegetative compatibility group to which the US biocontrol agent *Aspergillus flavus* AF36 belongs is also endemic to Mexico. *J. Appl. Microbiol.* 120: 986–998.

Otsuki, T., J.S. Wilson, and M. Sewadeh. 2001. What price precaution? European harmonization of aflatoxin regulations and African groundnuts exports. *Eur. Rev. Agric. Econ.* 28: 263–284.

Pal, K.K., and B.M. Gardener. 2006. Biological Control of Plant Pathogens. *Plant Health Instruct.* doi: 10.1094/PHI-A-2006-1117-02.

Palumbo, J.D., T.L. O'Keeffe, and H.K. Abbas 2008. Microbial interactions with mycotoxigenic fungi and mycotoxins. *Toxin. Rev.* 27: 261–285.

Pfohl-Leszkowicz, A., and R.A. Manderville. 2007. Ochratoxin A: An overview on toxicity and carcinogenicity in animals and humans. *Mol Nutr Food Res.* 51: 61–99.

Palumbo, J.D., T.L. O'Keeffe, and J.A. McGarvey. 2011. Incidence of fumonisin B_2 production within *Aspergillus* section *Nigri* populations isolated from California raisins. *J. Food Prot.* 74: 672–675.

Palumbo, J.D., T.L. O'Keeffe, Y.S. Ho, and C.J. Santillan. 2015. Occurrence of ochratoxin A contamination and detection of ochratoxigenic *Aspergillus* species in retail samples of dried fruits and nuts. *J. Food Prot.* 78: 836–842.

Papa, K.E. 1984. Genetics of *Aspergillus flavus*: Linkage of aflatoxin mutants. *Can. J. Microbiol.* 30: 68–73.

Payne, G.A., J. Yu, W.C. Nierman, M. Machida, D. Bhatnagar, T.E. Cleveland et al. 2008. A first glance into the genome sequence of *Aspergillus flavus*. In: S. Osmani, and G. Goldman (eds), The *ASPERGILLI: Genomics, Medical Aspects, Biotechnology and Research Methods*, vol. 26. Boca Raton, FL: CRC Press, pp. 15–23.

Peraica, M., B. Radić, A. Lucić, and M. Pavlović. 1999. Toxic effects of mycotoxins in humans. *Bull. World Health Organ.* 77: 754–766.

Pereira, P., A. Nesci, C. Castillo, and M. Etcheverry. 2010. Impact of bacterial biological control agents on fumonisin B_1 content and *Fusarium verticillioides* infection of field-grown maize. *Biol. Contr.* 53: 258–266.

Petersson, S., and J. Schnurer. 1998. *Pichia anomala* as a biocontrol agent of *Penicillium roqueforti* in high-moisture wheat, rye, barley, and oats stored under airtight conditions. *Can. J. Microbiol.* 44: 471–476.

Petersson, S., M.W. Henson, K. Axberg, K. Hult, and J. Schnurer. 1998. Ochratoxin A accumulation in cultures of *Penicillium verrucosum* with the antagonistic yeast *Pichia anomala* and *Saccharomyces cerevisiae. Mycol. Res.* 102: 1003–1008.

Pildain, M.B., J.C. Frisvad, G. Vaamonde, D. Cabral, J. Varga, and R.A. Samson. 2008. Two novel aflatoxin-producing *Aspergillus* species from Argentinean peanuts. *J. Syst. Evol. Microbiol.* 58: 725–735.

Probst, C., H. Njapau, and P.J. Cotty. 2007. Outbreak of an acute aflatoxicosis in Kenya in 2004: Identification of the causal agent. *Appl. Environ. Microbiol.* 73: 2762–2764.

Puel, O., G. Pierre, and I.P. Oswald. 2010. Biosynthesis and toxicological effects of patulin. *Toxins 2*: 613–631. doi:10.3390/toxins2040613

Rheeder, J.P., W.F. Marasas, and H.F. Vismer. 2002. Production of fumonisin analogs by *Fusarium* species. *Appl. Environ. Microbiol.* 68: 2101–2105.

Riley R.T., E. Enongen, and K.A.Voss, W.P. Norred, F.I. Meredith, R.P. Sharma, D.Williams, and A.H. Jr. Merrill. 2001. Sphingolipid perturbations as mechanisms for fumonisin carcinogenesis. *Environmental Health Perspectives* 109: 301–308.

Robens, J. 2008. Aflatoxin-recognition, understanding, and control with particular emphasis on the role of the Agricultural Research Service. *Toxin Rev.* 27: 143–169.

Samson, R.A., J.A.M.P. Houbraken, A.F.A. Kuijpers, J.M. Frank, and J.C. Frisvad. 2004. New ochratoxin A or sclerotium producing species in *Aspergillus* section *Nigri. Stud. Mycol.* 50: 45–61.

Sorrenti, V., C. Di Giacomo, R. Acquaviva, I. Ignazio Barbagallo, M. Bognanno, and F. Galvano. 2013. Toxicity of ochratoxin A and its modulation by antioxidants: A review. *Toxins* 5: 1742–1766.

Stockmann-Juvalla, H. and K. Savolainen. 2008. A review of the toxic effects and mechanisms of action of fumonisin B1. *Human & Experimental Toxicology*. 27: 799–809.

Storari, M., L. Bigler, C. Gessler, and G.A. Broggini. 2012. Assessment of the ochratoxin A production ability of *Aspergillus tubingensis*. *Food Addit. Contam*. 29: 1450–1454.

Trucksess, M.W., and P.M. Scott. 2008. Mycotoxins in botanicals and dried fruits: A review. *Food Addit. Contam.* 25: 181–192.

Tsitsigiannis, D. I., M. Dimakopoulou, P. P. Antoniou, and C. T. Eleftherios. 2012. Biological control strategies of mycotoxigenic fungi and associated mycotoxins in Mediterranean basin crops. *Phytopath. Medit*. 51: 158–174.

Van Egmond, H.P., R.C. Schothorst, and M.A. Jonker. 2007. Regulations relating to mycotoxins in food: Perspectives in a global and European context. *Anal. Bioanal. Chem.* 389: 147–157.

Varga, J., J.C. Frisvad, and R.A. Samson. 2010. A reappraisal of fungi producing aflatoxins. *World Mycotoxin. J.* 2: 263–277.

Verheecke, C., T. Liboz, P. Anson, Y. Zhu, and F. Mathieu. 2015. *Streptomyces-Aspergillus flavus* interactions: Impact on aflatoxin B accumulation. *Food Addit. Contam.* 32: 572–576.

Visagie, C.M., J. Varga, J. Houbraken, M. Meijer, S. Kocsube, N. Yilmaz, R. Fodetar, K.A. Seifert, J.C. Frisvad, and R.A. Samson. 2014. Ochratoxin production and taxonomy of the yellow aspergilli (*Aspergillus* section *Circumdati*). *Stud. Mycol.* 78: 1–61.

Wild, C.P., Y.Y. Gong. 2009. Mycotoxins and human disease: A largely ignored global health issue. *Carcinogenesis* 31: 71–82.

Wogan, G.N. 2000. Impacts of chemicals on liver cancer risk. *Sem. Cancer Biol.* 10: 201–210.

Wu, F., D. John, J.D. Groopman, and J.J. Pestka. 2014. Public health impacts of foodborne mycotoxins. *Annu. Rev. Food Sci. Technol.* 5: 351–372.

Yazar, S., and G.Z. Omurtag. 2008. Fumonisins, trichothecenes and zearalenone in cereals. *Int. J. Mol. Sci.* 9: 2062–2090.

Yin, Y., T. Lou, L. Yan, T.J. Michailides, and Z. Ma. 2009. Molecular characterization of toxigenic and atoxigenic *Aspergillus flavus* isolates, collected from peanut fields in China. *J. Appl. Microbiol.* 107: 1857–1865.

Yu, J., Chang, P.K., Ehrlich, K.C., Cary, J.W., Bhatnagar, D., T.E. Cleveland, G.A. Payne, J.E. Linz, C.P. Woloshuk, and J.W. Bennett. 2004. Clustered pathway genes in aflatoxin biosynthesis. *Appl. Environ. Microbiol.* 70: 1253–1262.

Zhang, H.Z., G.F. Jin, and H.B. Shen. 2012. Epidemiologic differences in esophageal cancer between Asian and Western populations. *Chin J. Cancer* 31: 281–266.

Zhang, F., Z. Guo, H. Zhong, S. Wang, W. Yang, Y. Liu, and S. Wang. 2014. RNA-Seq-based transcriptome analysis of aflatoxigenic *Aspergillus flavus* in response to water activity. *Toxins (Basel)* 6: 3187–3207.

7 Bacterial Toxins

Waldemar Dąbrowski, Alicja Dłubała, and Izabela Helak

CONTENTS

7.1 INTRODUCTION

Food products contain many human pathogens. The alimentary tract is an impassable barrier for a lot of them, which prevents them from penetrating the whole body. Examples include infections of the upper respiratory tract, especially purulent tonsillitis caused by staphylococci or streptococci, which turn tonsils into bacteria cultures. The bacteria use swallowed saliva to reach the alimentary tract, but they cannot survive there and make the infection develop. Some of them can cross the physiological and morphological barrier and infiltrate other organs, where the infection develops, but with no visible symptoms from the alimentary tract; these include *Salmonella typhi*, bovine *Mycobacterium tuberculosis* (*M. bovis*), *Francisella tularensis*, *Yersinia pseudotuberculosis*, and *Brucella* bacteria.

Another group of microorganisms includes bacteria for which the alimentary tract is not an obstacle and they grow in it, producing such symptoms as vomiting, diarrhea, abdominal pain, and sometimes fever. The intestinal epithelium, and sometimes intestinal walls, is usually damaged to a different extent, which is manifested as ulcerations and abscesses. However, there are no data on whether the presence of their toxins in water or in food presents any threat. The environmental conditions in food may not favor the production of toxins. A separate group of microorganisms transmitted with food includes those whose presence in the alimentary tract does not induce any disease symptoms; instead, they produce toxins in food, and it is not until its consumption that disease symptoms develop. Such microorganisms are listed in Table 7.1.

TABLE 7.1
Pathogens in the Human Alimentary Tract

	Group	Microorganisms
1	Microorganisms that cross the alimentary tract barrier and that do not cause enterocolitis	*Salmonella typhi*—causes typhoid fever, constipation or diarrhea, enlargement of the spleen, possible development of meningitis, and/or general malaise
		Salmonella paratyphi A and B—causes typhoid fever
		Mycobacterium bovis—symptoms similar to those produced by
		Francisella tularensis—tularemia
		Yersinia pseudotuberculosis—fever and right-sided abdominal pain mimic appendicitis
		Brucella abortus—infection through milk and dairy products—weakness, muscle pain, fever
		Listeria monocytogenes—listeriosis of the central nervous system and other organs
		Clostridium botulinum—botulism in new-born babies
		Clostridium baratii—botulism in new-born babies
		Clostridium butyricum—botulism in new-born babies
2	Microorganisms that grow in the alimentary tract and produce disease symptoms in it—enterocolitis and gastroenteritis	Salmonella, different serotypes—diarrhea
		Shigella—causes dysentery
		Escherichia coli—diarrhea of various intensity depending on the serotype; particularly dangerous vero cytotoxin-producing *Escherichia coli* (VTEC) O157, enterohemorrhagic
		Campylobacter spp.—mild diarrhea
		Yersinia enterocolitica—yersiniosis
		Helicobacter pylori—gastric ulcer
		Listeria mono cytogenes—diarrhea
		Clostridium difficile—severe enteric infections, especially following antibiotic therapy
		Clostridium perfringens—antibiotic-associated diarrhea, epidemic diarrheas
		Vibrio cholerae (causes cholera)
		V. parahaemolyticus, *V. vulnificus*—gastroenteritis following consumption of seafood
3	Microorganisms that produce toxins outside the human body—in food	*Clostridium botulinum*—botulism
		Bacillus cereus group—vomiting, diarrheal illness
		Staphylococcus group—diarrheal illness

7.2 *CLOSTRIDIUM BOTULINUM*

7.2.1 Introduction

Clostridium botulinum is a spore-forming bacillus, which grows only in anaerobic conditions and at pH above 4.6. Cells, rounded at the ends and ciliated peritrichally, exhibit gram-positive staining. The cell size depends on the strain and culturing conditions and ranges from 3.4 to 8.6 μm. Endospores are formed subterminally, causing specific cell swelling.

Clostridium botulinum are ubiquitous in the natural environment, they occur in the soil, in animal alimentary tract, in bottom deposits, and in coastal waters, from where they can contaminate food products. Production of botulinum toxin in food products is accompanied by specific changes, that is, the appearance of a specific smell of rancid fat and the production of large amounts of gas (swelling of tin cans).

Each microorganism able to produce one of the seven botulinum toxins (A, B, C, D, E, F, G) can be regarded as *C. botulinum*. Contemporary researchers classify *Clostridium* bacteria into four groups (I–IV) (Grenda and Kwiatek 2009):

Group I comprises proteolytic strains of *C. botulinum* capable of producing A, B, and F type toxins, as well as nontoxin-producing strains of *C. sporogenes*.
Group II comprises nonproteolytic strains of *C. botulinum* capable of producing toxins of A, B, and E type.
Group III comprises proteolytic and nonproteolytic strains of *C. botulinum* capable of producing toxins of C and D type, as well as strains of *C. novyi* of the A type.
Group IV comprises strains of *C. botulinum* which produce toxin type G (classified as a distinct species *C. argentinense*), and without a toxin-producing potential of *C. subterminale* and *C. hastiforme*.

Botulinum toxin can also be produced by nonproteolytic strains of *C. butyricum* (type E toxin) and *C. barati*, which can produce type F toxin, which are not classified as *C. botulinum* (Grenda and Kwiatek 2009).

Currently, there is no uniform clinical classification of botulism. Usually, six forms of such poisonings are identified in the literature: foodborne botulism, wound botulism, infant botulism, inhalational botulism, iatrogenic botulism, and botulism with no established source. The form of the disease depends on how food containing the botulinum toxin of a spore of *C. botulinum* got into the body.

Foodborne botulism is a consequence of consuming food containing botulinum toxin. Symptoms of poisoning usually appear 12–36 hours after consuming the food. Acute bilateral neuropathy of cranial nerves develops, with consequent dryness in the mouth and difficulty in swallowing, slurred speech, dropping eyelids, and ophthalmoplegia. Failure to start therapy will result in paralysis of breathing muscles and consequent death.

Infant botulism affects children under 12 years. The disease develops as a result of the consumption of food, usually honey or powdered milk for infants, contaminated with spores of *C. botulinum*; toxins are produced during germination in the alimentary tract (Kizerwetter-Świda and Binek 2010).

Wound botulism is recorded relatively rare. Disease occurs when it gets into a wound spore of *C. botulinum*, which enters the bloodstream and with the blood goes to other parts of the body. Neurological symptoms are the same as in the case of botulism tract, lack only the symptoms of the gastrointestinal tract (Kizerwetter-Świda and Binek 2010).

Iatrogenic botulism is an extremely rare form of the disease caused by botulinum toxin getting into the body with an injection. Symptoms are usually limited to generalized muscle weakness, usually accompanied by slight dropping of eyelids, double vision, dryness of the mucous membrane of the oral cavity, dysphagia, and dysarthria (Shapiro et al. 1998).

Inhalational botulism, along with iatrogenic botulism, virtually never occurs naturally. It happens when an individual is exposed to an aerosol containing botulinum toxin.

Cases of botulism, which failed to identify the source of the bacteria or toxins in food, are classified by the Centres for Disease Control and Prevention as cases of "undetermined origin." They occur in adults and children above the age 12 months (equivalent to infant botulism). It is noted in patients undergoing surgery or gastrointestinal tract are treated with antibiotics and may be the result of disruption of the natural balance of intestinal microflora, which results in the alimentary tract being colonized by *C. botulinum* (Kizerwetter-Świda and Binek 2010).

7.2.2 *Clostridium* Toxins

C. botulinum and *C. tetani* produce the most potent of the known biological toxins. Neurotoxins produced by *Clostridium* bacteria include tetanus toxin (TeNT) and seven different botulinum neurotoxins (BoNT, i.e., A, B, C, D, E, F, G) (Rao et al. 2005) with nearly identical pharmacological action but with different antigen structure (Reis and Mierzejewski 2004). Botulinum toxin (BoNT) is commonly regarded as the most potent toxic substance that occurs naturally in the environment. An amount ranging from 0.2 to 2.0 μg/kg of body weight is regarded as a lethal dose for a person (Sharma and Whiting 2005). Most toxin-producing strains of *Clostridium* are capable of producing one type of toxin, but there have been literature reports on strains which can produce two types of toxins: Ab, Ba, Af, Bf (a capital letter denotes a toxin produced in the larger amount); Ba and Bf *Clostridium* strains produce 10 times more of the B toxin than the A or F toxin (Parasion et al. 2007).

Botulism in people is usually caused by A, B, E neurotoxins, which cause 99% of all the cases of the disease on record. BoNT/C and BoNT/D toxins induce botulism in household and wild animals (Humeau et al. 2000), whereas the G toxin is produced by bacteria isolated from the soil.

Neurotoxins produced by *Clostridium* bacteria are synthesized as a single chain of a biologically inactive protein with a molecular weight of about 150 kDa which, following post-translation processing—assuming a two-chain structure with a 50-kDa light chain (LC) and a 100-kDa heavy chain (HC). Both parts are bound by a noncovalent bond and a single disulfide bridge (Brunger and Rummel 2009). There are three 50 kDa functional domains within botulinum toxins: (1) zinc-dependent metalloprotease (LC), (2) a domain which facilitates toxin transport through the presynaptic membrane, and (3) a domain which binds the toxin on the surface of the presynaptic membrane receptor, which consists of two subdomains (HC HN and HC C) (Parasion et al. 2007).

The HC plays an important role in binding a neurotoxin to a receptor on a nerve cell surface and translocation of the LC to the cell interior. Binding a neurotoxin to a receptor is made possible by the presence of an N-terminal HC-N domain, which in BoNT/A and BoNT/B consists of two β-sheets bound by a α-helix. Translocation of the LC through the vesicular membrane into the cytosol is effected by the C-terminal domain HC-C. In BoNT/A and BoNT/B, it consists of two long α-helixes and one long loop—a "translocation belt," which surrounds the LC (Parasion et al. 2007).

The LC plays the role of a metalloprotease. The substrate binds at the catalytic site, located in a deep crevice on the surface of the protein molecule, with an anion channel leading to it. It has a zinc-binding motive consisting of two molecules of histidine and glutamate residues (His-Glu-x-x-His) (Parasion et al. 2007).

Botulinum toxins are accumulated in cytosol of bacterial cells and are excreted during the process of cell autolysis (Simpson 1981). No additional proteins are bound to tetanus toxin and neurotoxins of *C. botulinum* are excreted as "progenitor toxins," stabilized by noncovalent bonds. They consist of BoNT and nontoxic neurotoxin-associated proteins (NAPs) (Sharma and Whiting 2005), which do or do not possess the hemagglutination capability (hemagglutinin and nonhemagglutinin, respectively). NAPs in protoxins probably protect toxins against inactivation at low pH of gastric juice and the action of proteases in the alimentary tract (Arndt et al. 2005). Protoxins also stabilize botulinum toxins when they are produced for therapeutic purposes (Callaway et al. 2002).

Three forms of progenitor toxins have been identified in supernatants of *C. botulinum* cultures:

1. M-toxin (*medium toxin*) with a molecular weight of 300 kDa (sedimentation constant 12S) (Schiavo et al. 2000). A complex of M-toxin comprises one molecule of the BoNT toxin (150 kDa) and a molecule of nontoxic nonhemagglutinin protein (NTNH) (Arndt et al. 2005). It is produced by all types of *C. botulinum* except for the G type.
2. L is a toxin with a molecular weight of 500 kDa and a sedimentation constant of 16S, which consists of a single molecule of BoNT, NTNH, and hemagglutinin-type proteins, comprising four subunits: HA1, HA2, HA3a, and HA3b. Components HA1 and HA3b are able to actively bind to erythrocytes, but at least three HA components are needed for full hemagglutination activity: HA1, HA2, HA3b. "A" type L-toxins bind to the small intestine by means of galactose residues. They are produced by type A, B, C, D *C. botulinum*.
3. LL-toxin (*extralarge toxin*) with a molecular weight 900 kDa (sedimentation constant 19S) consists of two L subunits with a molecular weight of 900 kDa (sedimentation constant 19S). It is produced by A type strains of *C. botulinum* (Grenda and Kwiatek 2009).

BoNT/A occurs in three forms (M, L, and LL) and BoNT/B, BoNT/C, BoNT/D, and BoNT/F in two (M and L), whereas BoNT/F exists only in the M form. The number of NAP molecules is different in all serotypes of *C. botulinum*: there are seven of them in serotypes A and B and only one in serotype E (Sharma and Whiting 2005).

Production of toxins by strains of *Clostridium* is largely affected by bacteriophages, and the toxin-forming potential of the third group strains depends on the type of bacteriophages which infect them. Moreover, bacteriophages can transform nontoxic strains into toxic forms with the different antigen nature of the toxins they produce.

After they get into the body, botulinum toxins or tetanus toxin spread with body fluids to the presynaptic membrane of the cholinergic endings (Schiavo et al. 2000). A nerve impulse is transmitted through the nerve–muscle connection; it opens calcium channels in the presynaptic membrane. Calcium ions infiltrate the cell interior through the channels and bring about fusion of synaptic vesicles containing acetylcholine to the nerve cell membrane and its release to the gap between the synapse and a muscle. Acetylcholine binds to the muscle cell receptor, which results in a muscle contraction (Arnon et al. 2006). Botulinum toxin does not allow fusion of the synaptic vesicle and the neuron membrane, which prevents secretion of acetylcholine and results in flaccid paralysis of muscles.

The mechanism of action of *Clostridium* neurotoxins, regardless of their type, can be divided into three stages. During the first stage, the toxin binds specifically to nerve cell membranes, which happens if there are appropriate receptors on their surface. Different types of toxins bind to specific protein receptors, with an important role in the process being played by gangliosides (GT1b and GD1a) or glycoprotein 2 (SV2) (Montecucco et al. 2004). Tetanus toxin binds to the glycosylphosphatidylinositol (GPI)-anchored protein—Thy-1, whereas type A, B, E, G botulinum neurotoxins interact with synaptogamin I and II.

At stage II, BoNT infiltrates cytosol of a poisoned cell, a synaptic vesicle is formed, and a toxin molecule is absorbed into the neuron by endocytosis. A bisulfide bridge between HC and LC is broken by trypsin or by endogenous enzymes of the body. Owing to the acidic environment, HC forms pores in the membrane of the synaptic vesicle, through which LC is translocated to cytoplasm. Botulinum toxin is inactive when both chains—LC and HC—are bound by a disulfide bridge, because the active site of metalloprotease is obscured by the translocating domain of the HC. Therefore, the last stage involves reduction of the disulfide bridge which connects the HC and LC of the neurotoxin. The LC becomes a metalloprotease, which targets the SNARE complex (N-ethylmaleimide-sensitive factor attachment-protein receptor), connecting the synaptic vesicles containing neurotransmitters with the nerve cell membrane. Degradation of any of those proteins enables connection of the synaptic vesicle with the presynaptic membrane and releasing acetylcholine to the presynaptic space.

Clostridium perfringens is commonly known to cause gas gangrene. It is much less known that it is an important pathogen causing acute diarrheas in the United States and the United Kingdom, where it is regarded as the third most important bacterial pathogen responsible for food poisonings. This bacterium occurs commonly in soil and in sewage. There can be as many as 30% people who are healthy carriers (Sobel et al. 2005). The bacteria produce a range of toxins, among which enterotoxin is responsible for food poisonings, antibiotic-associated diarrhea (AAD) and sporadic diarrheas. It is believed that 6% of *C. perfringens* isolates produce the toxin when vegetative cells form spores. It is important that the bacteria can neutralize the acidic pH in the stomach by producing ammonia from arginine in a process catalyzed by arginine deiminase (Myers et al. 2006). It is very important that these are very rapidly multiplying microorganisms, because the duration of one generation is 6.3 min. Owing to these features, bacteria transported in contaminated food can cross the gastric barrier to the intestines where they multiply very quickly and produce enterotoxin, which results in acute diarrhea and abdominal pain appearing after 8 to 24 hours (Borriello 1995). It cannot be ruled out that enterotoxin can be produced in food, all the more so that it is not susceptible to the action of proteolytic enzymes (Smedley et al. 2004).

7.2.3 *Clostridium botulinum* Toxins in Food

As *C. botulinum* and its spores occur commonly in the environment, practically any food can be contaminated with botulinum bacilli. If such food is not treated to destroy the bacteria spores or if it is not subjected to thermal treatment to inactivate botulinum toxin before it is consumed, then botulism can develop. The limiting conditions for the proteolytic strains (group I) are: pH 4.6, minimum growth temperature 10°C–12°C, concentration of NaCl 10%, and spores resistance to heating >15 min ($D_{100°C}$). In the case of nonproteolytic strains (group II), the respective values are as follows: pH 5, minimum growth temperature 3°C, concentration of NaCl 5%, resistance of spores to heating <0.1 min ($D_{100°C}$); it is significant, however, that they usually occur in fish products (Peck and Stringer 2005).

Contrary to what is suggested by the Latin name (botulus—sausage), poisonings can originate not only from meat products but also from vegetables or fish. Botulinum toxin has been found in many different foods, such as fish and meat products, poultry products, canned meat, ham, sausage, stuffed eggs, lobsters, smoked and salted fish, canned maize, pepper, beans, honey, mushrooms, and olives (Abgueguen et al. 2003; Lindström et al. 2006). The most unusual cases of botulism occurred in prisoners in several prisons in the United States, which was caused by the consumption of illegally produced alcohol, called pruno or prison wine. This indicates that botulinum toxin can be produced in alcohol fermentation.

The number of cases of botulism in different countries varies, but in general it is smaller than for other intoxications and food toxoinfections. In Europe, poisonings with botulinum toxin are believed to originate from homemade meat products, whereas in the United States they originate from homemade products prepared from plant raw materials contaminated with spores of *C. botulinum.*

It is assumed that food prepared in an improper manner at home is a source of *C. botulinum* more frequently than that available in mass distribution. However, the number of cases of botulinum poisonings following consumption of industry-made food has been growing in recent years, which is caused by some changes in the methods of food production (Peck 2006). Consumers expect food products to be as little processed as possible and free of preservatives. Therefore, production technology is often limited to securing a product by refrigerating and packaging it in a modified atmosphere containing carbon dioxide. Refrigerators used during the process of food distribution and in consumers' homes frequently ensure a temperature of 10°C, at which spores of *C. botulinum* in Group II can germinate to vegetative forms. The atmosphere of CO_2 used in the modified atmosphere packaging technology helps botulinum bacilli to survive. Moreover, heat treatment of food in a temperature range, which is not lethal to *C. botulinum*, allows them to survive during the food processing stage. According to literature reports, botulism following the consumption of food produced in food factories is caused by nonproteolytic strains of *C. botulinum* of Group II.

Food stored properly and in proper conditions is not a carrier of *C. botulinum*. Unlike nonproteolytic strains, proteolytic strains do not grow at refrigeration temperatures. The number of spores in meat, including poultry, is rather small, much larger numbers have been recorded in fish meat.

Growth of *C. botulinum* requires an appropriate composition of the culturing medium, temperature, gas conditions, pH, redox potential of the environment (E_h), and water activity (a_w). The toxin is usually produced only in the optimum, or close to optimum, growth conditions. The nutritional requirements of *C. botulinum* are complex, and they include availability of amino acids, vitamins B, and minerals in the medium. Nonproteolytic strains of B and F type *C. botulinum* grow in liquid medium and produce toxins at the temperature of 4°C, but the toxin production in crab meat is minimal and it does not take place until a temperature of 26°C (Alberto et al. 2003). Water activity at which *C. botulinum* grow fluctuates between 0.94 (type B) and 0.97 (type E). The actual ability of *C. botulinum* strains to grow largely depends on the chemical compound which was used to adjust a_w of the medium.

The ability of *C. botulinum* to grow is also affected by other microorganisms present in the food. Growth of botulinum bacilli and production of neurotoxins at low pH is promoted by yeast. A synergistic effect has also been observed between *Clostridium* bacteria and lactic acid bacteria (LAB). Since they produce bacteriocins, LAB can also inhibit growth of *C. botulinum*. Such properties are exhibited by *Lactobacillus*, *Lactococcus*, *Streptococcus*, and *Pediococcus* (Rodgers et al. 2003). Growth of *C. botulinum* can be inhibited by the presence of other *Clostridium* spp., for example, *C. sporogenes* and *C. perfringens*. A similar relationship has been observed in the genus *Paenibacillus* and *Bacillus* (Girardin et al. 2002).

7.2.4 Detection of Botulinum Toxins

A biological test on mice with neutralization using antitoxins is a conventional method used to detect neurotoxins; its features include high specificity and sensitivity, and it can be used to determine the type of botulinum neurotoxins. However, the method has a number of limitations caused by the use of laboratory animals, consumption of large amounts of time (observation of animals every 4 days), which undoubtedly makes it difficult to start a targeted therapy promptly. The biological test can also give false-positive results caused by the presence of endotoxins of G (–) bacteria, tetanus toxin, or a large number of *C. botulinum* spores, which can produce botulinum neurotoxin *in vivo* (Lindström and Korkeala 2006).

Since suspected poisoning with botulinum toxin requires rapid diagnostics, laboratory confirmation of botulism is increasingly often done by molecular biology methods, polymerase chain reaction (PCR) techniques, and its modification (multiplex PCR, real-time PCR [qPCR], reverse transcription [RT]-PCR) (Dahlenborg et al. 2001). Molecular biology-based methods are highly sensitive and specific, and a result can be obtained within a short time. Since a positive result of a PCR reaction is only a sign of the potential for neurotoxin production (the presence of a gene encoding a neurotoxin), no conclusion can be drawn on the actual presence of BoNT in a sample. It is another issue that positive results can be obtained from material which contains dead cells of *C. botulinum*. In such a case, RT-PCR should be used, which detects a fragment of the BoNT gene only in live cells. qPCR enables quantitative measurement of the sought sequences of the BoNT gene, which reflects the content of the organism being detected in a sample. In recent years, several other genetic methods have been adapted to detect fragments of the *C. botulinum* genome, such as pulsed-field gel electrophoresis (PFGE), rybotyping, amplified DNA fragment length polymorphism (AFLP), random amplification of polymorphic DNA (RAPD), and repetitive element sequence-based PCR (Rep-PCR).

Shortening the time of diagnosis to a few hours is also made possible by methods based on immunological reactions: immune-enzymatic (ELISA, enzyme-linked immunosorbent assay), indirect hemagglutination test (HAp), or immunofluorescence-adsorption test (IFOA). Their advantages include a short time needed for such a test, while their disadvantages are low sensitivity and specificity. The sensitivity of the conventional ELISA method is 10 to 100 times lower than that of the biological test (Lindström et al. 1999).

Certain problems are encountered in detecting *C. botulinum*, both by molecular, biological, and immunoenzymatic methods in such samples as feces, blood, and food samples. Bile acid salts, immunoglobulins, blood, fats, and proteins can inhibit DNA reactions or reduce their sensitivity considerably (Kizerwetter-Świda and Binek 2010).

7.3 *STAPHYLOCOCCUS* GROUP

7.3.1 Introduction

Genus *Staphylococcus*, which belongs to the family Staphylococcaceae, order *Bacillales*, class *Bacilli*, phylum *Firmicutes*, is represented by gram-positive bacteria with a cell diameter of 0.5–1.5 μm which are relatively anaerobic, immobile, nonspore-forming mesophiles (Euzéby 2015). Their name is associated with their being typically arranged in irregular bunches (Greek *staphyle* = grapes). In the natural environment, they can also occur as single cells, diplococci, quadruple cocci, or short chains (Fischetti et al. 2000).

The majority of staphylococci can grow at temperatures ranging from 7°C to 48°C, pH 4–10, and at $a_w = 0.86$. Their characteristic features include high resistance to various physical and chemical factors. They grow in culturing media containing 40% of bile and 15% of sodium chloride. They die at a temperature of 60°C but only after being heated for half an hour. They are also resistant to drying, and they can survive for a long time outside an organism provided they have access to protein (Schmitt et al. 1990).

Genus *Staphylococcus* comprises 51 species and 27 subspecies. Bacteria of this group are a component of natural, physiological flora in people and animals. A number of species prefer being in specific places on the body, for example, on the skin (*S. epidermidis*), mucous membranes (e.g., in the nasopharynx—*S. aureus*), sweat glands (*S. hominis*, *S. aureus* subsp. *anaerobius*, *S. haemolyticus*), head skin (*S. capitis*), or the face skin (*S. saccharolyticus*) (Szewczyk 2011). Apart from the presence on the skin and mucous membranes in people and animals, staphylococci have been isolated from samples of soil, water, air, and different kinds of food (Ruaro et al. 2013). Among the 78 identified *Staphylococcus* species/subspecies, 31 have been associated with specific human and/or animal diseases, and some of them have been associated with cases of food poisonings. The most potent human pathogens include *S. aureus*, *S. epidermidis*, *S. haemolyticus*, *S. saprophyticus*, and *S. lugdunensis* (Veras et al. 2008).

7.3.2 *Staphylococcus* Toxins

Staphylococcus aureus is the best-known human and animal pathogen staphylococcus. The pathogenicity of *S. aureus* strains is affected by toxin-like enzymes, toxins, and components of external covers (Haveri et al. 2007).

Toxin-like enzymes damage cells and promote the spread of toxins. There are five enzymes produced by *S. aureus*: hyaluronidase, coagulase and fibrinolisin, lipase, and nuclease (Kaneko and Kamio 2003).

Toxins produced by *S. aureus* include six types of cytolytic toxins: α-hemolysin, β-hemolysin, γ-hemolysin, δ-hemolysin, leukocidins, and Panton–Valentine leukocidin (PVL) as well as a large group of toxins, which comprises exotoxins in pyrogenic groups with superantigenic properties (PTSAgs—*pyrogenic toxin superantigens*). This includes the toxic shock syndrome toxin-1 (TSST-1), enterotoxins SEs (*S. enterotoxins*) and four types of exfoliatin (ETA, ETB, ETC, and ETD) (Dinges et al. 2000).

Pathogenicity of staphylococci depends on the presence of specific cell structures, such as the capsule, peptidoglycan, and teichoic acids. The capsule inhibits chemotaxia, phagocytosis, proliferation of neutrophils as well as facilitates adhesion to surfaces. Peptidoglycan also inhibits phagocytosis, but it mainly ensures the osmotic stability of cells and stimulates the production of puss-forming agents. The presence of teichoic acids helps to bind to fibronectin. *S. aureus* exhibits the ability to excrete surface proteins that facilitate adhesion to host cells. *S. aureus* bacteria also produce proteins that bind to proteins and blood cells (protein A, clumping factor—CF), which blocks the immune response and plays an important role in initiation and/or intensification of the inflammation (Foster and Hook 1998).

α-Hemolysin (Hla, α-toxin, toxin A)—consists of 293 amino acids with a molecular weight of 33 kDa and pI of about 8.5. The amino acids of the polypeptide do not include cysteine. Mature protein consists mainly of a β-sheet (65%) and α-helix, which comprises 10% of the secondary structure (Dinges et al. 2000; Gurnev and Nestorovich 2014).

α-Hemolysin is encoded by the *hla* gene, which was cloned and sequenced in 1984 by Gray and Kehoe (1984). Expression of the toxin is regulated by a two-component regulatory system—accessory gene regulator (agr) and a signal transduction system—saeR/S. It has cytotoxic, hemolytic, and dermonectoric properties and affects a wide range of human cells, including erythrocytes, monocytes, lymphocytes, macrophages, and epithelial cells. A lethal dose of α-hemolysin is small—approx. 1 μg in an intravenous injection for a rabbit. The toxin can also induce aggregation of human thrombocytes with neutrophils. Selectivity of the α-toxin toward cells of different species, as well as specific cells, is associated with expression of the recently discovered cellular receptor ADAM10 (Disintegrin and Metalloproteinase Domain-containing protein 10) (Berube and Wardenburg 2013).

β-Hemolysin (neutral sphingomyelinase, SPH, "hot-cold" hemolysin) is a monomeric surface-secreted protein, with a molecular weight of 35 kDa in *S. aureus* and 33.5 kDa in *S. intermedius* and pI > 9 (Szymańska and Buczek 1999; Huseby et al. 2007). β-Hemolysin has a toxic effect on human monocytes, leukocytes, keratinocytes, and lymphocytes, and even if it does not cause directly cell lysis, it makes them sensitive to other toxins, such as phenol-soluble modulins (PSMs) (Salgado-Pabón et al. 2014).

γ-Hemolysins (HlγA, HlγB, and HlγC) called gamma-toxins, PVL (LukS-PV and LukF-PV) and different variants of leukocidins (LukM, LukE, LukD) are two-component exotoxins of the family of proteins with the structure of a β-barrel. Active proteins comprise two formed, but not initially bound polypeptide chains—S component (HlγA, HlγC, LukS-PV, LukM, LukE) and F component (HlγB, LukF-PV, LukD), which have affinity to cell membranes. S class proteins are the first to bind to the membranes of sensitive cells; they are followed by F class proteins. Subsequently, Ca^{2+} ions flow out, pores are formed, and ethidium flows in, which causes cell death (Alessandrini et al. 2013; Alonzo and Torres 2014). γ-Hemolysins exhibit a cytotoxic effect on rabbit, human, and sheep erythrocytes and also on human neutrophils. P-V leukocidin is leukotoxic, but it does not exhibit hemolytic activity (Taylor and Bernheimer 1974).

δ-Hemolysin (δ-toxin, δ-lysin) is an amphipathic polypeptide with a small molecular weight of 2.9 kDa with a α-helix structure, consisting of 26 amino acids (Pokorny et al. 2008). It belongs to a family of PSMα (Otto 2014) and is produced by nearly all *S. aureus* as well as by some coagulase-negative staphylococci (e.g., *S. epidermidis*, *S. haemolyticus*, *S. hominis*, *S. lugdunensis*, and *S. warnerii* and also, to a lesser extent, by *S. cohnii*, *S. sciuri*, *S. saprophyticus*, and *S. xylosus* (Verdon et al. 2009). This toxin is encoded by the *hld* gene, which is a structural element of the RNAIII molecule of the agr regulatory system, whose function includes global regulation of both cell surfaces and secretion of the virulence agents. The mechanism of toxin action on the host's cell membranes depends on its toxin concentration in the environment. When the concentration is lower than the boundary concentration, the toxin aggregates and adheres to the surface, disturbing its two-layer form and opens the channels when the concentration increases slightly: small channels in the form of octamers or large channels made up of oligomers. When the toxin concentration is high, above the boundary value, it acts as a surfactant and disrupts the two-layer structure of a cell membrane, which results in immediate cell lysis (Verdon et al. 2009). δ-Hemolysin has the hemolytic effect on erythrocytes of many mammal species and other mammalian cells, as well as on membrane-covered cellular structures.

Exfoliative toxins produced by *S. aureus* are classified as serine proteases. To date, there are four serotypes of exfoliative toxins (ETA, ETB, ETC, and ETD), three of which are linked with human infections. The best known are two types of exfoliative toxins ETA and ETB, which are species specific and which affect cells of humans, monkeys, mice, and hamster, but they do not affect cells of the rat, rabbit, dog, hedgehog, vole, or hen. Both toxins have been identified and sequenced (their sequence is homologous in 40%). ETA and ETB consist of 242 and 246 amino acids, and their molecular weights are 26.950 and 27.274 Da, respectively (Papageorgiou et al. 2000). The *eta* gene is chromosomally encoded while *etb* is plasmid encoded. ETA is a thermally stable toxin, which retains its exfoliating effect even after it is heated at 60°C for 30 minutes. However, ETB is a thermally labile toxin (Ladhani et al. 1999).

Exfoliatins A and B cause staphylococcal scalded skin syndrome (SSSS) and bullous impetigo. Scalded skin syndrome, also known as Ritter's disease, manifests itself as large, flat blisters, whose covers are disrupted after a short time, exposing vast areas of skin without the epidermis (Bukowski et al. 2010). Exfoliatins damage desmoglobin-1 (Dsg-1), which occurs in connections between keratinocytes (desmosomes). Damage to Dsg-1 results in the separation of keratinocytes, with consequent exfoliation of the epidermis and formation of blisters and the bacteria infiltrate deeper layers of the epidermis. SSSS occurs mainly in new-born babies and in small children, because desmoglein is present only in the skin of young mammals (Amagai et al. 2000; Onuma et al. 2011).

The TSST-1 is a water-soluble exotoxin, made up of 234 amino acids with a molecular weight of 22.000 Da and pI 7.2. It does not have cysteine residues, and it is resistant to high temperatures and the action of proteolytic enzymes. TSST-1 can be boiled for more than 1 hour without losing its biological activity. Its properties do not change after prolonged exposure to trypsin. TSST-1 is chromosomally encoded by the *tst* gene (Dinges et al. 2000). It is responsible for inducing toxic shock syndrome (TSS). This disease usually affects women who use tampons during their menstruation, but it can also affect nonmenstruating women or men and it can be associated with local foci, such as abscesses or burns.

The SEs are members of the super antigen family, which stimulate a large population of T cells (Pinchuk et al. 2010). They are called thus because they induce vomiting after being given orally to primates. Several SEs have been separated and called SE-like (SEl), because they either do not induce vomiting or their vomit-inducing activity has not been confirmed. Twenty-three serotypes of enterotoxins have been identified so far: five classical ones—SEA, SEB, SEC1-2-3, SED, SEE and 18 new ones, that is, SEG, SEH, SlE, SElJ, SElK, SElL, SElM, SElN, SElO, SElP, SElQ, SER, SES, SET, SElU, SElU2, SElV, SElX (Wilson et al. 2011; Hennekinne et al. 2013; Podkowik et al. 2013). The genes which encode SEs and SEls are located both in the chromosomal DNA (*seb, seg, seh, sei, selm, seln, selo, selu, selv, selx*) and on different moveable elements, that is, prophages (*sea, see, selp*), transposons (*seh*), plasmids (*seb, sed, selj, ser, ses,* and *set*), and pathogenicity islands (*seb, sec, selk, sell, selq*). There are also *se* genes that are coregulated within the *egc* (enterotoxin gene cluster) operon, that is, *seg, sei, selm, seln, selo, selu,* and *selv* (Gencay et al. 2010; Hennekinne et al. 2013; Hu and Nakane 2014).

Both classical enterotoxins and enterotoxin-like toxins (SE-*like*) are water-soluble and physiological-saline-soluble proteins, made up of—depending on the toxin—168–257 amino acids, with the molecular weight of 19–28 kDa (Hu and Nakane 2014). These are thermostable compounds, active within a wide range of pH. Studies of enterotoxicity of staphylococci, which have dealt mainly with *S. aureus*, have confirmed that different enterotoxins can be produced in a wide range of temperatures (10°C–45°C), a_w (0.85–0.99), and pH (4–9.6). The optimum conditions for such production are: $T = 37°C–45°C$, $a_w = 0.98$, and pH 7–8 (Hennekinne et al. 2013; Qi and Miller 2000). It is a common feature of SEs that they are highly resistant to proteolytic enzymes, that is, pepsin and trypsin.

7.3.3 Enterotoxins in Food Products

Source data on staphylococci confirm their frequent occurrence and diverse composition in terms of species present and their cell count in different products (Erkan et al. 2008; Goja et al. 2013; Ruaro et al. 2013). However, the mere presence of staphylococci in food does not have to mean that a consumer's health is at risk. Such risk is posed by toxin-producing strains whose count in food exceeds 10^5 cfu/g/cm^3 (Bhatia and Zahoor 2007).

Vegetative cells of staphylococci are killed during thermal treatment at temperatures exceeding about 65°C. SEs are resistant to thermal treatment, they can retain their biological activity even after pasteurization, boiling, or smoking. It has been shown that the thermal resistance of enterotoxins depends on their type, concentration, and the type of food they are in. Enterotoxin B is the most heat resistant (it can withstand sterilization at the temperature of 121°C for 20 minutes). The risk of food poisonings caused by enterotoxins is intensified by the fact that they do not change the taste, smell, or appearance of food products (Niścigorska 1999).

According to valid regulations, only coagulase-positive strains, mainly *S. aureus*, but also *S. intermedius* and *S. hyicus.*, are regarded as being capable of producing enterotoxins and causing food poisonings. However, recent literature reports suggest that some coagulase-negative staphylococci can also produce enterotoxins. These species include *S. caprae*, *S. chromogenes*, *S. cohnii*, *S. epidermidis*, *S. haemolyticus*, *S. lentus*, *S. saprophyticus*, *S. sciuri*, *S. warneri*, *S. xylosus* (Cremonesia et al. 2005; Jay et al. 2005), *S. simulans*, *S. equorum*, *S. capitis* (Vernozy-Rozand et al. 1996), *S. carnosus* and *S. piscifermentans* (Zell et al. 2008).

The following four conditions must be met for a staphylococci-induced food poisoning to occur (Hennekinne et al. 2010):

- The presence of a source containing an enterotoxic staphylococcus strain, for example, a human as a carrier,
- Transferring staphylococcus from a source to food, for example, owing to a lack of hygiene,
- Favorable conditions for multiplication and production of enterotoxins, that is, the right pH, temperature, a_w, and time,
- Consumption of food containing a specific amount of enterotoxins (20–100 ng).

Food poisoning caused by staphylococci usually occurs after eating confectionery products with cream, milk and dairy products, fish or meat products, salads and vegetable products, or ice cream.

Enterotoxin A and, less frequently B and C, are responsible for the largest portion of food poisonings. Enterotoxin(s) consumed with food produces symptoms of food poisoning—depending on the type and dose of the toxin—0.5 to 8 hours after it was consumed. The symptoms usually include: nausea, vomiting, abdominal pain and diarrhea, and very rarely fever (Satora 2008). The duration of the symptoms usually ranges from 24 to 48 hours. Deaths following the consumption of food contaminated with enterotoxin are very rare (1 per 3000) and occur mainly in children and individuals with vascular issues.

Staphylococci are one of the major causes of food poisonings on a global scale. According to a report prepared by the European Food Safety Authority (EFSA) and European Centre for Disease Prevention and Control (ECDC) (2013), staphylococci were responsible for 386 focal food poisonings (3203 cases) in the European Union (EU) countries in 2013. Compared with 2012 (346 foci/2532 cases), the number of poisonings foci with this cause increased by as much as 11.6%. In the 12 EU countries from which epidemiological statistical data are available for 2013, the largest number of staphylococci-caused food poisonings was recorded in France and Spain. No deaths were recorded. Poisonings usually happened after eating "mixed foods" (19.1%) and "vegetables and juices and other related products" (12.8%). With 103 cases on record, Poland ranked sixth in terms of food poisonings caused by staphylococcal toxins.

7.3.4 Detection of Staphylococcal Toxins

The ability to produce toxins and the genes encoding the toxins in staphylococci can be detected by different methods. These can be classified as: biological, genetic, immunological, indirect, and physicochemical.

Biological (in vivo) methods, due to their low sensitivity and ethical limitations, are used to detect toxins decreasingly often, but simple methods are still used in routine diagnostic tests (in vitro), for example, to asses hemolytic activity. The simplest method (described in 1973) of differentiating hemolysins: α, β, γ, δ and leukocidins is one based on the difference of sensitivity of cells isolated from different animal species (Thelestam et al. 1973; Prevost et al. 1995).

Another group of methods used to detect only the presence of the toxin-encoding genes includes molecular biology techniques that employ different variants of the PCR reaction (e.g., multiplex-PCR, real-time PCR). The techniques are based on amplification of nucleic acids in the PCR reaction using specific DNA starters that are complementary to the sequence. These methods can be used to detect the presence of toxin-encoding genes, that is, hemolysin (*hla*, *hlb*, *hld*, *hlg*, and hlg_v), leukocidin (lukS-PV, LukF-PV, lukS-I, LukF-I, lukM, lukED, lukGH/AB), exfoliative toxins (*eta*, *etb*, *etc*, and *etd*), TSST-1 (*tst*), and genes which encode individual enterotoxins (*sea*, *seb*, *sec*1-2-3, *sed*, *see*, *seg*, *seh*, *sei*, *selj*, *selk*, *sell*, *selm*, *seln*, *selo*, *selp*, *selq*, *ser*, *ses*, *set*, *selu*, *selu2*, *selv*, *selx*). Moreover, some toxins (e.g., PVL) can be identified at the RNA level, for example, by the RT-PCR method (Bronner et al. 2000;

Deurenberg et al. 2004). Genetic methods are widely applied in detecting toxins because they are specific, sensitive, and rapid. However, they have some limitations, the main ones being isolation of a strain from the environment and that the result only gives information about the presence of a gene and not about its expression.

The third group of methods of detecting toxins is immune techniques, which include: immunofluorescent techniques, immunochromatographic tests, and—the most widely used—the ELISA test (Genestier et al. 2005; Rainard 2007; Badiou et al. 2010). These tests can be used to detect hemolysins, leukocidins, and also enterotoxins. Apart from ELISA, enterotoxins can be detected by the enzyme-linked fluorescent assay (ELFA) or reverse passive latex agglutination (RPLA) methods. However, these are methods of low sensitivity and specificity and because antibodies against only some types of staphylococcal toxins are available for economic reasons, the tests can be used only to detect five types of enterotoxins SEA–SEE or, with RPLA, only four SEA–SED (Vasconcelos and Cunha 2010).

To fully characterize the ability to produce toxins, immunological, molecular, and other techniques are increasingly often combined.

There is a separate group of methods—indirect methods—which are hard to classify into one of the groups mentioned above, because they are combinations of different techniques of detection. These are mainly colorimetric methods, in which certain structures are stained and the resulting changes are observed under a microscope (optical, fluorescent, confocal, or TEM—transmission electron microscope). Such methods include: tests of cytotoxicity (test of incorporation of neutral red) (Rainard et al. 2003), tests based on reduction of tetrasole salts (Chung et al. 1993), determination of fragmentation of leukocyte DNA (TUNEL method), flow cytometry (Gauduchon et al. 2001), and observation of changes in morphology of cells stained by the methods of: May–Grünwald, Wright, Giemsa, Hoechst 33342 and by the immunofluorescent method (Genestier et al. 2005; Barrio et al. 2006).

Due to certain limitations of the tests mentioned above, using the methods from the latter group, based on physicochemical techniques, has been attracting growing attention. The largest interest has been attracted by mass spectrometry (MS), especially MALDI-TOF (matrix-assisted laser desorption/ ionization time-of-flight mass spectrometry) (Ritz and Curtis 2012). Currently, this is the most sensitive and rapid method of qualitative and quantitative analysis of samples in regard to the presence of toxins. However, due to high costs and the need to prepare the material in a specific manner, it is a supplementary method in detailed analyses.

7.4 *BACILLUS CEREUS* GROUP

7.4.1 Introduction

The genus *Bacillus* comprises spore-forming bacteria with various temperature-related requirements, pathogenic potential, and importance and ranges from strains used as plant growth promoters, biopesticides, and probiotics to strains responsible for infections/food poisonings in humans (Messelhäusser et al. 2010). Currently, the *B. cereus* group, referred to as *B. cereus* sensu lato, which comprises the following seven, closely-related species, is identified within the genus *Bacillus*, which includes

270 species (Euzéby 2012): *B. anthracis*, *B. thuringiensis*, *B. mycoides*, *B. pseudomycoides*, *B. weihenstephanensis*, *B. cereus* sensu stricto, and *B. cytotoxicus* sp. novel (Lamberet et al. 2013). A comparative analysis of the sequence of genomes of the species emphasizes the great similarity between these bacteria, which makes their species identification difficult.

It is a characteristic feature of *Bacillus* bacteria that they are capable of forming ellipsoidal endospores, with central or subterminal arrangement in a cell, which are highly resistant to heating (in some cases, light thermal treatment can stimulate spore germination, which creates the risk of food poisoning caused by *B. cereus*), drying, disinfectants, ionizing, and ultraviolet (UV) radiation.

7.4.2 *Bacillus* spp. and Their Toxins in Food

Bacillus cereus sensu lato are common in the environment, that is, in soil, sewage, water, dust, fertilizers, fodders, and they can be present in food of different origin and at different levels of processing as primary or secondary contamination. *Bacillus cereus* has been isolated from plant products (pasta, rice, vegetables, fruit, spices, nuts) (Subramanian et al. 2006). Spores of those bacteria frequently contaminate milk as a result of soiling udders with dirt, fodder, or animal feces (Anadon et al. 2006). They have been isolated from products of marine origin, meat products, and infant formulas.

The pathogenicity of *B. cereus* is determined by a range of toxins and toxin-like enzymes. The expression of the majority of pathogenicity factors in *B. cereus* depends on the presence of the global pleiotropic regulator PlcR, encoded by the *plcR* gene (Slamti et al. 2004). PlcR is responsible for the positive regulation of the expression of such genes as those of phospholipase C—phosphatidyl inositol hydrolase (Lereclus et al. 1996) and phosphatidylcholine hydrolase and SPH, three-component toxins hemolysin BL (HBL) and NHE, RNase, S-layer proteins (Agaisse et al. 1999), cell wall hydrolase (Økstad et al. 1999), at least five proteases, cereolysin, cytotoxin K, and thuringolysin (Slamti et al. 2004). Promoters of the genes that encode the virulence factors mentioned above have a characteristic sequence upstream of the transcription initiation site, which is responsible for binding PlcR. These genes do not create a common operon or "an island of pathogenicity," and genes regulated by PlcR are spread around different sites of a chromosome. It is believed that the regulon consists of at least 100 genes (Slamti et al. 2004), with the function of some of them still unknown. Transcription of genes regulated by PlcR occurs during the stationary phase of growth as a result of the quorum-sensing mechanism (Slamti and Lereclus 2002).

B. cereus is generally regarded as the causative factor in gastrointestinal disorders. The most frequently produced *B. cereus* sensu lato toxins include phospholipases C, hemolysins, enterotoxins, a range of extracellular protein toxins, and toxin-like enzymes. Moreover, *B. cereus* sensu stricto and *B. weihenstephanensis* can produce cereulide (emetic toxin) (Thorsen et al. 2006).

Hemolysins produced by *B. cereus* bring about lysis of erythrocytes as a result of synergistic action of phospholipase C (PC-PLC) dependent on phosphatidylcholine (PC) and SPH, which make up a biological complex known as cereolysin AB (CerAB) (Gilmore et al. 1989).

CerAB causes hemolysis by enzymatic degradation of the cell membrane, but it does not form pores. Pore-forming hemolysins of *B. cereus* include: hemolysin I (cereolysin O, CLO), hemolysin II, hemolysin III, and hemolysin IV, commonly known as cytotoxin K.

Since the specificity of hemolysins of *B. cereus* is low, they cause lysis of erythrocytes, but they also damage most eukaryotic cells (Stachowiak and Bielecki 2000). Hemolysin IV seems to be the fastest acting and the most common hemolysin in filtrates from *B. cereus* cultures, which indicates that it may be an important virulence factor (Fagerlund et al. 2004).

Hemolysin is a toxin produced by *B. cereus*, *B. thuringiensis*, and *B. anthracis*, and it is referred to as CLO, thuringolysin O (TLO), and anthrolysin O (ALO), respectively (Shannon et al. 2003). It is a cholesterol-dependent cytotoxin (CDC) (Alouf et al. 2005), which brings about lysis of different types of cells, including erythrocytes under in vitro conditions.

Hemolysin II (Hly II) is common in *B. cereus* bacteria, including *B. thuringiensis* (Budarina et al. 1994), and it does not require the presence of cholesterol for its activity (Sinev et al. 1993). It is thermolabile and susceptible to the action of proteolytic enzymes. It is one of pore-forming toxins β-PFT, which is typical of gram-positive bacteria.

Hly exhibits hemolytic and cytotoxic activity toward human cell lines (Andreeva et al. 2006), but its role in the microorganism virulence has not been determined. Hemolytic activity of the toxin toward rabbit blood cells is more than 15 times stronger than that of α-toxins of *Staphylococcus* (Miles et al. 2006). It has been suggested that it is inactivated by trypsin in the small intestine (Stenfors et al. 2008); therefore, it has not been associated with diarrheas caused by *B. cereus*. Moreover, it has been shown that regulation of production of HlyII depends on the redox potential of the environment; the toxin accumulates at a high redox potential (Clair et al. 2010). Due to a low redox potential of the intestinal environment (anaerobic conditions), HlyII will not be a factor of virulence with a role in etiology of the gastrointestinal system diseases.

Hemolysin III (Hly III) is another hemolysin of *B. cereus*. It attacks the erythrocyte membrane as a monomer, and it is not until a number of monomers accumulated on the erythrocyte surface that lysis occurs. Toxin binding to the erythrocyte surface seems to be temperature dependent (Baida and Kuzmin 1996). It is an example of what is known as the multi-impact mechanism, typical of streptolysin O, and theta-toxin of *C. perfringens* (Baida and Kuzmin 1996). The amino acid sequence of the toxin does not contain any typical signal peptides (Baida and Kuzmin 1995).

Strains of *B. cereus* can produce collagenase that degrades soluble and insoluble forms of collagen, gelatin, and bradykinin to small peptides. Its production is dependent on the strain and the culture medium; also, it is more intensive in anaerobic than in aerobic conditions (Kotiranta et al. 2000). Proteases produced by *B. cereus* probably play a significant role in parenteral infections. Proteases isolated from virulent strains of *B. cereus* were able to hydrolyze hemoglobin, albumin, and casein (Sierecka 1998).

7.4.3 Epidemiological and Medical Importance of *Bacillus* Toxins

According to data from EFSA and ECDC , based on epidemiological reports from 11 and 10 EU member states for the years 2011 and 2012, respectively, toxin-producing *Bacillus* were the causative factor in 220 and 259 focal infections/food poisonings with 2307 and 2518 cases, respectively, of which 174/231 required hospitalization and 1/3 ended with the patient's death (EFSA 2013, 2014). Interestingly, the number of focal food poisonings caused by *B. cereus* increased by 122% in 2011 as compared with 2010 (EFSA 2012). Both the number of cases of poisoning caused by the bacteria and the portion of toxin-forming *Bacillus*-caused focal infections/food poisonings in the EU—3.9% in 2011 and 4.8% in 2012 and incidence—0.04/100,000 in 2011 and 0.05/100,000 in 2012—has been increasing in recent years.

According to epidemiologists, statistical data regarding cases of infections/food poisonings per year provide only approximate data on their number, and they are strongly understated for such pathogens as, for example, toxin-producing *Bacillus* spp. (CDC 2011). Among the possible causes for this, there are such factors as mild course of infections caused by the bacteria, which does not usually require medical intervention, attributing symptoms to other causal factor present in the product-carrier or, in the case of atypical *B. cereus*, classifying them as cases of unknown etiology.

B. cereus is capable of producing two main types of toxins responsible for food poisonings, that is, enterotoxins and the emetic (vomit-inducing) toxin. Enterotoxins are commonly produced by populations of *B. cereus* bacteria; however, the ability to produce the emetic toxin has been detected in *B. cereus* sensu stricto (Ehling-Schulz 2006b) and in individual strains of *B. weihenstephanensis* (Thorsen et al. 2006), which are phenotypically closer to psychrophilic *B. mycoides* than in *B. cereus* (Thorsen et al. 2006).

According to reports, food poisonings with vomiting are most commonly caused by *B. cereus* consumed with starch products, whereas diarrheal poisonings are caused by such products as meat, vegetables, and dairy products.

B. cereus-induced diarrheal food poisonings are caused by two different protein enterotoxins, that is, HBL (Beecher and MacMillan 1991) and nonhemolytic enterotoxin (NHE) (Lund and Granum 1996). Each enterotoxin consists of three protein components. They are produced by vegetative *B. cereus* cells in human small intestine during the logarithmic phase of growth. Higher enterotoxin activity is observed in strains capable of fermenting lactose (Giffel et al. 1997).

The HBL toxin is commonly regarded as the main factor that causes *B. cereus* sensu lato-induced diarrheal food poisonings. The thermostable three-component HBL enterotoxin consists of three protein components: B, L_1i L_2 (Gilois et al. 2007) with the molecular weight of 37, 38, and 46 kDa, respectively. Each of the protein component of HBL is genome-encoded, and one DNA sequence corresponds to one component. Components of toxin HBL are transcribed from operon *hbl* (Ryan et al. 1997), on which four genes have been found, that is, *hblC*—which encodes protein L_2, *hblD*—which encodes protein L_1, *hblA*—which encodes protein B, and *hblB*—which encodes protein B′ (probably a substitute of protein B), homologous in 73% to protein B (Granum et al. 1999). All the components are necessary to induce symptoms of a disease (Beecher and Wong 1994), but not all strains are capable of producing the three protein components of the toxin (Veldin't et al. 2001). This can be associated with the fact that operon *hbl* is situated in an unstable part of the chromosome of *B. cereus* (Granum et al. 1999).

The latest literature reports present two mechanisms of cell lysis induced by enterotoxin HBL. According to one of them, binding the lytic components (L1 and L2) to a cell is preceded by joining of the binding factor B (Beecher and MacMillan 1991). Beecher and Wong (2000) showed that the independently binding toxin components make up a complex that attacks a cell membrane. A cell is destroyed as a result of internalization in the membrane of at least one of the lytic components of the toxin, which leads to osmotic lysis (Beecher and Wong 1997). None of the components of toxin HBL individually is biologically active, but in combination they make up a lytic system that affects permeability of cell membranes, with cytotoxic, hemolytic, dermonecrotic, and enterotoxic effect (Beecher and Wong 1997). HBL activates enteric adenylate cyclase, which affects conversion of adenosine triphosphate (ATP) to cyclic adenosine monophosphate (cAMP), which increases permeability of cell membranes, thereby causing secretion of liquids in the intestines (diarrhea).

HBL is secreted by about 45%–65% of *B. cereus* strains (Moravek et al. 2006). However, the percentage of strains capable of producing the toxin depends on the environment in which the strains are isolated, and it ranges from 43% (environmental strains) to 81% (clinical strains).

The nonhemolytic toxin NHE was first isolated from the *B. cereus* strain responsible for the outbreak of food poisoning in Norway (Lund and Granum et al. 1996). It is believed to be secreted by 100% of *B. cereus* strains (Moravek et al. 2006).

The NHE consists of three protein components: NheA with the molecular weight of 41 kDa, NheB with the molecular weight of 39 kDa, and NheC with the molecular weight of 105 kDa (Ryan et al. 1997). Like with enterotoxin HBL, all the components are necessary to produce a cytotoxic effect; moreover, they have the maximum toxic effect on Vero cells when the ratio of the components concentration is 10:10:1 (NheA:NheB:NheC) (Lindbäck et al. 2004).

The NHE is chromosomally encoded. Operon *nhe* in *B. cereus* contains three open frames for readout of *nheA*, *nheB*, and *nheC*. The first two of them encode two components of the nonhemolytic toxin—NheA and NheB, the role of *nheC* remains unknown. According to literature reports, protein NheC can be a specific catalyst that joins the other two components, or it can accelerate conformational changes (Lindbäck et al. 2004).

Cytotoxin K is a protein cytotoxin with the molecular weight of 34 kDa with necrotic, cytotoxic, and hemolytic properties, first described by Beecher and Wong (2000). The toxin was first isolated, cloned, sequenced from the strain of *B. cereus* 391/98 NVH (Lund et al. 2000). The strain was the cause of a focus of food poisoning, and the toxin caused the death of three people with diagnosed necrotic gastritis (Lund et al. 2000). Currently, the strain has been classified as a new, seventh species in *B. cereus* group: *B. cytotoxicus* (Guinebretière et al. 2012). Not much is known about the action of CytK at the cellular level. In vitro studies have shown high toxicity toward Vero and CaCo-2 cells (Hardy et al. 2001). Pores formed by the toxin are weakly anion selective. It is assumed that the minimum diameter of cytK pores is about 7Å (Hardy et al. 2001), while the stoichiometry and structure of the pores remains unknown. The conductivity of channels formed by CytK-2 is smaller than those formed by CytK-1.

Two types of cytotoxin K have been identified with 89% similarity of their amino acid composition. Variant 2 (CytK-2), which is more frequent, also exhibits hemolytic and toxic activity toward human intestinal cells as well as Caco-2 and Vero cell lines. However, the first of them (CytK-1) is more toxic toward human intestinal cells and Caco-2 and Vero cell lines. According to source data, genes of cytotoxin K are common in different strains of *B. cereus* (Rosenquist et al. 2005), with cytK-2 being particularly common in mesophilic groups of *B. cereus* (phylogenetic group III and IV), and uncommon or absent in psychrotolerant or moderately psychrotolerant strains (groups VI, II, and V). The *cytK* gene has not been found in strains of group I.

The key role in infections with diarrhea is played by spores of enterotoxic strains of *B. cereus* consumed with food. Between 10^3 and 10^7 spores/bacteria/g is regarded as an infective dose (Granum and Lund 1997). In virulent and highly adhesive strains, symptoms can be induced by 200 spores/g of food consumed. After reaching the small intestine, spores cling to the walls of epithelial cells, where they germinate and produce enterotoxins. Bacteria fixed to intestinal epithelium cells can cause cytotoxicity. In addition, enterotoxins activate adenylate cyclase, which converts ATP to cAMP, which, in effect, increases secretion of liquids in the intestine. Apart from diarrhea, nonspecific symptoms can occur, such as abdominal pain and nausea. They appear 8–20 hours after consuming food contaminated with *B. cereus* sensu lato bacteria, and they usually persist for 12–24 hours. The course of infection is usually mild; more severe cases are rare.

The emetic toxin (cereulide) has the form of a ring (dodecadepsipeptide) made up of three replications of four amino acids and/or oxyacids: $[\text{D-O-Leu-D-Ala-L-O-Val-L-Val}]_3$ with the molecular weight of 1.2 kDa, and it is close to potassium ionophore (valinomycin) (Agata et al. 1994). The emetic toxin is thermo- and acid-resistant, soluble in methanol, it does not have an antigenic action, it is not proteolyzed by pepsin or trypsin, it does not have an isoelectric point, and it is stable at the temperature of 121°C for 90 minutes at pH 2–11 (Andersson et al. 1998). The emetic toxin is highly thermostable, and it is not destroyed during conventional thermal processing of food. One of the mechanisms of controlling cereulide production is quorum sensing, which explains why the toxin is not produced in shaken cultures (Rajkovic et al. 2007), when local communication between bacteria is disturbed. The presence in the growth environment of such amino acids as L-valine and L-leucine stimulates production of cereulide but only when they are available in the nonbound form (Jääskeläinen et al. 2004).

Emetic strains of *B. cereus* differ from the others by some biochemical features (absence of amylase, poor hemolytic activity), different thermal requirements, and small differences in thermal resistance. The emetic strains exhibit slightly higher resistance to heating but lower activity at lower temperatures (Carlin et al. 2006), hence they pose a risk in heated food, which is kept at the room temperature (restaurants, bars). Refrigerated food should not pose any health risk in regard to these strains.

The emetic toxin is produced extracellularly during the stationary phase of growth. Like other antibiotics and bioactive peptides typical of *B. cereus* sensu lato, cereulide is produced by the NRPS (nonribosomal peptide synthetases) system (Horwood et al. 2004). This multifunctional complex of enzymatic peptide synthetases, which occurs in all strains of *B. cereus*, is genomically encoded, and it can manifest slight differences in the nucleotide sequence in the emetic and nonemetic strains.

The protein-encoding genes associated with production of the emetic toxin are located in the *ces* operon. It consists of a cluster of seven genes of cereulide synthetase: *cesH*, *cesP*, *cesT*, *cesA*, *cesB*, *cesC*, *cesD*. The product of the *cesH* gene, with the molecular weight of 31 kDa, is probably hydrolase/acylotransferase; the *cesP* gene probably encodes 4′- phosphopantetheinyl transferase (28.9 kDa), which takes part in synthesis of gramicidin S and sulphactin in *B. subtilis*; and the *cesT*, with the molecular weight of 27.6 kDa, is an alleged type II thioesterase. The structural genes of cereulide synthetase are encoded by *cspA* (10 kpz) and *cesB* (8 kpz). However, *cesC* and *cesD* genes probably encode the ABC transporter (Ehling-Schulz et al. 2006a). The modules of cereulide synthesis mentioned above are probably responsible for the formation of cyclic dodecadepsipeptide.

According to literature data, production of the emetic toxin largely depends on the *B. cereus* strain and the environmental conditions, that is, composition of the growth medium, pH, temperature, and availability of oxygen (Rajkovic et al. 2006). Production of the toxin starts at the end of the phase of logarithmic growth of the bacteria and is independent of the process of sporulation (Häggblom et al. 2002).

Production of the emetic toxin in static cultures was observed at temperatures of 22°C and 30°C. Finlay et al. (2000) did not record production of the toxin at the temperature of 37°C, and they regarded 15°C–30°C as the optimum temperature for its production. However, Häggblom et al. (2002) recorded small amount of cereulide in cultures maintained at 8°C and 40°C. This can indicate that production of cereulide by strains of *B. cereus* in the human body is unlikely and vomiting can be caused by consumption of the toxin already present in food. The amount of the emetic toxin in food, which induced vomiting, ranged from 0.02 to 1.28 μg cereulide/g (Agata et al. 1996). Rice and rice products make a favorable environment for production of cereulide by *B. cereus*. Meanwhile, emetic food poisonings, mainly following consumption of food with rice, has usually been recorded in Japan (Nichols et al. 1999).

The emetic toxin is produced mainly by strains of *B. cereus* of the ciliated serovar H-1; this potential is manifested to a lesser extent by strains of serovars H-3, H-5, and H-12. However, diarrheal strains (which do not produce cereulide) are usually ones of serotypes H-2, H-6, H-8, H-9, and H-10 (Mikami et al. 1994). So far, two emetic strains have been identified which are not *B. cereus* sensu stricto, but, most probably, *B. weihenstephanensis*, whose phenotype was closer to the psychrophilic strains of *B. mycoides* than *B. cereus*. Apart from these exceptional species, the ability to produce the emetic toxin is attributed to *B. cereus* sensu stricto (Ehling-Schulz et al. 2006b). The emetic toxin acts like an ionophore that transports K^+ ions to mitochondria according to the gradient of concentrations and the electric gradient. This mechanism resembles the action of valinomycin, whose chemical structure is similar. The action of cereulide inactivates mitochondria, in which the redox processes discontinue, which manifests as a change of the motility of sperm in the microscopic picture (Rajkovic et al. 2006). Cereulide has an inhibiting effect on human cytotoxic white blood cells (killer cells), whereby it can affect the immune system. Vomiting is a result of a combination of the emetic toxin with the 5-HT3 receptor and stimulation of the vagus nerve (Agata et al. 1995). Cereulide is also responsible for inhibiting oxidation of fatty acids in mitochondria of hepatocytes, which results in liver damage (Mahler et al. 1997).

It is assumed that 10^5–10^8 bacteria/spores/g of *B. cereus* can produce enough toxin for the disease symptoms to develop. The amount of the emetic toxin that induces the disease symptoms fluctuated between 0.02 and 1.28 μg cereulide/g of food. It has been suggested that the clinical dose of cereulide is approx. 10 μg/kg of body weight (Paananen et al. 2002). Symptoms of poisoning appear 0.5–6 hours after consumption of food contaminated with cereulide, and they persist for 6–24 hours. The symptoms are usually similar to poisoning with a staphylococcal toxin, that is, vomiting, nausea, and they are usually mild. Two known cases of death were caused by liver damage as a result of a large dose of the emetic toxin (Dierick et al. 2005).

7.5 EVALUATION OF HEALTH HAZARDS CAUSED BY BACTERIAL TOXINS

Opinions of epidemiologists have confirmed that the actual number of food poisonings caused by microorganisms per year is very high, and as much as 30% of the population may be affected. In the United States, diseases caused by foodborne bacteria affect about 14 million people a year, with 2.2% of them requiring hospitalization. A comparison of the number of cases caused by pathogens of different groups that require hospitalization shows that bacteria pose the biggest threat for human health and life.

It is believed that in the nearest future the number of disease cases caused by foodborne pathogens can increase considerably. Globalization of the food supply is going to play an important role in the process. Importing food from other countries can expose consumers to other, specific strains of microorganisms. Moreover, eating habits of societies have changed in recent years. Now that the interest in ready-to-eat-food (RTEF), including refrigerated processed food of extended durability (REPFED) is growing, presence of pathogens on such carriers, including toxin-producing and psychrotolerant bacteria can pose a real threat to consumers of such food. Mild thermal processing eliminates only vegetative forms of microorganisms. If the material is contaminated with *B. cereus* or *C. botulinum*, this can stimulate them to germinate. Depending on the conditions and the individual features of strains that contaminate the product, the process of slow cooling down can stimulate their multiplication in refrigerated storage. An increase in production output of convenient food is followed by increasing international trade in such food products. Combined with a growing percent of people from risk groups, including elderly people or ones with decreased immunity, this can mean that the health risk from “new pathogens,” which include toxin-producing, psychrotolerant *B. cereus* sensu lato, is growing.

New strains of pathogens appear more and more frequently, which are formed by mutation or adaptation to new environmental conditions, which previously inhibited their growth effectively.

REFERENCES

Abgueguen, P., V. Delbos, J.M. Chennebault, S. Fanello, O. Brenet, P. Alquier, J.C. Granry, and E. Pichard. 2003. Nine cases of foodborne botulism type B in France and literature review. *Eur. J. Clin. Microbiol. Infect. Dis.* 22: 749–752.

Agaisse, H., M. Gominet, O.A. Økstad, A.B. Kolstø, and D. Loreclus. 1999. PlcR is a pleiotropic regulator of extracellular virulence factor gene expression in *Bacillus thuringiensis. Mol. Microbiol.* 32: 1043–1053.

Agata, N., M. Mori, M. Ohta, S. Suwan, I. Ohtani, and M. Isobe. 1994. A novel dodecadepsipeptide, cereulide, isolated from *Bacillus cereus* causes vacuole formation in Hep-2 cells. *FEMS Microbiol. Lett.* 121: 31–34.

Agata, N., M. Ohta, and M. Mori. 1996. Production of an emetic toxin, cereulide, is associated with a specific class of *Bacillus cereus. Curr. Microbiol.* 33: 67–69.

Agata, N., M. Ohta, M. Mori, and M. Isobe. 1995. A novel dodecadepsipeptide, cereulide, is an emetic toxin of *Bacillus cereus. FEMS Microbiol. Lett.* 129: 17–20.

Alberto, F., V. Brousole, D.R. Mason, F. Carlin, and M.W. Peck. 2003. Variability in spore germination response by strains of proteolytic *Clostridium botulinum* types A, B and F. *Lett. Appl. Microbiol.* 36: 41–45.

Alessandrini, A., G. Viero, S.M. Dalla, G. Prevost, and P. Facci. 2013. Gamma-hemolysin oligomeric structure and effect of its formation on supported lipid bilayers: An AFM investigation. *Biochim. Biophys. Acta.* 1828: 405–411.

Alonzo, F., and V.J. Torres. 2014. The bicomponent pore-forming leucocidins of *Staphylococcus aureus. Microbiol. Mol. Biol. Rev.* 78: 199–230.

Alouf, J.E., S.J. Billington, and B.H. Jost. 2005. Repertoire and general features of the family of cholesterol-dependent cytolysins. In: J.E. Alouf and M.R. Popoff (eds) *The Comprehensive Sourcebook of Bacterial Protein Toxins*, 3rd edn. London: Academic Press, pp. 643–658.

Amagai, M., N. Matusuyoshi, A.J.R. Stanley, and Z.H. Wang. 2000. Toxin in bullous impetigo and staphylococcal scalded-skin syndrome targets desmoglein 1. *Nat. Med.* 11(6): 1275–1277.

Anadon, A., M.R. Martinez-Larranga, and M.M. Aranzazu. 2006. Probiotics for animal nutrition in the European Union. Regulation and safety assessment. *Regul. Toxicol Pharmacol.* 45: 91–95.

Andersson, A., P.E. Granum, and U. Rönner. 1998. The adhesion of *Bacillus cereus* spores to epithelial cells might be an additional virulence mechanism. *Int. J. Food Microbiol.* 39: 93–99.

Andreeva, Z., V.F. Nesterenko, I.S. Yurkov, Z.I. Budarina, E.V. Sineva, and A.S. Solonin. 2006. Purification and cytotoxic properties of *Bacillus cereus* hemolysin II. *Prot. Express. Purif.* 47: 186–193.

Arndt, J.W., J. Gu, and L. Jaroszewski. 2005. The structure of the neurotoxin-associated protein HA33/A from *Clostridium botulinum* suggests a reoccurring beta-trefoil fold in the progenitor toxin complex. *J. Mol. Biol.* 346(4): 1083–1093.

Arnon, S.S., R. Schecter, and S.E. Maslanka. 2006. Human botulism immune globulin for the treatment of infant botulism. *N. Engl. J. Med.* 354: 462–471.

Badiou, C., O. Dumitrescu, N. George, A.R. Forbes, E. Drougka, K.S. Chan, N. Ramdani Bouguessa, H. Meugnier, M. Bes, F. Vandenesch, J. Etienne, L.Y. Hsu, M. Tazir,

I. Spiliopoulou, G.R. Nimmo, K.G. Hulten, and G. Lina. 2010. Rapid detection of *Staphylococcus aureus* Panton-Valentine leukocidin in clinical specimens by enzyme-linked immunosorbent assay and immunochromatographic tests. *J. Clin. Microbiol.* 48: 1384–1390.

Baida, G.E., and N.P. Kuzmin. 1995. Cloning and primary structure of a new hemolysin gene from *Bacillus cereus. Biochim. Biophys. Acta.* 1264: 151–154.

Baida, G.E., and N.P. Kuzmin. 1996. Mechanism of action of hemolysin III from *Bacillus cereus. Biochim. Biophys. Acta.* 1284: 122–124.

Barrio, M.B., P. Rainard, and G. Prévost. 2006. LukM/LukF′-PV is the most active *Staphylococcus aureus* leukotoxin on bovine neutrophils. *Microbes Infect.* 8: 2068–2074.

Beecher, D.J., and A.C.L. Wong. 1994. Improved purification and characterization of hemolysin BL, a hemolytic dermonecrotic vascular permeability factor from *Bacillus cereus. Infect. Immunol.* 62: 980–986.

Beecher, D.J., and A.C.L. Wong. 1997. Tripartite hemolysin Bl from *Bacillus cereus*. Hemolytic analysis of component interactions and a model for its characteristic paradoxical zone phenomenon. *J. Biol. Chem.* 272: 233–239.

Beecher, D.J., and A.C.L. Wong. 2000. Cooperative, synergistic and antagonistic haemolytic interactions between haemolysin BL, phosphatidylcholine phospholipase C and sphingomyelinase from *Bacillus cereus. Microbiology* 146: 3033–3039.

Beecher, D.J., and J.D. MacMillan. 1991. Characterization of the components of hemolysin BL from *Bacillus cereus*. *Infect. Immunol.* 59: 1778–1784.

Berube, B.J. and J.B. Wardenburg. 2013. *Staphylococcus aureus* alpha-toxin: nearly a century of intrigue. *Toxins (Basel)* 5: 1140–1166.

Bhatia, A., and S. Zahoor. 2007. *Staphylococcus aureus* enterotoxins: a review. *J. Clin. Diag. Res.* 1: 188–197.

Borriello, S.P. 1995. Clostridial disease of the gut. *Clin. Infect. Dis.* 20: 242–250.

Bronner, S., P. Stoessel, A. Gravet, H. Monteil, and G. Prevost. 2000. Variable expressions of *Staphylococcus aureus* bicomponent leucotoxins semiquantified by competitive reverse transcription-PCR. *Appl. Environ. Microbiol.* 66: 3931–3938.

Brunger, A.T., and A. Rummel. 2009. Receptor and substrate interactions of clostridial neurotoxins. *Toxicon* 54: 550–560.

Budarina, Z.I., M.A. Sinev, S.G. Mayorov, A.Y. Tomashevski, I.V. Shmelev, and N.P. Kuzmin. 1994. Hemolysin II is more characteristic of *Bacillus thuringiensis* than *Bacillus cereus. Arch. Microbiol.* 161: 252–257.

Bukowski, M., B. Wladyka, and G. Dubin. 2010. Exfoliative toxins of *Staphylococcus aureus. Toxins* 2(5): 1148–1165.

Callaway J.E., C.J. Arezzo, and A.J. Grethlein. 2002. Botulinum toxin type B: An overview of its biochemistry and preclinical pharmacology. *Dis. Mon.* 48(5): 367–383.

Carlin, F., M. Fricker, A. Pielaat, S. Heisterkamp, R. Shaheen, M. Salkinoja Salonen, B. Svensson, C. Nguyen-The, and. M. Ehling-Schulz. 2006. Emetic toxin-producing strains of *Bacillus cereus* show distinct characteristics within the *Bacillus cereus group. Int. J. Food Microbiol.* 109: 132–138.

Cato, E.P., W.L. George, and S.M. Finegold. Genus Clostridium, Prazmowski, 1880, [w:] Sneath P. H. A., Mair N. S., Sharpe M. E., and Holt J. G. 1986. *Bergey's Manual of Systematic Bacteriology*, vol 2. Baltimore, MD: Williams & Wilkins, pp. 1141–1200.

CDC. 2011. Vital signs: incidence and trends of infection with pathogens transmitted commonly through food-foodborne diseases active surveillance network, 10 U.S. sites, 1996–2010. *MMWR Morb. Mortal. Wkly. Rep.* 60(22): 749–755.

Chung, W.B., L. Backstrom, J. Mcdonald, and M.T. Collins. 1993. The (3-(4,5-dimethylthiazol-2-yl)-2,5-diphenyltetrazolium) colorimetric assay for the quantification of *Actinobacillus pleuropneumoniae* cytotoxin. *Can. J. Vet. Res.* 57: 159–165.

Clair, G., S. Roussi, J. Armengaud, and C. Duport. 2010. Expanding the known repertoire of virulence factors produced by *Bacillus cereus* through early secretome profiling in three redox conditions. *Mol. Cell. Proteomics* 9: 1486–1498.

Cremonesia, P., M. Luzzanaa, M. Brascab, S. Morandib, R. Lodib, Ch. Vimercatic, D. Agnellinia, G. Caramentid, P. Moronic, and B. Castiglionie. 2005. Development of a multiplex PCR assay for the identification of *Staphylococcus aureus* enterotoxigenic strains isolated from milk and dairy products. *Mol. Cell Probes*. 19: 299–305.

Dahlenborg, M., E. Borch, and P.L. Ridström. 2001. Development of combined selection and enrichment PCR procedure for *Clostridium botulinum* types B, E and F and its use to determine prevalence in fecal samples from slaughtered pigs. *Appl. Environ. Microbiol.* 67: 4781–4788.

Deurenberg, R.H., C. Vink, M. Driessen, N. Bes, J. London, E.E. Etienne, and E.E. Stobberingh. 2004. Rapid detection of Panton-Valentine leukocidin from clinical isolates of *Staphylococcus aureus* strains by real-time PCR. *FEMS Microbiol. Lett.* 240: 225–228.

Dierick, K., E. VanCoillie, I. Swiecicka, G. Meyfrodit, H. Develieger, A. Maulemans, G. Hoedemaekers, L. Fourie, M. Heyndricky, and J. Mahillon. 2005. Fatal family outbreak of *Bacillus cereus*-associated food poisoning. *J. Clin. Microbiol.* 43: 4277–4279.

Dinges, M.M., P.M. Orwin, and P.M. Schlievert. 2000. Exotoxins of *Staphylococcus aureus*. *Clin. Microbiol. Rev*. 13: 16–34.

ECDC. 2012. Annual epidemiological report reporting on 2011 surveillance data and 2012 epidemic intelligence data.http://www.ecdc.europa.eu/en/publications/Publications/annual-epidemiological-report-2013.pdf 25.06.2014

EFSA. 2012. The European Union summary report on trends and sources of zoonoses, zoonotic agents and foodborne outbreaks in 2010. *EFSA J.* 10(3): 2597.

EFSA. 2013. The European Union summary report on trends and sources of zoonoses, zoonotic agents and foodborne outbreaks in 2011. *EFSA J.*11(4): 3129.

EFSA. 2014. The European Union summary report on trends and sources of zoonoses, zoonotic agents and foodborne outbreaks in 2012. *EFSA J.* 12(2): 3547.

EFSA and ECDC. 2013. The European Union summary report on trends and sources of zoonoses, zoonotic agents and foodborne outbreaks in 2013. *EFSA J.* 13(1): 133–136.

Ehling-Schulz, M., B. Svensson, M.H. Guinebretiere, T. Lindbäck, M. Andersson, A. Schulz, M. Fricker, A. Christiansson, P.E. Granum, E. Märtlbauer, C. Nguyen-The, M. Salkinoja-Salonen, and S. Scherer. 2006a. Emetic toxin formation of *Bacillus cereus* is restricted to a single evolutionary lineage of closely related strains. *Microbiol.* 151: 183–197.

Ehling-Schulz, M., M.H. Guinbretiere, A. Monthan, O. Berge, M. Fricker, and B. Svensson. 2006b. Toxin gene profiling of enterotoxic and emetic *Bacillus cereus*. *FEMS Microbiol. Lett*. 260: 232–240.

Erkan, M.E., A. Vural, and T. Özekinci. 2008. Investigating the presence of *Staphylococcus aureus* and coagulase-negative staphylococci (CNS) in some leafy green vegetables. *Res. J. Biol. Sci.* 3: 930–933.

Euzéby, J.P. 2012. List of prokaryotic names with standing in nomenclature. http://www.bacterio.net/index.html.

Euzéby, J.P. 2015. List of Prokaryotic names with standing in nomenclature.

Fagerlund, A., O. Ween, T. Lund, S.P. Hardy, and P.E. Granum. 2004. Genetic and functional analysis of the cytK family of genes in *Bacillus cereus*. *Microbiol.* 150: 2689–2697.

Finlay, W.J.J., N.A. Logan, and A.D. Sutherland. 2000. *Bacillus cereus* produces most emetic toxin at lower temperatures. *Lett. Appl. Microbiol.* 31: 385–389.

Fischetti, V.A., R.P. Novick, J.J. Ferretti, D.A. Portnoy, and J.J. Rood. 2000. *Gram-Positive Pathogens*. Washington, DC: American Society for Microbiology, pp. 96–104.

Foster, T. J., and M. Hook. 1998. Surface protein adhesions of *Staphylococcus aurues*. *Trends Microbiol.* 6: 484–488.

Gauduchon, V., S. Werner, G. Prévost, H. Monteil, and D.A. Colin. 2001. Flow cytometric determination of Panton-Valentine leucocidin S component binding. *Infect. Immun.* 69: 2390–2395.

Gencay, Y.E., N.D. Ayaz, and A. Kasımoglu-Dogru. 2010. Enterotoxin gene profiles of *Staphylococcus aureus* and other staphylococcal isolates from various foods and food ingredients. *Erciyes Üniv. Vet. Fak. Derg.* 7: 75–80.

Genestier, A.L., M.C. Michallet, G. Prévost, G. Bellot, L. Chalabreysse, S. Peyrol, F. Thivolet, J. Etienne, G. Lina, F.M. Vallette, F. Vandenesch, and L. Genestier. 2005. *Staphylococcus aureus* Panton-Valentine leukocidin directly targets mitochondria and induces Bax-independent apoptosis of human neutrophils. *J. Clin. Invest.* 115(11): 3117–3127.

Giffel, M.C., R.R. Beumer, S. Leijendekkers, and F.M. Rombouts. 1997. Incidence of *Bacillus cereus* and *Bacillus subtilis* in foods in the Netherlands. *Food Microbiol.* 13: 53–58.

Gilmore, M.S., A.L. Cruz-Rodz, M. Leimeister-Wächter, J. Kreft, and W. Goebel. 1989. A *Bacillus cereus* cytolytic determinant, cereolysin AB, which comprises the phospholipase C and sphingomyelinase genes: Nucleotide sequence and genetic linkage. *J. Bacteriol.* 171: 744–753.

Gilois, N., N. Ramarao, L. Bouillaut, S. Perchat, S. Aymerich, C. Nielsen-Leroux, D. Lereclus, and M. Gohar. 2007. Growth-related variations in the *Bacillus cereus* secretome. *Proteomics.* 7: 1719–1728.

Girardin, H., C. Albagnac, C. Dargaignaratz, C. Nguyen-The, and F. Carlin. 2002. Antimicrobial activity of foodborne *Paenibacillus* and *Bacillus* spp. against *Clostridium botulinum*. *J. Food Prot.* 65: 806–813.

Goja, A.M., T.A.A. Ahmed, S.A.M. Saeed, and H.A. Dirar. 2013. Isolation and identification of *Staphylococcus* spp. in fresh beef. *Pakistan J. Nutr.* 12: 114–120.

Granum, P. E., and T. Lund. 1997. *Bacillus cereus* and its food poisoning toxins. *FEMS Microbiol. Lett.* 157: 223–228.

Granum, P.E., K. OíSullivan, and T. Lund. 1999. The sequence of the non-haemolytic enterotoxin operon from *Bacillus cereus. FEMS Microbiol. Lett.* 177: 225–229.

Gray, G. S., and M.Kehoe. 1984. Primary sequence of the a-toxin gene from *Staphylococcus aureus* Wood 46. *Infect. Immun.* 46: 615–618.

Grenda, T., and K. Kwiatek. 2009. *Clostridium botulinum*—charakterystyka i znaczenie epidemiologiczne. *Med. Wet.* 65: 743–746.

Guinebretière, M H., S. Auger, N. Galleron, M. Contzen, B. De Sarrau, M. L. De Buyser, G. Lamberet, A. Fagerlund, P. E. Per Einar Granum, D. Lereclus, P. De Vos, C. Nguyen-The, and A. Sorokin. 2012. *Bacillus cytotoxicus* sp. novel is a new thermotolerant species of the *Bacillus cereus* Group occasionally associated with food poisoning. *Int. J. Sys. Evol.* 10: 14–30.

Gurnev, P., and E. Nestorovich. 2014. Channel-forming bacterial toxins in biosensing and macromolecule delivery. *Toxins* 6: 2483–2540.

Häggblom, M.M., C. Apetroaie, M.A. Andersson, and M.S. Salkinoja-Salonene. 2002. Quantitative analysis of cereulide, the emetic toxin of *Bacillus cereus*, produced under various conditions. *Appl. Environ. Microbiol.* 68: 2479–2483.

Hardy, S.P., T. Lund, and P.E. Granum. 2001. CytK toxin of *Bacillus cereus* forms pores in planar lipid bilayers and is cytotoxic to intestinal epithelia. *FEMS Microbiol. Lett.* 197: 47–51.

Haveri, M., A. Roslöf, L. Rantala, and S. Pyörälä. 2007. Virulence genes of bovine *Staphylococcus aureus* from persistent and nonpersistent intramammary infections with different clinical characteristics. *J. Appl. Microbiol.* 103: 993–1000.

Hennekinne, J.A, A. Ostyn, F. Guillier, S. Herbin, A.L Prufer, and S. Dragacci. 2010. How should staphylococcal food poisoning outbreaks be characterized? *Toxins* 2: 2106–2116.

Hennekinne, J.A., M.L. De Buyser, and S. Dragacci. 2013. *Staphylococcus aureus* and its food poisoning toxins: Characterization and outbreak investigation. *FEMS Microbiol Rev.* 36: 815–836.

Horwood, P.F., G.W. Burgess, and H.J. Oakey. 2004. Evidence for a non-ribosomal peptide synthetase production of cereulide (the emetic toxin) in *Bacillus cereus. FEMS Microbiol. Lett.* 236: 319–324.

Hu, D.L., and A. Nakane. 2014. Mechanisms of staphylococcal enterotoxin-induced emesis. *Eur. J. Pharmacol.* 722: 95–107.

Humeau, Y., F. Doussau, and N.J. Grant. 2000. How botulinum and tetanus neurotoxins block neurotransmitter release. *Biochimie* 82(5): 427–446.

Huseby, M., K. Shi, C. Brown, J. Digre, F. Mengistu, K. Seo, G. Bohach, P. Schlievert, D. Ohlendorf, and C. Earhar. 2007. Structure and biological activities of toxin from *Staphylococcus aureus. J Bacteriol.* 189: 8719–8726.

Jääskeläinen, E.L., M. Häggblom, M. Andersson, and M. Salkinoja-Salonen. 2004. Atmospheric oxygen and other conditions affecting the production of cereulide by *Bacillus cereus* in food. *Int. J. Food. Microbiol.* 96: 75–83.

Jay, J.M., M. Loessner, and D. Golden. 2005. *Staphylococcal Gastroenteritis (in) Modern Food Microbiology*. 7th edn. New York: Springer Science, pp. 545–567.

Kaneko, J., and Y. Kamio Y. 2003. Bacterial two—component and heteroheptameric pore—forming cytolytic toxins: structures, pore–forming mechanism and organizations of the genes. *Biosci. Biotechnol. Biochem.* 68(5): 981–1003.

Kizerwetter – Świda M., and M. Binek. 2010. Zatrucie jadem kiełbasianym—problem wciąż aktualny. *Post. Mikrobiol.* 40(2): 75–85.

Kotiranta, A., K. Lounatmaa, and K. Haapasalo. 2000. Epidemiology and pathogenesis of *Bacillus cereus* infections. *Mic. Infect.* 2: 189–198.

Ladhani, S., C. Joannou, D. Lochrie, R. Evans, and S. Poston. 1999. Clinical, microbial, and biochemical aspects of the exfoliative toxins causing Staphylococcal scalded-skin syndrome. *Clin. Microbiol. Rev.* 12: 224–242.

Lamberet, G., A. Fagerlund, P. Granum, and D. Lereclus. 2013. *Bacillus cytotoxicus* sp. nov. is a novel thermotolerant species of the *Bacillus cereus* group occasionally associated with food poisoning. *Int. J. Sys. Evol. Microbiol.* 63: 31–40.

Lereclus, D., H. Agaisse, M. Gominet, S. Salamitou, and V. Sanchis. 1996. Identification of a gene that positively regulates transcription of the phosphatidylinositol-specific phospholipase C gene at the onset of the stationary phase. *J. Bacteriol.* 178: 2749–2756.

Lindbäck, T., A. Fagerlund, M. Rødland, and P. Granum. 2001. Characterization of the *Bacillus cereus* NHE enterotoxin. *Microbiology* 150: 3959–3967.

Lindström, M., and H. Korkeala. 2006. Laboratory diagnostic of botulism. *Clin. Microbiol. Rev.* 19: 298–314.

Lindström, M., H. Jankola, S. Hielm, E. Hyytia, and H. Korkeala. 1999. Identification of *Clostridium botulinum* with API 20 A, Rapid ID 32 A and RapID ANA II. *FEMS Immunol. Med. Microbiol.* 24: 267–274.

Lindström, M., K. Kiviniemi, and H. Korkeala. 2006. Hazard and control of group II (non-proteolytic) *Clostridium botulinum* in modem food processing. *Int. J. Food. Microbiol.* 108: 92–104.

Lund, T., and P. Granum. 1996. Characterization of a non-haemolytic enterotoxin complex from *Bacillus cereus* isolated after a food borne outbreak. *FEMS Microbiol. Lett.* 141: 151–156.

Lund, T., M. de Buyser, and P. Granum. 2000. A new cytotoxin from *Bacillus cereus* that may cause necrotic enteritis. *Mol. Microbiol.* 38: 254–261.

Mahler, H., A. Pasi, J.M. Kramer, P. Schulte, A.C. Scoging, W. Bär, and S. Krähenbähl. 1997. Fulminant liver failure in association with the emetic toxin of *Bacillus cereus. J. Med.* 336: 1142–1148.

Messelhäusser, U., P. Kämpf, M. Fricker, M. Ehling-Schulz, R. Zucker, B. Wagner, U. Busch, and C. Höller. 2010. Prevalence of emetic *Bacillus cereus* in different ice creams in Bavaria. *J. Food. Prot.* 73(2): 395–399.

Mikami, T., T. Horikawa, T. Murakami, T. Matsumoto, A. Yamatawa, S. Murayama, S. Katagiri, K. Shinagawa, and M. Suzuki. 1994. An improved method for detecting cytostatic toxic (emetic toxin) of *Bacillus cereus* and its application to food samples. *FEMS Microbiol. Lett.* 119: 53–58.

Miles, G., H. Bayley, and S. Cheley. 2006. Properties of *Bacillus cereus* hemolysin II: A heptameric transmembrane pore. *Protein Sci.* 11: 1813–1824.

Montecucco, C., O. Rossetto, and G. Schiavo. 2004. Presynaptic receptor arrays for clostridial neurotoxins. *Trends Microbiol.* 12(10): 442–446.

Moravek, M., R. Dietrich, C. Buerk, V. Broussolle, M.H. Guinebretière, P.E. Granum, C. Nguyen-The, and E. Märtlbauer. 2006. Determination of the toxic potential of *Bacillus cereus* isolates by quantitative enterotoxin analyses. *FEMS Microbiol. Lett.* 257: 293–298.

Myers, G.S.A., D.A. Rasko, and J.K. Cheung. 2006. Skewed genomic variability in strains of the toxigenic bacterial pathogen, *Clostridium perfringens*. *Genome Res.* 16: 1031–1040.

Nichols, G.L., C.L. Little, V. Mithani, and J. de Louvois. 1999. The microbiological quality of cooked rice from restaurants and take-away premises in the United Kingdom. *J. Food. Prot.* 62: 877–882.

Niścigorska, J. 1999. Zatrucie enterotoksyną gronkowcową [w:] Choroby odzwierzęce przenoszone drogą pokarmową. *PZWL*. Warszawa: 63–65.

Økstad, O.A., M. Gominet, B. Purnelle, M. Rose, D. Lereclus, and A.B. Kolstø. 1999. Sequence analysis of three *Bacillus cereus* loci carrying PlcR-regulated genes encoding degradative enzymes and enterotoxins. *Microbiol.* 145: 3129–3138.

Onuma, K., T. Tanabe, and H. Sato. 2011. Development of a high-expression system for staphylococcal exfoliative toxin genes. *J. Vet. Med. Sc.* 73(8): 1051–1057.

Otto, M. 2014. *Staphylococcus aureus* toxins. *Curr. Opin. Microbiol.* 17: 32–37.

Paananen, A., R. Mikkola, T. Saraneva, S. Matkainen, M. Hess, M. Andersson, I. Julkunen, M.S Salkinoja-Salonene, and T. Timonen. 2002. Inhibition of human killer cell activity by cereulide, an emetic toxin from *Bacillus cereus*. *Clin. Exp. Immunol.* 129: 420–428.

Papageorgiou, A.C., L.R. Plano, C.M. Collins, and K.R. Acharya. 2000. Structural similarities and differences in *Staphylococcus aureus* exfoliative toxins A and B as revealed by their crystal structures. *Protein. Sci.* 9: 610–618.

Parasion, S., M. Bartoszcze, and R. Gryko. 2007. Struktura i mechanizm działania neurotoksyn bakterii rodzaju *Clostridium*. *Przegl. Epidemiol.* 61:519–527.

Peck, M.W. 2006. *Clostridium botulinum* and the safety of minimally heated, chilled foods: an emerging issue? *J. Appl. Microbiol.* 101: 556–570.

Peck, W., and S. C. Stringer. 2005. The safety of pasteurised in-pack chilled meat products with respect to the foodborne botulism hazard. *Meat. Science.* 70: 461–475.

Pinchuk, I.V., E.J. Beswick, and V.E. Reyes. 2010. Staphylococcal enterotoxins. *Toxins* 2: 2177–2197.

Podkowik, M., J.Y. Park, K.S. Seo, J. Bystroń, and J. Bania. 2013. Enterotoxigenic potential of coagulase-negative staphylococci. *Int. J. Food. Microbiol.* 163: 34–40.

Pokorny, A., E.M. Kilelee, D. Wu, and P.F.F. Almeida. 2008. The activity of the amphipathic peptide δ-lysin correlates with phospholipid acyl chain structure and bilayer elastic properties. *Biophys. J.* 95(10): 4748–4755.

Prevost, G., B. Cribier, P. Couppie, P. Petiau, G. Supersac, V. Finck-Barbancon, H. Monteil, and Y. Piemont. 1995. Panton-Valentine leukocidin and gamma hemolysin from *Staphylococcus aureus* ATCC 49775 are encoded by distinct genetic loci and have different biological activities. *Infect. Immun.* 63: 4121–4129.

Qi, Y., and K.J. Miller. 2000. Effect of low water activity on staphylococcal enterotoxin A and B biosynthesis. *J. Food. Prot.* 63: 473–478.
Rainard, P. 2007. *Staphylococcus aureus* leucotoxin LukM/F′ is secreted and stimulates neutralising antibody response in the course of intramammary infection. *Vet. Res.* 38: 685–696.
Rainard, P., J.C. Corrailes, M. B. Barrio, T. Cochard, and B. Pautrel. 2003. Leucotoxic activities of Staphylococcus aureus strain isolated from cows, ewes, and goats with mastitis: Importance of LukM/LukF0 -PV leukocidin. *Clin. Diagn. Lab. Immunol.* 10: 272–277.
Rajkovic, A., M. Uyttendaele, and J. Debevere. 2007. Computer aided boar semen motility analysis for cereulide detection in different food matrices. *Int. J. Food. Microbiol.* 114: 92–99.
Rajkovic. A., M. Uyttendaele, S.A. Ombregt, E. Jääskelainen, M. Salkinoja-Salonen, and J. Debevere. 2006. Influence of type of food on the kinetics and overall production of *Bacillus cereus* emetic toxin. *J. Food. Pro.* 69: 847–852.
Rao, K.N., D. Kumaran, and T. Binz. 2005. Structural analysis of the catalytic domain of tetanus neurotoxin. *Toxicon.* 45(7): 929–939.
Reiss, J., and J. Mierzejewski. 2004. Toksyna botulinowa—aspekty zagrożenia biologicznego. *Mikrobiol. Med.* 2(39): 24–35.
Ritz, N., and N. Curtis. 2012. The role of Panton–leukocidin in *Staphylococcus aureus* musculoskeletal infections in children. *Pediatr. Infect. Dis. J.* 31: 514–518.
Rodgers, S., P. Peiris, and G. Casadei. 2003. Inhibition of nonproteolytic *Clostridium botulinum* with lactic acid bacteria and their bacteriocins at refrigeration temperatures. *J. Food. Prot.* 66: 674–678.
Rosenquist, H., L. Smidt, S.R. Andersen, G.B. Jensen, and A. Wilcks. 2005. Occurrence and significance of *Bacillus cereus* and *Bacillus thuringiensis* in ready-to-eat food. *FEMS Microbiol. Lett.* 250: 129–136.
Ruaro, A., C. Andrighetto, S. Torriani, and A. Lombardi. 2013. Biodiversity and characterization of indigenous coagulase-negative staphylococci isolated from raw milk and cheese of North Italy. *Food. Microbiol.* 34: 106–111.
Ryan, P.A., J.M. Macmillan, and B.A. Zilinskas. 1997. Molecular cloning and characterization of the genes encoding the L1 and L2 components of hemolysin BL from *Bacillus cereus. J. Bacteriol.* 179: 2551–2556.
Salgado-Pabón, W., A. Herrera, B.G. Vu, C.S. Stach, J.A. Merriman, A.R. Spaulding, and P.M. Schlievert. 2014. *Staphylococcus aureus* beta-toxin production is common in strains with the beta-toxin gene inactivated by bacteriophage. *J. Infect. Dis.* 210: 784–792.
Satora, P. 2008. *Staphylococcus* w żywności—charakterystyka, detekcja, zwalczanie. *Laboratorium* 8: 36–41.
Schiavo, G., M., Matteoli, and C. Montecucco. 2000. Neurotoxins affecting neuroexocytosis. *Physiol. Rev.* 80(2): 717–766.
Schmitt, M., U. Schuler-Schmid, and W. Schmidt-Lorenz. 1990. Temperature limits of growth, TNase and enterotoxin production of *Staphylococcus aureus* strains isolated from foods. *Int. J Food. Microbiol.* 11: 1–2.
Shannon, J.G., C.L. Ross, T.M. Koehler, and R.F. Rest. 2003. Characterization of anthrolysin O the *Bacillus anthracis* cholesterol-dependent cytolysin. *Infect. Immun.* 71: 3183–3189.
Shapiro, R.L, C. Hatheway, and D.L. Swerdlow. 1998. Botulism in the United States: A clinical and epidemiologic review. *Ann. Intern. Med.* 129: 221–228.
Sharma, S.K., and R.C. Whiting. 2005. Methods for of *Clostridium botulinum* toxin in foods. *J. Food. Prot.* 68: 1256–1263.

Sierecka, J.K. 1998. Purification and partial characterization of a neutral protease from a virulent strain of *Bacillus cereus*. *Int. J. Biochem. Cell Biol.* 30: 579–595.
Simpson, L.L. 1981. The origin, structure, and pharmacological activity of botulinum toxin. *Pharmacol. Rev*. 33: 155–188.
Sinev, M.A., Z.I. Budarina, I.V. Gavrilenko, A.I. Tomashevskiĭ, and N.P. Kuzmin. 1993. Evidence of the existence of hemolysin II from *Bacillus cereus*: Cloning the genetic determinant of hemolysin II. *Mol. Biol.* 27: 1218–1229.
Slamti, L., S. Perchat, M. Gominet, G. Vilas-Bôas, A. Fouet, M. Mocka, V. Sanchis, J. Chaufaux, M. Gohar, and D. Lereclus. 2004. Distinct mutations in PlcR explain why some strains of the *Bacillus cereus* group are nonhemolytic. *J. Bact.* 186: 3531–3538.
Slamti, L., and D. Lereclus. 2002. A cell-cell signaling peptide activates the PlcR virulence regulon in bacteria of the *Bacillus cereus* group. *EMBO J.* 21: 4550–4559.
Smedley, J.G., D.J. Fisher, G. Chakrabarti, and B.A. McClane. 2004. Enteric toxins of *Clostridium perfringens*. *Rev. Physiol. Biochem. Pharmacol.* 52: 183–204.
Sobel, J., C.G. Mixter, P. Kolhe, A. Gupta, J. Guarner, S. Zaki, N. HoQman, J.G. Songer, M. Fremont-Smith, M. Fischer, G. Killgore, P.H. Britz, and C. MacDonald. 2005. Necrotizing enterocolitis associated with *Clostridium perfringens* type A in previously healthy North American adults. *J. Am. Coll. Surg.* 201: 48–56.
Stachowiak, R., and J. Bielecki. 2000. Hemolizyny bakteryjne. *Post. Mikrobiol.* 39: 253–270.
Stenfors, A.L.P., A. Fagerlund, and P.E. Granum. 2008. From soil to gut: *Bacillus cereus* and its food poisoning toxins. *FEMS Microbiol. Rev*. 32: 579–606.
Subramanian, S.B., A.S. Kamat, K.K. Ussuf, and R.D. Tyagi. 2006. Virulent gene based DNA probe for the detection of pathogenic *Bacillus cereus* strains found in food. *Pro. Bioch.* 41: 783–788.
Szewczyk, E. 2011. Diagnostyka bakteriologiczna. *PWN*, 20–27.
Szymańska, K., and J. Buczek. 1999. Charakterystyka mechanizmów chorobotwórczości gronkowców. *Med. Wet.* 55 (9): 590–594.
Taylor, A. G., and A.W. Bernheimer. 1974. Further characterization of staphylococcal gamma-hemolysin. *Infect. Immun.* 10: 54–59.
Thelestam, M., R. MoDlby, and T. Wadstrom. 1973. Effects of staphylococcal alpha-, beta-, delta-, and gamma-hemolysins on human diploid fibroblasts and HeLa cells. Evaluation of a new quantitative assay for measuring cell damage. *Infect. Immun.* 8: 938–946.
Thorsen, L., B.M. Hansen, K.F. Nielsel, N.B. Hendriksen, R.K. Phipps, and B.B. Budde. 2006. Characterization of emetic *Bacillus weihenstephanensis*, a new psychrotolerant cereulide producing bacterium. *Appl. of Env. Mic.* 72: 170–176.
Vasconcelos, N.G., and M.R. Cunha. 2010. Staphylococcal enterotoxins: Molecular aspects and detection methods. *J. Public. Health. Epidemiol.* 2: 29–42.
Veldin't, P.H., W.S. Ritmeester, E.H.M Delfgou-van Asch, J.B. Dufrenne, K. Wernars, E. Smit, and van F.M. Leusden. 2001. Detection of genes encoding for enterotoxins and determination of the production of enterotoxins by HBL blood plates and immunoassays of psychrotrophic strains of *Bacillus cereus* isolated from pasteurized milk. *Int. J. Food. Microbiol.* 64: 63–70.
Veras, J., L.S. Carmo, L.C. Tong, J.W. Shupp, C. Cummings, D.A. Dos Santos, M.M. Cerqueira, A. Cantini, J.R. Nicoli, and M. Jett. 2008. A study of the enterotoxigenicity of coagulase-negative and coagulase-positive staphylococcal isolates from food poisoning outbreaks in Minas Gerais, Brasil. *Int. J. Infect. Dis.* 12: 410–415.
Verdon, J., N. Girardin, C. Lacombe, J.M. Berjeaud, and Y. Héchard. 2009. Delta-hemolysin, an update on a membrane-interacting peptide. *Peptides.* 30: 817–823.
Vernozy-Rozand, C., C. Mazuy, C. Prevost, C. Lapeyre, M. Bes, Y. Brun, and J. Fleurette. 1996. Enterotoxin production by coagulase-negative staphylococci isolated from goats milk and cheese. *Int. J. Food. Microbiol.* 30: 271–280.

Wilson, G.J., K.S. Seo, R.A. Cartwright, T. Connelley, O.N. Chuang-Smith, J.A Merriman, C.M. Guinane, J.Y. Park, G.A. Bohach, P.M. Schlievert, W.I. Morrison, and J. R. Fitzgerald. 2011. A novel core genome-encoded superantigen contributes to lethality of community-associated MRSA necrotizing pneumonia. *PLoS. Pathog.* 7: 1–16.

Zell, C., M. Resch, R. Rosenstein, T. Albrecht, C. Hertel, and F. Götz. 2008. Characterization of toxin production of coagulase-negative staphylococci isolated from food and starter cultures. *Int. J. Food. Microbiol.* 127: 246–251.

8 Pesticide, Fertilizer, and Antibiotic Residues in Food

Hassan Abdel-Gawad

CONTENTS

8.1 INTRODUCTION

Pest control in intensive agriculture involves treatment pre- and postharvests with a variety of synthetic chemicals generically known as pesticides. These chemicals can be transferred from plants to animals via the food chain. Furthermore, breeding animals and their accommodation can be sprayed with pesticide solution to prevent pest infestations. Consequently, both these contamination routes can lead to bioaccumulation of persistent pesticides in food products of animal origin. The soil is receiving pesticides either directly through repeated and sometimes heavy applications of pesticides or indirectly by runoff from treated leaves and stems of the plants. Dispersion of pesticides and their transformation products within the soil to other environments is influenced not only by properties of the pesticides and soil but also by the prevailing climatic conditions. Pesticides may remain on the surface of plants or may penetrate the cuticle of leaves, fruits, stem, and roots by virtue of their lipophilicity. Plant metabolism studies of pesticides are very important for predicting the degradation behavior of the parent pesticide and determining the nature and extent of the metabolites as well as assessing the potential human, animal, and environmental hazards. Pollution by persistent chemicals is potentially harmful to the organisms at higher trophic levels in the food chain. Humans are mainly exposed to these chemicals through ingestion. The chronic effects of pesticides from food intake on human health are not well defined, but there is increasing evidence of carcinogenicity and genotoxicity, as well as disruption of hormonal functions (Baranowska et al. 2006; Fontcuberta et al. 2008).

8.2 BOUND PESTICIDE RESIDUES IN FOOD

When a xenobiotic (pesticide) is applied to a plant, to an animal, or to any component of the environment, a variety of chemical reactions including oxidation, hydrolysis, and/or conjugation of the parent compound or its degradation products take place. The resulting products may be excreted, stored, or subsequently metabolized. For studying bound pesticide residues (BRs) in a living organism, nuclear techniques proved a versatile and valuable tool. Radioisotopes can be used to determine: total quantities of residues present, the nature of the residue (i.e., both undecomposed parent material and its metabolites), rates of breakdown of the chemical, and loss and distribution of the chemical and its transformation products in any component of the environment. This information is essential for health and regulatory authorities to maintain and establish level of tolerance standards for protecting the health of the consumers.

BR in soils, plants, and food may be defined as chemical species originating from pesticides, used according to good agricultural practice, that are unextracted by methods that do not significantly change the chemical nature of these residues (Roberts 1984). In the analysis of residues of pesticides in soil and food samples, methanol is widely used to remove the extractable residues of pesticides. BR is operatively defined as parents or metabolites of pesticides left in sample when the sample was extracted by Soxhlet apparatus with methanol for 24 hours (IAEA 1986). The existence of BR was documented only after using the radiotracer techniques. Quantitation of the radioactive pesticide residues has revealed that classical methods of extraction do not remove the total radioactive residues. Initially, poor recovery in extracts was assumed to be the result of bad technique or improper extraction. Nonextractable residues may be the result of binding of the radioactive species to plant, soil, or food matrices. They may be further metabolized and become incorporated into natural products. BR may be associated with plant, soil, or food matrices by different types of interaction, including Van der Waals forces, covalent, ionic, hydrogen bonding, or hydrophilic binding. The radioactive BR can only be determined by combusting in a sample oxidizer followed by counting the collected $^{14}CO_2$ in liquid scintillation counter. The critical questions in connection with BR are concerned with their significance especially their bioavailability and toxicity. Soil organic matter especially humic substances play a vital role in the formation of BR. Experimental results indicate that parent molecules or metabolites are bound to the humic substances either by covalent bonding, ionic bonding, charge transfer complexes, ligand exchange, hydrogen bonding, Van der Waals forces, hydrophobic sorption, or entrapment due to sequestration reactions. It has been argued that theoretically a "truly bound" residue is one that is covalently bonded in the soil, that is, usually through C–C, C–O, C–N, or N–N bonding between the pesticide and soil humic substances. The type of interactions between the organic chemicals and humic substances is dependent on the molecular structure and properties of organic chemicals and the type of soils. The BRs of pesticides in soil have impact not only on nontarget animals or plants but also on human health by food chains. Therefore, it is important to assess the potential hazards of BR in soil to nontarget animals or plants.

8.3 EXTRACTION METHODS FOR BR

8.3.1 Introduction

Currently, there is a range of techniques available to assist with the characterization of nonextractable residues. They include solvent extraction, hydrolysis, derivatization of functional groups, model compound investigations, pyrolysis, and thermal desorption. New extraction technologies such as ultrasonication, microwave extraction, supercritical fluid extraction (SFE), and accelerated solvent extraction (ASE) enhance the extraction kinetics of organic compounds in comparison to Soxhlet extraction techniques. High-temperature distillation (HTD) and SFE techniques have been used for releasing the BR from biological samples. Dupont and Khan (1992) found that BRs were released from the extracted plant samples by HTD and supercritical acetone extraction (SAE) in their study on bound (nonextractable) ^{14}C-residues in soybean treated with ^{14}C-metribuzin. The distillates or the extracts were subjected to thin-layer chromatography, gas chromatography, and high-performance liquid chromatography for identification. Free ^{14}C-metribuzin and conjugated residues were shown to be present in the bound fraction of the roots and shoots of both varieties.

8.3.2 High-Temperature Distillation

Each solvent-extracted sample containing bound ^{14}C-residues was placed in a quartz tube and subjected to HTD. Weighed subsamples of approximately 1 g of roots or 2 g of shoots each were heated to 600°C in the quartz tube under a flow of helium

(50 mL/min). The volatilized material was trapped in three methanol traps. An additional trap containing Carbosorb was used to absorb and quantitate any $^{14}CO_2$ produced in the process.

SFE can be effectively applied to the extraction of BR in a variety of matrices including soil, plants, and wheat grains. Extraction of the BR increased with extraction temperature and pressure and by addition of methanol as a modifier. The SFE method did not appear to result in thermal degradation of the residues.

8.3.3 SAE

Weighed root (1 g) or shoot (2 g) subsamples of the solvent extracted plants containing bound ^{14}C residues were placed directly in the sample holder (empty liquid chromatography column). Supercritical acetone (250°C, 150 bars) was pumped through the apparatus at 1 mL/min for 3 hours. The extracts were collected and analyzed. The extracts were concentrated and radioassayed.

8.3.4 Spectroscopic Methods

Spectroscopic techniques such as electron spin resonance (ESR), Fourier transform infrared (FTIR), fluorescence, and nuclear magnetic resonance (NMR) are used for analysis of BR. The combination of the above techniques is undoubtedly a powerful tool for the analysis, characterization, and further study of BR. However, factors such as cost are always an important consideration, as are time and availability of the technique (including training of competent operators). For more detailed information, the above techniques for determination of organic bound residues are discussed by Northcott and Jones (2000). BR is most often investigated by the methods outlined previously. These are time consuming and can be very expensive. Enzyme immunoassay (EIA) techniques are becoming popular for the determination of pesticides as they are relatively easy to perform and less expensive than traditional chromatographic methods. An EIA technique has also been used to analyze benomyl residues in food commodities and different crop samples containing field-bound residues (Lavin et al. 1996).

8.4 BR IN SOIL

The extent of binding of pesticides to soil may depend on temperature, humidity, length of the incubation period as well as on the type of the soil. Binding was also reported to be probably related to the activity of soil microorganisms since sterilization resulted in a high reduction of bound ^{14}C-residues (Abdelhafid et al. 2000a, 2000b). Several researchers have reported on the ability of plants grown in soils containing BR to take up a portion of these residues. Printz et al. (1995) observed that the amendment of maize straw to soil led to significantly enhanced degradation and mineralization of [phenyl-U-^{14}C] methabenzthiazuron (MBT) and promoted the formation of BR. They also observed that the dissipation of the pesticide, formation of BR, and the metabolite demethyl-MBT were enhanced at higher temperatures. Increasing temperatures and the amendment of maize straw both promote the microbial activity in the soil. Repeated applications of some insecticides are known to increase the degradation of insecticides (Buhler et al. 1992). The dissipation half-live of monocrotophos in tropical soil was reported to be 2 weeks (Guth 1994; Laabs et al. 2002). Menon et al. (2004) found that the organophosphorus chlorpyrifos was moderately stable in both loamy and sandy loam soil with a half-life of 12.3 and 16.4 days, respectively. The rapid dissipation of the insecticide from the soil post application might have resulted from low sorption due to the alkalinity of the soil and its low organic matter content. Fast top soil dissipation is possible by volatilization and photochemical degradation possibly aided by the low water solubility, limited vertical mobility due to confinement of residues to the upper 15-cm soil layers, and microbial mineralization and nucleophilic hydrolysis. Menon and Gopal (2003) found that the movement of carbaryl was limited to 15-cm depth in the loamy sand soil. It was detected until 120 days, and its t_{50} was calculated as 14.39 days after application. Rapid dissipation of carbaryl could result from physical dissipation. The primary hydrolysis product of carbaryl in soil is 1-naphthol which can be metabolized by soil microorganism (Rajagopal et al. 1984). The persistence of carbaryl in soil is considered to be low to moderate, depending on the environmental factors such as pH and temperature, as well as the rate of application, chemical formulation, and frequency of application (Howard 1991). The half-life of carbaryl in soils is 8–15 days, depending on the aeration status of the soil. Zayed et al. (2002) reported that under aerobic conditions, organochlorine pesticide U-ring labeled 2, 4-D (2,4-dichlorophenoxy acetic acid) was mineralized in clay loam soil more readily than under aerobic condition (19% and 10%) within 90 days, respectively. However, incubation of ^{14}C-lindane with loamy sand and sandy soils under anaerobic conditions for 90 days indicates a slow rate of pesticide mineralization in soil that did not exceed 5.5% (Farghaly et al. 1998). The mineralization of ^{14}C-ring labeled pirimiphosmethyl in clay loam soil was determined in 3-month laboratory incubation period under anaerobic and aerobic conditions. The unextractable pesticide residues gradually increased with time, and the highest binding capacity of about 11%–13% was observed after 90 days of incubation (Zayed et al. 2006). Incubation of ^{14}C-carbofuran in clay loam soil under aerobic and anaerobic condition for 90 days. A maximum binding of about 5.3% and 13% of the applied dose was observed (Mahdy and Soliman 2005).

8.5 BR IN PLANTS

Residues of pesticides and/or metabolites in plants may be classified into three categories (Kacew et al. 1996). Freely extractable residues (primary metabolites), extractable conjugates (secondary metabolites), and unextractable residues bound to natural constituents of plants.

Early experiments indicated pesticide incorporation into proteins, lignins, pectins, and hemicelluloses in plants (Huber and Otto 1983; Roberts 1984; Pillmoor and Roberts 1985). A cell-wall fractionation procedure developed by Langebartels and Harms (1985) has been applied in numerous literature studies. This procedure has confirmed that proteins, lignins, hemicelluloses, and pectins can all act as major conjugation partners (Schmidt 1999; Sandermann et al. 2001). However, assignment to these macromolecules was only on the basis of solubilization behavior. In addition to the solubilization steps of the Langebartels/Harms procedure (1985), BRs have also been solubilized with specific enzymes such as cellulase, hemicellulose, and pectinase (Pillmoor and Roberts 1985; Skidmore et al. 1998). In addition, the cutin component of leaf surfaces has been shown to act as a covalent binding partner (Riederer and Schoenherr 1986).

By 1981, ^{1}H and ^{13}C-NMR spectroscopy had identified the benzylamine structure of lignin conjugates of chloroanilines (Still et al. 1981; Trenck et al. 1981). This structural assignment has recently been confirmed using more sophisticated NMR techniques (Lange et al. 1998). The linkage types for pectin and hemicellulose were derived from circumstantial evidence, but ester linkages to hemicelluloses were recently documented for phenoxyacetic acids (Laurent and Scalla 1999, 2000). Pectins are known to contain energy-rich methyl ester groups where nucleophilic substitution by nitrogenic ligands can occur (Daniel et al. 1994). Plant cuticles can contain reactive epoxide groups that have been proposed to bind xenobiotic carboxylic acids. Further proposed linkage types are photochemical addition reactions and to protein amino and sulfhydryl groups (Jahn and Schwack 2001).

Several investigations using radiolabeled compounds indicated that a considerable portion of pesticide residues may become bound in plants. Dry seeds of soybean from ^{14}C-carbofuran treated plants contained about 1% of the originally applied radioactivity (Zayed et al. 1998). The foliar treatment of soybean plants with ^{14}C-pirimiphos-methyl lead to appearance of ^{14}C-residues in the mature seeds. These amounted to 0.37% of the applied dose (Zayed et al. 2003). The ^{14}C-residues in dry maize seeds obtained from ^{14}C-chlorfenvinphos treated plants amounted to 0.12% of the originally applied radioactivity (Mahdy and El-Maghraby 2010).

Supercritical carbon dioxide modified with methanol improved the recovery of bound ^{14}C- residues from soil and plant samples. Supercritical methanol was found to be less efficient than supercritical carbon dioxide or methanol-modified supercritical carbon dioxide for the extraction of BRs. Analysis of the extracts indicated that the ^{14}C- BR in soil, plants, and wheat samples were present in the form of parent compounds and/or metabolites (Table 8.1) (Khan 1995).

The extracted plant tissue containing bound ^{14}C likely contained mainly lignin, carbohydrate, and denatured protein. The lignin extracted comprises free and bound lignin. The latter is bound to the carbohydrate of the cell wall and could only be extracted by boiling with dioxane-HC1 under N_2.

8.6 BIOAVAILABILITY OF BR IN PLANTS

The BR can in principle be digested in animals and humans and so release toxic fragments into the blood stream. Radioactivity in urine and in bile needs to be determined to judge animal exposure from BR through the blood stream as well as enterohepatic circulation. Urinary and/or biliary excretion of a compound or its metabolites signifies that the material is bioavailable. However, quantitative fecal elimination without biliary excretion indicates that a material is not bioavailable. The currently proposed linkage types indicate that xenobiotics are typically present as exterior substituents ("spikes") of dietary fiber macromolecules. This exposed location could facilitate the attack by stomach-pH, by digestive enzymes, and by

TABLE 8.1
Bound ^{14}C-Residue Levels of Pesticides in Soil, Plant, and Wheat Sample

Sample	Pesticide	Treatment		Treatment Time	Bound ^{14}C (%)
		^{14}C (μCi/g)	ppm		
Organic soil	Prometryn	0.047	12	1 year	57
	Deltamethrin	0.017	10	6 months	20
	Atrazine	0.006	25	1 year	54
Mineral soil	Atrazine[a]	0.012	10	9 year	50
	Diuron	0.322	10	6 months	20
	2,4-D	0.226	10	3 months	14
Wheat	Deltamethrin	0.050	5	168 days	12
	Pirimiphos-methyl	0.100	5	28 weeks	10
Beans	Pirimiphos-methyl	0.140	10	6 months	4
Onion	fonofos[b]	0.067	10	130 days	22
Radish	dieldrin[c]	0.005	10	21 days	24
Canola	Atrazine[d]	0.006	4	10 days	44

[a] Soil samples were obtained from field plots treated with ^{14}C-atrazine.
[b] Onion samples were obtained from field plots treated with ^{4}C-dyfonate.
[c] Radishes were grown in sand pots containing 0.005 μCi/mL ^{14}C-dieldrin in Hoagland nutrient solution.
[d] Canola was grown in Hoagland nutrient solution containing 0.006 μCi/mL ^{14}C-atrazine.

intestinal microorganisms. BR may therefore be much more digestible than their matrix molecules. It has been proposed that the bioavailability of BR depends on the digestibility of the macromolecule to which the pesticides are bound (Mathew et al. 1998). Mahdy and El-Maghraby (2010) found the BR of ^{14}C-chlorfenvinphos in maize was found to be considerably bioavailability. After feeding rats for 5 days with the cake, a substantial amount of ^{14}C-residues was eliminated in the urine (59.5%), while about 20% excreted in the feces. About 15% of the radioactive residues were distributed among various organs. Abdel-Gawad and Hegazi (2010) reported that in rats fed the extracted cake of canola seeds for 72 hours, the BR was found to be bioavailable. The main excretion route was via the expired air (42%), while the ^{14}C-residues excreted in urine and feces were 30% and 11%, respectively. The radioactivity detected among various organs accounted to 7.5%. Chromatographic analysis of urine indicated the presence of prothiofos oxon, *O*-ethyl phosphoric acid and 2, 4-dichlorophenole as main degradation products of prothiofos in free and conjugated form. Abdel-Gawad and Taha (2011a) investigated the bioavailability of chlorpyrifos ^{14}C-BR from sunflower plants when fed to rats; the animals eliminated 46% of the radioactivity in urine, 25% in feces, and 10% in the expired air. A further bioavailable amount of 8% was found in selected organs indicating that the BR was highly bioavailable. Bioavailability of BR from soybean plants treated with ^{14}C-ethyl profenofos was studied by feeding the rats with the extracted soybean seeds for 72 hours. It was observed that the major part of residues was eliminated via expired air (45%)

while residues in urine and feces accounted for 18% and 12% of the applied dose, respectively. Appreciable amount of ^{14}C-residue (15%) were also detected in liver, kidney, blood, and fat of treated rats (Abdel-Gawad and Taha 2011b).

8.7 BR IN STORED GRAINS

8.7.1 Introduction

Harvested food crops are attacked by pests during storage and losses of 30% are currently common in large areas of the world particularly in tropical and subtropical areas. Chemical control procedures continue to have the advantage of effectiveness, simplicity, versatility, low cost, and immediate availability. Pesticide chemicals may be applied to control heavy infestations or to prevent infestations becoming established. As a result of such applications, substantial residues may remain in treated commodities. The amount of residues usually depends on the method of application, length of time between application and consumption, temperature and moisture content during storage, and physicochemical properties of the active constituents. Investigations of the magnitude and nature of residues resulting from postharvest insecticidal applications are essential to produce insect free and to provide requisite assurance of consumer safety (Table 8.2).

Postharvest treatment with pesticides is widely used to control insects and pest organisms that attack crops during storage. Chemical control procedures have the

TABLE 8.2
Bound Pesticide Residues in Various Stored Grains

Pesticide	Commodity	Storage Period (Weeks)	% Bound Residues
Dichlorvos	Soybeans	30	8–10
	Faba beans	30	9–11
Pirimiphos-methyl	Soybeans	30	6
	Wheat	28	10
Carbaryl	Faba beans	30	5
	Soybean	30	6
Malathion	Faba beans	30	17–18
	Milled rice	15	7
	Unmilled rice	15	12
	Maize	30	18
	Soybeans	30	8–9
Chlorpyriphos-methyl	Wheat	60	29
Carbofuran	Faba beans	30	3
	Soybeans	30	4
Chlorpyriphos	Faba beans	30	7–9
	Soybeans	30	9–11
Fenitrothion	Faba beans	30	17–18
	Soybeans	30	18–20

advantage of being effective, simple, versatile, and economical. However, they frequently have the disadvantage of leaving unwanted residues in treated commodities that may be of concern to health of the consumer. The amount of such residues usually depends on a number of factors including: type and nature of the pesticide, method of application of the pesticide, type of commodity, storage period, and condition of storage.

Nuclear technique proved a valuable tool in tackling chemical residue problems of unstored products (Neskovic et al. 1989). They are superior and unique in identifying, detecting, and quantifying pesticide residues. The rate of breakdown, loss, distribution, and metabolism of a labeled pesticide can be followed specifically in the presence of other pesticides including the one being studied. Possible chemical binding of pesticide residues in food materials can only be indicated and quantified by using nuclear techniques. Upon studying the stability of fenitrothion in stored rice grains and wheat, the insecticide decomposed after 12 months. The major metabolites in rice grains were desmethyl fenitrothion and 3-methyl-4-nitrophenol and dimethyl phosphorothioic acid, as determined by gas liquid chromatography (Takimoto et al. 1978; Abdel-Kader and Webster 1982).

8.7.2 Biological Effects of BR in Grains

The importance of grains to human nutrition on global basis, the necessity for protecting stored grains from various pests by the use of toxic chemicals, and the fact that BRs are often present as terminal residues in grain and grain-derived products call for investigations of the potential toxicological significance of these xenobiotics in through and timely manner. Before these pesticides are cleared for such purposes and recommended by national and international agencies, there are many data required; toxicity studies; long-term feeding trials; persistence of residues and where they are located, as well as metabolic studies to determine the fate of the compound both in the treated commodity and in the animals (including humans) that may consume the raw or processed foodstuff after storage (IAEA 1990). Critical questions in connection with BR concern the nature and identity of BR as well as their toxicological significance with regard to bioavailability and biological activity. Nonextractable residues may be present in grain at significant concentration, and, therefore, an assessment of their toxicological potential is necessary to determine any biological impact they may have.

Feeding experiments on rat showed that bound ^{14}C-malathion residues in wheat are fairly bioavailable. It was reported that about 48.7% and 16.8% of the bound ^{14}C-activity was eliminated in urine and expired air, respectively, within 3 days (Neskovic et al. 1989). The ^{14}C-malathion bound residues in faba beans after storage for 30 weeks were reported to be 18% of the applied dose. About 75% of these residues proved to be bioavailable to rats within 2 days; the major part being excreted in urine (60%) and expired air (8%). According to Neskovic et al. (1992), rats fed on wheat with bound residues of ^{14}C-chlorpyrifos-methyl, excreted 79% of this radioactivity in urine, and 7% in expired air during 3 days. Feeding rats with the soybeans containing ^{14}C-pirimiphos-methyl bound residues for 72 hours revealed that these residues were bioavailable. The main excretion route was the urine (40%) and feces (18%), whereas a small amount (6%) could be detected in the expired air. About 25% of the administered radioactivity was detected among various organs of the rat (Mahdy 2003). Feeding studies on rats revealed that bound residues of both chemicals were bioavailable. Rats fed ^{14}C-bound malathion residues had about one-third of the administered radioactivity distributed among various organs. The main portion of radioactivity was eliminated via expired (15%) and urine (41%). The ^{14}C-activity of ^{14}C-bound carbofuran residues fed to rats was mainly eliminated in urine and in expired air as well (Farghaly et al. 2002). Feeding rats with the soybeans ^{14}C-dichlorvos bound residues for 72 hours revealed that these residues were bioavailable. The main excretion route was via the expired air (45%), whereas the ^{14}C-residues were excreted in urine and feces in nearly equal proportion. The radioactivity detected among various organs accounted to 15% (Mahdy and Taha 2007). Table 8.3 shows the distribution of released ^{14}C-activity in rat following feeding with ^{14}C-BRs on faba beans for 72 hours.

Feeding rats for 3 days was bound ^{14}C-fenitrothion residues; the main portion of radioactivity was eliminated via expired air (42%), urine (20%), and feces (11.5%). About 15% of the administrated radioactivity was distributed among various organs as, liver, kidney, lung, fat, intestine, blood, heart, and brain. ^{14}C-BR is readily bioavailability to rat. Therefore, the presence of BR can no longer be ignored in the evaluation of toxicological hazards.

To determine the biological activity and asses potential hazards of BR in grain for human health, subchronic feeding studies on mice for 90 days are to be conducted. Bound tetrachlorvinphos residues in faba beans proved to be of toxicological significance. Thus, feeding mice with these residues for 90 days led to an apparent decrease in the rate of body weight gain. The plasma cholinesterase was

TABLE 8.3
Distribution of Released ^{14}C-Activity in Rat Following Feeding with ^{14}C-Bound Pesticide Residues on Faba Beans for 72 Hours

	% of Activity Administered Dose					
Sample	Chlopyrifos	Dichlorvos	Pirimifos-methyl	Malathion	Carbaryl	Carbofuran
CO_2	50	35	7	60	2	12
Urine	15	20	46	8	60	35
Feces	10	11	15	3	10	15
	75	66	68	71	72	62
Fat	5	4	4	1	5	4
Blood	3	5	10	.2	6	11
Liver	3	7	7	2	3	7
Kidney	1	2	1	0	1	1
	12	18	22	3.2	15	22
Total released	87	84	90	74.2	87	85

significantly inhibited after feeding mice with bound residues for 2 months. Upon feeding rats on a diet containing bound malathion residues for 90 days, the blood cholinesterase activity was obviously inhibited in comparison with control ones. Both male and female rats revealed an increase in alkaline phosphatase, while a statistically significant increase in hemoglobin concentration was noted only in the males (Neskovic et al. 1989). Feeding mice with the bound malathion residues affected liver and kidney functions and inhibited cholinesterase activity (Zayed et al. 1992). The same authors in their study on stored soybeans found that the level of malathion BR was 8% of the applied dose 30 weeks following the application of the insecticide (Zayed et al. 1993). Since insects are the target species for the parent compounds, it seems probable that the type of chronic toxicological effects likely to be exhibited by nonextractable residues might be most readily demonstrated in insects. BR of chlorpyrifos-methyl in wheat caused a reduction in a number of adult of *Tribolium castaneum* reaching maturity. This is probably associated with the trichloropyridinol metabolite of chlorpyrifos-methyl that has been shown to comprise 60% of the nonextractable residues (Matthews 1992). However, there was no effect on the same insect in the tests involving the nonextractable residues of malathion. Subchronic feeding experiments on mice for 90 days with a diet containing the bound pirimiphos-methyl residues at a dose 1.6 (μg/g)/day/mouse caused no significant symptoms of toxicity during the period of the experiment. Both plasma and erythrocyte cholinesterases suffered a slight inhibition during the first 15 days. The blood picture and liver function enzymes showed no significant difference from control values. A significant increase in the level of blood urea nitrogen was observed, whereas creatinine clearance showed only a slight increase as compared with controls (Mahdy 2003). Feeding experiments on mice for 90 days with a diet containing the ^{14}C- BR at a dose of 0.91 and 2.39 (μg/g)/day/mouse for carbofuran and malathion, respectively, caused nonsignificant symptoms of toxicity during the period of the experiment. A slight inhibition in plasma and erythrocyte choline esterase activities was observed during the second and third months in both treated mice fed on carbofuran of malathion. Liver enzymes, total protein, albumin, cholesterol, triglycerides, and kidney functions showed nonsignificant differences from control values in case of mice fed on ^{14}C-bound carbofuran residues. However, these mentioned blood parameters showed only slight increase, as compared with controls, in treated mice fed on ^{14}C-bound malathion residues (Mahdy and Taha 2005). Subchronic feeding experiments on mice for 90 days with a diet containing the bound dichlorvos residues at a dose 1.7 (μg/g)/day/mouse caused a slight inhibition of both plasma and red blood cells cholinesterase activity. The maximum inhibition was observed after 2 months and amounted to 29% and 25%, respectively (Table 8.4).

However, the activity of the liver enzymes alanine amino transferase, aspartate amino transferase, and alkaline phosphatase showed a low significant increase in the treated group after 3 months of experiments compared with the control group. A moderate increase in blood urea concentration and slight increase in creatinine concentration was observed in the treated groups at the end of the experimental period (Table 8.5). All the blood parameters returned to the control values after a 1-month recovery period (Mahdy and Taha 2007). Toxicity of bound residues of ^{14}C-fenitrothion

TABLE 8.4
Cholinesterase Activity of Mice Fed for 90 Days on Extracted Soybeans Containing Bound Dichlorvos Residues

Treatment Period (days)	Plasma Cholinesterase Control X ± SD		Plasma Cholinesterase Treated X ± SD		Inhibition (%)	Erythrocte Cholinesterase Control X ± SD		Erythrocte Cholinesterase Treated X ± SD		Inhibition (%)
1	0.28	0.02	0.23	0.07	7	1.4	0.02	1.35	0.07	4
7	0.29	0.08	0.30	0.07	12	1.5	0.07	1.30	0.07	2
15	0.28	0.06	0.24	0.06	16	1.5	0.08	1.30	0.06	14
30	0.29	0.05	0.22	0.07	25	1.6	0.06	1.20	0.05	20
60	0.30	0.08	0.22	0.07	29	1.5	0.06	1.1	0.07	25
90	0.31	0.09	0.25	0.08	20	1.6	0.07	1.3	0.05	14
Recovery	0.31	0.08	0.29	0.07	6	1.6	0.09	1.5	0.08	5

TABLE 8.5
Effect of Feeding on Extracted Faba Beans Containing Bound Dichlorvos Residues on Liver and Kidney Function for 3 Months

Function	Sample	Feeding Period: One Month X ± SD		Two Month X ± SD		Three Month X ± SD		Recovery X ± SD	
Alanine amino transferase (units per liter)	C	51.50	3.53	52.25	2.86	55.50	1.25	55.80	3.20
	T	56.25	4.66	59.5	5.50	64.75	5.31	57.20	2.10
Aspartate amino transferase (units per liter)	C	92.50	5.89	94.00	6.22	93.50	3.39	94.5	3.40
	T	96.25	7.10	105.3	5.09	110.8	4.60	95.76	3.10
Alk. phosphatase	C	13.00	0.22	12.88	0.36	12.80	0.23	12.90	0.18
	T	14.00	0.39	14.04	0.17	15.30	0.25	13.20	0.22
Creatinine (mg/dL)	C	0.80	0.04	0.82	0.01	0.80	0.11	0.78	0.01
	T	0.84	0.02	0.86	0.02	0.93	0.03	0.80	0.01
Urea (mg/dL)	C	60.00	2.69	62.00	2.45	64.00	1.83	65.00	1.92
	T	67.00	2.59	76.00	1.87	83.00	3.02	70.00	2.20

in stored soybeans was studied in mice through feeding experiments for 3 months at a concentration of 1.9 mg/kg. The maximum inhibition in plasma and erythrocyte cholinesterase activity was observed 23%, 19%, 9%, 9% after 1 and 7 days, respectively. The obtained results showed a slight significant elevation after 3 months in the activity of liver enzymes alanine amino transferase, aspartate amino transferase, and alkaline phosphatase. A moderate increase in blood urea nitrogen and creatinine concentration was observed in the treated groups at the end of the experimental period.

8.8 DISSIPATION OF PESTICIDE RESIDUES IN FOOD

8.8.1 Washing

Table 8.6 gives details on the effect of various processing techniques on pesticide residue dissipation of different food commodities.

Washing is the most common form of processing, which is a preliminary step in both household and commercial preparation. Loosely held residues of several pesticides are removed with reasonable efficiency by varied types of washing processes (Street 1969). Chlorpyrifos and its breakdown product 3, 5, 6-trichloro-2-pyridinol were recovered from fortified rice grains in the levels of 456 and 3.4 ng/g, respectively. Washing rice grains with water removed approximately 60% of the chlorpyrifos residues (Lee et al. 1991). Washing of mango fruits by dipping in water for 10 minutes reduced residues to 66%–68% for dimethoate and fenthion as against 21%–27% for fenvalerate and cypermethrin simply by washing treatment (Awasthi 1993). The initial diazinon residue

TABLE 8.6
Effect of Processing Techniques on Pesticide Residue Dissipation

Processing	Commodity	Pesticide	% Residue Dissipations	Reason
Washing (twice)	Soybeans	Endosulfan	80–90	Sprayed pesticides remain as microparticles on the surface of the soybeans and are easily removed by mechanical stirring in water.
Washing	Golden delicious apples	Phosalone	30–50	Reduction on account of dissolution of phosalone in water.
Washing acetic acid solution	Tomatoes	HCB	51	Effectiveness of washing in removing residues depends upon four factors.
		Lindane	47	First, location of residue. Second, the age of the residue. Third, the water solubility of the pesticide.
		p, p-DDT	34	Lastly, the temperature and type of wash also affect residue removal.
		Dimethoate	92	Effectiveness of washing may be improved further by detergent.
		Profenofos	86	
		Pirimiphos methyl	94	
Washing with tap water	Tomatoes	HCB	10	
		Lindane	15	
		p, p-DDT	9	
		Dimethoate	19	
		Profenofos	23	
		Pirimiphos methyl	16	

(*Continued*)

TABLE 8.6 (*Continued*)
Effect of Processing Techniques on Pesticide Residue Dissipation

Processing	Commodity	Pesticide	% Residue Dissipations	Reason
Washing with sodium chloride (at 10% NaCl)	Tomatoes	HCB Lindane p, ′p-DDT Dimethoate Profenofos Pirimiphos methyl	43 46 27 91 82 91	Effectiveness of washing in removing residues depends upon four factors. First, location of residue. Second, the age of the residue. Third, the water solubility of the pesticide. Lastly, the temperature and type of wash also affect residue removal. Effectiveness of washing may be improved further by detergent.
Peeling	Mango	Fenthion Dimethoate Cypermethrin Fenvalarate	Complete removal	Peeling off fruit skin removed the residues absolutely at all the stages reflecting that accumulation of residues in fruit pericarp only and no movement to fruit pulp.
Cooking 30 minutes (boiling)	Potato Cabbage mash	Dimethoate Dimethoate	37–53 56–86	Disappearance of residues from boiling extract due to decomposition by effect of heat, the stronger adsorption of pesticide onto plant tissues, and/or the poor solubility of pesticides in water.
Cooking at 100°C Sterilization at 121°C for 15 minutes	Tomato homogenates	Maneb Ethylenethio-urea (ETU) Maneb ETU	74 28 ND 32	Processes involving heat can increase volatilization, hydrolysis, or other chemical degradation and thus reduce residue levels.
Juicing	Tomatoes	HCB Lindine p, ′p-DDT Dimethoate Profenofos Pirimiphos-methyl	73–78	The residue levels in juices from fruit or must from grapes depend on partitioning properties of pesticide between the fruit skins/pulp and the juice. The pulp or pomace often include skin, retain a substantial proportion of lipophilic residues.
Canning (processing tomato to paste)	Tomato	Dimethoate Profenofos Pirimiphos methyl HCB Lindane p,′p- DDT	71–82 31–35	The levels of reduction of organochlorines were lower than the organophosphates due to the high stabilities of organochlorines to heat treatments.

(*Continued*)

TABLE 8.6 (*Continued*)
Effect of Processing Techniques on Pesticide Residue Dissipation

Processing	Commodity	Pesticide	% Residue Dissipations	Reason
Canning	Cherries	Tetrachlorvinphos	95	Processes involving heat can increase volatilization, hydrolysis, or other chemical degradation and thus reduce residue levels.
Sunlight drying	Apricot fruit	Bitertanol	50	This reduction due to photodegradation.
Oven drying	Raisins	Dimethoate	81	The decrease in dimethoate was attributed to heat that could cause evaporation and degradation.
Fermentation process	Meat products (fermented sausage)	DDT	10	Fermentation process in meat products reduced the pesticide residues, and these reductions were due to the activity of meat starter.
		Lindane	18	
Milling and storage for 365 days	Wheat	Phoxim-methyl	8–10	During milling, residues accumulate in the bran fractions and reduced in white flour.
12 months of storage in an open basket	Maize grains	Malathion	64	These high losses were explained by volatilization and possible settling of pesticide dust formulation to the bottom and on the sides of basket during storage in the open and windy tropical laboratory.
	Beans		47	

level (0.8 μg/g) on cucumbers was decreased by 22.3% by washing for 15 seconds by rubbing under running water (Cengiz et al. 2006). Captan residues in apples washed for 10–15 seconds with continuous hand rubbing were 50% lower than in those apples that received no postharvest washing (25.5–5100 ng/g) (Rawn et al. 2008).

8.8.2 Peeling

Peeling is an important step in the processing of most fruits and vegetables. Chemical peeling (mostly lye peeling), mechanical peeling (mainly abrasion peeling), steam peeling, and freeze peeling are conventional methods for peeling in the processing of fruits and vegetables. A majority of the insecticides or fungicides applied directly to crops undergo very limited movement or penetration of the cuticle. It, therefore, follows that residues of these materials are confined to the outer surfaces where they are amenable to removal in peeling, hulling, or trimming operations.

The peeling process had a significant effect on the elimination of pesticide residues from tomato contaminated at level of 1 μg/g, the losses of Hexachlorobenzene, lindine, p,p-Dichlorodiphenyltrichloroethane (DDT), dimethoate, profenofos, and pirimiphos- methyl residues ranged from 80% to 89% (Abou-Arab 1999). Peeling of potatoes reduced 91%–98% chlorpropham residues from an initial concentration of 3.8 μg/g in individual tubers 10 days post application (Lentza-Rizos and Balokas 2001). Abdel-Gawad et al. (2008) found that on their study distribution and degradation of ^{14}C-ethyl prothiofos in potato plant and the effect of processing, the residues of prothiofos insecticide were mainly located in the peels of potato tubers (peeling process removed 85% of the total residue after 1 month of the treatment). The initial procymidone residue level (0.86 μg/g) on tomatoes was decreased 77% by the peeling procedure (Cengiz et al. 2007).

8.8.3 Cooking

Cooking of apples (processing apple to sauce) significantly reduced the levels of azinphos-methyl residue. About 96% of azinphos-methyl was removed when the unwashed apples were processed into sauce. The total amount of residue on the control unwashed fruit was determined to be 0.67 μg/g (Ong 1996). Blanching and frying of eggplant for 5 minutes completely removed the profenofos residues that were initially present at level of 0.27 μg/g (Radwan et al. 2005). Hence, processes involving heat can increase volatilization, hydrolysis, or other chemical degradation and thus reduce residue levels (Holland et al. 1994). Potatoes are processed in three ways: frying, boiling, and baking, which is simulated in home preparation. The amount of prothiofos residues was found to decrease on boiling (70%) and further on baking (82%) and frying (100%). The results indicated that frying is the most effective method for reducing the amount of pesticide residues (Abdel-Gawad et al. 2008).

8.8.4 Drying and Fermentation

Drying has been found to reduce the pesticide residues considerably. Drying of grapes lead to 64%–72% losses of methamidophos possibly due to evaporation of the pesticide during the process (Athanasopoulos et al. 2005). Abdel-Gawad et al. (2011) investigated the effect of drying process on ethion residues in chamomile flowers. Ethion residues were decreased by sun drying of chamomile flowers. The percentage of removal was 18%–47%.

Fermentation has been studied for reduction in pesticide residues. The fermentation in meat products (fermented sausage) reduced the pesticide residues by 10% and 18% of DDT and lindane after 72 hours from an initial level of 5 and 2 μg/g, respectively. The results confirmed that fermentation process in meat products reduced the pesticide residues, and these reductions were due to the activity of meat starter (Abou-Arab 2002). Malolactic fermentation resulted in significant reduction in chlorpyrifos concentrations, which were reduced by 70% (at levels 1 and 0.1 μg/g). The total dicofol concentration was reduced by more than 30% (at levels 5.0 and 2 μg/g). These reductions of pesticide concentrations could possibly be due to the absorption onto the bacterial cell walls, rather than chemical or biological degradation (Ruediger et al. 2005).

8.8.5 Storage

Grains are frequently stored long term (3–36 months) at ambient temperatures in bulk silos where insecticides may be applied postharvest to reduce losses from storage pests (Holland et al. 1994). Grain-based foods therefore have the potential to be a major source of residues in the diet for these insecticides. Studies on grain following post-harvest treatments with insecticides have generally shown that residues only decline rather slowly. Residues of the more lipophilic materials tend to remain on the seed coat, although a proportion can migrate through to the bran and germ that contain high levels of triacylglycerols (Holloland et al. 1994). The mean concentration of chlorpropham in individual potato tubers stored at 5°C in dark was 3.8 μg/g/10 days post application, which decreased to 2.9 μg/g/28 days post application and became 2.2 μg/g after 65 days of application (Lentza-Rizos and Balokas 2001). Overall disappearances of 64% and 47% of initial dose of malathion from maize grains (initial 7.7 μg/g) and beans (initial 7.5 μg/g), respectively, were obtained, after 12 months of storage in an open basket. These high losses were explained by volatilization and possible settling of the pesticide dust formulation to the bottom and on the sides of basket during storage in the open and windy tropical laboratory (Lalah and Wandiga 2002). The initial dimethyl 2,2-dichlorovinyl phosphate (DDVP) residue level (1.7 μg/g) in cucumber samples was decreased 48% (0.9 μg/g) by storage at 4°C for 3 days and 71% (0.5 μg/g) by the storage procedure at 4°C for 6 days (Cengiz et al. 2006). The dynamics of incurred pesticide residues in apples, variety Melrose, was monitored during their cold storage at 1°C–3°C for 5 months. Only six fungicides (captan, cyprodinyl, dodine, pyrimethanil, tebuconazole, tolyfluanid) and one insecticide (phosalone) were detected at the time of harvest. Successive decrease of residues occurred during storage period, after 5 months only fungicide dodine and insecticide phosalone were detected (Ticha et al. 2008).

8.9 DISSIPATION OF BR

The formation of BR decreases the toxicity and the bioavailability of pesticides. Soil microorganisms are believed to play an important role in the release (dissipations) and further degradation of BR. Mineralization is the ability of soil microorganism for biodegradation of pesticides to CO_2 and inorganic components (chloride and phosphate), for example, the mineralization of dichlorvos as shown in Figure 8.1.

The dissipation of (O-methyl-^{14}C) monocrotophos and U-ring labeled ^{14}C-carbaryl was monitored for over 2 years in the absence and presence of other insecticides using

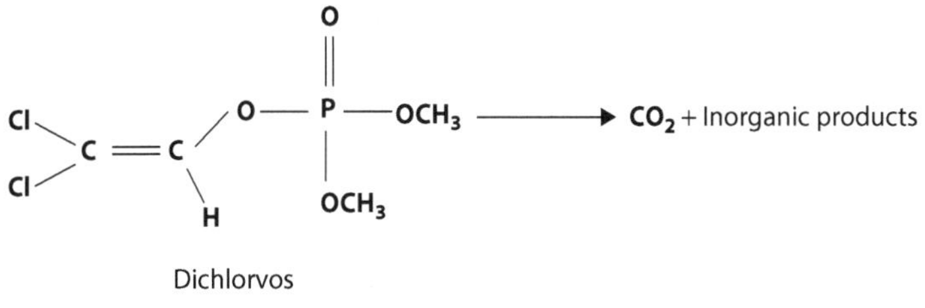

Dichlorvos → CO_2 + Inorganic products

FIGURE 8.1 Dissipation of ^{14}C-dichlorvos.

in situ soil columns. The dissipation of ^{14}C-monocrotophos from soil treated with methomyl and carbaryl showed a faster rate of downward movement than in a control column tagged with the labeled insecticide alone. The same trend was observed in experiments with ^{14}C-carbaryl that dissipated more readily in soil treated with nonlabeled monocrotophos and methomyl. In the presence of other insecticides, the percentage of BR was generally lower than in control experiments. The BR at the top of the column is released at a low rate under conditions prevailing in the field. The overall time required for dissipation of 50% of monocrotophos and carbaryl (t_{50}) as estimated from control experiment was approximately 20 and 24 weeks, respectively (Figures 8.2 and 8.3). The data indicate that repeated applications of pesticides might enhance the release of ^{14}C-bound residues (Zayed et al. 2008).

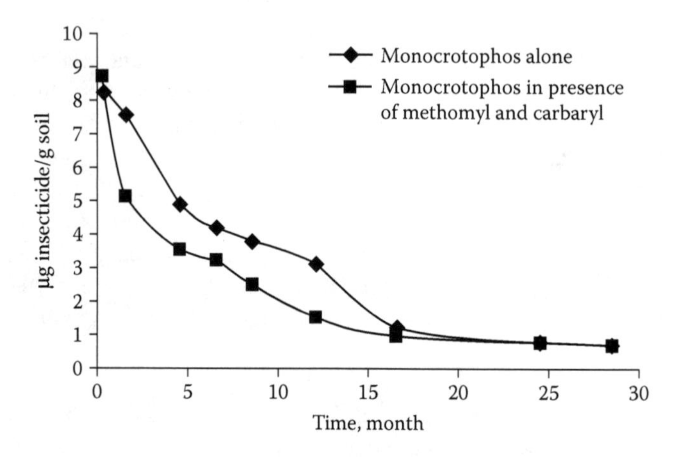

FIGURE 8.2 Dissipation of ^{14}C-monocrotophos in the absence and presence of methomyl and carbaryl in soil columns during two successive years. ◆ ^{14}C-monocrotophos only (control) ■ ^{14}C-monocrotophos in the presence of methomyl and carbaryl.

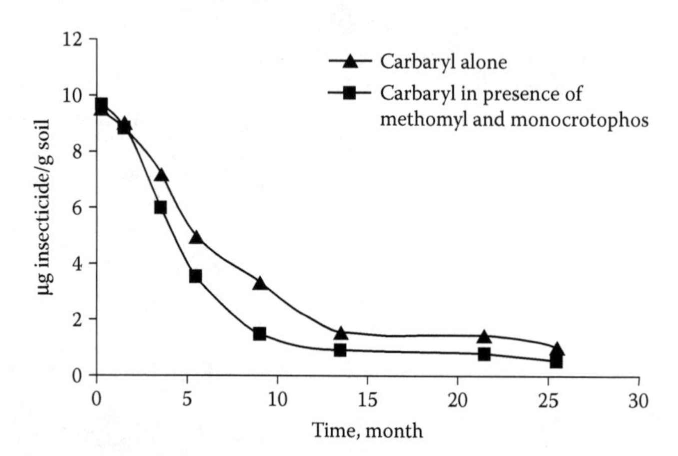

FIGURE 8.3 Dissipation of ^{14}C-carbaryl in the absence and presence of methomyl and monocrotophos in soil columns during two successive years. ▲ ^{14}C-carbaryl only (control) ■ ^{14}C-carbaryl in the presence of methomyl and monocrotophos.

The release of BR includes microbial and physicochemical release (Hayar et al. 1997), bioavailability (Mathew et al. 1998), plant uptake (Haque et al. 1982; Gevao et al. 2001; Han et al. 2009), or earthworm's uptake (Haque et al. 1982; Gevao et al. 2001). Release, bioavailability, and uptake by plants or earthworms only represent a small percentage of the total amounts of BR. Ionic modifications and the addition of nitrogen to the soil can induce a partial release of some BR, as demonstrated for chloro–aniline bound pesticide, which was released by addition of N-ammonic fertilizers (Saxena and Bartha 1983) and for prometryn bound pesticide, which was released by addition of N-ammoniac and N-nitrate (Yee et al. 1985). The release of BR also occurs by changing in agricultural practices and the introduction of certain chemicals that may change the chemistry of the soil. This reintroduces the compounds into the soil solution, which may eventually lead to their uptake by plants. Although soil-BR is highly stabilized, they can be released from the soil particles and be degraded by soil microorganisms, plants, or physical and chemical modifications of the soil (Dec et al. 1990; El-Hamady et al. 2008). Persistence of several insecticides in grains and beans stored under typical conditions has been studied in a number of countries using radiotracer techniques (IAEA 1990; Holland et al. 1994). Extractable residues of parent malathion after storage periods of 3–9 months ranged from 16% to 65% of the applied doses. Considerable amounts of hydrolysis products were also present and BR comprised 5%–20% of the applied dose. Chlorpyrifos-methyl, fenvalerate, and pirimiphos-methyl were generally more persistent than malathion (Holland et al. 1994). An attempt to study the effect of cooking on ^{14}C-carbaryl and ^{14}C-chlorpyrifos residues in stored faba beans was carried out by Mahdy (2002, 2003). The results show that a considerable portion of radioactivity (4%–7%) and (7%–9%) was associated with the seeds as BR for both insecticides, respectively. Cooking of faba beans did not affect the amount of "bound" carbaryl and chlorpyrifos residues.

8.10 FERTILIZERS

There are different types of fertilizers such as organic manures and fertilizers, inorganic fertilizers, nitrogen fertilizers, phosphate fertilizers, potassium fertilizers, calcium fertilizers, magnesium fertilizers, sulfur fertilizers, iron fertilizers, manganese fertilizers, boron fertilizers, zinc fertilizers, copper fertilizers, molybdenum fertilizers, fluid mixed fertilizers, and fertilizer-pesticide mixtures.

Organic fertilizers can be divided into two categories according to the addition to soil: solid fertilizers and liquid fertilizers. Solid fertilizers can add to soil by spreading on its surface or by handing or by using special machines. These fertilizers must be mixed with the soil and not leave on the surface prevent them from losing in the atmosphere. Liquid fertilizers can be added by irrigation machines or by using special machines to inject them directly to soil.

Fertilizers may affect food in different aspects listed below:

- Adequate supply of N increases protein quality and quantity (more of the essential amino acids) and some vitamins.
- Excessive N supply tends to increase amide content, resulting in bad flavor after cooking, or in raising the nitrate content to unacceptable levels, especially in vegetables grown under protected culture systems.

- Low N causes premature ripening, whereas high N causes delayed ripening.
- High amounts of N and K decrease dry matter and starch content and affect the quality of starch in potatoes; low K affects the coloration of fried potatoes negatively and causes black spots in fresh potatoes.
- Adequate Ca supply leads to high quality of different fruits and vegetables. Ca deficiency causes low-quality banana fruits (fruit peels and splits at ripening).
- Sulfur increases the protein content in grain and the oil content of oil-seed crops.

8.11 ANTIBIOTIC RESIDUES IN FOOD

8.11.1 INTRODUCTION

The use of antibiotics in animals shortly followed their use in humans for the purpose of disease prevention and treatment (Gustafson 1993). Today, antimicrobial drugs are used to control, prevent, and treat infection and to enhance animal growth and feed efficiency. Currently, approximately 80% of all food-producing animals receive medication for part or most of their lives. The most commonly used antimicrobials in food-producing animals are the β-lactams, tetracyclines, aminoglycosides, lincosamides, macrolides, pleuromutilins, and sulfonamides (Figure 8.4) (Lee et al. 2001).

The use of antibiotics in food-producing animals may leave residues in foodstuffs of animal origin like meat, milk, and eggs. The occurrence of these residues may be due to any one of the following: a failure to observe the withdrawal periods of each drug, extralabel dosages for animals, contamination of animal feed with the excreta of treated animals, or the use of unlicensed antibiotics (Paige 1994).

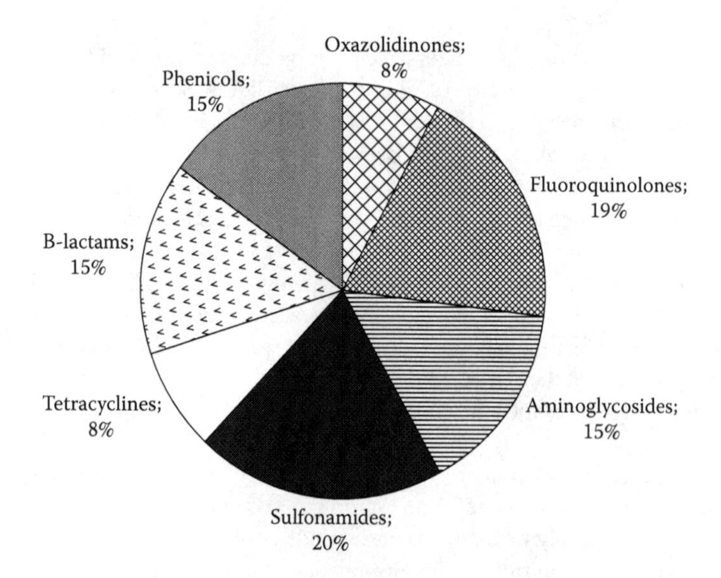

FIGURE 8.4 Distribution of the antibiotic families determined in food.

Antibiotic residues in foods of animal origin may be the cause of numerous health concerns in humans. These problems include toxic effects, transfer of antibiotic resistant bacteria to humans, immunopathological effects, carcinogenicity (e.g., sulphamethazine, oxytetracycline, and furazolidone), mutagenicity, nephropathy (e.g., gentamicin), hepatotoxicity, reproductive disorders, bone marrow toxicity (e.g., chloramphenicol), and allergy (e.g., penicillin) (Nisha 2008).

8.11.2 Occurrence of Antibiotic Residues in Foods

The main use of antibiotics in animal rearing was for the treatment and prevention of diseases. Indeed, antibiotics have been used for the treatment of mastitis, arthritis, respiratory diseases, gastrointestinal infections, and other infectious bacterial diseases (Draisci et al. 2001).

More recently, antibiotics have been used for improved growth, especially in broilers and fatteners. Indeed, antibiotics may improve growth rate by the following means: the thinning of mucous membranes in the gut, which facilitates absorption; alteration of gut motility, which enhances assimilation; production of favorable conditions for beneficial gut microbes by destroying harmful bacteria; and partitioning of proteins for muscle growth via cytokine suppression. Antibiotics also favor growth by decreasing the activity of the immune system, reducing the waste of nutrients, and reducing toxin formation. In most cases, however, only young growing animals and poultry are responsive to antibiotic-mediated health maintenance; this approach actually is problematic as these feed additives are usually used without prescription and for very long periods, in both large and small doses, which leads to drug residues entering animal-derived food. As we can see in Figure 8.4, seven antibiotic families have been employed as veterinary drugs in recent years, sulfonamides and fluoroquinolones being the most used.

In many African countries, antibiotics may be used indiscriminately for the treatment of bacterial diseases or they may be used as feed additives for domestic animals and birds. The ongoing threat of antibiotic contamination is one of the biggest challenges to public health that is faced not only by the African people, but also by the human population worldwide (Cars et al. 2008). Such residues are spreading rapidly, irrespective of geographical, economical, or legal differences between countries.

The most important screening approaches to detect antibiotic residues in food samples (i.e., immunoassays, microbiological tests, and biosensors). Their main advantages are short analysis time, high sensitivity and selectivity for immunoassays, simplicity and low cost for microbiological tests, and automation and the possibility of *in situ* analysis for biosensors. Moreover, it is important to note a great increase in the number of commercial kits (Cháfer-Pericás et al. 2010).

8.11.3 Recommendations for the Reduction of Antibiotic Contamination in Food in African Countries

There is no doubt that neither humans nor animals can live without antibiotics as they are some of the most effective antimicrobial treatments. However, at the same time, the misuse of antibiotics may result in the aforementioned health hazards. Thus, the reduction of antibiotic use constitutes a challenge for the world.

To achieve such a reduction, the following 10 steps should possibly be considered with regard to all antibiotics:

- The effective prevention of infectious diseases and the adoption of strict hygiene standards and rearing skills may reduce our need for antibiotics, particularly in the veterinary field.
- The use of alternatives to antibiotics, such as plant-derived antimicrobial substances and probiotics, may represent a promising option; vaccination against some bacterial diseases may be of great value in the near future.
- The reduction of unnecessary antibiotic use in animals in captivity should be pursued, as should antibiotic use for the treatment of viral disease in animals; the reduction of prophylactic antibiotic use should also be considered.
- Strict national legislation must be passed around the world to avoid the unnecessary use of antibiotics. In 2006, the European Union banned the use of antibiotics for the purpose of livestock health maintenance (Carlet et al. 2012).
- National monitoring of antibiotic residues in foods and updating of the maximum permissible limits of these residues for each country should be undertaken.
- Antibiotics use in feed additives should be ceased.
- Avoid using antibiotics in the veterinary field without a veterinarian's prescription (in some African countries veterinarian or even human medical formulas are sold in supermarkets).
- Strict observation of antibiotic cessation times should be made; the avoidance of antibiotics lacking clearly documented pharmacokinetic and pharmacodynamic properties must be considered.
- The heat treatment of meat, milk, and eggs may inactivate antibiotic contaminants in feedstuffs.
- The freezing of animal-derived foods may also contribute to the reduction of some antibiotic contamination.

8.12 CONCLUSIONS

- The BR represents compounds in soils, plants, or animals, which persist in the matrix in the form of the parent substance or its metabolite(s) after extraction. The extraction method must not substantially change the compounds themselves or the structure of the matrix.
- Soil pesticide interactions include ionic, hydrogen and covalent bonding, Van der Waals forces, ligand exchange, charge-transfer complexes, and hydrophobic partitioning.
- Methods to identify the chemical nature of bound residues as chromatographic techniques, HTD, thermoanalytical methods, supercritical methanol or carbon dioxide extraction, alkaline hydrolysis, spectrometric methods as NMR, and degradative techniques.
- Plants grown in soils containing bound residues to take up a portion of these residues. A portion of these residues may again become within plant tissues.

- Chlorinated hydrocarbons form the lowest portion of bound residues, and higher percentage are formed from phenol and nitrogen containing compounds plant growth conditions have an important influence on the formation of bound residues. Under good growth conditions, high crop yields with high level of bound residues.
- Most of BRs were shown to be localized in lignin and to identify the chemical nature of these residues hydrolytic, or pyrolytic degradation methods have been developed. The extracted plant tissue containing bound likely contained mainly lignin, carbohydrate, and denatured protein.
- The soil-bound residues are absorbed and translocated in plant tissues; they may be present in three possible forms:
    - Freely extractable residues.
- Extractable conjugated bound to natural components of plants.
- Unextractable or bound residues incorporated into plant constituents.
- The BR in grains is readily bioavailable to rats. Therefore, the presence of BRs can no longer be ignored in the evaluation of toxicological hazards.
- The hepatic and renal lesions may be taken as indices for the toxicological significance of pesticide residues.
- The important matter is not so much how the residue is defined, but the question of the reversibility between unavailable and available forms of the residues and their biological availability. Accounting for potential biological effects may lead to improved risk assessments.
- Pesticide residues in food are influenced by storage, handling, and processing, which is postharvest of raw agricultural commodities but prior to consumption of prepared foodstuffs. Extensive literature review demonstrates that in most cases processing leads to large reductions in residue levels in the prepared food, particularly through washing, peeling, and cooking operations.
- Washing with water and various chemical solutions for domestic and commercial use are necessary to decrease the intake of pesticide residues.
- Freezing as well as juicing and peeling are necessary to remove the pesticide residues in the skins.
- Cooking of food products helps to eliminate most of the pesticide residues.
- Residues of postharvest insecticide treatment on stored grains generally decline only rather slowly. However, even in those processing into foods results in large losses. Removal of residues in food by processing is affected by type of food, insecticide type and nature, and severity of processing procedure used. Hence, a combination of processing techniques would suitably address the current situation in food safety.
- In a developing country like Egypt there is a great need to regulate the use of pesticides where the extensive use of pesticides is causing serious health and alarming environmental problems. To minimize the risk of pesticides on health, different processing operations are applied on fruit and vegetable crops that reduce the pesticide residues below the risk level. It is further concluded that treatment of vegetables with acidic and alkaline solutions can effectively minimize the pesticide residues. There is a need to educate the consumers through media.

- New legislation and an institutional commitment to environmental governance are becoming extremely important. Creating regulatory systems to face the new challenges and to be updated regularly is the major task that Arab countries should start with. Although some countries perform better than others, all face issues that have to be tackled at the regional level and not merely the country level. Many countries have resources and capacities for a better performance if a commitment to greater environmental sustainability and food safety is made.
- Governments should develop effective extension programs to teach farmers about proper methods for the use and handling of agrochemicals and adopt modern laws concerning the use of fertilizers and pesticides.
- In addition, governments should consider institutional reforms and support the establishment of laboratories to ensure the safety of the food consumed, produced, and exported from the region.

8.13 FUTURE SCOPE

The progress in this topic is steadily increasing all over the world. It is of high significance to expand in application of natural pesticides particularly pyrethroids that enhance low environmental persistence and low mammalian toxicity. Moreover, we should improve our research realms as possible to decrease the amount of bound residues to save human health and money.

There is need to optimize the processing techniques with regard to pesticide residue dissipation and nutrient content. Substantial attention needs to be focused on addressing optimization of the processing techniques in a manner that leads to considerable pesticide residue dissipation but preserves most of the essential food nutrients, thereby addressing the delicate balance between the two important parameters of food quality and safety.

Finally, further understanding of BR formation and long-term behavior is essential for the development of meaningful quality criteria, regulatory limits and risk assessment criteria for organic chemicals in soil, sediment, and food.

REFERENCES

Abdel-Gawad, H., and B. Hegazi. 2010. Fate of ^{14}C-ethyl prothiofos insecticide in canola seeds and oils. *J. Environ. Sci. Health B* 45: 116–122.

Abdel-Gawad, H., and H. Taha. 2011a. Bioavailability and toxicological potential of sunflower-bound residues of 14C-chlorpyrifos insecticide in rats. *J. Environ. Sci. Health B* 46(8): 683–690.

Abdel-Gawad, H., and H. Taha. 2011b. Fate of ^{14}C-ethyl profenofos in soybean seeds and oils, residue removal, bioavailability, toxicity and protective action of cinnamon extract towards experimental animals. *Egypt. J. Chem.* 54(2): 155–174.

Abdel-Gawad, H., R.M. Abdelhameed, A.M., Elmesalamy, and B. Hegazi. 2011. Distribution and elimination of ^{14}C-ethion insecticide in chamomile flowers and oil. *Phosphorous Sulfur Silicon Relat. Elem.* 186: 2122–2134.

Abdel-Gawad, H., R.M. Abdel-Hameed, L.M. Affi, and B. Hegazi. 2008. Distribution and degradation of ^{14}C-ethoxy prothiofos in potato plant and the effect of processing. *Phosphorous Sulfur Silicon Relat. Elem.* 183: 2734–2751.

Abdelhafid, R., S. Houot, and E. Barriuso. 2000a. Dependence of atrazine degradation on C and N availability in adapted and non-adapted soils. *Soil Biol. Biochem.* 32: 389–401.
Abdelhafid, R., S. Houot, and E. Barriuso. 2000b. How increasing availabilities of carbon and nitrogen affect atrazine behaviour in soils. *Biol. Fertil. Soils* 30: 333–340.
Abdel-Kader, M.H.K., and G.R.B. Webster. 1982. Analysis of fenitrothion and metabolites in stored wheat. *Int. J. Environ. Anal. Chem.* 11: 153–165.
Abou-Arab, A.A.K. 1999. Behavior of pesticides in tomatoes during commercial and home preparation. *Food Chem.* 65: 509–514.
Abou-Arab, A.A.K. 2002. Degradation of organochlorine pesticides by meat starter in liquid media and fermented sausage. *Food Chem. Toxicol.* 40: 33–41.
Athanasopoulos, P.E., C. Pappas, N.V. Kyriakidis, and A. Thanos 2005. Degradation of methamidophos on soultanina grapes on the vines and during refrigerated storage. *Food Chem.* 91: 235–240.
Awasthi, M.D. 1993. Decontamination of insecticide residues on mango by washing and peeling. *J. Food Sci. Technol.* 30(2): 132–133.
Baranowska, I. H. Barchanska, and E. Pacak, 2006. Procedures of trophic chain samples preparation for determination of triazines by HPLC and metals by ICP-AES methods. *Environ. Pollut.* 143: 206–211.
Buhler, W.G., A.C. York, and R.F. Turco. 1992. Effect of enhanced biodegradation of carbofuran on the control of striped cucumber beetle (Coleoptera: Chrysomelidae) on muskmelon. *J. Econ. Entomol.* 85: 1910–1918.
Carlet, J., V. Jarlier, S. Harbarth, A. Voss, H. Goossens, and D. Didier Pittet. 2012. Ready for a world without antibiotics? The pensières antibiotic resistance call to action. *Antimicrob. Resist. Infect. Control* 1: 11.
Cars, O., L.D. Hogberg, M. Murray, O. Nordberg, S. Sivaraman, C.S. Lundborg, A.D. So, and G. Tomson. 2008. Meeting the challenge of antibiotic resistance. *B.M.J.* 337: 14–38.
Cengiz, M.F., M. Certel, B. Karakas, and H. Gocmen. 2006. Residue contents of DDVP (Dichlorvos) and diazinon applied on cucumbers grown in greenhouses and their reduction by duration of a pre-harvest interval and post-harvest culinary applications. *Food Chem.* 98: 127–135.
Cengiz, M. F., M. Certel, B. Karakas, and H. Gocmen. 2007. Residue contents of captan and procymidone applied on tomatoes grown in greenhouses and their reduction by duration of a pre-harvest interval and post-harvest culinary applications. *Food Chem.* 100: 1611–1619.
Cháfer-Pericás, C., Á. Maquieira, and R. Puchades. 2010. Fast screening methods to detect antibiotic residues in food samples. *Trends Anal. Chem.* 29(9): 1038–1049.
Daniel, J.R., A.C.J. Voragen, and W. Pilnik. 1994. Starch and other polysaccharides. In: B. Elvers, S. Hawkins, and W. Russey (eds), *Ullmann's Encyclopedia of Industrial Chemistry*, vol A25, 5th edn, Weinheim, Germany: VCH Verlagsgesellschaft, pp. 1–62.
Dec, J., K.L. Schuttleworth, and J.M. Bollag. 1990. Microbial release of 2,4-dichlorophenol bound to humic acid or incorporated during humification. *J. Environ. Qual.* 19: 546–551.
Draisci, R., F. delli Quadri, L. Achene, G. Volpe, L. Palleschi, and G. Palleschi. 2001. A new electrochemical enzyme-linked immunosorbent assay for the screening of macrolide antibiotic residues in bovine meat. *Analyst* 126: 1942–1946.
Dupont, S., and S.U. Khan. 1992. Bound (nonextractable) carbon-14 residues in soybean treated with [14C]metribuzin. *J. Agric. Food Chem.* 40: 890–893.
El-Hamady, S.E., R. Kubiak, and A.S. Derbalah. 2008. Fate of imidacloprid in soil and plant after application to cotton seeds. *Chemosphere* 71: 2173–2179.
Farghaly, M., F. Mahdy, and S.M.A.D. Zayed, 2002. Bioavailability to rats of bound residues of ^{14}C-malathion and ^{14}C-carbofuran in soybean seeds. *Bull. NRC, Egypt.* 27: 351–359.
Farghaly, M., S.M.A.D. Zayed, F. Mahdy, and M. S. Soliman. 1998. Lindane degradation and effects on soil microbial activity. *Biomed. Environ. Sci.* 11: 218–225.

Fontcuberta, M., J.F. Arques, J.R. Villalbi, M. Martinez, F. Centrich, E. Serrahima, L. Pineda, J. Duran, and C. Casas. 2008. Chlorinated organic pesticides in marketed food: Barcelona, 2001–06. *Sci. Total Environ.* 389: 52–57.

Gevao, B., C. Mordaunt, K.T. Semple, T.G. Piearce, and K. C. Jones. 2001. Bioavailability of nonextractable (bound) pesticide residues to earthworms. *Environ. Sci. Technol.* 35: 501–507.

Gustafson, R. 1993. Historical perspectives on regulatory issues of antimicrobial resistance. *Vet. Hum. Toxicol.* 35: 2–5.

Guth, J.A. 1994. Monocrotophos—environmental fate and toxicity. *Rev. Environ. Contam. Toxicol.* 139: 75–136.

Han, A., L. Yue, Z. Li, H. Wang, Y. Wang, Q. Ye, L. Lu, and J. Ga. 2009. Plant availability and phytotoxicity of soil bound residues of herbicide ZJ0273, a novel acetolactate synthase potential inhibitor. *Chemosphere* 77(7): 955–961.

Haque, A., I. Schuphan, and W. Ebing. 1982. Bioavailability of conjugated and soil-bound [^{14}C]"hydroxymonolinuron"-β-D-glucoside residues to earthworms and ryegrass. *Pestic. Sci.* 13: 219–228.

Hayar, S., C. Munier-Lamy, T. Chone, and M. Schiavon. 1997. Physico-chemical versus microbial release of ^{14}C-atrazine bound residues from a loamy clay soil incubated in laboratory microcosms. *Chemosphere* 34: 2683–2697.

Holland, P.T., D. Hamilton, B. Ohlin, and M.W. Skidmore. 1994. Pesticides report 31: Effects of storage and processing on pesticide residues in plant products (Technical Report). IUPAC Reports on Pesticides (31). *Pure Appl. Chem.* 66(2): 335–356.

Howard, P.H. 1991. *Handbook of Environmental Fate and Exposure Data for Organic Chemicals.* Chelsea, MI: Lewis Publishers.

Huber, R., and S. Otto. 1983. Bound pesticide residues in plants, in IUPAC Pesticide chemistry, human welfare and the environment. In: Miyamoto J. and Kearney P.C. (eds) *Proceeding of the fifth International Congress of Pesticide Chemistry*, vol 3. Oxford: Pergamon Press, pp. 357–362.

IAEA. 1986. *Quantification, Nature and Bioavailability of Bound ^{14}C- Residues in Soil, Plant and Food.* Vienna: IAEA, pp. 177–185.

IAEA. 1990. *Panal Proceeding Series, STI/PUB/822, Studies of the Magnitude and Nature of Pesticide Residues in Stored Product Using Radiotracer Techniques.* Vienna: IAEA, p. 73.

IAEA. 1990. *Studies of the Magnitude and Nature of Pesticide Residues in Stored Products, Using Radiotracer Techniques.* Vienna: IAEA.

Jahn, C., and W. Schwack. 2001. Determination of cutin-bound residues of chlorothalonil by immunoassay. *J. Agric. Food Chem.* 49: 1233–1238.

Kacew, S., M.H. Akhtar, and S.U. Khan. 1996. Bioavailability of bound pesticide residues and potential toxicologic consequences—an update. *Proc. Soc. Exp. Biol. Med.* 211: 62–68.

Khan, S.U. 1995. Supercritical fluid extraction of bound pesticide residues from soil and food commodities. *J. Agric. Food Chem.* 43: 1718–1723.

Laabs, V., W. Amelung, G. Fent, W. Zech, and R. Kubiak. 2002. Fate of ^{14}C-labeled soybean and corn pesticides in tropical soils of Brazil under laboratory conditions. *J. Agric. Food Chem.* 50: 4619–4627.

Lalah, J.O., and S.O. Wandiga. 2002. The effect of boiling on the removal of persistent malathion residues from stored grains. *J. Stored Prod. Res.* 38: 1–10.

Lange, B.M., R. Hertkorn, and H. Sandermann. 1998. Chloroaniline/lignin conjugates as model system for nonextractable pesticide residues in crop plants. *Environ. Sci. Technol.* 32: 2113–2118.

Langebartels, C., and H. Harms. 1985. Analysis for nonextractable (bound) residues of pentachlorophenol in plant cells using a cell wall fractionation procedure. *Ecotoxicol. Environ. Safety* 10: 268–279.

Laurent, F.M.G., and R. Scalla. 1999. Metabolism and cell wall incorporation of phenoxyacetic acid in soybean cell suspension culture. *Pestic. Sci.* 55: 3–10.

Laurent, F.M.G., and R. Scalla. 2000. Phenoxyacetic acid residue incorporation in cell walls of soybean (*Glycine max.*). *J. Agric. Food Chem.* 48: 4389–4398.

Lavin, L., B.S. Young, and T.D. Spittler. 1996. Analysis of benomyl residues in commodities by enzyme immunoassay: extraction, conversion, and high-performance liquid chromatography validations. *ACS Symposium Series* 621: 150–166.

Lee, H.J., M.H. Lee, and P.D. Ruy. 2001. Public health risks: Chemical and antibiotic residues—review. *Asian-Aust. J. Anim. Sci.* 14: 402–413.

Lee, S.R., C.R. Mourer, and T. Shibamoto. 1991. *J. Agric. Food Chem.* 39(5): 906–908.

Lentza-Rizos, C., and A. Balokas. 2001. Residue levels of chlorpropham in individual tubers and composite samples of postharvest-treated potatoes. *J. Agric. Food Chem.* 49(2): 710–714.

Mahdy, F. 2002. Effects of cooking on ^{14}C-carbaryl residues in faba beans. *Bull. NRC, Egypt* 27(2): 165–173.

Mahdy, F. 2003. Bioavailability to rat and toxicity of bound pirimiphos methyl residues in stored soybeans. *Bull. NRC, Egypt.* 28: 403–413.

Mahdy, F., and S. El-Maghraby. 2010. Effect of processing on ^{14}C-chlorfenvinphos residues in maize oil and bioavailability of its cake residues on rats. *Bull. Environ. Contam. Toxicol.* 84: 582–586.

Mahdy, F., and S.M. Soliman. 2005. Mineralization of ^{14}C-carbofuran in soil under aerobic and anaerobic conditions. *Bull. NRC, Egypt.* 30: 265–277.

Mahdy, F., and H. Taha. 2005. Bound residues of ^{14}C-carbofuran and ^{14}C-malathion in stored soybeans seeds and their toxicological effects on mice. *Isotope Rad. Res.* 37: 383–393.

Mahdy, F., and H. Taha. 2007. Toxicity of bound ^{14}C-dichlorovos residues in stored soybean and their bioavailability in rats. *Bull. NRC, Egypt.* 32: 125–137.

Mathew, R., S. Kacew, and S.U. Khan. 1998. Bioavailability in rats of bound pesticide residues from tolerant or susceptible varieties of soybean and canola treated with metribuzin or atrazine. *Chemosphere* 36: 589–596.

Matthews, W.A. 1992. The biological activity of bound residues of ^{14}C-chlorpyrifos-methyl and ^{14}C-malathion on treated wheat in a stored product insect. *J. Environ. Sci. Health B* 27: 419–426.

Menon, P., and M. Gopal. 2003. Dissipation of ^{14}C carbaryl and quinalphos in soil under a groundnut crop (Arachis hypogaea L.) in semi-arid India. *Chemosphere* 53: 1023–1031.

Menon, P., M. Gopal, and R. Prasad. 2004. Dissipation of chlorpyrifos in two soil environments of semi-arid India. *J. Environ. Sci. Health B* 39: 517–531.

Neskovic, N.K., V. Karan, M. Budimir, V. Vojinovic, S. Gasic, and S.J. Vitorocic. 1992. Bioavailability and biological activity of wheat-bound chlorpyrifos-methyl residues in rats. *J. Environ. Sci. Health B* 27: 387–397.

Neskovic, N.K., V. Karan, S. Vitorocic, V. Vojinovic, and M. Budimin. 1989. *Second FAO/IAEA coordination meeting on biological activity and bioavailability of bound pesticide residues using nuclear techniques*, Vienna, Austria.

Neskovic, N.K., V.Z. Karan, V. Sabovijevic, and S. Vitorovic. 1989. Toxic effects of pirimiphos-methyl residues on rats. *J. Biomed. Environ. Sci.* 2: 115–130.

Nisha A. R. 2008. Antibiotic residues—A global health hazard. *Vet. World* 1(12): 375–377.

Northcott, G.L., and K.C. Jones. 2000. Experimental approaches and analytical techniques for determining organic compound bound residues in soil and sediment. *Environ. Pollut.* 108: 19–43.

Ong, K.C., J.N. Cash, M.J. Zabik, M. Saddiq, and A.L. Jones. 1996. Chlorine and ozone washes for pesticide removal from apples and processed apple sauce. *Food Chem.* 55(2): 153–160.

Paige, J.C. 1994. Analysis of tissue residues. *FDA Vet.* 9: 4–6.

Pillmoor, J.B., and T.R. Roberts. 1985. Approaches to the study of nonextractable (bound) pesticide residues in plants. In: D.H. Hutson and T.R Roberts (eds) *Progress in Pesticide Biochemistry and Toxicology*, vol 4. Chichester: Wiley, pp. 85–101.

Printz, H., P. Burauel, and F. Fuhr. 1995. Effect of organic amendment on degradation and formation of bound residues of methabenzthiazuron in soil under constant climatic conditions. *J. Environ. Sci. Health B* 30: 435–456.

Radwan, M.A., M.M. Abu-Elamayem, M.H. Shiboob, and A. Abdel-Aal. 2005. Residual behaviour of profenofos on some field-grown vegetables and its removal using various washing solutions and household processing. *Food Chem. Toxicol.* 43: 553–557.

Rajagopal, B.S., G.P. Barhmaprakash, B.R. Reddy, U.D. Singh, N. Sethunathan, F.A. Gunther, and J.D. Gunther. 1984. *Residue Rev.* 93: 87–203.

Rawn, D.F.K., S.C. Quade, W. Sun, A. Fouguet, A. Belanger, and M. Smith. 2008. Captan residue reduction in apples as a result of rinsing and peeling. *Food Chem.* 109: 790–796.

Riederer, M., and J. Schoenherr. 1986. Covalent binding of chlorophenoxyacetic acids to plant cuticles. *Arch. Environ. Contam. Toxicol.* 15: 97–105.

Roberts, T.R. 1984. Non-extractable pesticide residues in soils and plants. *Pure Appl. Chem.* 56: 945–956.

Ruediger, G. A., K.H. Pardon, A.N. Sas, P.W. Godden, and A. P. Pollnitz. 2005. Fate of pesticides during the winemaking process in relation to malolactic fermentation. *J. Agric. Food Chem.* 53: 3023–3026.

Sandermann, H., N. Hertkorn, R.G. May, and B.M. Lange. 2001. Bound pesticide residues in crop plants: chemistry, bioavailability, and toxicology. In: J. Hall, R.E. Hoagland, and R.M. Zablotowicz (eds) *Pesticide Biotransformation in Plants and Microorganisms: Similarities and Divergences*, ACS Symposium Series No 777. Washington, DC: American Chemical Society, pp. 119–128.

Saxena, A., and R. Bartha. 1983. Microbial mineralization of humic acid-3,4-dichloroaniline complexes. *Soil Biol. Biochem.* 15: 59–62.

Schmidt, B. 1999. Non-extractable residues of pesticides and xenobiotics in plants: A review. *Recent Res. Agric. Food Chem.* 3: 329–354.

Skidmore, M.W., G.D. Paulson, H.A. Kuiper, B. Ohlin, and S. Reynolds. 1998. IUPAC reports on pesticides (40), Bound xenobiotic residues in food commodities of plant and animal origin. *Pure Appl. Chem.* 70: 1423–1447.

Still, G.G., H.M.. Balba, and E.R. Mansager. 1981. Studies on the nature and identity of bound chloroaniline residues in plants. *J Agric. Food Chem.* 29: 739–746.

Street, J.C. 1969. Methods of removal of pesticide residues. *CMAJ* 100: 154–160.

Takimoto, Y., M. Ohshima, and J. Miyamoto. 1978. Degradation and fate of fenitrothion applied to harvested rice grains. *J. Pestic. Sci.* 3: 277–290.

Ticha, J., J. Hajslova, M. Jech, J. Honzicek, O. Lacina, J. Kohoutkova, V. Kocourek, M. Lansky, J. Kloutvorova, and V. Falta. 2008. Changes of pesticide residues in apples during cold storage. *Food Cont.* 19: 247–256.

Trenck, K.T., D. Hunkler, and H. Sandermann. 1981. Incorporation of chlorinated. Anilines into lignin. *Z. Naturforsch.* 36c: 714–720.

Yee, D., P. Weinberger, and S.U. Khan. 1985. Release of soil-bound prometryne residues under different soil pH and nitrogen fertilizer regimes. *Weed Sci.* 33: 882–887.

Zayed, S.M.A.D., M. Farghaly, and F. Mahdy. 1998. Effect of commercial processing procedures on carbofuran residues in soybean oil. *Food Chem.* 62: 265–268.

Zayed, S.M.A.D., M. Farghaly, and F. Mahdy. 2003. Efficiency of the refining processes in removing ^{14}C-pirimiphos-methyl residues in soybean oil. *Bull NRC Egypt* 28: 567–575.

Zayed, S.M.A.D., M. Farghaly, and H. Taha. 2002. Mineralization of ^{14}C-ring labelled 2,4-D in Egyptian soils under aerobic and anaerobic conditions. *Biomed. Environ. Sci.* 15: 306–314.

Zayed, S.M.A.D., M. Farghaly, and I.Y. Mostafa. 1992. Bioavailability to rats and toxicological potential in mice of bound residues of malathion in beans. *J. Environ. Sci. Health B* 27: 341–346.

Zayed, S.M.A.D., M. Farghaly, F. Mahdy, and S.M. Soliman. 2008. *J. of Environ. Sci. and Health Part B* 43: 595–604.

Zayed, S.M.A.D., M. Farghaly, and S. El-Maghraby. 2006. Mineralization of ^{14}C-Pirimiphos-methyl in soil under aerobic and anaerobic conditions. *Arab. J. Nucl. Sci. Appl.* 39: 233–241.

Zayed, S.M.A.D., S.M. Amer, M.F. Nawito, M. Farghaly, H.A. Amer, M.A. Fahmy, and F. Mahdy. 1993. Toxicological potential of malathion residues in stored soybean seeds. *J. Environ. Sci. Health B* 28: 711–729.

9 Toxic Microelements in Food

Mikołaj Protasowicki

CONTENTS

9.1 INTRODUCTION

Foods of animal and plant origin contain many chemical elements, which combine to form the building materials of proteins, lipids, carbohydrates, vitamins, and other complex compounds. Among these elements, carbon, hydrogen, nitrogen, and oxygen form the largest group. In addition to these, tissues of organisms contain many elements that, depending on their amount, are termed either macro- or microelements (the latter are also known as trace elements [C, N, H, O]).

Macroelements, as well as basic elements, are essential for plant and animal organisms. They are the building materials that support tissue, teeth, skin, and hair play an important role in water-electrolyte management and pH regulation, and are parts of many active compounds vital for metabolic processes.

Microelements are important because for two aspects:

- Some microelements are essential for the normal functions of organisms. They participate in numerous important life processes, for example, enzymatic reactions (Zn, Co, Ni, Mn, Fe, Cr, Al), glycolysis (Mn, Zn), nucleotide synthesis (Mg, Fe), erythropoiesis (Fe, Cu), organic acid transformation (Fe, Zn, Ni, Mn), nitrogen exchange (Fe, Mo, Cu, Mn, V, Co), and photosynthesis (Fe, Ti, Mg, Mn), and their lack or excess may be a cause of many serious diseases.
- Trace elements, which are not considered essential, may cause severe poisonings if administered in amounts equal to or higher than the minimal dose.

Determination of the role of microelements and the human daily requirements can be very difficult due to their low concentrations in the human body and problems connected with the elimination of their constant inflow. Throughout the evolution process, the human organism developed mechanisms to regulate the absorption of microelements and balance their levels within required ranges. Therefore, human bodies are adjusted to the natural levels at which those elements are present in the nonpolluted environment and noncontaminated foodstuffs. However, human industrial and economic activities are frequently and widely disturbing the environmental balance and leading to contamination of the environment, including foods, with trace elements.

The content of trace elements in foods depends on their concentration in raw materials and additives used in food production. In addition, trace elements may be transmitted to food from the equipment used during food processing and from the packaging material during storage.

Trace elements include heavy metals, some of which have recently received particular attention. Many definitions of "heavy metals" have been put forward. The simplest and most precise describes heavy metals as all metal compounds of atomic weight over 20. Other definitions are based on the specific weight, and give the lower limits for heavy metals as 4.5, 5, or even 6 g per cm^3. Due to toxicity of some heavy metals and the possibility of environmental contamination, the potential for high risk is linked to Hg, Cd, Pb, As, as well as Cu, Zn, Sn, Cr, and Ni. All mineral elements are present in the environment (and also in plant and animal organisms, and in water and food) as salts or as metal-organic compounds, and only in such forms are they biologically active.

To limit the possibilities of food poisonings in humans caused by ingestion of excessive amounts of microelements via food and water, maximum levels (MLs) for trace elements are recommended. The Joint Food and Agriculture Organization/World Health Organization (FAO/WHO) Expert Committee on Food Additives makes global recommendations for general norms, and publishes values of provisional tolerable weekly intake (PTWI) for particular toxic metals based on the results of actualized study results.

9.2 MERCURY

Mercury has been known since ancient times. As early as in 7 BC, Assyrian medics applied it to cure skin diseases. Mercury compounds were also used by Arabs in 6 BC for therapeutic reasons. Mercury was mentioned by Aristotle and Hippocrates (4 BC), who described cinnabar (HgS) as a dye. Mercury and its compounds have also been used in appropriate ways much more recently. The application of cinnabar to color rinds of cheese in England in the nineteenth century serves as an example, while the first agricultural application of mercury compounds (seeds treated with phenylmercury) took place in Germany in 1914 (Krenkel 1973).

Toxic properties of some mercury compounds have been known for a long time. There are theories that mercury compounds were used to poison Ivan the Terrible, Napoleon Bonaparte, and Charles II of England. Improper handling and treatment of samples during the synthesis of organic mercury compounds was the cause of lethal poisonings of chemists in the nineteenth and twentieth centuries.

The first outbreak of food poisoning caused by mercury compounds was reported in 1953 in Japan. The outbreak was caused by the ingestion of fish containing significant amounts of methylmercury. As the outbreak affected the population living at the Minamata Bay, the disease was named Minamata disease, the name now frequently used as a general name for any foodborne form of mercury poisoning. Other outbreaks of Minamata disease, also of fish origin, have been reported in Japan (Kurland et al. 1960; Harada 1995). However, the most tragic outbreaks happened in Iraq, from 1955 to 1960, and later from 1971 to 1972. A total number of about 8000 people became sick after ingestion of bread prepared from grain treated with methylmercury. Similar cases were reported in Guatemala, Pakistan, and Ghana (Al-Tikriti and Al-Mufti 1976). A surprising case of mercury poisoning occurred in the Aland Islands, Finland. The patient affected was a female who had consumed merganser eggs that contained significant amounts of methylmercury.

Most cases of mercury poisoning led to handicap, chronic disease, or death. The most frequent symptoms include numbness of limbs, lips and tongue, speech abnormalities, limb function disorders, visual acuity disorders, deafness, and muscular atrophy. Insomnia, hyperactivity, and coma have also been reported. Methylmercury penetrates the blood–brain barrier and causes central nervous system injuries. Mercury also has a teratogenic effect, leading to congenital abnormalities or congenital Minamata disease.

Mercury has been always present in the environment, and as a result, mercury is naturally found in living organisms, where it can occur in methylmercury form. In the case of aquatic organisms, methylmercury may comprise up to 100% of total mercury content. The range of natural mercury content that is observed in food of animal and plant origin from nonpolluted environments has been measured as from <0.001 to about 0.05 μg/g. Fish are the exception, where the amount of mercury in muscles, even in noncontaminated environments, may reach up to 0.2 μg/g.

Despite the significant decrease during past decades of the anthropogenic emission of mercury into the environment (due to the restrictions or prohibition of its application), there is still a need for control of mercury levels in food. This is because of the significant toxicity of its compounds and their high mobility in the environment. Therefore, in European countries the highest admissible level of mercury in fish muscle, fish products, and crustaceas is 0.5 μg/g, exception 1.0 μg/g for some predators fish (EC 2006, 2011).

The Joint FAO/WHO Expert Committee determined that PTWI for mercury via all possible physiological routes should not exceed 4 μg per kg body weight, and only 1.6 μg per kg body weight may be in the form of a methyl derivative (JECFA 2011).

9.3 CADMIUM

Cadmium was isolated for the first time in 1817 by Strohmeyer. In nature, cadmium is usually present in the form of sulfides accompanying zinc and copper ores. The application of cadmium in various branches of industry started at the beginning of the twentieth century. It was widely used in metallurgy (as a component of alloys and to coat surfaces of other metals), and electrotechnics, and in production of pigments, plastics (as a stabilizer), gum, and pesticides. Now the use of cadmium and its compounds have been restricted, and their use in the production of pesticides is totally prohibited. This industrial use leads to food contamination via the ecosystem contamination. Other sources of cadmium contamination include the burning of coal, oil, and waste. Significant amounts of cadmium are also found in some mineral fertilizers, as well as in industrial and municipal waste used as manure (McLaughlin et al. 1996).

The toxicity of cadmium compounds has been known since the first publication by Marmé in 1867. Although acute cadmium poisonings are usually rare, chronic diseases caused by a long-term exposure occur quite frequently. Symptoms include nausea, vomiting, stomachache, headache, and lowered body temperature. Poisoning leads to acute gastroenteritis, as well as renal, liver, testicle, and prostate disorders. Anemia, hypertension, cardiovascular changes, pregnancy complications, and bone decalcification are reported. Cadmium is also suspected to be a factor increasing the frequency of prostate cancer, although its carcinogenic effect has not been confirmed. In tests on animals poisoned with cadmium during pregnancy, congenital defects in fetuses were observed.

Toxicity of cadmium increases in case of zinc deficiency, due to the zinc substitution in biological systems, which leads to functional disorders. Cadmium reduces assimilation of vitamins C and D. However, a large amount of those vitamins in diet will decrease the toxicity of cadmium through the reduction of its absorption from the intestinal tract (McLaughlin et al. 1999).

Many cases of foodborne cadmium poisonings were reported in the 1940s in England, France, New Zealand, the United States, the USSR, and other countries. They were caused by consumption of lemonade, coffee, wine, and other products that have been prepared or stored in cadmium-coated containers, or in refrigerators with cadmium-coated freezers.

The Japanese disease "itai-itai" (ouch-ouch) is a particular syndrome caused by chronic cadmium poisoning. It leads to fractures of long bones due to decalcification, and to muscular dystrophy. The first time the disease was reported after World War II, within a population in the lower basin of the Jintzu River, Japan. It was caused by consumption of rice that contained cadmium at a level of 0.6–1.1 μg/g. Undoubtedly, other plants that are cultivated in environments highly contaminated with cadmium may also be the cause of poisonings, as would foods of animal origin.

Cadmium poisonings are particularly dangerous as the daily excretion of assimilated cadmium is minimal (0.5% of total intake). The biological half-life of cadmium is very long, about 33 years. Cadmium is therefore accumulated in humans throughout their whole lifetimes. Although only 5–10% of cadmium is absorbed from the gastrointestinal tracts of adults, a daily dose of 66–132 μg is sufficient to result in a critical value of 6 μg/g in the kidneys at the age of 50. These factors cause the high level of concern regarding the risks for human health posed by cadmium—cadmium is considered more dangerous than mercury and lead.

The amounts of cadmium found in food from noncontaminated areas do not exceed 0.05 μg/g of products. Exceptions are the livers and, especially, kidneys of slaughtered animals, which may contain even up to a few microgram per gram.

European legislation sets limits for the maximum amount of cadmium in food, depending on the kind of food products, within a range from 0.005 to 3.0 μg/g. Extremely high contents of cadmium are allowed only in fungi, kidneys, mollusks, and cephalopods (1 μg/g), and food supplements of dried seaweed or molluscs or derived from seaweed (3 μg/g) (EC 2011, 2014). The European Food Safety Authority suggests that PTWI for cadmium should not exceed 2.5 μg per kg of body weight (EFSA 2009).

9.4 LEAD

Lead was known and mined in the ancient times, and its ease to use promoted its wide application. Lead was used for water-supply systems first, in the ancient Greece, and later in the Roman Empire. Wealthy Romans used lead wine cups, kitchen utensils, decorations, and other paraphernalia, and it is suggested that this might have led to chronic poisoning (Gilfillan 1965). Although toxic properties of lead had already been known in ancient Greece, Egypt, and Rome, where lead poisoning was known as "saturnism," the metal was not identified as a toxic component of food until the eleventh century (Mahaffey 1990). Despite this knowledge, in England in the nineteenth century, candies were colored with lead chromate and white lead, and the use of lead for water pipes has survived up to the present time. Tea was also regenerated using lead chromate, and minium (Pb_3O_4) was applied to cheese to make the rind red.

At present, lead is used for production of accumulators, crystal glass, and hunting ammunition (with arsenic). It is also applied in chemical, rubber, textile, and ceramic industries and in many other branches of human economic activity (McLaughlin et al. 1996).

To date there is no proof for the inevitability of lead for plant and animal organisms (including humans), whereas toxic activity is widely known. More reported poisonings involved lead than other elements (Philip and Gearson 1994a,b). As early as in 1774, Lind noted that lemon juice stored in lead-enameled containers may cause poisoning. A special royal commission was appointed to study the problem 4 years later.

Food contamination may result from transmission of lead from glaze, enamel, or tinning on kitchen dishes, or from the lead on surfaces of containers or pipes used for storage, processing, and transportation of food products. The occurrence of lead in food can also result from environmental contamination, as plants and animals may assimilate lead during growth and incorporate it into their tissues. The level of lead found in plant tissues is proportional to its concentration in the environment, and in cases of animals, the feed and water supplies also play important roles (Sedki et al. 2003).

Symptoms of lead poisoning occur after a daily dose of 2–4 mg is ingested for a period of a few months, while daily doses of 8–10 mg will cause poisoning after only 3–4 weeks.

At the onset of poisoning, symptoms include chronic headaches, hyperactivity, muscle tremor, lead colic, and lead line (1–2 mm) on gums. Hyperactivity and intelligence-quotient decrease are observed in cases of chronic poisoning in children. Lead poisonings result in anemia due to hemoglobin synthesis disorders.

Neurological, encephalopathic, enzymatic, and mutagenic changes, as well as liver, kidney, spinal medulla, and brain damage, are also observed. Lead may be transmitted from the blood of pregnant women to their fetuses, which may result in congenital defects (teratogenic effect). Lead compounds may also exert carcinogenic effects (Silbergeld 2003).

All food products contain some lead. They usually do not exceed the level of 0.1–0.2 μg/g, although venison may contain up to several microgram per gram due to its contamination via ammunition.

In order to lower lead intake, the highest allowed concentrations have been established for various food products, within a range from 0.020 μg/g (milk) to 1.5 μg/g (mussels). For most products, the values are set between 0.1 and 0.3 μg/g (EC 2006, 2011).

The Joint FAO/WHO Expert Committee calculated that lead PTWI should not exceed 25 μg per kg of body weight (JECFA 2011). It is particularly important that infants and children should be protected against the possibility of lead uptake.

9.5 ARSENIC

Arsenic is a metalloid, yet it is still classified as a heavy metal. Arsenic compounds have also been known since ancient times, but were described for the first time by Albert the Great in the thirteenth century (Sullivan 1969). Auripigment and realgar were used as yellow paints, and arsenic was one of the most widely known and widely used poisons.

Pure arsenic is presently used as a component of alloys (e.g., with lead to produce hunting ammunition). Arsenic compounds are also used in the chemical, pharmaceutical, and tanning industries, in the manufacture of glass and ceramic (Nriagu and Azcue 1990). They were also used in agriculture and fruit farming (pesticides), but currently arsenic compounds are not used as pesticides.

The toxicity of arsenic action depends on types of bonds present: nonorganic compounds are significantly more toxic than organic ones, whereas As^{+3} salts are more toxic than As^{+5} salts. Small amounts of arsenic exert a stimulating effect on human and animal organisms. Antagonistic properties of this element against selenium and iodine have been also revealed. Hypersensitivity to arsenic, or arsenicphagia, which is typical of miners and consumers of sea fish (who get used to the presence of arsenic), has been described.

Excessive amounts of arsenic can cause skin, lung, and heart diseases, and gastrointestinal disorders, and it is known to have carcinogenic influence. As^{+3} compounds, which are bound by erythrocytes, affect the activity of numerous enzymes—especially those involved in respiratory processes (Cebrian et al. 1983; JECFA 2011).

Over 80% of the total arsenic content of aquatic organisms is present as organic compounds. During digestion of such organic arsenic compounds, arsenic is not released or is only released gradually. This explains why no cases of arsenic poisonings have been reported among seafood consumers despite the high levels observed in seafood (Lawrence et al. 1986).

The levels of arsenic in food do not generally exceed 0.1 μg/g, although higher amounts (even up to several microgram per gram) have been found in kidneys and livers of slaughter animals and in fish. According to a decision of the EU Commission published as the annex to Regulation (EC) No 1881/2006, the maximum permissible levels of arsenic in rice products (only) are within the range of 0.10–0.30 μg/g (EC 2015). There are no MLs for other foodstuffs. However, the Joint FAO/WHO Expert Committee suggests that PTWI for arsenic of 15 μg per kg of body weight is not appropriate and should be changed (JECFA 2011).

9.6 COPPER

Copper is inseparably linked to the history of human civilization. According to suggested standards, the daily physiological demand of copper is from 1.5 to 2.7 mg per person (Ziemlański 2001). The basic physiological importance of copper is connected with erythropoetic processes and tissue respiration. Copper is essential for catalysis of processes of food-originated iron binding into organic bonds. It stimulates maturation of reticulocytes and their transformation into erythrocytes, and is a constituent of oxidation enzymes, such as polyphenoloxidase, lactase, tyrosinase, ascorbinase, and cytochrome C oxidase. Copper acts similarly to insulin—diabetics administered copper salts from 0.5 to 1 μg daily demonstrated clear evidence of improvement.

Copper exerts an effect on the activity of excretory glands, increases the phagocytic properties of leukocytes, therefore promoting human immunity, and also boosts antibiotic activity.

Animal tests have proven that copper is essential for the growth of organisms. If insufficient doses of copper are administered with food, the inhibition of growth is observed.

Large amounts of copper are found in liver, larger amounts in young individuals than in old. In case of copper deficiency, anemia, hair discoloration, and other pathological symptoms have been observed. Increased levels of copper, which result from defense mechanism actions of the immune system, have been reported in infectious and cancer diseases (Sarkar 1995).

Despite the positive effects of optimal levels of copper, deleterious effects may occur if a threshold level is exceeded. Wilson's disease (hepatolenticularic degeneration) is one of the diseases linked to the excess of copper in body. It results from a dysfunction of the copper transmission process, which occurs due to a lack of suitable enzyme to catalyze the process of copper deletion from detached bonds with albumins and binding to ceruloplasma. The condition leads to neuron degradation, liver cirrhosis, and occurrence of colorful rings on the cornea (DiDonato and Sarkar 1997).

Foodborne poisonings due to copper and its compounds can be caused by the improper use of copper dishes (Müller et al. 1998). They may also be caused by breaches of carency period after the application of copper-based pesticides.

Copper is usually present in food at levels of 1–2 μg/g; higher levels are found in animal livers. The highest levels of copper are present in shellfish, because copper is a component of their blood pigment, hemocyanin.

A copper complex of chlorophyll in amounts not higher than 1 μg/g of product is used for coloring preserved vegetables. Nonorganic copper compounds were used in the past for food coloration; in the nineteenth century in England, copper salts were used to color food products and condiments.

Symptoms of copper poisoning include metallic taste, salivation, stomachaches, blue vomiting, diarrhea, reduced blood tension, and tachycardia. Acute cases may also include symptoms of paralysis of the central nervous system, cardiovascular failure, hepatitis, anemia, and uremia.

The Joint FAO/WHO Expert Committee recommends that PTWI should not exceed 3.5 mg per kg of body weight (WHO 1982).

9.7 ZINC

Alloys of zinc were used for brass production as early as in the ancient times. Trials of zinc production were conducted in Europe in the sixth century; however, it had been produced earlier in China and India. Zinc is widely applied, that is, in metallurgy, electrotechnics, printing, rubber production, production of articles of daily use, paints, drugs, disinfectants, and impregnates, as well as microfertilizers and pesticides.

Zinc is a microelement essential for a proper functioning of the human body. The level of daily demand for zinc was established as 13–16 mg (Ziemlański 2001). Zinc plays a role in protein and carbohydrate metabolism and is a component of over 60 metaloenzymes, including alkaline phosphatase, pancreatic carboxypeptidases A and B, alcoholic and lactic dehydrogenases, carbonate anhydrase, and proteases. It also forms bonds with nucleic acids—which is very important for their function (Prasad 1983).

Human food, both plant and animal, usually contains satisfactory amounts of zinc to cover the requirement for this metal, which is present within the range of a few to several microgram per gram of product. Zinc deficiencies are usually caused by a reduction of its absorption in the gastrointestinal tract rather than by its lack. Reduction in absorption may be caused by antagonistic activity of cadmium, calcium, or phytates. A decrease in assimilation of zinc is also observed among alcoholics.

Zinc deficiency causes growth inhibition, depigmentation of dark hair, balding, corneous and thick epithelium, and skin desquamation. Acute deficiencies of zinc lead to testicular atrophy and to sterility (Shils et al. 1994).

An excess of zinc will cause problems in humans. Excessive doses can lead to biochemical control system damage, while doses slightly higher than optimal can cause disorders in iron and copper metabolism, resulting in incurable anemia, decrease in activity of zinc protein enzymes, and pancreas and kidney damage (Boularbah et al. 1999). Increased levels of zinc have been observed in nuclei of neoplastic cells and in cases of acute dental caries; however, its role in these diseases has not been explained.

Zinc poisonings may occur after consumption of products stored in zinc-coated containers. For instance, a dish of curried poultry, which was a source of zinc poisoning, was found to contain 1 mg/g. Poisoning may be also caused if the carency period after application of zinc pesticides is not observed.

Symptoms of acute zinc poisoning include acute gastroenteritis, vomiting, diarrhea, dizziness, and heaviness in chest.

The Joint FAO/WHO Expert Committee recommends PTWI should not exceed 7 mg per kg of body weight (WHO 1982).

9.8 TIN

Tin, similar to copper, had been already known in the Bronze Age, and it is still widely used today. Tin compounds were used in production of plastics, antifouling paints, pesticides, wood impregnates, and antiparasitic drugs for animals (Ebdon et al. 1998). Now tin compounds are not used in production of pesticides and antifouling paints. In some countries, inorganic tin compounds ($SnCl_2$) are added to vegetable preserves packed in glass jars to preserve the natural colors of vegetables. Tin-coated metal cans, used for packing foods, may lead to food contamination. Tin compounds may be leached from the tin coating if the food has a low pH.

If ingested, inorganic salts are poorly assimilated and are almost completely excreted from the human body via stools and so their toxicity is low. Organic compounds display higher toxicity, and alkyl derivatives, for example, tributyltin (TBT), are particularly dangerous. The toxicity therefore depends on the type of tin compound (Forsyth et al. 1994). After the consumption of large quantities of tin, enzymatic and ingestion processes are distorted. A long-term exposure to organic tin derivatives leads to sexual gland atrophy and to changes in the nervous system (Ghaffari and Motlagh 2011).

It is estimated that the average daily tin uptake per adult is approximately 4 mg; however, tin is not accumulated in the body. So far, the role of tin in the human body has not been completely understood, although some data lead to the conclusion that it is involved in oxidation-reduction processes. Some authors suggest that the lack of tin in the fodder of test animals causes reduced growth and tooth depigmentation (Schwartz et al. 1970).

At present standards limit the content of tin only in canned food products, and in fruit and vegetable juices, and other canned dietary foods for special medical purposes intended specifically for infants (EC 2006). The content of tin in products intended for children up to the age of 3 must not exceed 50 μg/g, and for other products it must not exceed 100 μg/g (canned beverages, including fruit juices and vegetable juices) or 200 μg/g (for food other than beverages). The Joint FAO/WHO Expert Committee established the PTWI value for tin as 14 mg per kg of body weight (JECFA 2006).

9.9 THE INFLUENCE OF TECHNOLOGICAL PROCESSES ON THE CHANGES OF MICROELEMENTS IN FOOD PRODUCTS

Although the levels of toxic microelements in raw materials and processed foods are widely examined, studies on the effects of technological treatment on the levels of these elements have so far focused much less attention.

Meat of slaughter animals and fish are usually processed in various ways before consumption. Most often, heat treatments are applied, such as cooking, roasting, frying, and grilling. Fish processing may also include salting and marination, and in the production of canned fish, also adding vinegar and steaming, while in the production of fish meals and concentrates, also drying. Studies on the effects of these processes on mercury levels in final fish products were undertaken in the 1970s. The studies revealed that none of the processes reduced considerably mercury content in fish products compared to its content in raw fish, and during drying, mercury content increased relatively in proportion to water loss (Protasowicki 1980). Some other studies on the procedures used in fish processing showed that occasionally only small reduction or increase in the levels of Cd, Pb, Cu, and Zn occurred, but the changes were always below 20% (Protasowicki 1987). Similarly, cooking of beef (steak, neck, brisket, loin, and rump) with and without salt addition also contributed to minimal changes in the levels of toxic microelements (Lidwin-Kaźmierkiewicz et al. 2006).

Processes such as blanching, freezing, and cooking of vegetables and fruits were reported to noticeably reduce the content of Cd, Pb, and Zn (Fik and Surówka 1994). Abou-Arab and Abou Donia (2000) revealed that considerable amounts of metals pass to the water extract during boiling of medicinal plants, and that boiling leads to the extraction of higher amounts of metals than immersing the plants in the hot water. Equally large losses of Cd and Pb were observed in mussels, when mussel cellular structure was destroyed by heating (Bastías at al. 2015).

The effect of heat treatment on the levels of arsenic, cadmium, lead, and mercury in various foodstuffs was studied by, for example, Perelló et al. (2008). Heat treatment (frying, grilling, roasting, and cooking) of fish, beef, pork, lamb, poultry, string bean, potato, rice, and olive oil had just a minimal reducing effect on the levels of the studied toxic microelements. Water evaporation during heat treatment was often reported to increase meal levels (Kalogeropoulos et al. 2012; Czerwonka and Szterk 2015). Recent studies on fish frying, grilling, and cooking have revealed that these processes effectively reduce mercury levels in fish products (Mieiro et al. 2016).

9.10 CONCLUSIONS

Studies on the content of heavy metals in food are conducted in the majority of countries worldwide. Toxic heavy metals attract particular attention. Studies carried out on a range of foods and on daily food intakes have revealed that the amounts of heavy metals found in foods in Poland are within acceptable limits and do not exceed values observed in other European countries. The present daily uptake of heavy metals has decreased when compared with the values reported in the 1980s.

Alarmingly, higher uptake of lead and cadmium (when compared to PTWI) has been observed in children, especially in industrial areas, and in people who require high food intakes (e.g., manual workers). The PTWI for cadmium and lead may also be exceeded due to consumption of foods containing the highest concentration of these toxic metals.

In conclusion, heat processing of animal raw materials, unless cell structures are damaged, does not considerably affect the levels of toxic metals, and is mainly associated with water losses. While in the case of plant raw materials, cooking contributes to passing of large amounts of these elements into the aqueous phase.

REFERENCES

Abou-Arab, A.A.K., and M.A. Abou Donia. 2000. Heavy metals in Egyptian spices and medicinal plants and the effect of processing on their levels. *J. Agric. Food Chem.* 48: 2300–2304.

Al-Tikriti, K., and A.W. Al-Mufti. 1976. An outbreak of organomercury poisoning among Iraqi farmers, *Bull. WHO* 53: 15–21.

Bastías, J.M., J. Moreno, C. Pia, J. Reyes, R. Quevedo, and O. Muñoz. 2015. Effect of ohmic heating on texture, microbial load, and cadmium and lead content of Chilean blue mussel (*Mytilus chilensis*). *Innov. Food Sci. Emerg. Technol.* 30: 98–102.

Boularbah, A., G. Bitton, and J.L. Morel. 1999. Assessment of metal and toxicity of leachates from teapots. *Sci. Total Environ.* 227: 69–72.

Cebrian, M.E., A. Albores, M. Aguilar, and E. Blakeley 1983. Chronic arsenic poisoning in the North Mexico. *Human Toxicol.* 23: 121–133.

Czerwonka, M., and A. Szterk. 2015. The effect of meat cuts and thermal processing on selected mineral concentration in beef from Holstein-Friesien bulls. *Meat Sci.* 105: 75–80.

DiDonato, M., and B. Sakar 1997. Review. Copper transport and its alterations in Menkes and Wilson diseases. *Biochim. Biophys. Acta* 1360: 3–16.

Ebdon, L., S.J. Hill, and C. Rivas. 1998. Organotin compounds in solid waste: a review of their properties and determination using high-performance liquid chromatography. *Trends Anal. Chem.* 17(5): 278–288.

European Commission. 2006. Commission Regulation No 1881/2006 of 19 December 2006 setting maximum levels for certain contaminants in foodstuffs. *Off. J. Eur. Union L.* 364: 5–24.

European Commission. 2011. Commission Regulation No 420/2011 of 29 April 2011 amending Regulation (EC) No 1881/2006 setting maximum levels for certain contaminants in foodstuffs. *Off. J. Eur. Union L.* 111: 3–6.

European Commission. 2014. Commission Regulation No 488/2014 of 12 May 2014 amending Regulation (EC) No 1881/2006 as regards maximum levels of cadmium in foodstuffs. *Off. J. Eur. Union L.* 138: 75–78.

European Commission. 2015. Commission Regulation 2015/1006 of 25 June 2015 amending Regulation (EC) No 1881/2006 as regards maximum levels of inorganic arsenic in foodstuffs. *Off. J. Eur. Union L.* 161: 14.

EFSA. 2009. Cadmium in food. Scientific Opinion of the Panel on Contaminants in the Food Chain. *EFSA J.* 980: 1–139.

Fik, M., and J. Surówka. 1994. Effect of technological processes on the content of Cd, Pb and Cu in selected vegetables and their concentration in some frozen fruit-vegetable products. *Zeszyty Naukowe Akademii Rolniczej w Krakowie. Technologia Żywności* 6: 53–65. [in Polish].

Forsyth, D.S., W.F. Sun, and K. Dalglish. 1994. Survey organotin compounds in blended wines. *Food Add. Contam.* 11: 343–350.

Ghaffari, M.A., and B. Motlagh. 2011. In vitro effect of lead, silver, tin, mercury, indium and bismuth on human sperm creatine kinase activity: a presumable mechanism for men infertility. *Iran. Biomed. J.* 15(1/2): 38–43.

Gilfillan, S.C. 1965. Lead poisoning and the fall of the Roman empire. *J. Occup. Med.* 7: 53–60.

Harada, M. 1995. Minamata disease: methylmercury poisoning in Japan caused by environmental pollution. *Crit. Rev. Toxicol.* 25: 1–24.

JECFA. 2006. Evaluation of certain food additives and contaminants, 64th Report of Joint FAO/WHO Expert Committee on Food Additives, *Technical report series 930*, Geneva.

JECFA. 2011. Evaluation of certain food additives and contaminants, 72nd Report of Joint FAO/WHO Expert Committee on Food Additives, *Technical report series 959*. Geneva.

Kalogeropoulos, N., S. Karavoltsos, A. Sakellari, and S. Avramidou. 2012. Heavy metals in raw, fried and grilled Mediterranean finfish and shelfish. *Food Chem. Toxicol.* 50: 3702–3708.

Krenkel, P.A. 1973. Mercury: environmental considerations. Part I. Statement of the problem. *CRC Crit. Rev. Environ. Contr.* 5: 303–373.

Kurland, L.T., S.N. Faro, and H. Seidler. 1960. Minamata disease. *World Neurol.* 1(5): 370–395.

Lawrence, J.F., P. Michalik, G. Tam, and H.B.S. Conacher. 1986. Identification of arsenobetain and arsenocholine in Canadian fish and shellfish by high-performance liquid chromatography with atomic absorption detection and confirmation by fast atom bombardment mass spectrometry. *J. Agric. Food Chem.* 34: 315–319.

Lidwin-Kaźmierkiewicz, M., M. Rajkowska, and M. Protasowicki. 2006. Effect of cooking beef on the content of Cd, Cu, Hg, Pb, Zn. *Roczniki Naukowe Polskiego Towarzystwa Zootechnicznego* 2 (1): 127–132 [in Polish].

Mahaffey, K.R. 1990. Environmental lead toxicity: nutrition as a component of intervention. *Environ. Health Perspect.* 89: 75–78.

McLaughlin, M.J, D.R. Parker, and J.M. Clarke. 1999. Metals and micronutrients—food safety issues. *Field Crops Res.* 60: 143–163.

McLaughlin, M.J., K.G. Tiler., R. Naidu, and D.P. Stevens. 1996. Review: the behavior and environmental impact of contaminants in fertilizers. *Aust. J. Soil. Res.* 34: 1–54.

Mieiro, C.I., J.P Coelho, M. Dolbeth, M. Pacheco, A.C. Duarte, and M.A. Pardal. 2016. Fish and mercury: influence of fish filet culinary practices on human risk. *Food Control* 60: 575–581.

Müller, T., W. Müller, and H. Feichtinger. 1998. Idiopathic copper toxicosis. *Am. J. Clin. Nutr., Suppl.* 67: 1082–1086.

Nriagu, J.O., and J.M. Azcue. 1990. *Arsenic in the Environment. Part 1: Cycling and Characterization*. John Wiley and Sons, New York.

Perelló, G., R. Martí-Cid, J.M. Llobet, and J.L. Domingo. 2008. Effects of various cooking processes on the concentrations of arsenic, cadmium, mercury, and lead in foods. *J. Agric. Food Chem.* 56(23): 11262–11269.

Philip, A., and B. Gearson. 1994a. Lead poisoning—part 1: incidence, etiology, and toxicokinetics. *Clin. Lab. Med.* 14: 423–439.

Philip, A., and B. Gearson. 1994b. Lead poisoning—part 2: effects and assay. *Clin. Lab. Med.* 14: 651–666.

Prasad, A.S. 1983. The role of zinc in gastrointestinal and liver disease. *Clin. Gastroenterol.* 12: 713–741.

Protasowicki, M. 1980. Effect of some technological operations on Hg content in fish flesh. Model studies. *Zesz. Nauk. AR Szczec.* 82: 163–181. [in Polish].

Protasowicki, M. 1987. Processing effect on the level of Cd, Pb, Cu and Zn in the meat herring, XVIII Sesja Nauk. Kom. Technol. i Chem. Żywn. PAN nt. Technologia Żywności—Operacje i Procesy Jednostkowe oraz Aspekty Chemiczne, Gdańsk 1987, 18 [in Polish].

Sarkar, B. 1995. Copper, in Seiber, H.G., et al., eds. *Handbook of Metals in Clinical and Analytical Chemistry*. Marcel Dekker, New York, 339–347.

Schwartz, K., D.B. Milne, and E. Vinyard. 1970. Growth effects of tin compounds in rats maintained in a trace element-controlled environment. *Biochem. Biophys. Res. Comm.* 40: 22–29.

Sedki, A., N. Lekouch, S. Gamon, and A. Pineau. 2003. Toxic and essential trace metals in muscle, liver and kidney of bovines from a polluted area of Morocco. *Sci. Total Environ.* 317: 201–205.

Shils, M.E., J.A. Olson, and M. Shike. 1994. *Modern Nutrition in Health and Disease*. Lea and Febiger, Malvern, PA.

Silbergeld, E.K. 2003. Review. Facilitative mechanisms of lead as a carcinogen. *Mutation Res.* 533: 121–133.

Sullivan, R.J. 1969. Preliminary air pollution survey of arsenic and its compounds. *National Air Pollution Control Administration Publication,* No. APTD 69-26, Raleigh.

WHO. 1982. Toxicological evaluation of certain food additives: copper, zinc. *WHO Food Additives Series*, No. 17.

Ziemlański, S. 2001. *Standards of Human Nutrition.* Wyd. Lek. PZWL, Warsaw, Poland [in Polish].

10 Cyanogenic Compounds and Estrogen Disruptors

Błażej Kudłak, Monika Wieczerzak, and Jacek Namieśnik

CONTENTS

10.1 ENDOCRINE DISRUPTORS AS XENOBIOTICS IN FOODS

To understand what endocrine disrupting chemicals (EDCs) are and how they act, one has to understand that hormonal or endocrine systems are a communication one. In multicellular organisms the communication between cells is essential to work in coordinated manner. These communication and integration of information are induced by chemical stimuli. The adjacent cells are connected by surface molecules and specialized junctions, while communication between cells that are remote is performed through the secretion of chemical messengers, hormones, which activate target cells by interacting with specific receptors (see Table 10.1 for details).

Hormones can act like enzymes, by a direct action on any particular chemical reaction, or they may act on the target cell binding to a specific receptor. Here, the mode of action will depend on the type of receiver:

- Membrane receptors: located on the membrane of cells. Receptor binding with the membrane can cause alterations in the permeability of the membrane (e.g., the basis of the transmission of nerve impulse to the neurons, thus also acting insulin and the glucocorticoids). It can also cause a change in an intracellular second messenger (cyclic adenosine monophosphate [CAM] and cyclic guanosine monophosphate [CGM]).
- Intracellular receptors: hormone-activated and transported into the nucleus where they give the order to synthesize a new effect or protein.

TABLE 10.1
Four Types of Hormone Secretion

Autocrine: the target cell is the secretory cell itself (e.g., the EGF or epidermal growth factor).
Paracrine: target cell is adjacent to the secreting cell (e.g., prostaglandins in diffuse neuroendocrine system).
Endocrine: target cells are removed from the secretory cells and are transported through the blood.
Synapse: a direct communication between two cells, characteristic of the nervous system. The secretory cell, in this case a neuron, is in direct contact with the target cell (e.g., another neuron, a muscle cell) and activates this through a neurotransmitter chemical messenger that can be shared with the endocrine system. As can be deduced, this transmission is almost instantaneous.

The system used to transport chemical messengers to the target cells is the circulatory one. Anatomical organization of the endocrine system consists of the cells (termed endocrine cells) whose main function is to secrete chemical messengers (hormones) and can be found in three anatomical locations:

- Endocrine cells grouped to form an organ or unskilled endocrine gland,
- Endocrine cells forming small groups within other organs (ovary, testis, pancreas),
- Endocrine cells individually dispersed among other cells of epithelial tissues, especially the digestive and respiratory systems, referred to collectively as the diffuse neuroendocrine system.

Hormones regulate many different functions and very different levels of complexity, and can:

- Act as simple transmitters of information
- Check to lower/upper limits of metabolic functions
- Act as a feedback control
- Control complex systems such as the menstrual cycle
- Regulate the development of mammary glands
- Alter regular metabolic rates
- Alter embryonic development

EDCs, environmental estrogens, xenoestrogens, endocrine modulators, ecoestrogens, environmental hormones, hormonally active compounds, and phytoestrogens all describe endocrine disruptors, chemicals that can alter the hormonal balance and the regulation of embryonic development and, therefore, are capable of causing adverse health effects in an organism or its progeny. They are able to interfere with some synthetic human hormone system chemicals known since the 1940s, when people began to use the diethylstilbestrol drug (DES) to prevent spontaneous abortions. However, the term endocrine disruptor—taken from "Endocrine Disrupting Chemical (EDC)"—was coined 50 years later, in 1991, at the Wingspread Conference, where a group of experts in endocrinology, reproductive and developmental biology, toxicology, marine biology, ecology, and psychiatry gathered to assess the causes of the adverse effects observed in epidemiological studies of people and wild animals in the Northern Hemisphere, including damage to the reproductive and immune system and hormone-dependent cancers in organs among others (Bern et al., 1992).

The term endocrine disruptor defines a diverse and heterogeneous group of exogenous chemicals capable of altering the synthesis, release, transport, metabolism, binding action, or elimination of natural hormones in the body (Kavlock et al., 1996).

The catalogue of endocrine disruptors is vast and growing every day, ranging from chemicals synthesized by man to substances found naturally in the environment.

The EDCs are considered as "chameleon substances" because the same EDC may have different modes of action depending on its concentration level.

Thus, high doses of dioxin can kill, but very low concentrations (similar to ones the human population is exposed to through ingestion of contaminated food) increase the risk of reproductive abnormalities in women. High (nM) levels of hexachlorobenzene (HCB) suppress androgen activity in prostate cells, whereas low doses (<1 nM) increase androgen activity (Hursh et al., 2007; Vandenberg, 2012).

Uterine exposure of mice to 100 μM doses of DES causes the mice adults too thin; however, at exposure to 1 μM, the adult organisms of mice are obese.

EDCs may also have different modes of operation depending on the specific stage of development of the tissue in contact: for an uterotrophic response in an adult mouse, it is necessary to administer 100 mg/kg/day of bisphenol A (BPA). However, administration of only 25 ng/kg/day of BPA during the period of gestation is capable of eliciting the response of ductal breast tissue. And the adverse effect caused may vary depending on the time of exposure as well as the hormonal balance of the exposed person, as we have seen it depends on the age and sex among other factors (Colborn, 2004).

The time of exposure in the developing organism is crucial to determine the nature, severity, and subsequent evolution/appearance of the EDC effect. The effects of EDC are different on the embryo, fetus, perinatal organism, or adult organism. If they act during a critical period (e.g., the early stages of life characterized by rapid cell differentiation and organogenesis), they may cause irreversible lesions. There is ample evidence on the exquisite sensitivity of the developing organism to chemicals that may interfere in hormonal activity during critical stages of organogenesis during uterine development. In many cases, this impact is irreversible and remains on during the rest of his life organism (Fernández, 2011). Moreover, there may be a long period of latency between the time of exposure and the time when the effects become manifest. Exposure to biologically active chemicals (at concentration levels at which natural body hormones act) can lead to a set of side effects that vary progressively along the different developmental stages. These effects may be different from the effects of the same substance when administered in high doses, or when the individual is fully developed (Soto and Sonnenschein, 2010). When exposed *in utero* to EDCs, the effects are not expressed in the birth; they can remain latent for some years, or could appear in descendants instead of the person who was exposed to EDCs. Because of that, the consequences of the exposure to EDCs are more probably that they appear in the children than in the exposed parent. Therefore, the consequences of EDC exposure occur most frequently in children than in the parent exposed.

The effects of exposure to EDCs in one generation can be passed on to future generations through the mechanisms involved in gene activity, called epigenetic changes programming. Examples include:

- The action of chemicals capable of interfering with androgen action during the male programming in fetal life; this includes androgen receptor antagonists, such as certain pesticides and phthalates. Some of the results of the decrease of androgen action in experimental animals become apparent only in adulthood, including malformations of the reproductive organs. Most of the effects are irreversible.
- Epidemiological studies demonstrate that exposure to dioxin (e.g., TCDD) during the perinatal period has a negative impact on semen quality, while exposure during adulthood does not affect semen quality.
- Estradiol and estrogenic substances can interfere with the peptide system in rodents during the neonatal period, influencing the age of onset of puberty.
- The development of the female reproductive system is programmed during fetal development and can be interrupted at this stage by improper signaling caused by chemicals such as DES, with multiple and irreversible consequences.
- It is believed that many hormonal cancers such as breast, prostate, testicular, ovarian, and endometrial cancers may originate in fetal life and at puberty. During these stages of life, there is a high sensitivity to chemical exposure involved in these cancers.
- The action of thyroid hormones during uterine development of various organs is essential, including brain development and neuroendocrine system. The action of thyroid disruption by exposure to chemicals at this stage of development can have detrimental and irreversible effects.
- There are many examples of vulnerable stages of many animals, including grasshoppers, amphibians, and reptiles that are extremely sensitive to exposure to EDCs.

10.2 CYANOGENIC COMPOUNDS AS NATURAL XENOBIOTICS IN FOOD

Xenobiotics can penetrate into foods at many stages of cultivation, production, preparation, thermal treatment, and storage of food and their ingredients. If present in foods, they might be of external origin, for example, heavy metals, pesticides, antibiotics, bacteria, viruses, and fungi, which enter foods from polluted environment or contaminated production lines. Additionally some of the "foreign" compounds are intentionally added to prevent rapid deterioration of foods (preservatives), to improve taste (flavor enhancers, e.g., monosodium glutamate), and food dyes (tartrazine), and so on (Jacobs et al., 2014).

Certain xenobiotics, particularly in plant products are synthesized by plants themselves as secondary metabolites, as it happens in the case of cyanogenic compounds. The basic function of those compounds is protection against pests, pathogens, and herbivores.

Small amounts of hydrogen cyanide are formed during synthesis of ethyne in plants from ACC (1-aminocyclopropane-1-carboxylic acid); additionally hydrogen cyanide can also form in plant tissues from glyoxylate and hydroxylamine—indirect products of photorespiration and nitrate reduction pathway (Siegień, 2007).

Tissue damage causes the initiation of cyanogenesis resulting in release of HCN from cyanogenic glycosides (CGs) or lipids (CLs). Hydrogen cyanide and most of its salts are rapidly absorbed through the skin, lungs, and the gastrointestinal tract. Cyanide ions bind to ferric ions (Fe^{3+}) in red blood cells inhibiting the action of the enzyme cytochrome oxidase and preventing the use of oxygen by the cells. Toxicity of hydrogen cyanide involves the inhibition of enzyme activity in the mitochondrial respiratory chain and prevents the utilization of oxygen by the cells, resulting in suffocation at the cellular level (concentration of 1 mg/kg of body weight may prove to be fatal to human beings) (Anseeuw et al., 2013). Reduced use of oxygen in tissues is manifested by the accumulation of oxyhemoglobin in the blood of thrombosis (blood becomes bright red), which causes the skin and mucous membranes of people suffering from poisoning take characteristic red color. Hydrogen cyanide acts on the nervous system and causes heart rhythm disturbances. The decrease in blood pressure can lead to cardiogenic shock (Gracia and Shepherd, 2004).

10.3 CYANOGENIC COMPOUNDS

Cyanogenic compounds are found in more than 2500 species of plants primarily belonging to the Poaceae, Rosaceae, Liliaceae, Euphorbiaceae, and Scrophulariaceae families. A major source of cyan hydrogen in plant tissues are cyanogenic glycosides and in the case of certain species, for example, Sapindaceae and Hippocastanaceae-cyanogenic lipids. An important feature of all cyanogenic compounds is the possibility of releasing toxic HCN through the cyanogenesis processes (Lewis and Elvin-Lewis, 2003). All known cyanogenic glycosides are O-β-glycosides-α-hydroxynitrile derived from L-amino acids (valine, isoleucine, leucine, phenylalanine, and tyrosine), as well as non-protein amino acid cyclopentyl glycine. Examples of the most studied compounds are prunasin, lotaustralin, amygdalin, vicianin, linamarin, sambunigrin, and dhurrin (see Figure 10.1).

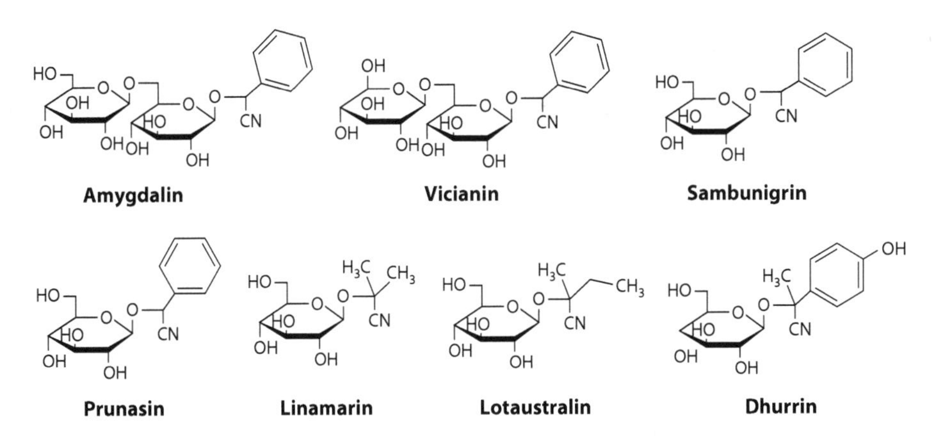

FIGURE 10.1 Molecular structures of cyanogenic glycosides present in plants.

10.3.1 Cyanogenic Glycosides in Plants, Their Role, Biosynthesis, and Hydrolysis

Biosynthesis of cyanogenic glycosides involves the transfer of uridyl group from uridine-5′-triphosphate (UTP) to a carbohydrate-1-phosphate forming UTP-carbohydrate-pyrophosphate, which is catalyzed by uridylyltransferase, followed by transfer of hydrocarbon to the corresponding aglycone catalyzed by glycolysis transferase (Ben-Yehoshua and Conn, 1964; Conn, 1979) (see Figure 10.2).

All plants may store cyanogenic glycosides in vacuoles. Mastication of plant tissues by herbivores while eating or damage caused by pests or pathogens leads to the release of glycosides to cytoplasm where glycosides are hydrolyzed by enzymes resulting in release of cyanides. Storing them in inactive form in the vacuole prevents damage to the plants under normal conditions.

Molecules of cyanogenic glycosides are hydrolyzed by enzymes called β-glucosidases, and synthesized by plants from two synthons: aglycone (cyanohydrin part) and glycon (carbohydrate part). Cyanohydrins are unstable and, depending on the pH (faster in alkaline medium), break down to carbonyl compounds and hydrogen cyanide. In the plant tissues (which have slightly acidic pH), enzymes like hydroxynitrile lyase accelerate this reaction even 20-fold. Table 10.2 summarizes the information about plant sources of cyanogenic glycosides and the products of their decomposition (Poulton, 1990; Vetter, 2000; Gleadow and Woodrow, 2002).

The best known example is the hydrolysis of amygdalin by β-glucosidase (emulsin) to gentiobiose and L-mandelonitrile. Gentiobiose further is hydrolyzed to glucose, and mandelonitrile is hydrolyzed to benzaldehyde and hydrogen cyanide (Lessner et al., 2015) (see Figure 10.3).

The amount of CGs in plants depends not only on the vegetation period but also on the climatic conditions and soil quality. During the germination of *Phaseolus lunatus* seeds, the amount of CGs is constant. While sorghum seeds do not contain CGs and birdsfoot trefoil (*Lotus corniculatus*) seeds contain small amounts of these compounds, their synthesis rate increases rapidly during germination. HCN accumulates in high concentrations in the organs of reproduction, such as seeds, fruits,

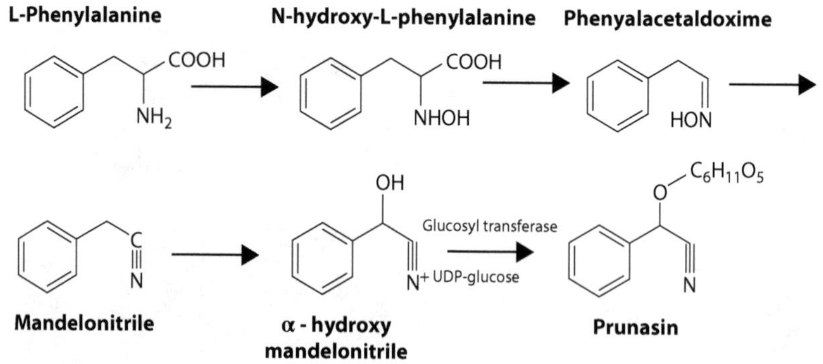

FIGURE 10.2 Prunasin biosynthesis starts with a phenylalanine as a precursor and the chiral center in mandelonitrile permits attachment of sugar molecule.

TABLE 10.2
Plant Sources of Cyanogenic Glycosides and Their Hydrolysis Products

Cyanogenic Compound	Plant Source	Products of Enzymatic Hydrolysis
Amygdalin	Rosaceae, particularly of the genus *Prunus,* Poaceae (grass), Fabaceae (legumes), flax seed and cassava, apricots (8%), peach (6%), bitter almonds (5%) and plums (2.5%)	-HCN, benzaldehyde, glucose
Prunasin	*Prunus japonica* or *Prunus maximowiczii* and *Amygdalus communis*. Leaves and stems of *Olinia ventosa, Olinia radiata, Olinia emarginata* and *Olinia rochetiana, Acacia greggii*	-HCN, benzaldehyde, glucose
Vicianin	Seeds of *Vicia angustifolia*	-HCN, benzaldehyde, glucose, arabinose
Linamarin	Leaves and roots of cassava, lima beans, and flax	-HCN, acetone, glucose
Lotaustralin	*Lotus australis, Manihot esculenta, Phaseolus lunatus, Rhodiola rosea* and *Trifolium repens*)	-HCN, acetone, glucose
Sambunigrin	Leaves, flowers, and seeds of elderberry (*Sambucus nigra, Sambucus canadensis*)	-HCN, benzaldehyde, glucose
Dhurrin	*Sorghum bicolor*	-HCN, benzaldehyde, glucose

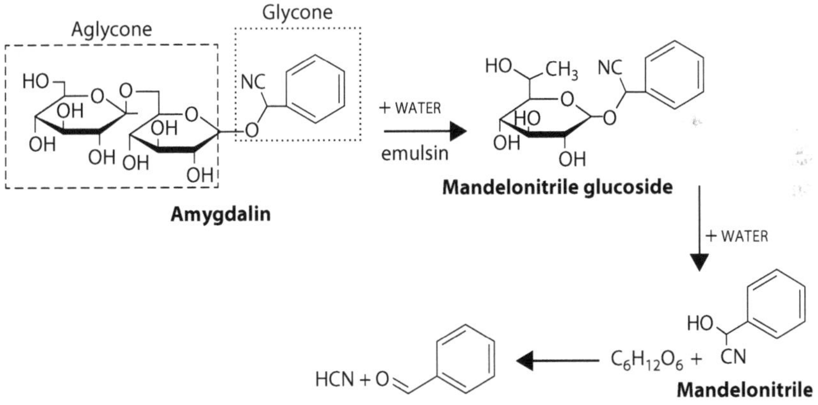

FIGURE 10.3 Hydrolysis of amygdalin.

flowers, and also young leaves and seedlings, in these tissues that, due to the function or stage of development, require special protection (Siegień, 2007).

10.3.2 Cyanogenic Lipids

CGs are widely distributed in the plants, while cyanogenic lipids (CLs) are limited almost entirely to the occurrence in the Sapindaceae, and in contrast to CGs, little is known about the metabolism of lipids cyanide. These substances consist of a hydroxynitrile, which is stabilized by esterification with a fatty acid. Removal of the fatty acid catalyzed by lipase results in unstable hydroxynitrile cleaved spontaneously or through catalysis of hydroxynitrile lyase to release HCN.

Most of CLs are esters of 1-cyano-2-methylprop-2-ene-1-ol with C:20 fatty acids and are stored in the seeds of *Ungnadia speciosa*, the only species present in the Sapindaceae family. During germination and seedling development, these lipids are completely consumed.

Studies suggest that CLs are used for synthesis of non-cyanogenic compounds. It is concluded that these lipids serve as storage for reduced nitrogen. Due to tissue injuries, cyanogenic lipids come into contact with the related hydrolytic enzymes (lipases) that hydrolyze the cyanogenic lipids. It results in dissociation of hydroxynitrile and liberation of HCN. However, there are still large gaps in knowledge about cyanogenesis and biosynthesis of CLs as well as about their functions and possible transformation routes into non-cyanogenic compounds. It turned out, however, that the repellent effect of cyanogens is weak or even negligible, and can have rather antifungal properties.

Balanced diet consists largely of plants containing cyanogenic compounds in the form of the more common cyanogenic glycosides and sometimes lipids. Maize, wheat, rye, apple, barley, oats, sugarcane, and yet many other plants consumed by humans contain cyanogenic compounds.

However, the risk of poisoning is negligible as it is very easy to remove the toxic HCN by grinding and drying in air or soaking in water, and an additional thermal treatment contributes to the denaturation of proteins (enzymes) that initiate the process of cyanogenesis. Furthermore, man is provided with a quite effective cyanide detoxifying mechanism, functioning effectively with adequate protein diet (Jones, 1998). In 1990, scientists suggested that the role of cyanogenic compounds can only come down to defense against fungi because their harmfulness is negligible (Selmar et al., 1990).

Since little evidences exist on possibility of cyanogenic compounds as direct EDCs, studies are needed to confirm possibility of their impact on hormonal action of higher animals due to binding with hormones, their degradation, or metabolic shifts after HCN release into circulation system.

ACKNOWLEDGMENT

This project was partially funded by the Polish National Science Centre based on decision number DEC-2013/09/N/NZ8/03247.

REFERENCES

Anseeuw, K., Delvau, N., Burillo-Putze, G., De Iaco, F., Geldner, G., Holmström, P., Lambert Y., and Sabbe, M. 2013. Cyanide poisoning by fire smoke inhalation: a European expert consensus. *Eur. J Emerg. Med.* 20(1): 2–9.

Ben-Yehoshua, S., and E.E. Conn. 1964. Biosynthesis of prunasin, the cyanogenic glucoside of peach. *Plant Physiol.* 39: 331–333.

Bern, H., P. Blair, S. Brasseur, T. Colborn, G.R. Cunha, W. Davis, K.D. Dohler, G. Fox, M. Fry, E. Gray, R. Green, M. Hines, T.J. Kubiak, J. McLachlan, J.P. Myers, R.E. Peterson, P.J.H. Reijnders, A. Soto, G. Van Der Kraak, F. vom Saal, and P. Whitten. 1992.

Statement from the work session on chemically-induced alterations in sexual development: the wildlife/human connection in Chemically-Induced Alterations, in *Sexual and Functional Development: The Wildlife/Human Connection.* Eds. T. Colborn and C. Clement. Princeton, NJ: Princeton Scientific Publishing.

Colborn, T. 2004. Commentary: setting aside tradition when dealing with endocrine disruptors. *ILAR J.* 45(4): 394–400.

Conn, E.E. 1979. Biosynthesis of cyanogenic glycosides. *Naturwissenschaften* 66: 28–34.

Fernández, M. 2011. Fundamentos De Toxicologia. Seminario de actualizaci6n en Toxicología Laboral. ISTAS, Madrid, Spain.

Gleadow, R.M., and I.E. Woodrow. 2002. Mini-Review: constraints on effectiveness of cyanogenic glycosides in herbivore defense. *J. Chem. Ecology* 28: 1301–1313.

Gracia, R., and G. Shepherd. 2004. Cyanide poisoning and its treatment. *Pharmacotherapy* 24(10): 1358–1365.

Hursh, D.W., C.A. Martina, H.B. Davis, and M.A. Trush. 2007. Does the dose make the poison? Extensive results challenge a core assumption in toxicology. Teaching Environmental Health to Children: An Interdisciplinary Approach, Springer.

Jacobs, D.R., J. Ruzzin, and D.H. Lee. 2014. Environmental pollutants: downgrading the fish food stock affects chronic disease risk. *J. Intern. Med.* 276(3): 240–242.

Jones, D.A. 1998. Why are so many food plants cyanogenic? *Phytochemistry* 47(2): 155–162.

Kavlock, R.J., Daston, G.P, DeRosa, C., Fenner-Crisp, P., Gray, L.E., Kaattari, S., Lucier, G., Luster, M., Mac, M.J., Maczka, C., Miller, R., Moore, J., Rolland, R., Scott, G., Sheehan, D.M., Sinks, T., and Tilson, H.A. 1996. Research needs for the risk assessment of health and environmental effects of endocrine disruptors: a report of the U. S. EPA-sponsored workshop. *Environ. Health Perspect.* 104: 715.

Lessner, K.M., Dearing, M.D., Izhaki, I., Samuni-Blank, M., Arad, Z., and Karasov, W.H. 2015. Small intestinal hydrolysis of plant glucosides: higher glucohydrolase activities in rodents than passerine birds. *J. Exp. Biol.* 218: 2666.

Lewis, W.H., and Elvin-Lewis, M.P. 2003. *Medical Botany: Plants Affecting Human Health.* John Wiley & Sons, New York.

Poulton, J.E. 1990. Cyanogenesis in plants. *Plant Physiol.*, 94: 401.

Selmar, D., Grocholewski S., and Seigler D.S. 1990. Cyanogenic Lipids, Utilization during Seedling Development of *Ungnadia speciosa. Plant Physiol.* 93: 631.

Siegień, I. 2007. Cyjanogeneza u roślin i jej efektywność w ochronie roślin przed atakiem roślinożerców i patogenów. *Kosmos* 56: 155–166.

Soto, A.M., and C. Sonnenschein. 2010. Environmental causes of cancer: Endocrine disruptors as carcinogens. *Nat. Rev. Endocrinol.* 6: 363–370.

Vandenberg, L. 2012. Opinion: "There are no safe doses for endocrine disruptors." *Environmental Health News*, http://www.environmentalhealthnews.org/ehs/news/2012/opinion-endocrine-disruptors-low-level-effects (accessed March 15, 2012).

Vetter, J. 2000. Plant cyanogenic glycosides. *Toxicon* 38: 11–36.

11 Phthalates

Tine Fierens, Mirja Van Holderbeke, Arnout Standaert, Isabelle Sioen, and Stefaan De Henauw

CONTENTS

11.1 INTRODUCTION

Phthalates is the common generic name for dialkyl or alkyl aryl esters of *ortho*phthalic acid or 1,2-benzene dicarboxylic acid (Figure 11.1). The environmental and biological behavior of this group of substances largely depends on the physicochemical properties of the individual compounds. Most phthalates are liquids at ambient temperature and their vapor pressure generally declines with increasing molecular mass or alkyl chain length. A similar decreasing trend with increasing alkyl chain length is observed for their solubility in water: dimethyl phthalate (DMP) dissolves best in water while di(2-ethylhexyl) phthalate (DEHP) is nearly water insoluble. On the contrary, the octanol–water partition coefficient, which is the ratio of a chemical's

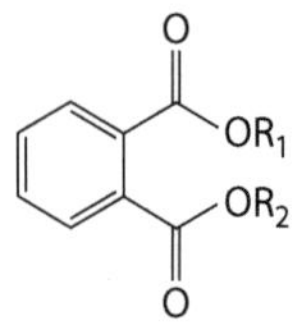

FIGURE 11.1 Generalized chemical structure of phthalates; R_1 and R_2 are the same or different alkyl or aryl groups.

equilibrium concentrations in an octanol–water system and typically used to predict the partitioning of a chemical between water and animal/plant lipids or between water and sediment/soil organic matter, generally increases with increasing alkyl chain length (Cousins et al., 2003).

To date, more than 30 different phthalate compounds are commercially available on the market. Among them, DEHP, diisononyl phthalate (DiNP), and diisodecyl phthalate (DiDP) are the most prevalent ones. The use of phthalates is very widespread and the type of application mostly depends on the length of the alkyl chain. Short-alkyl-chain phthalates (i.e., phthalates with one up to six carbon atoms in the alkyl chain) are generally used as solvents and can be present in adhesives, varnishes, resins, printing inks, personal care products, pharmaceuticals, pesticides, and food contact applications. Examples of such phthalates are diethyl phthalate (DEP), diisobutyl phthalate (DiBP), di-*n*-butyl phthalate (DnBP), and benzylbutyl phthalate (BBP). Long-alkyl-chain phthalates like DEHP, DiNP, and DiDP are mainly used as a plasticiser to soften polyvinyl chloride (PVC). Products that may contain these substances are, for example, furniture, building materials, gloves, food contact materials, and medical devices (ECPI, 2014).

As a consequence of their widespread use, people are extensively and continuously exposed to phthalates via different exposure routes. Numerous studies have indicated that dietary intake is the most important exposure route for the general population, especially for phthalates like DEHP and DiNP. Other pathways relevant to phthalate exposure are ingestion of dust and soil, inhalation of indoor and ambient air, mouthing objects (typically for young children), intake of enteric-coated tablets, and dermal contact with consumer products and medical devices (Hernández-Díaz et al., 2013; Rudel and Perovich, 2009; Wormuth et al., 2006).

Some phthalates and their metabolites are suspected to be endocrine-disrupting compounds. This means that they may alter the functioning of the endocrine system and consequently cause adverse health effects—even at background levels—in intact organisms, or their progeny, or (sub)populations (European Commission, 2014; Grandjean et al., 2006). Epidemiological studies have indicated the influence of (prenatal) phthalate exposure on, among others, birth weight, genital development, hormone production, semen quality, and the occurrence of allergic symptoms, obesity, and diabetes (Hoppin et al., 2013; Stahlhut et al., 2007; Swan, 2008).

Because of association of phthalates with adverse health effects in humans, authorities have established regulations regarding the use of these compounds in a wide range of applications. In Europe, for instance, DEHP, DiBP, DnBP, and BBP cannot be used or placed on the market anymore except if they are used in applications for which companies have been granted authorization (ECHA, 2015).

Furthermore, there are regulations specific to the use of certain phthalates in one specific type of application such as plastic food contact materials or toys and childcare articles (Official Journal of the European Union, 2005, 2011 and amendments).

11.2 LEVELS OF PHTHALATES IN FOOD PRODUCTS

Phthalates have been analyzed in food products for many years. To illustrate the concentration ranges of these substances in foods, Table 11.1 summarizes the concentrations of DiBP, DnBP, BBP, DEHP, and DiNP—five commonly monitored phthalate compounds—in different food categories as recently reported (i.e., from 2006 onward) by several authors. Comparing phthalate levels obtained from different monitoring studies needs to be done with caution, not only due to dissimilarities between the studies regarding sampling method, analytical procedure, and more, but also because of differences in legislation concerning the use of phthalates in the countries where the studies were conducted.

11.2.1 Fruits, Vegetables, and Nuts

Fruits, vegetables, and nuts have been monitored for the occurrence of phthalates by, among others, Chinese, European, and Canadian researchers. Ji et al. (2014) detected DnBP, BBP, and DEHP in 25 Chinese fruit and vegetable samples. Concentrations amounted to 1.0–22, 0.03–0.9, and 1.6–14 µg/kg, respectively. Sakhi et al. (2014) analyzed phthalates in jam and frozen vegetables purchased from the Norwegian market. The investigated jam contained 0.9 µg/kg DnBP, 9.5 µg/kg DEHP, and 4.0 µg/kg DiNP, whereas the frozen vegetables only contained quantifiable levels of DiNP, namely, 2.9 µg/kg. In Belgium, 47 fruit, vegetable, and nut samples were analyzed (Van Holderbeke et al., 2014). Concentrations ranged between undetectable and 480, 38, 58, and 1413 µg/kg for DiBP, DnBP, BBP, and DEHP, respectively. In the 41 Canadian samples under study, levels of DiBP and DnBP were all below the limit of quantification (Cao et al., 2015). However, measurable levels of BBP and DEHP up to 9.4 and 676 µg/kg, respectively, were observed.

11.2.2 Milk and Dairy Products

Yogurt, milk beverages, cheese, cream, and related products are by far the food group most investigated for the presence of phthalates. Measurement campaigns have been set up in Europe, China, and Canada. In the six European studies mentioned in Table 11.1, concentrations in milk and dairy products were situated between undetectable and 4400, 780, 50, 3000, and 3055 µg/kg for DiBP, DnBP, BBP, DEHP, and DiNP, respectively (Bradley et al., 2013a; Fierens et al., 2013; Peters, 2006; Sakhi et al., 2014; Sorensen, 2006; Van Holderbeke et al., 2014). The highest levels of DiBP, DnBP, BBP, and DEHP were found by Peters (2006) while the highest DiNP concentration was found in the British study of Bradley et al. (2013a). In China, at least four studies were conducted between 2011 and 2014 in

TABLE 11.1
Phthalate Levels in Different Food Categories (min–max; in µg/kg fresh weight)

Food Category (Study)	Country	*N*	DiBP	DnBP	BBP	DEHP	DiNP
					(In µg/kg fresh weight)		
Fruits, vegetables, and nuts							
(Ji et al., 2014)	China	25	–	1.0–22	0.03–0.9	1.6–14	–
(Sakhi et al., 2014)	Norway	2	ND	ND–0.9	ND	ND–9.5	2.9–4.0
(Van Holderbeke et al., 2014)	Belgium	47	ND–480	ND–38	ND–58	ND–1413	–
(Cao et al., 2015)	Canada	41	<5.0–<15	<6.1–<30	<0.6–9.4	<14–676	–
Milk and dairy products							
(Peters, 2006)	Europe	8	ND–4400	ND–780	ND–50	ND–3000	ND–660
(Sorensen, 2006)	Denmark	7	–	<9	<4	13–37	<5
(Li et al., 2011)	China	4	–	113–131	ND–24	–	–
(Yan et al., 2011)	China	5	–	ND–5.2	ND	–	–
(Guo et al., 2012)	China	11	1.2–59	2.4–226	ND–1.5	ND–134	–
(Bradley et al., 2013a)	UK	15	ND–186	ND	ND	ND–690	ND–3055
(Fierens et al., 2013)	Belgium	21	ND–24	ND–27	ND–19	4.7–287	–
(Ji et al., 2014)	China	27	–	0.6–5.0	0.003–0.2	0.7–3.7	–
(Sakhi et al., 2014)	Norway	4	ND–5.4	ND–31	ND	19–173	6.8–166
(Van Holderbeke et al., 2014)	Belgium	79	ND–116	ND–54	ND–48	ND–2385	–
(Cao et al., 2015)	Canada	14	<1.5–<15	<5.0–54	<2.4–18	32–223	–
Cereals and cereal products							
(Guo et al., 2012)	China	21	1.8–326	1.5–572	ND–17	ND–762	–
(Bradley et al., 2013a)	UK	34	ND–108	ND–60	ND	ND–365	ND
(Ji et al., 2014)	China	2	–	3.0–4.0	0.1–0.2	5.0–6.7	–

(*Continued*)

TABLE 11.1 (*Continued*)
Phthalate Levels in Different Food Categories (min–max; in µg/kg fresh weight)

Food Category	Country	*N*	DiBP	DnBP	BBP	DEHP	DiNP
(Study)					(In µg/kg fresh weight)		
(Sakhi et al., 2014)	Norway	5	1.0–24	1.3–16	ND–3.5	ND–60	ND–734
(Van Holderbeke et al., 2014)	Belgium	129	ND–1383	ND–106	ND–24	ND–2264	–
(Cao et al., 2015)	Canada	12	2.9–6.5	<6.1–24	<0.6–16	31–272	–
(He et al., 2015)	China	44	–	12–284	ND–63	43–1380	–
Meat and meat products							
(Peters, 2006)	Europe	10	ND–2300	ND–760	ND–17	ND–3300	ND–470
(Guo et al., 2012)	China	6	0.4–43	0.7–15	ND–2.3	37–184	–
(Bradley et al., 2013a)	UK	69	ND	ND–33	ND	ND–256	ND–1820
(Ji et al., 2014)	China	4	–	0.6–3.7	0.05–0.2	1.8–8.3	–
(Sakhi et al., 2014)	Norway	8	ND–12	ND–5.8	ND–78	ND–117	3.0–275
(Van Holderbeke et al., 2014)	Belgium	37	ND–36	ND–25	ND–18	10–850	–
(Cao et al., 2015)	Canada	13	<3.0–4.9	7.6–16	<1.2–<5.8	<27–330	–
(He et al., 2015)	China	4	–	18–61	0.2–1.8	103–400	–
Fish and fish products							
(Guo et al., 2012)	China	3	ND–65	1.6–12	ND	27–111	–
(Bradley et al., 2013a)	UK	74	ND–62	ND	ND	ND–2176	ND–11576
(Ji et al., 2014)	China	1	–	5.2	0.2	12	–
(Sakhi et al., 2014)	Norway	5	ND–3.2	ND–12	ND–32	ND–35	2.0–55
(Van Holderbeke et al., 2014)	Belgium	22	ND–13	ND–13	ND–8.0	ND–5932	–
(Cao et al., 2015)	Canada	4	<4.5–11	24–43	<5.8	<19–74	–
(He et al., 2015)	China	3	–	86–116	1.6–8.7	523–1500	–

(*Continued*)

TABLE 11.1 (*Continued*)
Phthalate Levels in Different Food Categories (min–max; in μg/kg fresh weight)

Food Category (Study)	Country	*N*	DiBP	DnBP	BBP	DEHP	DiNP
					(In μg/kg fresh weight)		
Fats and oils							
(Peters, 2006)	Europe	1	ND	ND	340	24,000	72
(Guo et al., 2012)	China	3	3.5–13	4.0–18	1.7–18	47–71	–
(Bradley et al., 2013a)	UK	24	ND–49	ND–141	ND–2084	ND–6447	ND–1500
(Sakhi et al., 2014)	Norway	2	ND	ND	ND	118-323	ND–15
(Van Holderbeke et al., 2014)	Belgium	34	ND–53	ND–203	ND–1127	ND–1827	–
(Cao et al., 2015)	Canada	1	<15	<14	1.9	63	–
Salty and sweet snacks							
(Guo et al., 2012)	China	3	ND–76	ND–83	ND–2.6	ND–172	–
(Sakhi et al., 2014)	Norway	2	6.2–7.7	ND–7.1	ND	56–76	88–362
(Van Holderbeke et al., 2014)	Belgium	29	ND–114	ND–65	ND–23	0.5–308	–
(Cao et al., 2015)	Canada	17	<3.5–40	9.5–208	<0.6–35	19–284	–
(He et al., 2015)	China	17	–	3.8–181	0.4–12	64–933	–
Condiments and sauces							
(Guo et al., 2012)	China	10	0.6–111	ND–236	ND–1.2	ND–14	–
(Sakhi et al., 2014)	Norway	2	0.8–2.2	ND–1.2	ND	ND–33	9.4–14
(Van Holderbeke et al., 2014)	Belgium	41	ND–155	ND–157	ND–388	ND–2154	–
(Cao et al., 2015)	Canada	5	<15–27	<14–<68	<1.8–51	<19–667	–
(He et al., 2015)	China	7	–	9.4–101	0.2–8.7	62–400	–

(*Continued*)

TABLE 11.1 (*Continued*)
Phthalate Levels in Different Food Categories (min–max; in µg/kg fresh weight)

Food Category	Country	*N*	DiBP	DnBP	BBP	DEHP	DiNP
(Study)					**(In µg/kg fresh weight)**		
Baby food							
(Sorensen, 2006)	World	8	–	<9	<4	10–138	<5–12
(Gärtner et al., 2009)	Germany	20	ND–1796	ND–100	ND	ND	–
(Bradley et al., 2013a)	UK	26	ND–13	ND	ND	ND–125	ND
(Van Holderbeke et al., 2014)	Belgium	17	0.1–16	0.1–32	ND–16	ND–67	–
(Cao et al., 2015)	Canada	9	2.4–<15	ND	<1.2–<8.7	<19–135	–
Beverages							
(Peters, 2006)	Europe	1	ND	ND	ND	ND	ND
(Bosnir et al., 2007)	Croatia	45	–	ND–133	ND–27	ND–136	–
(Guo et al., 2012)	China	17	0.01–107	ND–557	ND–0.4	ND–73	–
(Chatonnet et al., 2014)	France	130	ND–170	<4–2212	<4–122	<4–1522	ND
(Sakhi et al., 2014)	Norway	4	0.1–0.9	0.3–1.0	ND–0.2	0.2–0.7	ND–3.2
(Santana et al., 2014)	Portugal	11	ND–1.9	ND–6.5	–	ND–0.2	–
(Van Holderbeke et al., 2014)	Belgium	89	ND–2.0	ND–30	ND–21	ND–11	–
(Cao et al., 2015)	Canada	8	ND	<5.7–14	<2.4–7.9	<14–35	–
(He et al., 2015)	China	3	–	33–53	0.03–0.6	72–160	–

N: number of samples; ND: undetectable; –: not investigated; UK: United Kingdom.

which phthalates were determined in milk and dairy products (Guo et al., 2012; Ji et al., 2014; Li et al., 2011; Yan et al., 2011). DiBP was only analyzed in the 11 samples of Guo et al. (2012): concentrations between 1.2 and 59 µg/kg were found. DEHP was investigated in the two most recent Chinese studies: levels varied between undetectable and 134 µg/kg in the study of Guo et al. (2012) and between 0.7 and 3.7 µg/kg in the sampling campaign of Ji et al. (2014). All four studies analyzed DnBP (undetectable–226 µg/kg) and BBP (undetectable to 24 µg/kg) in milk and dairy products while DiNP was not investigated in any of the Chinese samples. Most recently, Cao et al. (2015) determined levels of DiBP, DnBP, BBP, and DEHP in 14 Canadian milk and dairy product samples. DiBP levels were unquantifiable, whereas levels of DnBP, BBP, and DEHP amounted up to 54, 18, and 223 µg/kg, respectively.

11.2.3 Cereals and Cereal Products

The food category "cereals and cereal products" includes products like bread, breakfast cereals, flour, rice, pasta, and starches; biscuits, pies, cakes, and crisps are handled within the category "salty and sweet snacks." The largest number of cereal samples has been investigated in a Belgian study (Van Holderbeke et al., 2014). In this study, flour contained the maximum concentration of DiBP (1383 µg/kg), bread the highest DnBP (106 µg/kg) and DEHP (2264 µg/kg) levels, and popcorn the highest BBP content (24 µg/kg). In addition, other European research groups investigated cereal products for the occurrence of phthalates. Bradley et al. (2013a) observed concentrations up to 108 µg/kg for DiBP, 60 µg/kg for DnBP, and 365 µg/kg for DEHP while the phthalates BBP and DiNP could not be detected in the 34 samples under study. Samples of bread, dry pasta, buns, breakfast cereals, and flour were analyzed by Sakhi et al. (2014). Besides detectable levels of DiBP, DnBP, BBP, and DEHP, also DiNP was found in the samples analyzed in this Norwegian study. The DiNP concentration ranged between undetectable and 734 µg/kg. Over the course of three measurement campaigns, DiBP, DnBP, BBP, and DEHP were analyzed in 67 cereal product samples purchased from the Chinese market (Guo et al., 2012; He et al., 2015; Ji et al., 2014). Concentrations amounted to 1.8–326, 1.5–572, undetectable–63, and undetectable–1380 µg/kg, respectively. Lastly, another 12 cereal products were sampled in a Canadian study (Cao et al., 2015). Concentrations were determined for DiBP (2.9–6.5 µg/kg), DnBP (<6.1–24 µg/kg), BBP (<0.6–16 µg/kg), and DEHP (31–272 µg/kg).

11.2.4 Meat and Meat Products

Phthalates have been analyzed in a total of 124 European meat and meat product samples (Bradley et al., 2013a; Peters, 2006; Sakhi et al., 2014; Van Holderbeke et al., 2014). The highest level was found for DEHP (3300 µg/kg), followed by DiBP (2300 µg/kg), DiNP (1820 µg/kg), DnBP (760 µg/kg), and BBP (78 µg/kg). Three Chinese studies examined the presence of DiBP, DnBP, BBP, and DEHP, but not DiNP in 14 meat and meat products as well (Guo et al., 2012; He et al., 2015; Ji et al., 2014). Observed concentrations were 0.4–43, 0.7–61, undetectable–2.3, and

37–400 μg/kg, respectively. The lowest levels were determined by Ji et al. (2014). In Canada, 13 meat samples were investigated (Cao et al., 2015). Veal cutlets turned out to contain the highest phthalate levels, namely, 4.9 μg/kg DiBP, 16 μg/kg DnBP, and 330 μg/kg DEHP. BBP could not be quantified and DiNP was not analyzed in this Canadian study.

11.2.5 Fish and Fish Products

The occurrence of phthalates in fish and related products has been examined, among others, by three Chinese research groups (Guo et al., 2012; He et al., 2015; Ji et al., 2014). In the 7 products investigated, concentrations were situated between undetectable and 65 μg/kg for DiBP, between 1.6 and 116 μg/kg for DnBP, between undetectable and 8.7 μg/kg for BBP, and between 12 and 1500 μg/kg for DEHP; DiNP was not analyzed. More or less comparable levels of DiBP, DnBP, and BBP were found in the European and Canadian studies (Bradley et al., 2013a; Cao et al., 2015; Sakhi et al., 2014; Van Holderbeke et al., 2014). However, levels of DEHP turned out to be much higher in fish products bought on the European food market: concentrations up to 2176 and 5932 μg/kg were observed by Bradley et al. (2013a) and Van Holderbeke et al. (2014), respectively. Two of the three European studies listed in Table 11.1 also measured DiNP in fish and fish product samples. Bradley et al. (2013a) examined 74 British samples. In these samples, the DiNP contents varied from undetectable to 11,576 μg/kg. Much lower DiNP levels were observed in the five Norwegian products of Sakhi et al. (2014), that is, levels between 2.0 and 55 μg/kg.

11.2.6 Fats and Oils

Phthalate contents reported for fats and oils seem to be much higher in Europe than in Canada or China. For instance, a maximum DnBP concentration of 203 μg/kg was observed in a vegetable oil sample purchased from a Belgian food shop (Van Holderbeke et al., 2014) compared to 12 μg/kg in cooking oil from China (Guo et al., 2012) and <14 μg/kg in a composite sample of cooking fats and salad oils sold in Canada (Cao et al., 2015). DiNP levels were only reported for European fats and oils: concentrations varied from undetectable to 1500 μg/kg (Bradley et al., 2013a; Peters, 2006; Sakhi et al., 2014).

11.2.7 Salty and Sweet Snacks

Between 2012 and 2015, at least two studies were conducted in China that explored the presence of DiBP, DnBP, BBP, and DEHP in salty and sweet snacks (Guo et al., 2012; He et al., 2015). In a set of 20 samples, levels varied between undetectable and 76, 181, 12, and 933 μg/kg, respectively. Similar concentration ranges of these four compounds were observed in two European studies and a Canadian one (Cao et al., 2015; Sakhi et al., 2014; Van Holderbeke et al., 2014). One of the European campaigns also analyzed DiNP in two sweet snack products: Norwegian chocolate spread contained 362 μg/kg DiNP, and the investigated biscuits sample contained 88 μg/kg DiNP (Sakhi et al., 2014).

11.2.8 Condiments and Sauces

The category "condiments and sauces" comprises food products like pesto, mayonnaise, mustard, ketchup, nutmeg, and basil. Phthalates have been analyzed in this food group by at least five research groups (Cao et al., 2015; Guo et al., 2012; He et al., 2015; Sakhi et al., 2014; Van Holderbeke et al., 2014). The highest concentrations of DiBP (155 μg/kg), BBP (388 μg/kg), and DEHP (3154 μg/kg) were measured in Belgian condiment samples (Van Holderbeke et al., 2014), whereas a Chinese condiment contained the utmost DnBP level (388 μg/kg). DiNP was only analyzed in two sauces bought from a Norwegian food shop: mayonnaise contained a bit more DiNP than the tomato sauce sample, namely, 14 compared to 9.4 μg/kg (Sakhi et al., 2014).

11.2.9 Baby Food

Sorensen (2006) investigated the presence of DnBP, BBP, DEHP, and DiNP in eight infant formula samples originating from different parts of the world. The DEHP and DiNP contents ranged between 10 and 138 μg/kg and between <5 and 12 μg/kg, respectively; DnBP and BBP were both unquantifiable. In addition, three European and one Canadian study analyzed phthalate levels in baby food (Bradley et al., 2013a; Cao et al., 2015; Gärtner et al., 2009; Van Holderbeke et al., 2014). DiNP could not be detected, whereas the concentrations of the other compounds were varying from undetectable to 1796 μg/kg for DiBP, 100 μg/kg for DnBP, 16 μg/kg for BBP, and 135 μg/kg for DEHP.

11.2.10 Beverages

The food group "beverages" consists of all types of water-based drinks, both alcoholic and nonalcoholic. None of the five phthalates of interest could be detected in the European orange juice sample of Peters (2006). Bosnir et al. (2007), however, observed detectable levels up to 133 μg/kg of DnBP, 27 μg/kg of BBP, and 136 μg/kg of DEHP in Croatian soft drinks and mineral waters. Bottled water, soft drinks, wine, and beer originating from China contained maximal DiBP, DnBP, BBP, and DEHP concentrations of 107, 557, 0.6, and 160 μg/kg, respectively (Guo et al., 2012; He et al., 2015). With the exception of BBP, these maximum levels are much higher than the ones observed in the corresponding Belgian, Norwegian, and Canadian beverage samples (Cao et al., 2015; Sakhi et al., 2014; Van Holderbeke et al., 2014). Santana et al. (2014) investigated the occurrence of DiBP, DnBP, and DEHP in drinking water consumed in Portugal. These researchers observed concentration ranges between undetectable and 1.9, 6.5, and 0.2 μg/kg, respectively. Lastly, Chatonnet and coworkers (2014) analyzed the 5 phthalates of interest in 130 different types of wines and spirits that were produced in France. DiNP could not be detected while measurable levels were found for the remaining compounds, specifically a range of undetectable or unquantifiable to 170 μg/kg for DiBP, 2212 μg/kg for DnBP, 122 μg/kg for BBP, and 1522 μg/kg for DEHP.

11.3 POSSIBLE CONTAMINATION SOURCES FOR PHTHALATES IN FOOD PRODUCTS

11.3.1 The Environment

Phthalates are not covalently bound in the products they are used in. As a consequence, they are constantly being released into the environment by direct release, migration, evaporation, leaching, and/or abrasion and thus may transfer into food products during cultivation (Wormuth et al., 2006). Du et al. (2010), for instance, studied the occurrence of DEHP in the atmosphere and in four vegetable crops cultivated on land surrounding a plastic production factory. The DEHP concentrations in air were the highest in close vicinity to the production site, namely, 9.4–12.8 μg/m^3 at 0.2-km distance compared to 0.04–0.27 μg/m^3 at 1.6-km distance. The same observation was done for the vegetable crops: DEHP contents in the northerly (downwind) direction reached 19.4–52.0 mg/kg dry weight at 0.2-km distance and decreased to 4.5–12.1 mg/kg dry weight at 1.6-km distance. Thus, DEHP has clearly been taken up by the vegetable crops as a result of atmospheric deposition.

Plant uptake via phthalate containing soil (pore water) was investigated by Yin et al. (2003). In their field experiment, capsicum seedlings were cultivated on soils of which the top layer (0–10 cm) was treated with DnBP and DEHP. After 90 days of cultivation, capsicum fruit, shoot, and root samples were collected and analyzed. DnBP concentrations in fruit, shoot, and root samples increased with rising soil-applied DnBP/DEHP contents. DEHP on the contrary, being a rather water-insoluble compound, was not transferred from soil pore water as it was not detected in any of the capsicum samples.

Plants, water, and soil contaminated with phthalates may be ingested by animals. As a consequence, phthalates can also enter animals and animal products due to environmental transfer. This was demonstrated by Fierens et al. (2012a) among others. This research group investigated potential environmental contamination pathways for phthalates in raw cow's milk by analyzing phthalate levels in groundwater, soil, feed (silage, pasture, and concentrate), and manually collected raw cow's milk (to avoid phthalate contamination via the mechanical milking process). An association was observed between the concentrations of DiBP and DEHP detected in the feed (i.e., silage and for DEHP also pasture) and in the milk.

Effects of pasture ingestion by ewes on total phthalate concentrations in milk were investigated in a Scottish study (Rhind et al., 2007). A distinction was made between ewes fed with pasture treated with sewage sludge (containing a total of about 100 mg phthalates/kg dry weight) and ewes fed with pasture treated with an inorganic fertilizer ("control"). Total phthalate concentrations in milk ranged from <200 to 20,000 μg/kg dry weight. No significant effect was seen between the milk of the two groups of ewes.

The distribution of phthalates (eight individual phthalate esters and five commercial isomeric mixtures) in a marine aquatic food web was studied by Mackintosh et al. (2004). In their study, phthalate concentrations were determined in 18 marine species representing approximately 4 trophic levels. The phthalates tested did not biomagnify in the studied food web. In fact, the direct exchange and partitioning of phthalates between the organisms and the water turned out to be the main exposure route in this food web.

11.3.2 Food Contact Materials

Phthalates can migrate to food products from phthalate-containing materials that are in contact with the foods during cultivation, transport, production, storage, or preparation at home or outdoors. For example, a Chinese study indicated that vegetables take up DEHP from plastic mulch films that are used during field cultivation. Such mulch films contain about 16.5% DEHP and are mainly used to reflect sunlight in glasshouses (Du et al., 2009).

Phthalates may also release from flexible tubings, as was demonstrated for DEHP in a Canadian study (Feng et al., 2005). In this study, several phthalates were analyzed in raw cow's milk that was milked both by hand and by machine. The mechanically obtained milk samples contained much higher DEHP levels than the manually obtained ones, namely, 215 μg/kg compared to 16 μg/kg. The same observation was done by other researchers as well (Fierens et al., 2012a; Sharman et al., 1994).

Chatonnet et al. (2014) investigated contamination sources of phthalates in French wines and grape spirits. During wine fermentation and aging, various potential phthalate-containing polymer-based materials are used for pumping, storing, and handling wines and spirits and thus remain in direct contact with the liquids for varying periods of time. The hoses used for pumping contained high concentrations of DEHP and DiNP, whereas high DnBP and DiBP levels were found in some types of epoxy resins used in the coatings on the storage and fermentation vats.

An example of phthalate-containing materials used during food preparation is PVC gloves. Based on the surveys of Tsumura et al. (2001a, 2001b), it was demonstrated that BBP and DEHP migrated from PVC gloves—containing up to 2.8% BBP and 41% DEHP—during the preparation of retail packed lunches. Observed BBP and DEHP concentrations ranged between 2 and 277 μg/kg and between 346 and 11,800 μg/kg, respectively. Two months after the prohibition of DEHP-containing PVC gloves for cooking purposes in Japan, BBP and DEHP levels varied between undetectable and 10 μg/kg and between 45 and 517 μg/kg, clearly lower than the previously determined pre-ban levels.

Packaging represents a special type of food contact material, since food products can be stored in it for extended periods before they are consumed. The use of phthalates in packaging materials is widespread. For instance, phthalates like DEHP, DiNP, and DiDP are added to PVC plastisols with typical concentrations between 20% and 31% by weight. These plastisols are used in the metal lids of glass jars to create a hermetic sealing. Migration of DiNP and DiDP from such metal lids has been confirmed in a Danish study (Pedersen et al., 2008). In this study, food products stored in glass jars with metal lids in which DiNP and DiDP were used as the principal plasticiser contained <1–99 mg/kg DiNP and <1–173 mg/kg DiDP, respectively.

Another application of phthalates is their use as a carrier for pigments in printing inks and adhesives. When such inks or adhesives are present on packaging materials, phthalates can migrate from the inks or adhesives through the packaging into the foods. This especially holds true if the packaging material is permeable as is the case for paper and cardboard (Castle, 2007). For instance, in a Belgian study, pasta and rice packed in printed packaging materials were examined for the presence of eight phthalates (Fierens et al., 2012b). When packaged in cardboard, pasta contained more DiBP and to a lesser degree also more DnBP, BBP, and DEHP than when packaged in plastic. Concerning the rice samples, DiBP, DnBP, BBP, and DEHP contents in loose rice were higher than in boil-in-bag rice indicating that the plastic boiling bag may act as a barrier to phthalate migration.

Finally, recycled packaging materials also form potential contamination sources for phthalates in foods since traces of phthalates can be present in these materials as a result of previous applications such as printing inks and adhesives. Bradley et al. (2013a) conducted a concentration depth profile of lasagne sheets packaged in recycled cardboard in order to determine contamination sources for DiBP. A DiBP concentration of 200–250 μg/kg was found in the lasagne sheet that had come into direct contact with the cardboard packaging (i.e., 0–0.3 cm from the packaging); the lasagne sheet that was situated in the middle (i.e., 2.0–2.3 cm from the packaging) contained 40–80 μg/kg DiBP. The migration of phthalates in foods packed in recycled paper and cardboard has also been demonstrated by other researchers like Gärtner et al. (2009) among others.

11.3.3 Heat Treatment Steps

Research has indicated that heat treatment steps such as frying and pasteurization during the production process of a foodstuff may enhance migration (Castle, 2007). Ishida (1993) investigated the effects of several cooking processes upon the persistence of DEHP in chicken eggs, liver, and breast meat. All processes created a DEHP reduction in the examined food products: reduction rates amounted to 21–41% for freeze-drying, 26–53% for roasting, 12–33% for boiling, and 11–44% for frying.

The influence of frying on phthalate levels in meat and fish has been investigated by Fierens et al. (2012b). Higher DiBP and DEHP contents were found when the meat or fish was fried in a nonstick frying pan without using margarine than when it was fried in a frying pan with margarine. According to the authors, this difference could be owing to the fact that DiBP and DEHP are lipophilic and, therefore, might have migrated to the margarine used. Another possible explanation of the difference in DiBP and DEHP contents in this study was the presence of these compounds in the coating of the nonstick frying pan. This has been observed by other researchers as well (Bradley et al., 2007). Also phthalate contents in starchy products (potatoes, pasta, and rice) before and after boiling have been examined in the study of Fierens et al. (2012b): levels of BBP and DEHP were significantly lower after boiling (p-value of 0.036 and 0.031, respectively) and—although not significant—the same trend was observed for DiBP, DnBP, and DEP (p-value of 0.059, 0.074, and 0.28, respectively).

In another study, Fierens and coworkers (2013) investigated the transfer of eight phthalates during the production process of milk powder. Median DEHP concentrations increased from 364 μg/kg fat in raw milk to 426 μg/kg fat in pasteurized milk. Once the cooled milk was concentrated, pasteurized, homogenized, and spray dried, the median DEHP concentration increased for a second time, namely, from 426 to 478 μg/kg fat. These increases were most likely caused by the migration of DEHP from the food contact materials used during the different heat treatment steps (e.g., tubings and sealants).

11.4 HUMAN DIETARY EXPOSURE TO PHTHALATES AND RISK ASSESSMENT

11.4.1 Dietary Exposure Studies

Dietary exposure to phthalates has been investigated by many research groups. In Table 11.2, an overview is given of the 50th, 95th, and/or 97.5th percentiles of various dietary intake studies conducted for DiBP, DiNP, BBP, DEHP, and/or DiNP during the last decade (Bradley et al., 2013b; Fromme et al., 2007; Guo et al., 2012; Heinemeyer et al., 2013; Ji et al., 2014; Sakhi et al., 2014; Schecter et al., 2013; Sioen et al., 2012). As can be noticed from this table, the exposure rates of all considered phthalates are higher in European population groups than in Chinese or American groups. Nonetheless, this comparison needs to be interpreted with caution as the food consumption surveys and the types of analyzed food samples used within these studies may differ. With the exception of the dietary exposure to DnBP investigated by Ji et al. (2014), exposure rates within a population are decreasing with age. This is owing to the fact that children have

TABLE 11.2
50th, 95th, and/or 97.5th Percentiles of Various Dietary Phthalate Intake Studies (in µg/kg bw/day)

Compound	Country	Age	Food Type	P50	P95	P97.5
(Study)				(In µg/kg bw/day)		
DiBP						
(Fromme et al., 2007)	Germany	14–60 y.	Duplicate diet	0.6	2.1	–
(Guo et al., 2012)	China	18+ y.	Total diet	0.25	–	–
(Sioen et al., 2012)	Belgium	2.5–6.5 y.	Retail	0.42	0.64	–
(Sioen et al., 2012)	Belgium	15–98 y.	Retail	0.14	0.28	–
(Bradley et al., 2013b)	UK	1.5–4.5 y.	Total diet	–	–	1.2–2.7
(Bradley et al., 2013b)	UK	4–18 y.	Total diet	–	–	0.6–1.8
(Bradley et al., 2013b)	UK	18+ y.	Total diet	–	–	0.6–1.0
(Schecter et al., 2013)	USA	0.5–1 y.	Retail	0.01	–	–
(Schecter et al., 2013)	USA	18+ y.	Retail	0.01	–	–
(Sakhi et al., 2014)	Norway	18–70 y.	Retail	0.03	0.07	–
DnBP						
(Fromme et al., 2007)	Germany	14–60 y.	Duplicate diet	0.3	1.4	–
(Guo et al., 2012)	China	18+ y.	Total diet	0.24	–	–
(Sioen et al., 2012)	Belgium	2.5–6.5 y.	Retail	0.20	0.30	–
(Sioen et al., 2012)	Belgium	15–98 y.	Retail	0.08	0.16	–
(Bradley et al., 2013b)	UK	1.5–4.5 y.	Total diet	–	–	0.4–1.0
(Bradley et al., 2013b)	UK	4–18 y.	Total diet	–	–	0.2–0.7
(Bradley et al., 2013b)	UK	18+ y.	Total diet	–	–	0.2–0.3

(Continued)

TABLE 11.2 (*Continued*)
50th, 95th, and/or 97.5th Percentiles of Various Dietary Phthalate Intake Studies (in µg/kg bw/day)

Compound	Country	Age	Food Type	P50	P95	P97.5
(Study)				**(In µg/kg bw/day)**		
(Schecter et al., 2013)	USA	0.5–1 y.	Retail	0.04	–	–
(Schecter et al., 2013)	USA	18+ y.	Retail	0.03	–	–
(Ji et al., 2014)	China	2–6 y.	Retail	0.18	–	–
(Ji et al., 2014)	China	7–17 y.	Retail	0.12	–	–
(Ji et al., 2014)	China	18+ y.	Retail	0.16	–	–
(Sakhi et al., 2014)	Norway	18–70 y.	Retail	0.03	0.06	–
BBP						
(Guo et al., 2012)	China	18+ y.	Total diet	0.01	–	–
(Sioen et al., 2012)	Belgium	2.5–6.5 y.	Retail	0.12	0.21	–
(Sioen et al., 2012)	Belgium	15–98 y.	Retail	0.05	0.12	–
(Bradley et al., 2013b)	UK	1.5–4.5 y.	Total diet	–	–	0.07–1.3
(Bradley et al., 2013b)	UK	4–18 y.	Total diet	–	–	0.03–0.9
(Bradley et al., 2013b)	UK	18+ y.	Total diet	–	–	0.03–0.5
(Schecter et al., 2013)	USA	0.5–1 y.	Retail	0.13	–	–
(Schecter et al., 2013)	USA	18+ y.	Retail	0.02	–	–
(Ji et al., 2014)	China	2–6 y.	Retail	0.002	–	–
(Ji et al., 2014)	China	7–17 y.	Retail	0.002	–	–
(Ji et al., 2014)	China	18+ y.	Retail	0.002	–	–
(Sakhi et al., 2014)	Norway	18–70 y.	Retail	0.02	0.16	–
DEHP						
(Fromme et al., 2007)	Germany	14–60 y.	Duplicate diet	2.4	4.0	–
(Guo et al., 2012)	China	18+ y.	Total diet	0.62	–	–
(Sioen et al., 2012)	Belgium	2.5–6.5 y.	Retail	3.5	5.4	–
(Sioen et al., 2012)	Belgium	15–98 y.	Retail	1.5	2.9	–
(Bradley et al., 2013b)	UK	1.5–4.5 y.	Total diet	–	–	5.7–9.9
(Bradley et al., 2013b)	UK	4–18 y.	Total diet	–	–	2.7–6.7
(Bradley et al., 2013b)	UK	18+ y.	Total diet	–	–	2.6–4.0
(Heinemeyer et al., 2013)	Germany	14–80 y.	Retail	10	29	–
(Schecter et al., 2013)	USA	0.5–1 y.	Retail	1.6	–	–
(Schecter et al., 2013)	USA	18+ y.	Retail	0.42	–	–
(Ji et al., 2014)	China	2–6 y.	Retail	0.15	–	–
(Ji et al., 2014)	China	7–17 y.	Retail	0.12	–	–
(Ji et al., 2014)	China	18+ y.	Retail	0.12	–	–
(Sakhi et al., 2014)	Norway	18–70 y.	Retail	0.38	0.78	–
DiNP						
(Sakhi et al., 2014)	Norway	18–70 y.	Retail	0.40	1.1	–

–: not available; Pxx: xxth percentile; UK: United Kingdom; USA: the United States of America.

higher food consumption rates per unit of body weight than adolescents or adults. In general, dietary exposure to DEHP is the most common, followed by exposure to DiBP, DnBP, BBP, and DiNP. The maximum 95th or 97.5th percentiles observed for these phthalates amount to 29 μg/kg bw/day in German adolescents and adults, 2.7 μg/kg bw/day in British preschool children, 1.4 μg/kg bw/day in Germans aged between 14 and 60 years old, 1.3 μg/kg bw/day in British pre-school children, and 1.1 μg/kg in Norwegian adults, respectively. Still, the exposure to these phthalates might change within the coming years as the plasticizer industry is substituting more and more phthalates like DEHP by other, less harmful (phthalate) compounds such as DiNP, DiDP, di(2-propyl heptyl) phthalate, or diisononyl cyclohexane dicarboxylate (ECPI, 2014).

11.4.2 Contribution of the Diet to Integral Phthalate Exposure

People can be exposed to phthalates via various routes. Depending on the phthalate compound and the population group considered, the contribution of every exposure route to integral phthalate exposure is different. Table 11.3 summarizes the contribution percentages of food ingestion to integral exposure to DiBP, DnBP, BBP, DEHP, and DiNP as estimated by several researchers (Clark et al., 2011;

TABLE 11.3
Contribution of Food Ingestion (in %) to Integral Phthalate Exposure in Several Population Groups

Population (Age)	Country	DiBP	DnBP	BBP	DEHP	DiNP	Study
Infants (0–0.5 y.)	Canada	–	13–46	<6	34–76	–	Clark et al. (2011)
Infants (0.5–1 y.)	Denmark	–	99	97	26	7	Müller et al. (2003)
Infants–toddlers (0–4 y.)	Europe	60	60–70	20	50	<2	Wormuth et al. (2006)
Toddlers (2 y.)	Korea	–	25–41	26–50	63–75	–	Lee et al. (2014)
Toddlers (2 y.)	Denmark	–	50	49	54	–	Lee et al. (2014)
Toddlers (1–6 y.)	Denmark	–	99	98	66	46	Müller et al. (2003)
Toddlers (2–6 y.)	China	–	49	88	74	–	Ji et al. (2014)
Children (4–10 y.)	Europe	85	60	73	90	<1	Wormuth et al. (2006)
Children (7–14 y.)	Denmark	–	95–99	98	82	92	Müller et al. (2003)
Children–Teenagers (7–17 y.)	China	–	44	90	78	–	Ji et al. (2014)
Teenagers (11–18 y.)	Europe	95	40–60	20	95	5	Wormuth et al. (2006)
Toddlers–adults (0.5–70 y.)	Canada	–	75	68–77	95	61–71	Clark et al. (2011)
Adults (15–80 y.)	Denmark	–	91–99	94	76	89	Müller et al. (2003)
Adults (18–80 y.)	Europe	95	80–90	60	98	5	Wormuth et al. (2006)
Adults (18+ y.)	China	<10	<10	–	30–100	–	Guo et al. (2012)
Adults (18+ y.)	China	–	53	89	79	–	Ji et al. (2014)
RANGE (%)		<10–95	<10–99	<6–98	26–100	<1–92	

Guo et al., 2012; Ji et al., 2014; Lee et al., 2014; Müller et al., 2003; Wormuth et al., 2006). With the exception of the Chinese study of Guo et al. (2012), integral DiBP exposure seems to be mainly caused by the ingestion of contaminated food: contribution percentages for DiBP via food ingestion amount to 60% for children below the age of 4 years old and to 85–95% for the older age categories. The contribution of food ingestion to integral DnBP exposure seems to be higher in European than in non-European countries. For instance, in Canadian infants, food is responsible for 13–46% of the total exposure to DnBP, whereas in Danish infants, DnBP exposure is for 99% caused by the ingestion of contaminated food products (Clark et al., 2011; Müller et al., 2003). With respect to BBP, it can be concluded that food contribution percentages vary considerably among the conducted studies: ranges between <6% and 98% have been reported. For DEHP, food ingestion can be seen as a major contributor, as was the case for DiBP. Estimated DEHP food contribution percentages are mostly higher than 75%, especially when considering older age categories. Regarding DiNP, contribution percentages are ranging between <1% and 92%. The DiNP percentages reported by Wormuth et al. (2006) are generally lower than those of Müller et al. (2003) and Clark et al. (2011) for corresponding population groups.

11.4.3 Risk Assessment

To assess the risks associated with phthalate exposure, estimated phthalate intake values have to be compared with exposure limit values. These values are estimates of the daily intake of a chemical that can occur over a lifetime without appreciable risk for human health (WHO, 2000). In Table 11.4, an overview is given of the tolerable daily intake (TDI) and oral reference dose (RfD) values of DnBP, BBP, DEHP, and DiNP as established by the European Food Safety Authority (EFSA, 2005a, 2005b, 2005c, 2005d) and the American Environmental Protection Agency (US EPA, 2007), respectively. Also the no-observed-adverse-effect-levels (NOAELs) observed in animals and the uncertainty factors that were used to derive these TDI and RfD values can be found in Table 11.4. As can be noticed, TDI and RfD values differ from each other since they are extrapolated from other NOAEL values obtained in toxicological studies and since other uncertainty factors were taken into account to extrapolate the data of the animal studies to human health. Moreover, the corresponding TDI and RfD values are based on other observed endpoints in animals: while the current TDIs of DnBP, BBP, and DEHP are based on developmental and/or reproductive effects observed in (multi)generation studies of mice or rats, the RfDs are based on altered growth and consumption rates, modified organ weights, or increased mortality observed in adult rats or guinea pigs (EFSA, 2005a, 2005b, 2005c; US EPA, 2007).

Food ingestion is not the only phthalate exposure route in humans. Therefore, it is important to take the contribution of the diet to integral phthalate exposure into account when comparing dietary phthalate intake estimates with exposure limit values. For the majority of the population groups studied (Table 11.2), no health risks are to be expected. However, depending on the population group (Table 11.2), contribution percentage (Table 11.3), and exposure limit (Table 11.4) considered,

TABLE 11.4
TDI and RfD Values of DnBP, BBP, DEHP, and DiNP Including the Information (Endpoints Observed in Animals, NOAELs, and Uncertainty Factors) Used to Establish These Values

Compound	Limit Value (µg/kg bw/day)	Endpoint Observed in Animals	NOAEL (µg/kg bw/day)	Uncertainty Factor	Reference
TDI					
DnBP	10	Developmental effects (germ cell development) in rats (offspring)	2000[a]	200	EFSA (2005a)
BBP	500	Developmental effects (decreased anogenital distance) in rats (multigeneration study)	50,000	100	EFSA (2005b)
DEHP	50	Testicular (decreased testis weight) and developmental (germ cell depletion) effects in rats (multigeneration study)	5000	100	EFSA (2005c)
DiNP	150	Hepatic (spongiosis hepatis, increased levels of liver enzymes, and increased liver weight) and renal (increased kidney weights) effects in rats (2-year chronic toxicity study)	15,000	100	EFSA (2005d)
RfD for chronic oral exposure					
DnBP	100	Increased mortality in adult rats (subchronic to chronic study)	125,000	1000	US EPA (2007)
BBP	200	Increased liver-to-body weight and liver-to-brain weight ratios in adult rats (6-month study)	159,000	1000	US EPA (2007)
DEHP	20	Increased relative liver weight in adult guinea pigs (subchronic to chronic study)	19,000[a]	1000	US EPA (2007)

[a] Lowest observed adverse effect level instead of NOAEL.

exceedances of the TDI and/or RfD might take place for DnBP, DEHP, and DiNP for a certain percentage of the population. For instance, Bradley et al. (2013b) calculated a 97.5th percentile of up to 9.9 μg/kg bw/day for dietary DEHP exposure in British children between 1.5 and 4.5 years old. This intake estimate corresponds to 50% of the RfD that was established for DEHP. This means that 2.5% of the British children are exposed to DEHP via food ingestion in a percentage close to or within the range of the contribution percentage range of the diet to integral DEHP exposure observed in European children (i.e., 50–90%). For BBP, even the most stringent dietary exposure limit value of 12 μg/kg bw/day – calculated as the minimum dietary intake contribution percentage (6%, see also Table 11.3) of the lowest exposure limit value (200 μg/kg bw/day, see also Table 11.4) – is not being exceeded by the population groups investigated in the dietary studies listed in Table 11.2. So, no negative health effects related to BBP exposure are to be expected. With regard to DiBP, no risk assessment could be performed as no exposure limit value is available for this phthalate. Considering that DiBP – just like DiNP – is classified as a Category 2 substance on the European priority list of chemicals with potentially endocrine disrupting activities (European Commission, 2014), it is currently unclear if any health risks related to the current levels of DiBP exposure are to be expected.

11.5 CONCLUSIONS

This chapter handled the occurrence of phthalates—one of the world's most used group of plasticizers—in food. More exactly, it discussed the occurrence of five commonly monitored phthalate compounds (DiBP, DnBP, BBP, DEHP, and DiNP) in food products, their possible contamination sources, and related dietary exposure in humans. At the moment, dietary exposure to DEHP is the most common, followed by exposure to DiBP, DnBP, BBP, and DiNP. As food ingestion is not the only exposure route in humans, it is important to take the contribution of the diet to integral phthalate exposure into account when comparing dietary phthalate intake estimates with exposure limit values like TDI or RfD values. In general, no health risks associated to dietary phthalate exposure are to be expected for the majority of the population. However, in specific situations, there might be a chance that exceedances of the TDI and/or RfD might take place for DnBP, DEHP, and DiNP for a certain percentage of the population. Furthermore, it should be noticed that no risk assessment could be done for DiBP even though this compound has also been suspected to be an endocrine-disrupting compound. So, for this phthalate, it is still unclear if health risks are to be expected.

REFERENCES

Bosnir, J., D. Puntaric, A. Galic, I. Skes, T. Dijanic, M. Klaric, M. Grgic, M. Curkovic, and Z. Smit. 2007. Migration of phthalates from plastic containers into soft drinks and mineral water. *Food Technol. Biotechnol.* 45: 91–95.

Bradley, E.L., R.A. Burden, I. Leon, D.N. Mortimer, D.R. Speck, and L. Castle. 2013a. Determination of phthalate diesters in foods. *Food Addit. Contam Part A Chem. Anal. Control Expo. Risk Assess.* 30: 722–734.

Bradley, E.L., R.A. Burden, K. Bentayeb, M. Driffield, N. Harmer, D.N. Mortimer, D.R. Speck, J. Ticha, and L. Castle. 2013b. Exposure to phthalic acid, phthalate diesters and phthalate monoesters from foodstuffs: UK total diet study results. *Food Addit. Contam Part A Chem. Anal. Control Expo. Risk Assess.* 30: 735–742.

Bradley, E.L., W.A. Read, and L. Castle. 2007. Investigation into the migration potential of coating materials from cookware products. *Food Addit. Contam.* 24: 326–335.

Cao, X.L., W.D. Zhao, and R. Dabeka. 2015. Di-(2-ethylhexyl) adipate and 20 phthalates in composite food samples from the 2013 Canadian total diet study. *Food Addit. Contam Part A Chem. Anal. Control Expo. Risk Assess.* 32: 1893–1901.

Castle, L. 2007. Chemical migration into food: an overview. In: Barnes, K.A., Sinclair, C.R. and Watson, D.H. (eds.), *Chemical Migration and Food Contact Materials*, Woodhead Publishing Limited, Cambridge, pp. 1–13.

Chatonnet, P., S. Boutou, and A. Plana. 2014. Contamination of wines and spirits by phthalates: types of contaminants present, contamination sources and means of prevention. *Food Addit. Contam Part A Chem. Anal. Control Expo. Risk Assess.* 31: 1605–1615.

Clark, K., R.M. David, R. Guinn, K.W. Kramarz, M.A. Lampi, and C.A. Staples. 2011. Modeling human exposure to phthalate esters: a comparison of indirect and biomonitoring estimations methods. *Hum. Ecol. Risk Assess.* 17: 923–965.

Cousins, I.T., D. Mackay, and T.F. Parkerton. 2003. Physical-chemical properties and evaluative fate modelling of phthalate esters. In: Staples, C.A. (ed.), *The Handbook of Environmental Chemistry: Phthalate Esters*, Springer, Berlin, Germany, pp. 57–84.

Du, Q.Z., J.W. Wang, X.W. Fu, and H.L. Xia. 2010. Diffusion and accumulation in cultivated vegetable plants of di-(2-ethylhexyl) phthalate (DEHP) from a plastic production factory. *Food Addit. Contam.* 27: 1186–1192.

Du, Q.Z., X.W. Fu, and H.L. Xia. 2009. Uptake of di-(2-ethylhexyl)phthalate from plastic mulch film by vegetable plants. *Food Addit. Contam.* 26: 1325–1329.

ECHA. 2015. Regulations—REACH. Helsinki, Finland, European Chemicals Agency. http://echa.europa.eu/regulations/reach.

ECPI. 2014. Plasticisers. Brussels, Belgium, European Council for Plasticisers and Intermediates. www.plasticisers.org

EFSA. 2005a. Opinion of the scientific panel on food additives, flavourings, processing aids and material in contact with food (AFC) on a request from the commission related to di-Butylphthalate (DBP) for use in food contact materials: Question N° EFSA-Q-2003-192. *The EFSA Journal* 242: 1–2.

EFSA. 2005b. Opinion of the scientific panel on food additives, flavourings, processing aids and materials in contact with food (AFC) on a request from the commission related to butylbenzylphthalate (BBP) for use in food contact materials: Question N° EFSA-Q-2003-190. *The EFSA Journal* 241: 1–2.

EFSA. 2005c. Opinion of the scientific panel on food additives, flavourings, processing aids and materials in contact with food (AFC) on a request from the commission related to Bis(2-ethylhexyl)phthalate (DEHP) for use in food contact materials: Question N° EFSA-Q-2003-191. *The EFSA Journal* 243: 1–2.

EFSA. 2005d. Opinion of the scientific panel on food additives, flavourings, processing aids and materials in contact with food (AFC) on a request from the commission related to Di-isononylphthalate (DINP) for use in food contact materials: Question N° EFSA-Q-2003-194. *The EFSA Journal* 244: 1–2.

European Commission. 2014. Endocrine disruptors. Brussels, Belgium, European Commission—Environment DG. http://ec.europa.eu/environment/chemicals/endocrine/index_en.htm

Feng, Y.L., J. Zhu, and R. Sensenstein. 2005. Development of a headspace solid-phase microextraction method combined with gas chromatography mass spectrometry for the determination of phthalate esters in cow milk. *Anal. Chim. Acta* 538: 41–48.

Fierens, T., M. Van Holderbeke, H. Willems, S. De Henauw, and I. Sioen. 2012a. Phthalates in Belgian cow's milk and the role of feed and other contamination pathways at farm level. *Food Chem. Toxicol.* 50: 2945–2953.

Fierens, T., G. Vanermen, M. Van Holderbeke, S. De Henauw, and I. Sioen. 2012b. Effect of cooking at home on the levels of eight phthalates in foods. *Food Chem. Toxicol.* 50: 4428–4435.

Fierens, T., M. Van Holderbeke, H. Willems, S. De Henauw, and I. Sioen. 2013. Transfer of eight phthalates through the milk chain—A case study. *Environ. Int.* 51: 1–7.

Fromme, H., L. Gruber, M. Schlummer, G. Wolz, S. Boehmer, J. Angerer, R. Mayer, B. Liebl, and G. Bolte. 2007. Intake of phthalates and di(2-ethylhexyl)adipate: Results of the integrated exposure assessment survey based on duplicate diet samples and biomonitoring data. *Environ. Int.* 33: 1012–1020.

Gärtner, S., M. Balski, M. Koch, and I. Nehls. 2009. Analysis and migration of phthalates in infant food packed in recycled paperboard. *J. Agric. Food Chem.* 57: 10675–10681.

Grandjean, P., J. Toppari, R. Sharpe, E. Gray, P. Foster, N.E. Skakkebaek, S. Swan, K. Main, A. Calafat, T. Schettler, F. Bro-Rasmusssen, and D. Gee. 2006. Possible effects of phthalate exposure in doses relevant for humans. *Int. J. Androl.* 29: 181–185.

Guo, Y., Z.F. Zhang, L.Y. Liu, Y.F. Li, N.Q. Ren, and K. Kannan. 2012. Occurrence and profiles of phthalates in foodstuffs from China and their implications for human exposure. *J. Agric. Food. Chem.* 60: 6913–6919.

He, M., C. Yang, R.J. Geng, X.G. Zhao, L. Hong, X.F. Piao, T. Chen, M. Quinto, and D.H. Li. 2015. Monitoring of phthalates in foodstuffs using gas purge microsyringe extraction coupled with GC-MS. *Anal. Chim. Acta* 879: 63–68.

Heinemeyer, G., C. Sommerfeld, A. Springer, A. Heiland, O. Lindtner, M. Greiner, T. Heuer, C. Krems, and A. Conrad. 2013. Estimation of dietary intake of bis(2-ethylhexyl)phthalate (DEHP) by consumption of food in the German population. *Int. J. Hyg. Environ. Health* 216: 472–480.

Hernández-Díaz, S., Y.-C. Sua, A.A. Mitchell, K.E. Kelley, A.M. Calafat, and R. Hauser. 2013. Medications as a potential source of exposure to phthalates among women of childbearing age. *Reprod. Toxicol.* 37: 1–5.

Hoppin, J.A., R. Jaramillo, S.J. London, R.J. Bertelsen, P.M. Salo, D.P. Sandler, and D.C. Zeldin. 2013. Phthalate exposure and allergy in the U.S. population: Results from NHANES 2005–2006. *Environ. Health Perspect.* 121: 1129–1134.

Ishida, M. 1993. Reduction of phthalate in chicken eggs, liver and meat by several cooking methods. *J. Food Hyg. Soc. Japan* 34: 529–531.

Ji, Y.Q., F.M. Wang, L.B. Zhang, C.Y. Shan, Z.P. Bai, Z.R. Sun, L.L. Liu, and B.X. Shen. 2014. A comprehensive assessment of human exposure to phthalates from environmental media and food in Tianjin, China. *J. Hazard. Mater.* 279: 133–140.

Lee, J., J.H. Lee, C.K. Kim, and M. Thomsen. 2014. Childhood exposure to DEHP, DBP and BBP under existing chemical management systems: a comparative study of sources of childhood exposure in Korea and in Denmark. *Environ. Int.* 63: 77–91.

Li, Z., F. Xue, L. Xu, C. Peng, H. Kuang, T. Ding, C. Xu, C. Sheng, Y. Gong, and L. Wang. 2011. Simultaneous determination of nine types of phthalate residues in commercial milk products using HPLC–ESI-MS–MS. *J. Chromatogr. Sci.* 49: 338–343.

Mackintosh, C.E., J. Maldonado, H.W. Jing, N. Hoover, A. Chong, M.G. Ikonomou, and F.A.P.C. Gobas. 2004. Distribution of phthalate esters in a marine aquatic food web: Comparison to polychlorinated biphenyls. *Environ. Sci. Technol.* 38: 2011–2020.

Müller, A.K., E. Nielsen, O. Ladefoged, and Institute of Food Safety and Nutrition. 2003. Human exposure to selected phthalates in Denmark. Soborg, Denmark, The Danish Veterinary and Food Administration.

Official Journal of the European Union. 2005. Directive 2005/84/EC of the European Parliament and of the Council of 14 December 2005 amending for the 22nd time Council Directive 76/769/EEC on the approximation of the laws, regulations and administrative provisions of the Member States relating to restrictions on the marketing and use of certain dangerous substances and preparations (phthalates in toys and childcare articles), No. L344, 40–43.

Official Journal of the European Union. 2011. Commission Regulation (EU) No 10/2011 of 14 January 2011 on plastic materials and articles intended to come into contact with food, No. L12, 1–89.

Pedersen, G.A., L.K. Jensen, A. Fankhauser-Noti, S. Biedermann-Brem, J.H. Petersen, and B. Fabech. 2008. Migration of epoxidized soybean oil (ESBO) and phthalates from twist closures into food and enforcement of the overall migration limit. *Food Addit. Contam.* 25: 503–510.

Peters, R.J.B. 2006. Man-made chemicals in food products. TNO-report 2006-A-R0095/B version 2. Apeldoorn, the Netherlands, TNO Built Environment and Geosciences.

Rhind, S.M., C.E. Kyle, C. Mackie, and G. Telfer. 2007. Effects of exposure of ewes to sewage sludge-treated pasture on phthalate and alkyl phenol concentrations in their milk. *Sci. Total Environ.* 383: 70–80.

Rudel, R.A., and L.J. Perovich. 2009. Endocrine disrupting chemicals in indoor and outdoor air. *Atmos. Environ.* 43: 170–181.

Sakhi, A.K., I.T.L. Lillegaard, S. Voorspoels, M.H. Carlsen, E.B. Loken, A.L. Brantsaeter, M. Haugen, H.M. Meltzer, and C. Thomsen. 2014. Concentrations of phthalates and bisphenol A in Norwegian foods and beverages and estimated dietary exposure in adults. *Environ. Int.* 73: 259–269.

Santana, J., C. Giraudi, E. Marengo, E. Robotti, S. Pires, I. Nunes, and E.M. Gaspar. 2014. Preliminary toxicological assessment of phthalate esters from drinking water consumed in Portugal. *Environ. Sci. Pollut. R.* 21: 1380–1390.

Schecter, A., M. Lorber, Y. Guo, Q. Wu, S.H. Yun, K. Kannan, M. Hommel, N. Imran, L.S. Hynan, D.L. Cheng, J.A. Colacino, and L.S. Birnbaum. 2013. Phthalate concentrations and dietary exposure from food purchased in New York state. *Environ. Health Perspect.* 121: 473–479.

Sharman, M., W.A. Read, L. Castle, and J. Gilbert. 1994. Levels of di-(2-ethylhexyl) phthalate and total phthalate esters in milk, cream, butter and cheese. *Food Addit. Contam.* 11: 375–385.

Sioen, I., T. Fierens, M. Van Holderbeke, L. Geerts, M. Bellemans, M. De Maeyer, K. Servaes, G. Vanermen, P.E. Boon, and S. De Henauw. 2012. Phthalates dietary exposure and food sources for Belgian preschool children and adults. *Environ. Int.* 48: 102–108.

Sorensen, L.K. 2006. Determination of phthalates in milk and milk products by liquid chromatography/tandem mass spectrometry. *Rapid Commun. Mass Spectrom.* 20: 1135–1143.

Stahlhut, R.W., W.E. van Wijngaarden, T.D. Dye, S. Cook, and S.H. Swan. 2007. Concentrations of urinary phthalate metabolites are associated with increased waist circumference and insulin resistance in adult U.S. males. *Environ. Health Perspect.* 115: 876–882.

Swan, S.H. 2008. Environmental phthalate exposure in relation to reproductive outcomes and other health endpoints in humans. *Environ. Res.* 108: 177–184.

Tsumura, Y., S. Ishimitsu, A. Kaihara, K. Yoshii, Y. Nakamura, and Y. Tonogai. 2001a. Di(2-ethylhexyl) phthalate contamination of retail packed lunches caused by PVC gloves used in the preparation of foods. *Food Addit. Contam.* 18: 569–579.

Tsumura, Y., S. Ishimitsu, Y. Nakamura, K. Yoshii, A. Kaihara, and Y. Tonogai. 2001b. Contents of eleven phthalates and di(2-ethylhexyl) adipate in retail packed lunches after prohibition of DEHP-containing PVC gloves for cooking purposes. *Shokuhin Eiseigaku Zasshi* 42: 128–132.

US EPA. 2007. Phthalates—TEACH chemical summary. Washington DC, US Environmental Protection Agency.

Van Holderbeke, M., L. Geerts, G. Vanermen, K. Servaes, I. Sioen, S. De Henauw, and T. Fierens. 2014. Determination of contamination pathways of phthalates in food products sold on the Belgian market. *Environ. Res.* 134: 345–352.

WHO. 2000. Hazardous chemicals in human and environmental health. Geneva, Switzerland, World Health Organization.

Wormuth, M., M. Scheringer, M. Vollenweider, and K. Hungerbuhler. 2006. What are the sources of exposure to eight frequently used phthalic acid esters in Europeans? *Risk Anal.* 26: 803–824.

Yan, H., X. Cheng, and B. Liu. 2011. Simultaneous determination of six phthalate esters in bottled milks using ultrasound-assisted dispersive liquid–liquid microextraction coupled with gas chromatography. *J. Chromatogr.* 879: 2507–2512.

Yin, R., X.G. Lin, S.G. Wang, and H.Y. Zhang. 2003. Effect of DBP/DEHP in vegetable planted soil on the quality of capsicum fruit. *Chemosphere* 50: 801–805.

12 Dioxins and Dioxin-Like Compounds in Food

Agata Witczak

CONTENTS

12.1 INTRODUCTION

The term “dioxins” commonly refers to a group of aromatic organochlorine compounds, such as polychlorinated dibenzo-*p*-dioxins (PCDDs) and polychlorinated dibenzofurans (PCDFs), which are highly toxic environmental pollutants widely distributed in all global ecosystems. There are 75 PCDDs and 135 PCDF congeners—7 and 10 of them, respectively, being specifically toxic. In these compounds, hydrogen atoms have been substituted with chlorine atoms at a number of positions (Figure 12.1). Additionally, due to similar properties and common mechanisms of action, the word “dioxins” refers also to 12 out of 209 congeners of polychlorinated biphenyls (PCBs)—those that do not have chlorine substitution in any *ortho* position or have maximum one (Fiedler 2003). All these compounds belong to the group of dangerous chemicals known as persistent organic pollutants (POPs).

12.2 PHYSICOCHEMICAL PROPERTIES

The toxic effect of dioxins and dioxin-like (DL) compounds results directly from their chemical structures as well as physicochemical properties.

Dioxins and furans are nonpolar compounds poorly soluble in water (from 419 ng/dm^3 for 2,3,7,8-Cl_4DF, 7.9 and 19.3 ng/dm^3 for 2,3,7,8-Cl_4DD to 0.074 ng/dm^3) but highly soluble in organic solvents. They have a great affinity for fat (solubility in organic/fatty matrices log K_{OW} ranges from 5.6 for Cl_4DF and 6.1/7.1 for Cl_4DD to 8.2 for Cl_8DD). Their thermal decomposition is possible only above 850°C. PCDDs and PCDFs may break down at 1000°C when the reacting gas contains dust to which they may absorb in the combustion process (Fiedler 2003). This is used in the thermal destruction of waste when high temperature and excess oxygen reduce emission of dioxins to the atmosphere (McKay 2002, Kulkarni et al. 2008).

Attaching halogen atoms in the positions 2,3,7, and 8 in molecules of PCDDs or PCDFs (there are 17 such compounds) makes them highly toxic. Therefore, 2,3,7,8-tetrachlorodibenzo-*p*-dioxin commonly known as TCDD is the most toxic one. It is

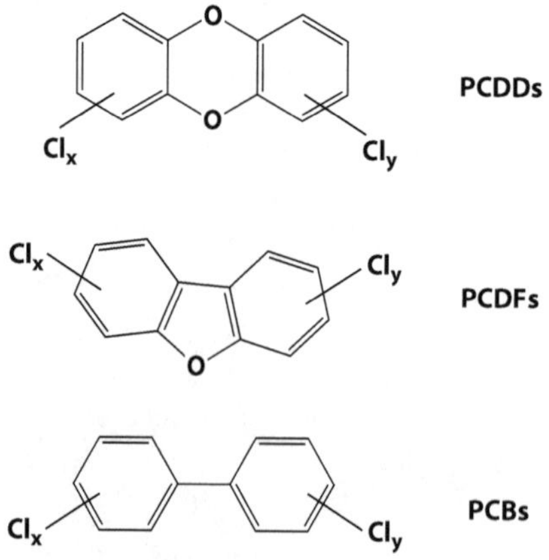

FIGURE 12.1 Structures of PCDDs, PCDFs, and PCBs.

highly resistant to temperature but UV radiation can easily break it down. Its photolysis was observed at the UV length of $\lambda = 290–300$ nm (Kim and O'Keefe 2000).

PCDFs frequently coexist with PCDDs. PCDFs may be formed from pyrolysis or combustion of chlorine-containing products or in the presence of chlorine donors (e.g., PCV) at temperature below 1200°C. PCDFs are low-volatile, colorless solid bodies with physicochemical and toxic properties similar to those of PCDDs.

As PCDD/Fs are persistent and lipophilic, they are absorbed strongly in soil or suspended dust. They biodegrade poorly and, thus, accumulate in sediments, sewage sludge, and both aquatic and terrestrial fauna—mainly their tetra-, penta-, hexa-, hepta-, and okta-isomers.

Dioxin traces were already found in samples originating several thousand years ago. Their natural sources are volcanic eruptions, forest fires, or atmospheric discharges. They are hazardous, however, mainly due to man's activities. The main sources of PCDD/Fs in the environment, generated as unintentional by-products, are as follows: combustion of organic chlorine-containing substances, for example, thermal processing of recyclable waste, uncontrolled incineration of industrial, municipal, and hospital waste in technologically obsolete incinerating plants and boiler rooms, combustion of heating and vehicle fuel, as well as coal and waste combustion in obsolete furnaces used for heating buildings. Such compounds are also present in ambient air as a result of traffic (tire wear and exhaust gases). Dioxins have never been produced intentionally and they have never had any technical applications.

In contrast to PCDD/Fs, PCBs have been used since the 1930s in a number of man's activities in closed applications (as a major component of dielectric fluids in transformers, capacitors, air conditioners, electromagnets), semi-closed applications (hydraulic fluids, heat transfer fluids, voltage regulators, vacuum pumps), and open-end applications (lubricants, adhesives, protective surface coatings, sealants, inks, paints, plasticizers). They were used so vastly because of their good physical and chemical properties, namely, thermal resistance, low combustibility, passivity, stability, and dielectric properties. They are resistant to acids and bases. Their solubility in water decreases, along with increasing chlorinity, from 1 to 5 mg/dm^3 for monochlorobiphenyls to 0.015 mg/dm^3 for decachlorobiphenyl (Giesy and Kannan 1998).

PCBs were manufactured from 1950 to the 1970s, as mixtures of 50–130 congeners, and at the peak, the PCB global production accounted for 100,000 tones/year. Due to some reports showing their toxic effect on living organisms, their production, sale, and usage were significantly reduced in Western Europe and North America (Swanson et al. 1995), while in Eastern Europe and Russia their production was carried on until the early 1990s (Dobson and van Esch 1993). PCBs are persistent and they do not biodegrade easily. At present, PCDDs, PCDFs, and PCBs may be still released into the environment and deposited in living organisms due to damaged equipment, improper storage and utilization of worked-out equipment, leakage from landfill waste, incineration, evaporation, or disposal of industrial waste. Moreover, bottom sediments of many rivers, lakes, and seas are a significant reservoir of PCBs. Some 60% of PCB global production was released into the seas and oceans, of which about 30% was accumulated in the coastal bottom sediments. PCBs transform in the environment very slowly, for years and decades, and their transformation rate depends on the number of chlorine atoms in the biphenyl skeleton. Half-lives of PCDD/Fs in marine sediments vary from 25 to 275 years.

There are two main differences between PCBs and PCDD/Fs to be mentioned. The first one refers to their sources in the environment and food, and the second one refers to higher vapor pressure of PCBs, thus, higher volatility. Moreover, PCBs bioaccumulate more easily in the trophic chain, particularly in the aquatic ecosystems.

The compounds having up to four chlorine atoms in the molecule have been shown to undergo partial biodegradation. They may be broken down by the microorganisms present in sewage. Some risk is combined with the fact that mezophilous and thermophilous fermentation can dechlorate PCBs to, dioxin-like congeners (Engwall et al. 2002).

12.3 HEALTH EFFECTS

12.3.1 Absorption, Accumulation, and Excretion of PCDD/Fs and DL-PCBs

PCDDs, PCDFs, and DL-PCBs contribute to dioxin toxicity in humans and wildlife after bioaccumulation through the food chain from the environment. Dioxin toxicity depends on the degree of chlorination and the species sensitivity of the exposed organisms.

Dioxins are absorbed by a human body through inhalation (8%), for example, by breathing air contaminated by smoke and dust to which they absorb, through dermal exposure (2%)—by epidermis, sebaceous glands, or hair bulbs, but primarily through ingestion (90%), especially of fatty food. Food rich in animal fat and breast milk for infants are the predominant sources of exposure to PCDD/PCDFs. The share of inhalation exposure in the general intake is rather small, but in highly industrialized areas with heavy traffic, inhaling dioxins may account for a higher percentage of the total intake. Some recent incidents of poisoning with these compounds are shown in Table 12.1.

The contaminants are rapidly absorbed from the gastrointestinal tract, and accumulate primarily in the liver, adipose tissues, and milk fat (Durand et al. 2008). It has been shown that 25–70% of 2,3,7,8-TCDD dose is accumulated in the liver. Dioxins bind to lipids and lipoproteins in the blood plasma; this way they are transported to the internal organs. A planar structure of chlorine atoms in the positions 2,3,7, and 8 increases dioxin ability to accumulate in the liver . Planar particles inhibit the activity of P-450 cytochrome, which results in a decreased rate of the body metabolism. The congeners with 5 and 6 chlorine atoms in the molecule have higher ability to accumulate in the liver than 2,3,7,8-TCDD (Diliberto et al. 1993). For all dioxin congeners, the metabolic transformation covers oxidative and reductive dechlorination and disruption of the oxygen bridge. Also conjugation with glutathione may undergo during the methabolic transformation, as evidenced by the presence of sulfur-containing glucuronide conjugates in the bile.

Dioxins are excreted from the human body mainly with feces and bile, as hydroxylic derivatives and conjugated compounds. In nursing mothers, however, lactation may be the main route of dioxin elimination from the body. At least 20% of the maternal body burden of some POPs may be excreted during the first 6 months of breast-feeding. The decrease in half-life is congener specific, and depends on the breast-feeding duration (Milbrath et al. 2009). Thus, on one hand, lactation promotes detoxification of the mother's body; on the other hand, it increases the risk posed to her child.

TABLE 12.1
Examples of Poisoning with PCDDs and PCBs

Year	Country	Product	Source
2000	Spain	Animal feed	PCP-contaminated sawdust as carrier in premixed choline chloride
2003	Germany	Animal feed	Use of waste wood for drying of the bakery waste
2004	Italy	Eggs, meat	Wood-shaving litter
2004	The Netherlands	Milk	Potato by-products (serving as animal feed) contaminated by kaolinitic clay
2006	The Netherlands	Pig feed	Waste fat contaminated by improperly filtered HCl used for gelatine production
2008	India	Guar gum	Use of pentachlorophenol
2008	Italy	Mozzarella from buffalo milk	Illegal waste burning
2008	Ireland	Pork and beef	PCB-contaminated fuel for direct drying of animal feed (bakery waste)
2008	Korea	Pork	Contaminated zinc oxide as feed ingredient from Chile
2008	The Netherlands	Feed additive	Brominated contaminants including brominated dioxins
2011	Germany	Animal feed	Fatty acids from a biodiesel company

Source: Based on Malisch, R. and A. Kotz, *Sci Total Environ*, 491–492, 2–10, 2014.

12.3.2 Mechanism of Action and Toxicity of PCDD/Fs and DL-PCBs

Dermal lesions, occurring mainly on the face and the nape of the neck, are caused by epidermal hyperplasia and hyperkeratosis around hair follicles, hyperkeratosis of hair follicles, and chloracne. Except for chloracne, when an organism is exposed to high concentration of dioxins, they also cause induction of microsomal enzymes, impaired breathing, conjunctivitis, and hepatomegaly. Acute exposure to dioxins leads to nausea, hyperhidrosis, dehydration, weight loss, irritation of eyes, skin and the respiratory system, fatty liver, cyanosis, as well as chloracne. Dioxins cause complex damage in the internal organs, endocrine, immunological, and reproductive systems, and they are strong promoters of tumor development (Fiedler 2003).

The mechanism of toxic action of PCDD/Fs and DL-PCBs is associated with forming complexes of dioxin and the cytosolic aryl hydrocarbon receptor (AhR), inducing the expression of genes that control the system of microsomal monooxygenases. The rate of induction is affected by the dose of ligand, size of ligand molecule, metabolism (that reduces affinity), planar structure of aromatic rings (opening a ring, thus loosing a planar structure reduces the affinity), chlorine substitution in minimum three positions (congeners with four chlorine substitutions are the most active) (Cuthill et al. 1991). AhR is very similar to the steroid hormone receptor in terms of structure and operation. The gene expression leads to forming a number of cytochrome P-450 forms, that is, the enzyme acting as a monooxygenase. The intense production of the cytochromes results in inducing in the liver such enzymes as aryl hydrocarbons hydroxylase (AHN) and ethoxyresorufin-*O*-deethylase (EROD).

Moreover, dioxins may induce or inhibit other genes. This leads to uncontrolled function of the genes and a number of toxic effects in living organisms (DeVito et al. 1995, Kato et al. 2007).

The carcinogen effects may be observed in people with chronic occupational exposure to high dioxin emissions or those who were in the vicinity of some accidents or chemical disasters resulting in TCDD/F and PCB releases. As examples may serve mass poisonings caused by contaminated rice bran oil—in Japan in 1968 (Yusho disease) and in Taiwan in 1979 (Yu-cheng disease) (Tsukimori et al. 2012). A severe disaster also occured in Seveso in 1976, where a reactor producing 2,4,5-trichlorophenol exploded releasing more than 1 kg of 2,3,7,8-TCDD to the atmosphere (Pesatori et al. 2009). As a result, first regulations on the control of major-accident hazards (Council Directive 96/82/EC) were enacted.

Xenobiotics may pose a serious risk to young organisms, infants, and babies. Dioxin compounds pass through the placental barrier what is particularly dangerous during the first trimester of pregnancy; as being teratogens, they cause fetal death and malformations. Infants born to mothers exposed to dioxins (e.g., Yusho women) were reported to have decreased birth weight (Tsukimori et al. 2012). Additionally, maternal breast milk contaminated with dioxins poses a serious health risk to breast-fed children due to, *inter alia*, neurotoxicity, endocrine disruption, immune system suppression, and adverse effects on psychomotor development and intellectual function.

The International Agency for Research on Cancer (IARC) has so far classified 2,3,7,8-TCDD, PCB 126 (3,4,5,3′,4′-pentachlorobiphenyl), and 2,3,4,7,8-PCDF, as Group 1: "Carcinogenic to humans" (Cogliano et al. 2011). In majority, tumors are detected in soft tissues, lungs, liver, thyroid, tongue, and lymphatic system. Dioxin-like compounds exert also xenoestrogenic and neurotoxic activity (Carpenter 2006).

Taking into account the omnipresence of dioxins, their long half-life in humans (6 years), and excretion taking 7–10 years (Fattore et al. 2008), long-term consumption of food even minimally contaminated will result in their accumulation in human tissues. Repeated exposure to small concentrations of dioxins may result in serious health problems of the future generations.

12.4 HEALTH RISK ASSESSMENT

12.4.1 TEQ Concept

In order to standardize the evaluation criteria, the concentrations of DL-PCBs, PCDDs, and PCDFs are expressed as toxic equivalents (TEQs). TEQ provides information on the toxicity of the chemical compounds in tested material; however, it takes into account only the toxic activity equivalent to the dioxin toxicity. According to the WHO (1998), toxic equivalency factor (TEF) values for individual congeners in combination with their chemical concentration can be used to calculate the total TCDD TEQs, contributed by all dioxin-like congeners in the mixture using the following Equation 12.1, which assumes dose additivity:

$$\mathrm{TEQ} = \Sigma_i\left(\mathrm{PCDD}_i \cdot \mathrm{TEF}_i\right) + \Sigma_i\left(\mathrm{PCDF}_i \cdot \mathrm{TEF}_i\right) + \Sigma_i\left(\mathrm{PCB}_i \cdot \mathrm{TEF}_i\right)\left(\mathrm{pg/kg}\right) \quad (12.1)$$

where:

TEQ—total 2,3,7,8-TCDD–like activity of the mixture,

$PCDD_i$, $PCDF_i$, PCB_i—concentration of the *i*th PCDD/PCDF/PCB congener,

TEF_i—toxic equivalency factor for PCDD, PCDF, PCB congeners in the reference to 2,3,7,8-TCDD (Table 12.2).

TABLE 12.2
WHO_{05} Toxic Equivalency Factors

Compound	$TEF_{WHO_{05}}$
PCDDs	
2,3,7,8-TetraCDD	1
1,2,3,7,8-PentaCDD	1
1,2,3,4,7,8-HexaCDD	0.1
1,2,3,6,7,8-HexaCDD	0.1
1,2,3,7,8,9-HexaCDD	0.1
1,2,3,4,6,7,8-HeptaCDD	0.01
1,2,3,4,6,7,8,9-OctaCDD	0.0003
PCDFs	
2,3,7,8-TetraCDF	0.1
1,2,3,7,8-PentaCDF	0.03
2,3,4,7,8-PentaCDF	0.3
1,2,3,4,7,8-HexaCDF	0.1
1,2,3,6,7,8-HexaCDF	0.1
2,3,4,6,7,8-HexaCDF	0.1
1,2,3,7,8,9-HexaCDF	0.1
1,2,3,4,6,7,8-HeptaCDF	0.01
1,2,3,4,7,8,9-HeptaCDF	0.01
1,2,3,4,6,7,8,9-OctaCDF	0.0003
PCBs	
3,3′4,4′-TetraCB (PCB 77)	0.0001
3,4,4′,5-TetraCB (PCB 81)	0.0003
2,3,3′,4,4′-PentaCB (PCB 105)	0.00003
2,3,4,4′,5-PentaCB (PCB 114)	0.00003
2,3′,4,4′,5-PentaCB (PCB 118)	0.00003
2′,3,4,4′,5-PentaCB (PCB 123)	0.00003
3,3′,4,4′,5-PentaCB (PCB 126)	0.1
2,3,3′,4,4′,5-HexaCB (PCB 156)	0.00003
2,3,3′,4,4′,5′-HexaCB (PCB 157)	0.00003
2,3′,4,4′,5,5′-HexaCB (PCB 167)	0.00003
3,3′,4,4′,5,5′-HexaCB (PCB 169)	0.03
2,3,3′,4,4′,5,5′-HeptaCB (PCB 189)	0.00003

Source: Van den Berg, M. et al., *Toxicol Sci*, 93, 223–241, 2006.

The TEQ application has its drawbacks owing to some simplifications made. One of them is the assumption that toxic action of the mixture components has an additive character, which results in neglecting the possibility of their synergistic and antagonistic interactions. Moreover, the toxicokinetic differences among individual congeners are not always taken into account. Also some health effects may remain undetected, as the endpoints of toxicity testing in animals may be inappropriate for detecting certain health effects. Nevertheless, no method with lesser uncertainty than the TEF/TEQ concept (Equation 12.1) has been developed so far (Van den Berg et al. 2006).

TEFs for PCDD/PCDF/PCB congeners are based on:

1. Structural similarity to dioxins,
2. Persistency and bioaccumulation in the food chain,
3. The capacity to bind to the Ah receptor and to elicit AhR-mediated biochemical and toxic responses at a short-term or a medium-term exposure.

Although the TEF scheme and the TEQ methodology became widely used, their use must be periodically reevaluated. The WHO has recommended their reevaluation approximately every 5 years to account for new scientific information (WHO 1998). The most recent review of the TEFs and TEQ methodology was completed by the WHO in 2005 (Van den Berg et al. 2006).

TEF values have so far been determined for 7 PCDDs, 10 PCDFs, and 12 coplanar PCBs that are regarded toxic (Table 12.2). In the scale of toxicity, the isomers 2,3,7,8-TCDD and 1,2,3,7,8-PCDD are the most toxic. The PCB-derived risk for living organisms results mainly from the toxicity of some PCB congeners, namely, non-*ortho* and mono-*ortho* compounds, which means PCBs having no chlorine substitution in *ortho* position or having maximum one (Table 12.2) (WHO 2000, Van den Berg et al. 2006).

The United States Environmental Protection Agency (US EPA) as well as several states, countries, and international agencies have adopted the WHO 2005 TEF scheme. Wide usage of the WHO 2005 TEF scheme will facilitate the comparison of environmental measurements to national and international databases.

The variability in relative toxicity of individual compounds listed in Table 12.2 may have an insignificant impact on an individual risk estimate. According to the US EPA draft reassessment, only five compounds (2,3,7,8-TCDD, 1,2,3,7,8-PentaCDD, 1,2,3,6,7,8-HexaCDD, 2,3,4,7,8-PentaCDF, and PCB 126) account for 70–80% of the TCDD TEQ in the human body and food products. Variability in the relative toxicity reported in the literature for these five compounds is much lower than for other compounds (US EPA 2003).

Risk assessment of dietary exposure to dioxins is usually determined as tolerable weekly intake (TWI) or tolerable daily intake (TDI). TDIs and TWIs are calculated on the basis of laboratory toxicity data, usually from studies in laboratory animals and sometimes also from human studies, to which TEFs are applied. The TWI for dioxins and DL-PCBs has been established by the Scientific Committee on Food (SCF) in the European Union as 14 pg WHO-TEQ/kg body weight.

Thus, the health risk posed by the chemicals depends on their dietary intake and increases when the TWI gets exceeded (CAC 2001, Commission Regulation (EC) No. 1881/2006 of 19 December 2006). The TDIs recommended by the WHO for dioxins and DL-PCBs are within 1–4 pg TEQ/kg body weight (Van Leeuwen et al. 2000).

Regarding the persistency of dioxin compounds, important is to assess also long-term risks to health posed by these substances. Total or average intake needs to be assessed over months, and the tolerable intake needs to be assessed over a period of at least 1 month. WHO (2010) has established for dioxins a provisional tolerable monthly intake (PTMI) of 70 pg/kg per month, which is the amount of dioxins that can be ingested over lifetime without detectable health effects.

12.4.2 Regulations

Regulations concerning toxic compounds in food will be discussed in Chapter 19. This section focuses on regulations concerning dioxins and dioxin-like compounds in food, as they are of importance for the issue of health risk assessment of these chemicals.

Under the Stockholm Convention of May 22, 2001, PCDDs, PCDFs, and PCBs have been classified as compounds highly toxic to the environment, so-called POPs.

Detailed EU standards of the maximum residue levels (MRLs) of PCDD/Fs and PCBs in foodstuffs are set in the Commission Regulation (EC) No. 1881/2006 of December 19, 2006. However, stricter maximum levels of PCDD/Fs and DL-PCBs were amended in another Commission Regulation (EC) No. 1259/2011 (Table 12.3), which has also distinguished a significant group of raw materials and foodstuffs intended for infants and young children (Table 12.3).

Outside the European Union, in various regions of the globe, also other dioxin exposure guidelines are defined on national and international levels (Table 12.4).

12.4.3 Problems with Assessing Health Risks

The problems with assessing health risks are frequently caused by:

1. Analytical difficulties associated with trace levels of these compounds,
2. Difficulty in assessing the threshold dose for a certain toxic effect,
3. Multiple directions in the action mechanisms of certain substances,
4. Transformations of xenobiotics both in the external environment and in human body leading to formation of new, frequently unknown, compounds with different toxicodynamic properties,
5. Toxic interactions (synergism, antagonism) in an organism,
6. Difficulty in translating the results of *in vivo* and *in vitro* laboratory research into actual conditions, and
7. Occurrence of adverse health effects in the future generations.

TABLE 12.3
MRLs of PCDDs, PCDFs, and DL-PCBs in Foodstuffs

	Maximum Levels		
Foodstuffs	**Total WHO-PCDD/F-TEQ**	**Total WHO-PCDD/F-PCB-TEQ**	**Total WHO-DL-PCB-TEQ**
Meat and meat products (excluding edible offal) of the following animals:			
• bovine animals and sheep	2.5 pg/g fat	4.0 pg/g fat	1.5 pg/g fat
• poultry	1.75 pg/g fat	3.0 pg/g fat	1.25 pg/g fat
• pigs	1.0 pg/g fat	1.25 pg/g fat	0.25 pg/g fat
Liver of bovine animals, sheep, poultry, and pigs, and derived products thereof	4.5 pg/g fat	10.0 pg/g fat	5.5 pg/g fat
Muscle meat of fish and fishery products and products thereof excluding wild caught eel. The maximum level for crustaceans applies to muscle meat from appendages and abdomen For crabs and crab-like crustaceans (*Brachyura* and *Anomura*) it applies to muscle meat from appendages[a]	3.5 pg/g wet weight	6.5 pg/g wet weight	3.0 pg/g wet weight
Muscle meat of wild caught freshwater fish with the exception of diadromous fish species caught in freshwater, and products thereof	3.5 pg/g wet weight	6.5 pg/g wet weight	3.0 pg/g wet weight
Muscle meat of wild caught eel and products thereof	3.5 pg/g wet weight	10.0 pg/g wet weight	8.0 pg/g wet weight
Fish liver and derived products thereof with the exception of marine oils from marine organisms[b]	–	20.0 pg/g wet weight[c]	
Marine oils intended for human consumption	1.75 pg/g fat	6.0 pg/g fat	4.25 pg/g fat
Raw milk and dairy products, including butter fat	2.5 pg/g fat	5.5 pg/g fat	3.0 pg/g fat
Hen eggs and egg products	2.5 pg/g fat	5.0 pg/g fat	2.5 pg/g fat
Fat of the following animals:			
• bovine animals and sheep	2.5 pg/g fat	4.0 pg/g fat	1.5 pg/g fat
• poultry	1.75 pg/g fat	3.0 pg/g fat	2.0 pg/g fat
• pigs	1.0 pg/g fat	1.25 pg/g fat	0.5 pg/g fat
Mixed animal fats	2.0 pg/g fat	3.0 pg/g fat	1.0 pg/g fat
Vegetable oils and fats	0.75 pg/g fat	1.5 pg/g fat	0.75 pg/g fat
Food for infants and young children[d]	0.1 pg/g wet weight	0.2 pg/g wet weight	0.1 pg/g wet weight

Source: Based on Commission Regulation (EC) No. 1881/2006 with amendments in the Commission Regulation (EC) No. 1259/2011 of February 2, 2011.

[a] Based on Commission Regulation (EC) No. 420/2011 of April 29, 2011.

[b] Based on Commission Regulation (EC) No. 565/2008 of June 18, 2008.

[c] For canned fish liver, the maximum permissible level applies to entire edible content of can.

[d] Based on the Commission Regulation (EC) No. 1259/2011 of December 2, 2011.

TABLE 12.4
Health Risk Assessment PCDDs, PCDFs, and DL-PCBs in Various Countries (A Comparison of Dioxin Risk Characterizations 2002)

Country or Public Health Authority	Exposure Guideline	Source
Canada	Tolerable daily intake, TDI 10 pg TEQ/kg bw/day	Health Canada, 1996
European Commission Scientific Committee on Food	TWI 14 pg TCDD/kg bw/day (converted to TDI 1–4 pg TEQ/kg bw/day)	European Commission Health and Consumer Protection Directorate-General Scientific Committee on Food, 2001
Japan	TDI 4 pg TEQ/kg bw/day	Ministerial Council on Dioxin Policy of Japan, 1999
Nordic Countries	TDI 5 pg TEQ/kg bw/day	Johansson and Hanberg 2000
US Agency for Toxic Substances and Disease Registry	Minimal risk level 1 pg TEQ/kg bw/day	US ATSDR, 2000
US Environmental Protection Agency (US EPA)	Reference dose RfD estimate 0.001 pg TEQ/kg bw/day	US EPA
Joint UN Food and Agricultural Organization /World Health Organization	Provisional tolerable monthly intake, PTMI 70 pg TEQ/kg bw/day (converted to 2.3 pg TEQ/kg bw/day)	JECFA, 2001

Source: Comparison of Dioxin Risk Characterizations. 2015. The Chlorine Chemistry Council® May 2002. Available online: http://www.dioxinfacts.org/dioxin_health/public_policy/dr.pdf.

12.5 CONCENTRATION IN FOODSTUFFS

12.5.1 Possible Food Contamination Pathways

Toxic chemicals may occur in food due to agricultural practices, industrial emissions, or natural occurrence. Airborne dioxins eventually settle into soil, water, and plants. They are accumulated along the food chain: air–grass–cattle–milk/meat–man. On plant surfaces, they can be deposited via wet deposition, via dry deposition of chemicals bound to atmospheric particles, or via diffusive transport of gaseous chemicals in the air to the plant surfaces.

Milk-producing animals absorb POPs mainly with food (feed, plants, water) and inhaled air. A small percentage may be taken in with soil from pastures by grazing ruminants. Organochlorine compounds accumulated in animals (their meat, liver, adipose tissues) are transferred to the products obtained from them. The compounds accumulate in dairy products mainly through the pathway: air/water–soil–plant–cattle–milk.

According to the bioaccumulation and biomagnification principles, increasing concentrations of dioxins and DL-PCBs accumulate in animals higher up the food

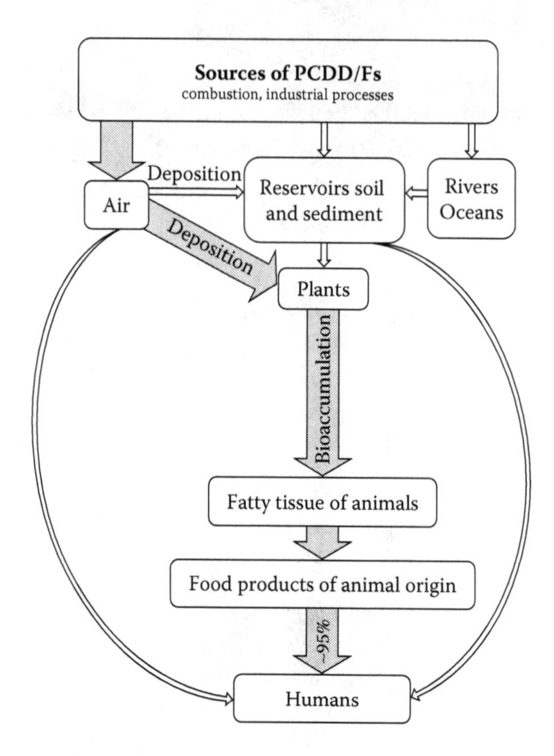

FIGURE 12.2 Dioxins in food chains.

chain. Products of animal origin are for humans a source of 90–95% total dietry intake of dioxins (Figure 12.2) (Perelló et al. 2012).

Thus, xenobiotics present in cattle feed affect greatly the level of PCB contamination of milk and dairy products. The PCB concentration in animal milk may vary depending on the season of the year, lactation, grass and soil contamination, vicinity of PCB sources, used feed, and feed additives such as root crops or cereals.

12.5.2 PCDDs, PCDFs, and DL-PCBs in Food Products

Human exposure to dioxins appears to come predominantly from meat, fish, and dairy products. Aquatic organisms are particularly susceptible to absorption, accumulation, and biomagnification of PCDD/Fs and DL-PCBs. The accumulation level depends on the concentration of these compounds in water, exposure time, trophic level, fish species, and fishing ground, while their bioaccumulation factors amount up to several thousands. The highest concentrations of DL-PCBs are usually found in seafood, mainly in fish, crustaceans, molluscs, fish products, and fish oil. The level of DL-PCBs has been decreasing gradually both in the environment and food. At the beginning (in the 1980s and 1990s), the decrease was very significant because the production and use of PCB containing products had been ceased.

The concentrations of TCDD/Fs and DL-PCBs in fish generally do not exceed the permissible amount of 8 pg TEQ/g wet weight (ww) specified by the European

Commission. According to Domingo and Bocio (2007), in Europe the amounts account for, at most, several pg TEQ/g ww. The exception is salmon caught in the Baltic Sea containing 8.8–17.4 pg $TEQ_{PCDD/F}$/g ww (Isosaari et al. 2006). In Baltic hering, the concentrations vary, but they are also relatively high, 3.5–12.0 pg $TEQ_{PCDD/F/DL\text{-}PCB}$/g ww (Shelepchikov et al. 2008, Godliauskienè et al. 2012). In Asia, dioxin concentrations in fish were noted to range within 0.003–5.0 pg $TEQ_{PCDD/F/DL\text{-}PCB}$/g ww (Sasamoto et al. 2006), and in Egypt, they were around 0.7–0.8 pg $TEQ_{PCDD/F/DL\text{-}PCB}$/g ww (Loutfy et al. 2007).

The highest mean levels of dioxins and DL-PCBs in food were observed for fish liver and products thereof (32.6 pg TEQ_{WHO98}/g whole weight basis). Significant differences in PCDD/Fs and DL-PCBs were observed for fish muscle and fish products excluding eel. The concentrations were ranging from 1.2 (farmed trout) to 8.0 (salmon) pg TEQ_{WHO98}/g whole weight basis (European Food Safety Authority 2010). The share of DL-PCBs in total TEQ for fish and fish products ranges from 35.6% for herring to 73% for farmed trout (Figure 12.3).

Lower concentrations are found in eggs, meat, and milk, and the lowest ones occur in vegetables and fruit (Malisch and Kotz 2014). Milk and dairy products had the highest share of DL-PCBs, namely, 57–66% in total TEQ (Figure 12.4). The share of PCDDs in total TEQ in goat meat and goat products was as big as 60% (Figure 12.4) (European Food Safety Authority 2010).

12.5.3 Dioxins and DL-PCBs in Milk and Dairy Products

Milk and dairy products constitute as much as 27–30% of foodstuffs, and they are basic foods in human diets all over the world. Based on the Food and Agriculture

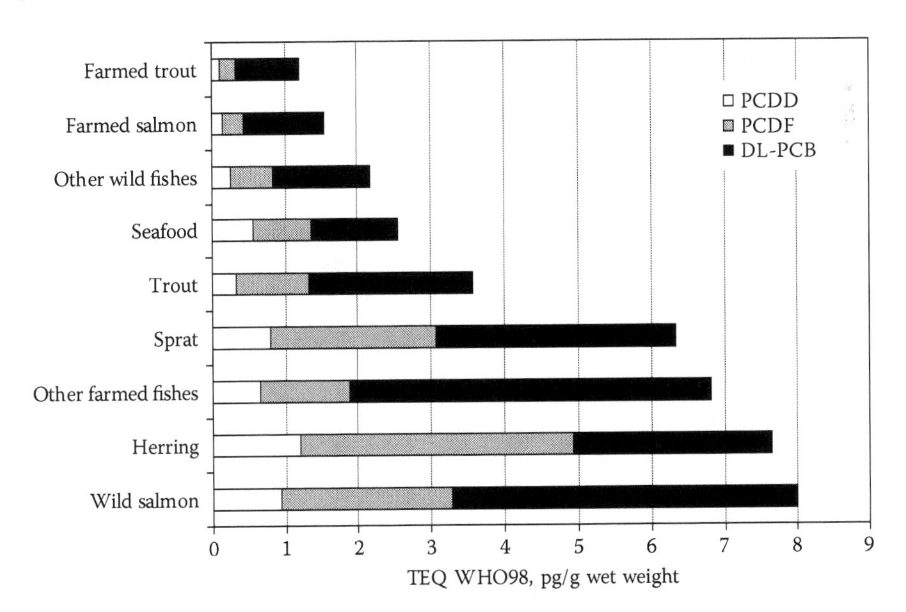

FIGURE 12.3 Concentrations of PCDD/Fs and DL-PCBs in fish muscle and fish products. (Based on European Food Safety Authority, *EFSA J*, 8, 1385, 2010.)

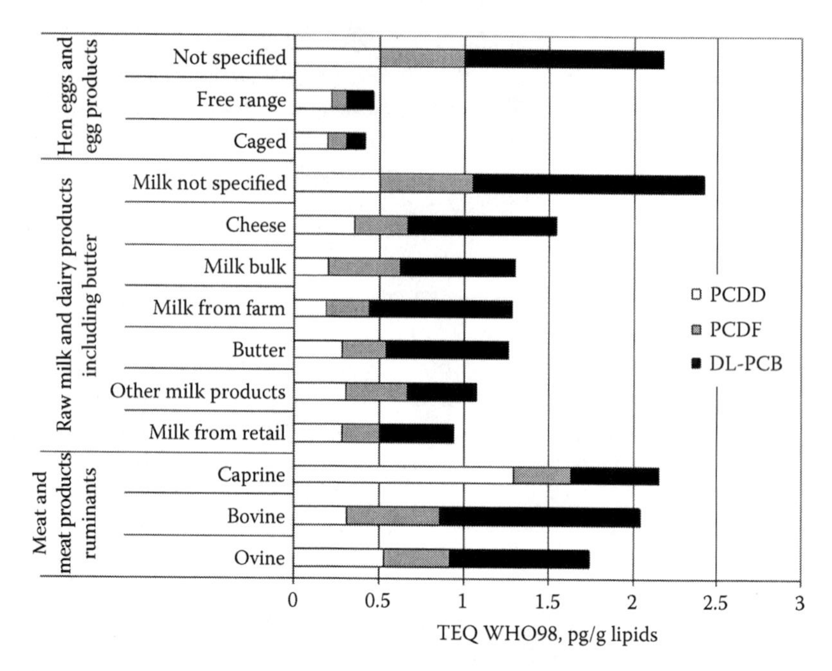

FIGURE 12.4 Concentrations of PCDD/Fs and DL-PCBs in selected products. (Based on European Food Safety Authority, *EFSA J*, 8, 1385, 2010.)

Organization (FAO) reports, at present the global milk production is about 800 million tones/year and increases annually by ca. 1.5–2%.

Milk and dairy products are potential sources of POPs, and they may serve as good bioindicators in the food chain. As early as in the 1980s, PCB residues in Belgian milk and dairy products were as high as 180–190 ng/g fat (Van Renterghem and Devlaminck 1980). In the mid-1990s, however, when the production of PCB-containing products had been ceased or limited considerably, reduced environmental pollution was reflected in decreased PCB concentrations in milk. Already in the 1990s in England, they were at 1.3–15.4 pg $TEQ_{non\text{-}ortho\ PCB}$/g fat (Krokos et al. 1996). In the US states, Panama, and Puerto Rico, milk contained 0.50 pg TEQ_{PCB}/g fat and 0.83 pg $TEQ_{PCDD/F}$/g fat (Lorber et al. 1998). Some years later, lower concentrations in Greek milk were recorded by Papadopoulos et al. (2004), 0.18 pg $TEQ_{non\text{-}ortho\ PCB}$/g fat and 0.39 pg $TEQ_{PCDD/F}$/g fat.

A gradual decrease in DL-PCB residues is also observed in butter to concentrations as low as 0.07–5.7 pg $TEQ_{PCDD/F/DL\text{-}PCB}$/g fat at the end of the 1990s (Santillo et al. 2003). Despite the highest total TEQs in the European and Mediterranean butter (particularly in the Spanish one), elevated levels were also recorded in the industrializing regions of Asia (India, China) and Latin America (Argentina) (Santillo et al. 2003) (Figure 12.5).

Regardless a clear global downward trend, the studies carried out in Egypt (Loutfy et al. 2007) revealed high levels of PCDD/Fs and PCBs in butter samples, 4.67 pg $TEQ_{PCDD/F}$/g fat and 4.47 pg $TEQ_{DL\text{-}PCB}$/g fat, that exceeded considerably the MRLs (Commission Regulation (EC) No. 1881/2006 of December 19, 2006),

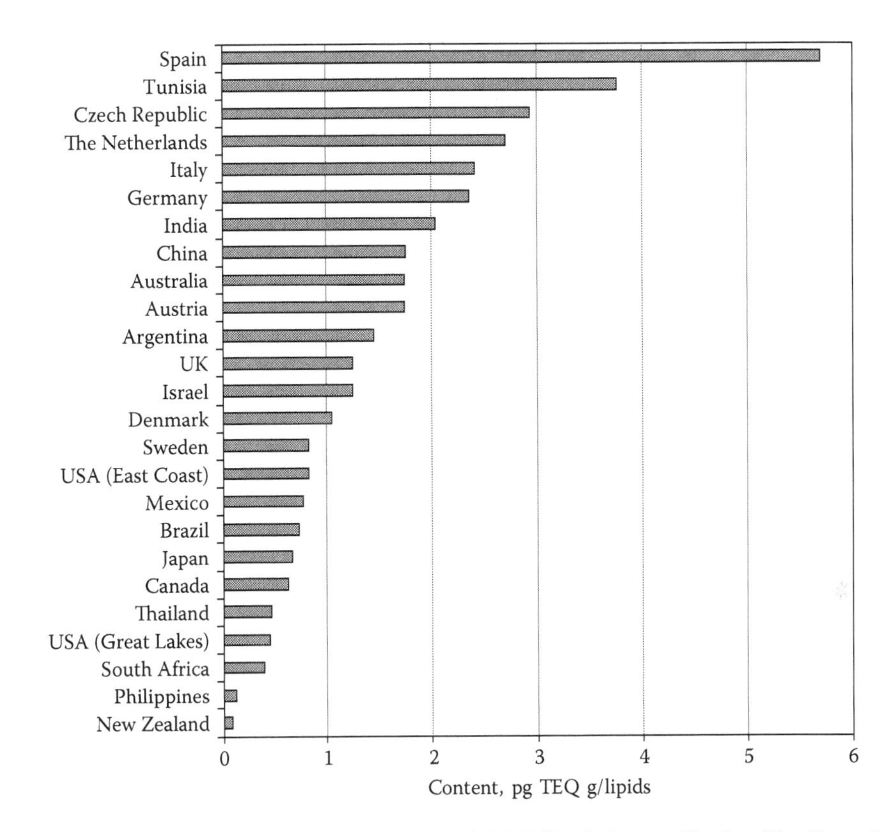

FIGURE 12.5 Concentration of PCDD/Fs and DL-PCBs in butter. (By Santillo, D. et al., *Food Addit Contam* 20, 281–290, 2003.)

and were higher compared to butter in Australia (mean 0.19 pg TEQ/g fat) or China (1.01 pg TEQ/g fat) (Müller et al. 2001, Santillo et al. 2003). According to Loutfy et al. (2007) such pollution could be mostly caused by waste incineration, and concentration levels in butter suggest a number of various pollution sources.

The gradual decrease is also recorded in other dairy products, for example, in cheese, dioxin residues in the last decade dropped to 0.09–0.17 pg TEQ/g fat (Papadopoulos et al. 2004, Llobet et al. 2008). Only Focant et al. (2002) found higher concentration of non-*ortho* PCBs in Belgian cheese, where high concentration of PCB 126 (15.8 pg/g fat) was recorded (Table 12.5).

In general, PCDD, PCDF, and DL-PCB residues found in the last several years in milk and dairy products were significantly lower than in the 1980s and 1990s, and stayed below 2 pg TEQ/g fat on average. There were, however, incidents of exceeded MRLs, for example, in Egypt (Loutfy et al. 2007) (Table 12.5). That confirms that despite the several decades for stopping the production of PCB-containing products, and lowered limits for emission of PCDD/Fs in most countries, the exposure to the most toxic congeners for PCDDs, PCDFs, and DL-PCBs taken in by humans with dairy products decreases very slowly, and such a problem may still exist for many years.

TABLE 12.5
Examples of PCDD/F and DL-PCB Concentrations in Cow's Milk and Dairy Products

			pg TEQ/g Fat		
Reference	**Country**	**Product**	**DL-PCB**	**PCDD/F/ DL—PCB**	**Non-*ortho* PCB**
Santillo et al. (2003)	England	Butter	0.79	0.07–5.69	
Focant et al. (2002)	Belgium	Butter		1.58–2.59	
Baars et al. (2004)	The Netherlands	Butter		1.26	
		Butter		1.64	
		Cheese		1.53	
Papadopoulos et al. (2004)	Greece	Butter			0.32
		Cheese			0.13
		Yogurt			0.41
		Milk			0.18
		Milk powder			0.04
Loutfy et al. (2007)	Egypt	Butter	4.47	9	
Hsu et al. (2007)	Taiwan	Milk, 3.4% fat	0.632	1.97	
Durand et al. (2008)	France	Milk	0.57	0.9	
Leondiadis et al. (2008)	Greece	Milk	0.29	0.7	
Ingelido et al. (2009)	Italy	Milk	0.52–2.9		
Ruoff et al. (2012)	Germany	Butter	0.463	0.63	

TABLE 12.6
Carryover Rate for Organochlorines Passing Through from Feed into Cows' Milk

Compounds	**Carryover Rate** (%)
Persistent PCDD/Fs	3–60
Other PCDD/Fs	<1–9
DL-PCBs	20–70
NDL-PCBs	2–9

Source: Based on Blüthgen, A., *Bull IDF*, 356, 43–47, 2000.

The intake of xenobiotics is also closely associated with their passage from contaminated feed into milk (carryover of xenobiotics). Blüthgen (2000) has defined the carryover rate as the percentage of the daily intake of a xenobiotic from feed (donor), which appears in the milk (or meat/fat) (accepting substrate) at a constant rate of uptake, metabolism, degradation, and excretion. The high carryover rates shown in Table 12.6 confirm that the risk of milk fat contamination is high.

Moreover, the data provided by many authors show that fat content in milk is not the only factor affecting the amount of accumulated contaminants. The level of environmental pollution and general conditions of milk cow husbandry may have a greater impact.

12.5.4 PCDDs, PCDFs, and DL-PCBs and Infants' Nutrition

12.5.4.1 Breast Milk

Infants are the most vulnerable group of consumers, and their basic food is based on breast milk. The presence of any toxic substances in their food may pose a risk to the infants' health. Relatively large amount of milk consumed by infants compared to their weight is another risk factor. Weisglas-Kuperus et al. (2000) emphasized that the presence of PCDDs, PCDFs, and DL-PCBs in breast milk strongly affects the development of infant's immunological system and brain.

Concentrations of PCDDs, PCDFs, and DL-PCBs in breast milk reflect environmental pollution. According to Noren and Meironytè (2000), concentrations of PCDD/Fs and DL-PCBs in breast milk of women living in Sweden decreased even by 70% from 1972 to 1997. High concentrations were reported by Bencko et al. (2004) in the Czech Republic (15.7 pg TEQ_{PCB}/g fat).

Costopoulou et al. (2006) reported 6.6 pg $TEQ_{DL\text{-}PCB}$/g fat and 7.3 pg $TEQ_{TCDD/Fs}$/g fat in breast milk of women living in Athens (Figure 12.6). Similar concentrations were also reported in the USA, 7.18 pg $TEQ_{PCDD/F}$/g fat and 4.61 pg TEQ_{PCB}/g fat. They were lower compared to the WHO data from various countries provided a few years earlier, when the smallest residues were recorded in Brazil (5.7 pg $TEQ_{TCDD/Fs/PCB}$/g fat), and the highest in Ukraine, 30 pg TEQ/g fat (Figure 12.6). A high contibution of TCDD/Fs (over 80%) to the total TEQ in breast milk of women living in Egypt should also be noticed (Figure 12.6). Lower concentrations of dioxin-like chemicals were reported by Harden et al. (2007) for breast milk of Australian women. Also Focant et al. (2013) reported a 40% reduction in breast milk concentrations of TCDD/Fs in France between 1998 and 2007.

The downward trend was confirmed by a study on breast milk carried out from 2009 to 2010 in a highly industrialized region of Belgium (Croes et al. 2012) that reported 5.9 ng $TEQ_{DL\text{-}PCB}$/g fat and 8.4 ng $TEQ_{PCDD/F}$/g fat in human milk.

The metabolism of PCB congeners leads to formation of OH-PCB congeners. They do not have any affinity for fat tissue, as the initial compounds do. But OH-PCB metabolites may be transferred to the fetal compartment. Para- or meta-substituted OH-PCB metabolites (with hydroxyl group adjacent to chlorine atoms) have a particularly high affinity for transthyretin (TTR), so when transferred via placenta they may pose a risk for disruption of the thyroid hormone system and adverse effects on neurological development. The compounds should also be included in the risk assessment of fetal exposure, as they are transferred to the fetal compartment more easily than the neutral PCBs (Park et al. 2007). Consequently, infants are posed to a considerable risk as they have immature detoxification mechanisms yet.

To estimate the cumulative intake (I) of PCDD/Fs and DL-PCBs for breast-fed infants, the following Equation 12.2 was proposed by Patandin et al. (1999) and modified by Ulaszewska et al. (2011):

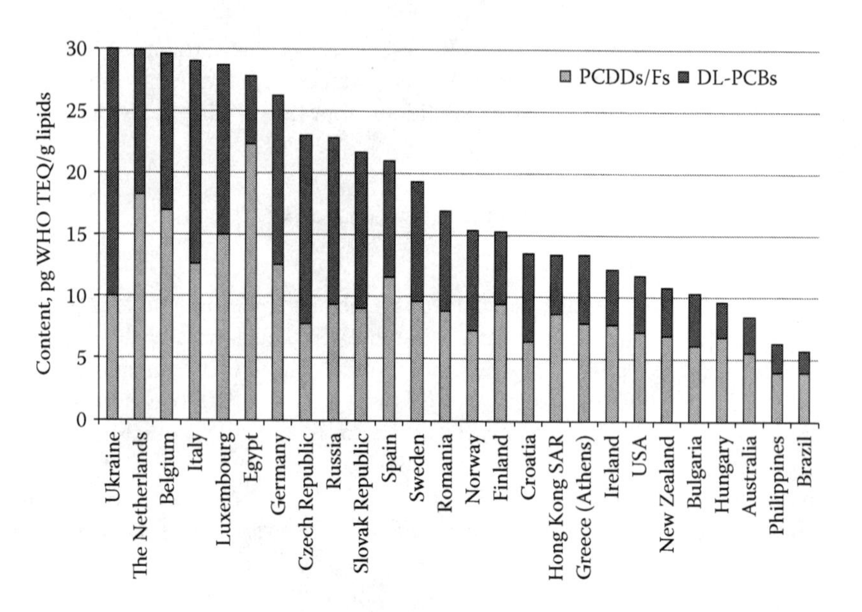

FIGURE 12.6 Mean concentrations of PCDD/Fs and dioxin-like PCBs in breast milk in different countries—data provided by WHO. (Based on Costopoulou, D. et al., *Chemosphere*, 65, 1462–1469, 2006.)

$$I = \left(0.95 \times V \times [\text{BMF}] \times [\text{TEQ}]_{\text{breastmilk}} \times \int_0^T e^{-0.017t}\,dt\right) \div 7(\text{pg/kg body weight}) \quad (12.2)$$

where:

0.95—fraction of intestinal absorption of PCDD/Fs and DL-PCBs in breast milk

V—weekly consumption of milk [cm^3]

BMF—milk fat concentration (3%)

T—duration of breast-feeding in weeks

TEQ—toxic equivalents of PCDD/Fs and DL-PCBs expressed as pg WHO$_{2005}$-TEQ/g fat

7—average infant's body weight (BW) in kg for a period of 12 months (detailed infant's weight: for Period 1 is 5.8 kg, for Period 2 is 8 kg, for Period 3 is 8.8 kg) (WHO Child Growth Standards)

0.017—percentage used to take into account a 1.7% weekly decrease in the PCDD/F and DL-PCB concentrations in the milk of the breast-feeding mother.

12.5.4.2 Infant Formulas

When infant feeding is concerned, the term "milk" is colloquially used also for infant formulas (IF), and follow-on formulas (FF). These foodstuffs were also reported to contain residues of undesirable compounds. As early as in the late 1970s, the total

PCB concentration reported for an infant formula sold in Belgium averaged 250 ng/g fat (Van Renterghem and Devlaminck 1980). A quarter century later, Pietrzak-Fiećko et al. (2005) reported 20-fold lower concentrations in infant formulas sold in Poland (on average 13 ng/g fat), but at the same time higher concentrations in cows' milk (35 ng/g fat) and several-fold higher in breast milk (218 ng/g fat).

Chovancova et al. (2005) reported for infant formula concentrations of non-*ortho* PCBs and mono-*ortho* PCBs of 0.30 pg TEQ/g fat and 0.04 pg TEQ/g fat, respectively. Significantly lower total non-*ortho* PCBs were reported by Papadopoulos et al. (2004), 0.01–0.08 pg $TEQ_{non\text{-}ortho\text{-}PCB}$/g lipids. The downward trend was also confirmed by Leondiadis et al. (2008), who assessed the concentration of non-*ortho* congeners in infant formulas at 0.04 pg TEQ/g fat, and mono-*ortho* congeners at 0.01 pg TEQ/g fat.

12.5.4.3 Analysis of Health Risks Based on DL-PCBs in Infant Formulas

When infant formulas based on cows' milk were tested by the author, the residues of DL-PCBs were found in virtually all of them. The mean total concentration of non-*ortho* PCBs in infant formulas (for babies over 6 months of age) ranged from 0.04 to 0.15 ng/g lipid. The dominant non-*ortho* congener was PCB 81, while PCB 126 was detected in only four products, and PCB 169 in 5 products.

Analysis of health risks of milk-based infant formulas revealed that $TEQ_{DL\text{-}PCB}$ values were low, in the range of 0.005–0.14 pg TEQ/g fat (equivalent to 0.0002–0.0046 pg TEQ/g ready-to-eat product), what after the conversion into diluted raw product gives minimum concentrations. Under the Commission Regulation (EC) No. 1259/2011 (OJ L 320, December 3, 2011), the residue levels detected were safe for health, as they remained well below the MRL of 0.1 pg TEQ_{PCB}/g ww. Despite the low TEQ values in infant formulas under study, the diet based on powder milk only, particularly in infants over 6 months of age, may lead to accumulation of these compounds in the body. Based on daily intake (DI) of DL-PCBs (0.02–0.46 pg TEQ/day) by infants, the data show that with the infant's diet limited to artificial food, the TDI value in any product was not exceeded, and DI/TDI ratios were 0.01–0.23% of TDI (Table 12.7).

However, dairy products represent about 30% of constituents of an average human diet, so they are not the only source of PCB residues. Moreover, assessing the total health risks to POPs in humans, based on the methodology, includes a wide range of tests involving also 7 PCDD congeners and 10 PCDF congeners in a number of foodstuffs. However, the share of DL-PCB congeners in assessing a total TEQ of milk and various dairy products may be even 80% (50–70% on average), what confirms the issue is very topical.

12.5.5 Conclusion

Reports of numerous authors indicate that concentrations of PCDDs, PCDFs, and DL-PCBs in milk and dairy products are usually significantly lower than in fish. However, taking into account the consumption of milk, which is a basic food right from the birth, and also an increasing consumption of other dairy products, there is a risk of a long-term accumulation of dioxin-like compounds in human bodies, and their negative impact on human organisms.

TABLE 12.7
Assessing the Daily Intake (DI) of DL-PCBs from Infant Formulas

Product	*a*	*b*	*c*	DP	LDP	DI_1	DI
1	4	4.6	5	92	23.4	0.68	0.10
2	6	4.9	3	88	19.2	0.37	0.04
3	7	5	3	105	20.5	0.32	0.04
4	7	4.9	2	69	13.9	0.29	0.03
5	6	4.6	5	138	35.2	0.17	0.03
6	6	5	3	90	20.7	0.13	0.02
7	4	4.3	5	86	23.8	3.03	0.47
8	6	4.5	3	81	19.1	2.71	0.33
9	7	4.7	2	65	14.1	0.47	0.05
10	4	4.3	5	86	20.7	1.74	0.27
11	6	4.7	3	85	17.9	1.06	0.13
12	4	5	5	100	26.5	0.88	0.14
13	6	5	3	90	16.6	1.84	0.23
14	6	5	2	60	12.9	1.56	0.16

Note: *a*, number of scoops; *b*, content of one scoop [g]; *c*, number of feedings; DP, daily portion [g dry weight]; LDP, amount of fat in DP [% fat in dry weight]; DI_1, daily intake of PCB [pg TEQ]; DI, daily intake of DL-PCB [pg TEQ/kg body weight]; assumed weight referred to formula use (1–3 months 6.5 kg, 6 months 8.2 kg, 12 months 10 kg).

Worldwide studies show a downward trend in the concentrations of TCDD/Fs and DL-PCBs in milk and dairy products. However, taking into account results reported in recent years, the MRLs were exceeded in some dairy products. (Milbrath et al. 2009) observed concentrations of the compounds in milk (2.9 pg TEQ/g fat) that in some cases were almost as high as the maximum residue levels.

A downward trend is also observed in the studies on breast milk. However, the reported breast milk concentrations are higher compared to cow's milk. Breast-fed infants are exposed to higher levels of dioxins and dioxin-like compounds than formula-fed infants due to higher contamination of maternal milk. Nevertheless, it has been confirmed that breast-fed infants develop better than those fed only formulas.

12.6 THE IMPACT OF TECHNOLOGICAL PROCESSES ON CHANGES IN THE CONCENTRATIONS OF DL-PCBs IN DAIRY PRODUCTS

12.6.1 Introduction

Taking into account even a 30% share of milk and dairy products in the diet of most people and a tendency to accumulate xenobiotics soluable in fat by them, the changes in DL-PCBs in butter, cream, curd cheese, and milk powder were tested in the course of manufacturing process. The raw material and semifinished products were sampled directly from the production lines at the creameries (Table 12.8).

TABLE 12.8
Characteristics of Material Sampled from Production Lines

Products	Raw Materials, Semifinished Products, End Products	Acidity, °SH	Fat Content in ww, %	Dry Weight Content, %
Butter 82%[b]	1. Raw milk	6.0	3.75 ± 0.05	12.0 ± 0.1
	2. Sweet cream[a]	5.0	38.3 ± 0.1	47.6 ± 0.4
	3. End product	1.4	82.0 ± 0.1	84.8 ± 0.2
Cream, pasteurized, homogenized, 18%[b]	1. Raw milk	6.0	3.75 ± 0.05	12.0 ± 0.03
	2. Sweet cream	5.0	38.3 ± 0.1	47.6 ± 0.4
	3. End product	28–29	18.0 ± 0.04	23.7 ± 0.4
Full-fat curd cheese[c]	1. Raw milk	6.4	4.00 ± 0.06	13.3 ± 0.1
	2. Skimmed milk used for standardization	6.2	0.10 ± 0.01	8.25 ± 0.04
	3. Pasteurized whole milk	6.0	3.79 ± 0.05	12.9 ± 0.1
	4. Curds for full-fat curd cheese production	36.6	3.66 ± 0.04	10.5 ± 0.05
	5. End product	64	8.47 ± 0.08	25.1 ± 0.1
Whole milk powder[d]	1. Raw milk	6.0	3.95 ± 0.07	12.0 ± 0.1
	2. Pasteurized whole milk	6.8	4.00 ± 0.04	12.1 ± 0,1
	3. Condensed milk from evaporator—concentrate	28.75	13.4 ± 0.1	48.5 ± 0.1
	4. Whole milk powder	6.8	3.20 ± 0.05	96.9 ± 0.1
	4a. Whole milk powder with lecithin	6.8–6.9	3.34 ± 0.06	98.1 ± 0.1

[a] Pasteurized at 95°C, 95 s.
[b] Creamery No 1.
[c] Creamery No 2.
[d] Creamery No 3.

12.6.2 Changes in DL-PCBs in the Course of Butter Production

Within the course of butter production, the loss of fat had mostly strong negative interrelations with concentrations of most dioxin compounds ($r_{fat} = -0.51$ to −0.95). The most significant changes occurred in the second phase of the technological process, which consists of, *inter alia*, cream maturing, churning, buttermilk separation, and butter rinsing (Table 12.8). The most dynamic decrease, by 39.8%, was recorded for PCB 156, while the loss of the remaining DL-PCBs ranged from 8.3% to 29.1%.

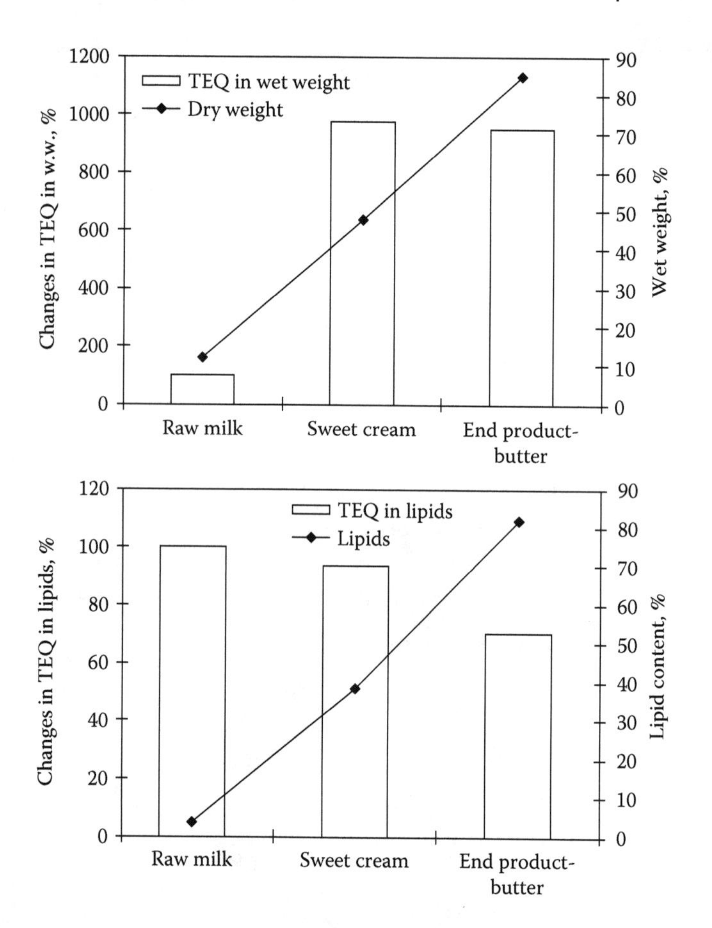

FIGURE 12.7 Changes in TEQ during butter production.

When butter was produced, a 17-fold increase in the TEQ in wet weight was observed, along with a 22-fold increase in the fat content in end product in comparison to raw milk. On fat basis, the TEQ significantly ($p < .05$) decreased by about 23%, of which a decrease by about 18% occurred in the second phase of butter production (Figure 12.7).

12.6.3 Changes in DL-PCBs in the Production of Pasteurized Homogenized Cream

In the production of pasteurized homogenized cream from sweet cream (phases 2 and 3), the loss in concentrations of PCB congeners was by 54–66% on average, with the loss in fat content by 53% and in dry weight by 50.2% (Table 12.8). The observed TEQ increase (3.5 times) was significant ($p < .05$). On lipid basis, however, TEQ decreased significantly, by 29%, and the greatest losses were noted

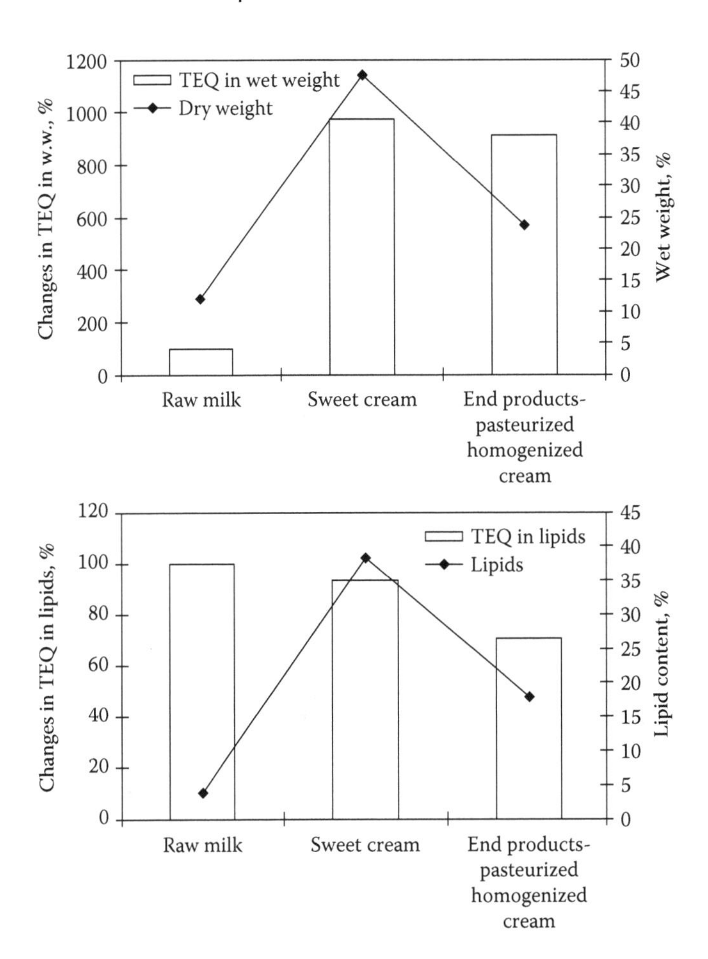

FIGURE 12.8 Changes in TEQ during the production of homogenized pasteurized cream.

after the second and third stages, when the cream got standardized to a specific butter fat content by the addition of skimmed milk (Figure 12.8).

12.6.4 Changes in DL-PCBs in the Full-Fat Curd Cheese Production

The production of full-fat curd cheese resulted in statistically significant ($p < .05$) changes in the concentrations of non-*ortho* and mono-*ortho* PCBs. With more than twofold increase in the fat content, the concentrations of PCB congeners in fat decreased, the decrease ranging from 1.7% to 59%, particularly during draining off the whey, and the curd rinsing. The TEQ was observed to decrease from 0.177 to 0.148 pg TEQ/g fat in all the production phases, but it was only a 17% decrease (Figure 12.9). If raw milk used for the curd cheese production has a higher concentration of DL-PCBs, such a decrease during production will not be sufficient.

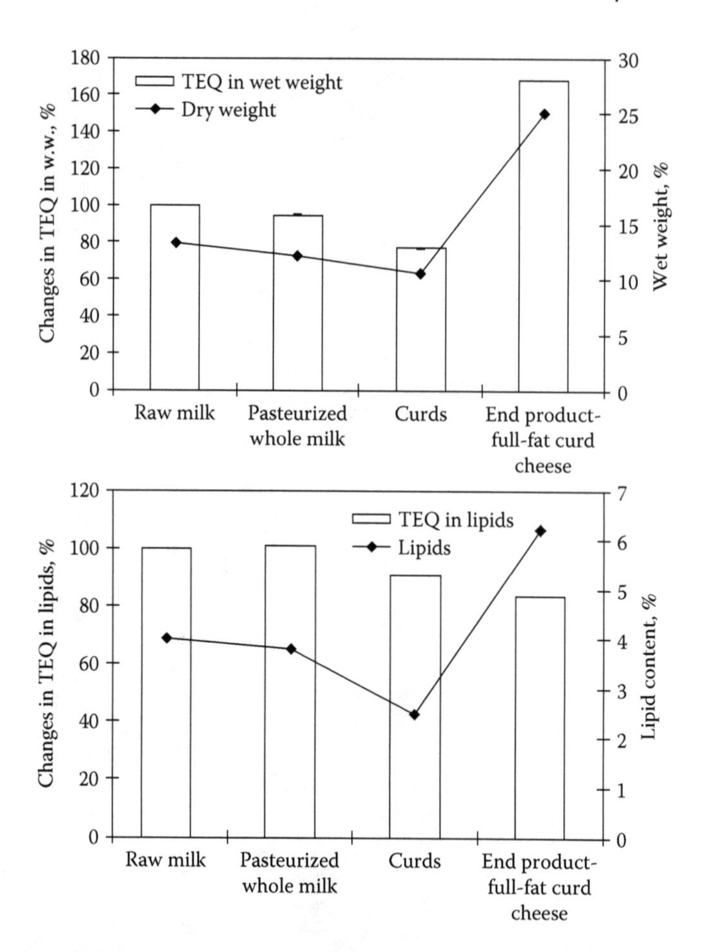

FIGURE 12.9 Changes in TEQ during the full-fat curd cheese production.

12.6.5 Changes in DL-PCBs in the Production of Whole Milk Powder

The processes of producing milk powder with and without lecithin were compared. Adding soya lecithin increases solubility of milk powder and allows to obtain a smooth texture.

The lecithinization process had no significant impact ($p < .05$) on the changes in the concentrations of DL-PCBs and their loss in production ranged from 22% to 43%. The data on DL-PCBs in the end product are given in ng/kg ww, taking into account the dilution of milk powder ready for drinking (13 g of powder in 100 cm^3 of water). In the production of whole milk powder, the dynamics in fat was rather weak, the highest dynamics was recorded for PCB 81 (total loss by 30.1%), the lowest in PCB 114 (loss by 4.1% on average). However, the pasteurization process had no significant impact on the changes on concentrations of PCB congeners in milk.

Analyzing certain phases in milk powder production, an insignificant 3% increase in TEQ ($p < .05$) was reported for a concentrate from the evaporator

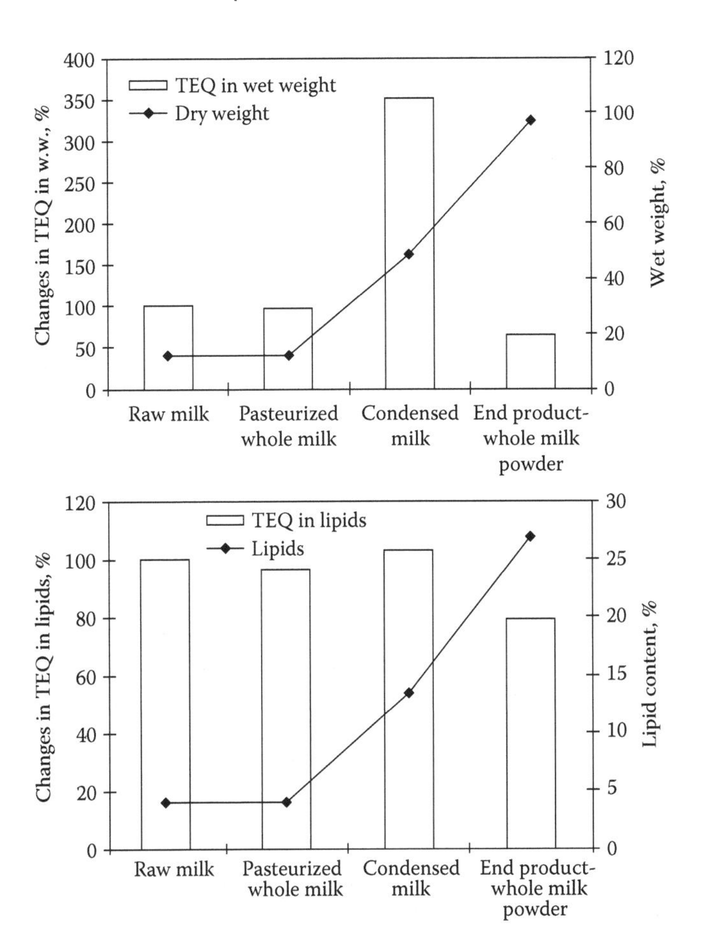

FIGURE 12.10 Changes in TEQ during the milk powder production.

(up to 0.263 pg TEQ/g fat). However, having had it dried up in a drying tower and then prepared for drinking, a significant ($p < .05$) 26% decrease in TEQ_{PCB} was reported (Figure 12.10).

12.6.6 Concluding Remarks

The quality assessment of food was based on the Commission Regulation (EC) No. 1259/2011, December 2, 2011). The TEQ_{PCB} values were determined with the use of TEF_{2005} (Van den Berg et al. 2006).

Some significant ($p < .05$) changes were reported in concentrations of both non-*ortho* and mono-*ortho* PCBs during the production of certain dairy products, and they were in strong positive correlation with the changes in fat content in wet weight of raw materials, semifinished products, and end products, while in the production of pasteurized homogenized cream and milk powder the correlations were weak or did not occur at all. The losses of most DL-PCB congeners in fat, that occurred in certain production phases, led to TEQ reduction, from 17% decrease in full-fat curd cheese up to 29% decrease in pasteurized homogenized cream.

Although technological processing reduces DL-PCB residues in dairy products, it will not provide consumers with safe products when raw milk with higher DL-PCB content is used for production. In such a case, the loss in DL-PCB concentrations will not be sufficient. Thus, more attention should be paid to conducting preliminary control of raw milk on a larger scale.

12.7 CONCLUSIONS AND PERSPECTIVES FOR FUTURE GENERATIONS

Food is a significant source of PCDD/Fs and DL-PCBs for humans. Therefore, according to the guidelines set by the WHO/FAO Codex Alimentarius Commission, health risk assessment is primarily based on testing the uptake of these compounds from foodstuffs.

In general, food in industrialized countries has more PCBs and dioxins than in less industrialized countries, which can be attributed to, both, greater present emissions of these chemicals, and their greater past production, use, and discharge. Prevention or at least reduction of human exposure may be best done using source-directed activities. Regarding the importance of environmental quality for producing safe food, especially important is to strictly control all industrial processes so that the formation of dioxins and their release to the environment get reduced as much as possible. Such controls should be the responsibility of national governments. Dioxin levels in foods and in human milk have been observed to generally decline in recent years. However, populations consuming much fish and seafood from contaminated waters have a high intake of some PCDD/Fs and DL-PCBs. What is worrying is that consumption of some fish oils as dietary supplements alone can sometimes result in an intake that exceeds the WHO TDI. The intake of PCDD/Fs and DL-PCBs by children may be higher, compared to adults, because children have comparatively higher food intake, and breast milk is often contaminated with these compounds. This is of concern regarding health impacts because infancy is a crucial time when physical and mental capabilities are developing. Therefore, the WHO, the FAO and the United Nations Environmental Programme (UNEP) have implemented the Global Environment Monitoring System's Food Contamination Monitoring and Assessment Programme (GEMS/Food), which delivers data on levels and trends of contaminants in food, their contribution to total human exposure, and significance with regard to public health and trade. Because of the continued release of these POPs into the environment, a potential still exists for their further severe impacts on the health of wildlife and humans, including effects on the developing stages of life, the unborn and nursing young. To prevent this risk and safeguard the health of future generations, necessary is to entirely eliminate the production, emission, and use of all POPs and implement clean production technologies.

Regarding globalization, incidents of serious contamination of food may have intenational repercussions. Presently there are many gaps in monitoring, and human exposure often occurs before the contamination is detected. The only way to address this problem is to prevent contamination at source, which means necessity of controls and practices during primary production of foodstuffs, their processing, distribution, and sale.

Consumers can minimize the risk of dietary exposure to dioxins by trimming fat from meat and consuming low-fat dairy products. Excessive exposure from a single source can also possibly be avoided through the use of a balanced diet that includes adequate amounts of fruits, vegetables, and cereals. This can help to reduce body burdens in a long-term perspective, and seems to be most relevant for girls and young women to reduce exposure of the developing fetus and when breast-feeding infants later on in life. However, consumers have little chance to considerably reduce their own exposure. The fact that the life span of women and men in developed countries is increasing in recent decades, indicating that long-term effects of POPs are generally well compensated by the development and wide use of new medical technologies and modern diagnostic methods. Also worldwide efforts to reduce environmental levels of various pollutants, including PCDD/Fs and DL-PCBs, result in a gradual, although very slow, reduction of dioxin residues in food, which is beneficial for human health.

REFERENCES

A Comparison of Dioxin Risk Characterizations. The Chlorine Chemistry Council® May 2002. Available online: http://www.dioxinfacts.org/dioxin_health/public_policy/dr.pdf, December 22, 2015.

Baars, A.J., M.I. Bakker, R.A. Baumann, P.E. Boon, J.L. Freijer, L.A. Hoogenboom, R. Hoogerbrugge, J.D. Klaveren van, A.K. Liem, W.A. Traag, and J. Vries de. 2004. Dioxins, dioxin-like PCBs and non-dioxin-like PCBs in foodstuffs: Occurrence and dietary intake in the Netherlands. *Toxicol Lett* 151: 51–61.

Bencko, V., M. Cerna, L. Jech, and J. Šmid. 2004. Exposure of breast-fed children in the Czech Republic to PCDDs, PCDFs, and dioxin-like PCBs. *Environ Toxicol Pharmacol* 18: 83–90.

Blüthgen, A. 2000. Contamination of milk from feed. *Bull IDF* 356: 43–47.

CAC 2001. Codex Alimentarius Commission. Joint FAO/WHO Food Standards Programme. Codex Committee on Food additives and Contaminants. XXXIII session, The Hague, the Netherlands, March 12–16, 2001.

Carpenter, D.O. 2006. Polychlorinated biphenyls (PCBs): Routes of exposure and effects on human health. *Rev Environ Health* 21(1): 1–23.

Chovancova, J., A. Kocan, and S. Jursa. 2005. PCDDs, PCDFs and dioxin-like PCBs in food of Animal origin (Slovakia). *Chemosphere* 61: 1305–1311.

Cogliano, V.J., R. Baan, K. Straif, Y. Grosse, B. Lauby-Secretan, F. El Ghissassi, V. Bouvard, L. Benbrahim-Tallaa, N. Guha, C. Freeman, L. Galichet, and C.P. Wild. 2011. Preventable exposures associated with human cancers. *J. Natl. Cancer Inst.* 103: 1827–1839.

Commission Regulation (EC) No 1881/2006 of 19 December 2006 setting maximum levels for certain contaminants in foodstuffs (Text with EEA relevance). *Official Journal of the European Union* L 364, p. 5.

Costopoulou, D., I. Vassiliadou, A. Papadopoulos, V. Makropoulos, and L. Leondiadis. 2006. Levels of dioxins, furans and PCBs in human serum and milk of people living in Greece. *Chemosphere* 65: 1462–1469.

Council Directive 96/82/EC of 9 December 1996 on the control of major-accident hazards involving dangerous substances. 1997. *Official Journal L 010*: P. 0013–P. 0033.

Croes, K., A. Colles, G. Koppen, E. Govarts, L. Bruckers, E. Van de Mieroop, V. Nelen, A. Covaci, A.C. Dirtu, C. Thomsen, L.S. Haug, G. Becher, M. Mampaey, G. Schoeters, N. Van Larebeke, and W. Baeyens. 2012. Persistent organic pollutants (POPs) in human milk: A biomonitoring study in rural areas of Flanders (Belgium). *Chemosphere* 89(8): 988–994.

Cuthill, S., A. Wihelmsson, and L. Poellinger. 1991. Role of the ligand in intracellular receptor function: Receptor affinity determines activation in vitro of the latent dioxin receptor to a DNA-binding form. *Mol Cell Biol* 11: 401–411.

DeVito, M.J., L.S. Birnbaum, W.H. Farland, and T.A. Gasiewicz. 1995. Comparisons of estimated human body burdens of dioxinlike chemicals and TCDD body burdens in experimentally exposed animals. *Environ Health Perspect* 103(9): 820–831.

Diliberto, J.J., L.B. Kedderis, J.A. Jackson, and L.S. Birnbaum. 1993. Effects of dose and routes of exposure on the disposition of 2,3,7,8-[3H]tetrabromodobenzo-p-dioxin (TBDD) in the rat. *Toxicol Appl Pharmacol* 120: 315–326.

Dobson, S., and G.J. van Esch. 1993. Polychlorinated biphenyls and terphenyls. In: *Environmental Health Criteria*, vol. 140, 2nd ed. World Health Organization, Geneva.

Domingo, J.L., and A. Bocio. 2007. Levels of PCDD/PCDFs and PCBs in edible marine species and human intake: A literature review. *Environ Int* 33(3): 397–405.

Durand, B., B. Dufour, D. Fraisse, S. Defour, K. Duhem, and K. Le-Barillec. 2008. Levels of PCDDs, PCDFs and dioxin-like PCBs in raw cow's milk collected in France in 2006. *Chemosphere* 70: 689–693.

Engwall, M., S. Stenlund, B. van Bavel, H. Olsman, and A. Schnurer. 2002. Fate of PCB (Clophen A50) during anaerobic treatment of organic household waste. *Organohalog Compd* 58: 61–64.

European Food Safety Authority. 2010. Results of the monitoring of dioxin levels in food and feed. *EFSA J* 8(3): 1385 (36 pp.). doi:10.2903/j.efsa.2010.1385. Available online: www.efsa.europa.eu.

Isosaari, P., A. Hallikainen, H. Kiviranta, P.J. Vuorinen, R. Parmanne, J. Koistinen, and T. Vartiainen. 2006. Polychlorinated dibenzo-p-dioxins, dibenzofurans, biphenyls, naphthalenes and polybrominated diphenyl ethers in the edible fish caught from the Baltic Sea and lakes in Finland. *Environ Pollut* 141: 213–225.

Fattore, E, R. Fanelli, E. Dellatte, A. Turrini, and A. di Domenico. 2008. Assessment of the dietary exposure to non-dioxin-like PCBs of the Italian general population. *Chemosphere* 73(1 Suppl): 278–283.

Fiedler, H. (ed.). 2003. Dioxins and Furans (PCDD/PCDF). Chapter 6 in *The Handbook of Environmental Chemistry* Vol. 3, *Part O Persistent Organic Pollutants*. Springer-Verlag, Berlin, Germany.

Focant, J.F., G. Eppe, C. Pirard, G. Eppe, C. Pirard, A.C. Massart, J.E. André, and E. De Pauw. 2002. Levels and congener distributions of PCDDs, PCDFs and non-ortho PCBs in Belgian foodstuffs: Assessment of dietary intake. *Chemosphere* 48(2): 167–179.

Focant, J.F., N. Fréry, M.L. Bidondo, G. Eppe, G. Scholl, A. Saoudi, A. Oleko, and S. Vandentorren. 2013. Levels of polychlorinated dibenzo-p-dioxins, polychlorinated dibenzofurans and polychlorinated biphenyls in human milk from different regions of France. *Sci Total Environ* 452–453: 155–162.

Giesy, J.P., and K. Kannan. 1998. Dioxin-like and non-dioxin-like toxic effects of polychlorinated biphenyls (PCBs): Implications for risk assessment. *Crit. Rev Toxicol* 28(6): 511–569.

Godliauskienė, R., J. Petraitisb, I. Jarmalaitėb, and E. Naujalisa. 2012. Analysis of dioxins, furans and DL-PCBs in food and feed samples from Lithuania and estimation of human intake. *Food Chem Toxicol* 50(11): 4169–4174.

Harden, F.A., L.M.L. Toms, R. Symons, P. Fürst, Y. Berry, and J.F. Müller. 2007. Evaluation of dioxin-like chemicals in pooled human milk samples collected in Australia. *Chemosphere* 67: S325–S333.

Hsu, M.S., K.Y. Hsu, S.M. Wang, U. Chou, S.Y. Chen, N.C. Huang, C.Y. Liao, T.P. Yu, and Y.C. Ling. 2007. A total diet study to estimate PCDD/Fs and dioxin-like PCBs intake from food in Tajwan. *Chemosphere* 67: S65–S70.

Ingelido, A.M., A. Abballe, A. Di. Domenico, I. Fochi, N. Iacovella, A. Saragosa, M. Spagnesi, S. Valentini, and E. De Felip. 2009. Levels and profiles of polychlorinated dibenzodioxins, polychlorinated dibenzofurans, and polychlorinated biphenyls in feedstuffs and milk from farms in the vicinity of incineration plants in Tuscany, Italy. *Arch Environ Con Tox* 57(2): 397–404.

Kato, S., Y. Fujii-Kuriyama, and F. Ohtake. 2007. A new signaling pathway of dioxin receptor ligands through targeted protein degradation. *AATEX* 14(Special Issue): 487–494.

Kim, M.K., and P.W. O'Keefe. 2000. Photodegradation of polychlorinated dibenzo-p-dioxins and dibenzofurans in aqueous solutions and in organic solvents. *Chemosphere* 41: 793–800.

Krokos, F., C.S. Creaser, C. Wright, and J.R. Startin. 1996. Levels of selected ortho and non-ortho polychlorinated biphenyls in UK retail milk. *Chemosphere* 32(4): 667–673.

Kulkarni, P.S., J.G. Crespo, and C.A.M. Afonso. 2008. Dioxins sources and current remediation technologies—A review. *Environ Int* 34: 139–153.

Leondiadis, L., D. Costopoulou, I. Vassiliadou, and A. Papadopoulos. 2008. Monitoring of dioxins and dioxin-like PCBs in food, feed, and biological samples in Greece. In: E. Mehmetli and B. Koumanova, (eds.), *The Fate of Persistent Organic Pollutants in the Environment*. Springer, the Netherlands, pp. 83–98.

Llobet, J.M., R. Martí-Cid, V. Castell, and J.L. Domingo. 2008. Significant decreasing trend in human dietary exposure to PCDD/PCDFs and PCBs in Catalonia, Spain. *Toxicol Lett* 178: 117–126.

Lorber, M.N., D.L. Winters, J. Griggs, R. Cook, S. Baker, J. Ferrario, C. Byrne, A. Dupuy, and J. Schaum. 1998. A national survey of dioxin-like compounds in the United States milk supply. *Organohalog Compd* 38: 125–129.

Loutfy, N., M. Fuerhacker, P. Tundo, S. Raccanelli, and M. Tawfic Ahmed. 2007. Monitoring of polychlorinated dibenzo-p-dioxins and dibenzofurans, dioxin-like PCBs and polycyclic aromatic hydrocarbons in food and feed samples from Ismailia city, Egypt. *Chemosphere* 66: 1962–1970.

Malisch, R., and A. Kotz. 2014. Dioxins and PCBs in feed and food—Review from European perspective. *Sci Total Environ* 491–492: 2–10.

McKay, G. 2002. Dioxin characterisation, formation and minimisation during municipal solid waste (MSW) incineration: Review. *Chem Eng J* 86: 343–368.

Milbrath, M.O., Y. Wenger, C.W. Chang, C. Emond, D. Garabrant, B.W. Gillespie, and O. Jolliet. 2009. Apparent half-lives of dioxins, furans, and polychlorinated biphenyls as a function of age, body fat, smoking status, and breast-feeding. *Environ Health Perspect* 117(3): 417–425.

Müller, J.F., J. Prange, C. Gaus, M.R. Moore, and O. Päpke. 2001. Polychlorinated dibenzodioxins and dibenzofurans in butter from different states in Australia. *Environ Sci Pollut Res Int* 8(1): 7–10.

Noren, K., and D. Meironyte. 2000. Certain organochlorine and organobromine contaminants in Swedish human milk in perspective of past 20–30 years. *Chemosphere* 40: 1111–1123.

Papadopoulos, A., I. Vassiliadou, D. Costopoulou, C. Papanicolaou, and L. Leondiadis. 2004. Levels of dioxins and dioxin-like PCBs in food samples on the Greek market. *Chemosphere* 57: 413–419.

Park, J.S., L. Linderholm, M.J. Charles, M. Athanasiadou, J. Petrik, A. Kocan, B. Drobna, T. Trnovec, A. Bergman, and I. Hertz-Picciotto. 2007. Polychlorinated biphenyls and their hydroxylated metabolites (OH-PCBs) in pregnant women from eastern Slovakia. *Environ Health Perspect* 115(1): 20–27.

Patandin, S., C.I. Lanting, P.G. Mulder, E.R. Boersma, P.J. Sauer, and N. Weisglas-Kuperus. 1999. Effects of environmental exposure to polychlorinated biphenyls and dioxins on cognitive abilities in Dutch children at 42 months of age, *J Pediatr* 134(1): 33–41.

Perelló, G., J. Gómez-Catalán, V. Castell, J.M. Llobet, and J.L. Domingo. 2012. Assessment of the temporal trend of the dietary exposure to PCDD/Fs and PCBs in Catalonia, over Spain: Health risks. *Food Chem Toxicol* 50: 399–408.

Pesatori, A.C., D. Consonni, M. Rubagotti, P. Grillo, and P.A. Bertazzi. 2009. Cancer incidence in the population exposed to dioxin after the "Seveso accident": Twenty years of follow-up. *Environ Health* 8: 39.

Pietrzak-Fiećko, R., K. Smoczyńska, and S. Smoczyński. 2005. Polychlorinated biphenyls in human milk, UHT cow's milk and infant formulas. *Pol J Environ Stud* 14(2): 237–241.

Ruoff, U., H. Karl, and H.G. Walte. 2012. Dioxins, dioxin-like PCBs and non-dioxin-like PCBs in dairy products on the German market and the temporal tendency in Schleswig-Holstein. *Journal für Verbraucherschutz und Lebensmittelsicherheit* 7(1): 11–17.

Santillo, D., A. Fernandes, R. Stringer, R. Alcock, M. Rose, S. White, K. Jones, and P. Johanston. 2003. Butter as an indicator of regional persistent organic pollutant contamination: Further development of the approach using polychlorinated dioxins and furans (PCDD/Fs), and dioxin-like polychlorinated biphenyls (PCBs). *Food Addit Contam* 20(3): 281–290.

Sasamoto, T., F. Ushio, N. Kikutani, Y. Saitoh, Y. Yamaki, T. Hashimoto, S. Horii, J. Nakagawa, and A. Ibe. 2006. Estimation of 1999–2004 dietary daily intake of PCDDs, PCDFs and dioxin-like PCBs by a total diet study in metropolitan Tokyo, Japan. *Chemosphere* 64: 634–641.

Shelepchikov, A.A., V.V. Shenderyuk, E.S. Brodsky, D. Feshin, L.P. Baholdina, and S.K. Gorogankin. 2008. Contamination of Russian Baltic fish by polychlorinated dibenzo-p-dioxins, dibenzofurans and dioxin-like biphenyls. *Environ Toxicol Pharmacol* 25: 136–143.

Stockholm Convention on Persistent Organic Pollutants (POPs). Geneva 2001, Secretariat of the Stockholm Convention. Available online: http://chm.pops.int.

Swanson, G.M., H.E. Ratcliffe, and L.J. Fischer. 1995. Human exposure to polychlorinated biphenyls (PCBs): A critical assessment of the evidence for adverse health effects. *Regul Toxicol Pharm* 21: 136–150.

Tsukimori, K., H. Uchi, C. Mitoma, F. Yasukawa, T. Chiba, T. Todaka, J. Kajiwara, T. Yoshimura, T. Hirata, K. Fukushima, N. Wake, and M. Furue. 2012. Maternal exposure to high levels of dioxins in relation to birth weight in women affected by Yusho disease. *Environ Int* 38: 79–86.

Ulaszewska, M.M., E. Zuccato, and E. Davoli. 2011. PCDD/Fs and dioxin-like PCBs in human milk and estimation of infants' daily intake: A review. *Chemosphere* 83: 774–782.

United States Environmental Protection Agency. 2003. Exposure and Human Health Reassessment of 2,3,7,8-Tetrachlorodibenzo-p-Dioxin (TCDD) and Related Compounds. Part III: Integrated Summary and Risk Characterization. National Academy of Sciences (NAS) Review Draft. December 2003. Available online: http://www.epa.gov/ncea/pdfs/dioxin/nas-review/pdfs/part3/dioxin_pt3_full_oct2004.pdf.

Van den Berg, M., L.S. Birnbaum, M. Denison, M. De Vito, W. Farland, M. Feeley, H. Fiedler, H. Hakansson, A. Hanberg, L. Haws, M. Rose, S. Safe, D. Schrenk, C. Tohyama, A. Tritscher, J. Tuomisto, M. Tysklind, N. Walker, and R. Peterson. 2006. The 2005 World Health Organization reevaluation of human and mammalian toxic equivalency factors for dioxins and dioxin-like compounds. *Toxicol Sci* 93(2): 223–241.

Van Leeuwen, F.X., M. Feeley, D. Schrenk, J.C. Larsen, W. Farland, and M. Younes. 2000. Dioxins: WHO's tolerable daily intake (TDI) revisited. *Chemosphere* 40: 1095–1101.

Van Renterghem, R., and L. Devlaminck. 1980. Polychlorinated biphenyl compounds in milk and dairy products. *Z Lebensm Unters Forsch* 170(5): 346–348.

Weisglas-Kuperus, N., S. Patandin, G. Berbers, T.C. Sas, P.G. Mulder, P.J. Sauer, and H. Hooijkaas. 2000. Immunologic effects of background exposure to polychlorinated biphenyls and dioxins in dutch preschool children. *Environ Health Persp* 108: 1203–1207.

WHO. 1998. Executive summary—Assessment of the health risks of dioxins: Re-evaluation of the Tolerable Daily Intake (TDI), WHO Consultation, May 25–29, 1998, Geneva, Switzerland. Available online: http://www.who.int/ipcs/publications/en/exe-sumfinal.pdf.

WHO. 2010. Dioxins and their effects on human health. Fact sheet No 225, May 2010. Available online: http://www.who.int/mediacentre/factsheets/fs225/en/index.html.

13 Epidemiological and Medical Impact of Food Contamination by Viruses Transmission via Food and Water

Elżbieta Kucharska and Joanna Bober

CONTENTS

13.1 MORPHOLOGICAL AND CULTURE DIFFERENCES BETWEEN VIRUSES AND BACTERIA

Until recently, the presence of viruses in water and food was questionable. The reason for that was the fact that viruses are able to multiply solely inside living cells. These could be cell cultures, animals—including people, or fertilized eggs. Water and food, especially subjected to heat treatment, are thus unfavorable environment, making the multiplication of viral molecules impossible. Partial change in the opinion was caused by the reported high resistance of viruses to external environmental conditions. It was observed that it is a group of micro-organisms that can survive not only during freezing but can also crystallize in unfavorable conditions. Thus, it was noted that even if the viruses do not multiply in outside cell environments, they can exist there. There have been philosophical considerations whether viruses are a form of life. The progress in molecular biology, the development of ribonucleic acids identification methods, followed by proteomics and metabolomics methods, put an end to this dispute, qualifying viruses as a form of life, even though it is known that their structure is different from that of bacterial cells. It is the virology dogma that the basic structures of viral molecules are genome, capsid, and lipid coat called an envelope. The latter is not an integral structure of the viruses, so they can be divided into enveloped and nonenveloped viruses.

However, the basic division is based on genome structure. Because viruses can have either DNA or RNA genome, they were divided into two families, and then, because both DNA and RNA can be present in the form of a single or double strand, ssRNA and dsRNA, and also ssDNA and dsDNA viruses are distinguished. The way the genome is folded, and then viral particle packed in proteins called capsomeres, together forming a capsid, decides on the shape of a virus. The morphological type can be helical, prolate, and icosahedral or near-spherical. Some viruses are additionally protected by a lipid envelope. Viruses possessing such an envelope are more resistant to environmental factors but are more susceptible to disinfectants having lipolytic activity (Rossmann 2013).

13.2 FOOD AND WATER AS POTENTIAL SOURCES OF VIRAL INFECTIONS

It was observed that consecutive natural disasters, floods or events of sewage system breakdown, especially in older cities, were accompanied by gastrointestinal infections, at the onset of which no pathogenic bacteria were cultured. Equatorial countries, with hot climate and with the access to clean drinking water still completely unresolved, are often places of gastrointestinal infections with diarrhea as the dominating symptom. It is estimated that due to that 2 million people from vulnerable age groups (children and elderly) die every year. It has been reported that gastrointestinal viral infections are the cause of 10–12% of children hospitalizations and the reason for major economic losses. For an infection to occur, in majority of cases only a small dose of viruses, 10–100 virions, is sufficient. The risk of infection via water and food does not only concern developing countries but also those economically developed (Leclerc et al. 2002). There are two routes of transmission: the most common is fecal–oral route, that is, the transfer of viruses through dirty hands from the contaminated source, for example, water, contaminated food not subjected to heat treatment: vegetable or food salads, appetizers. Second route is airborne—inhalation of viral particles spread in the air, for example, present from a vomit of a sick person or in the nasal and throat discharge. An average incubation period is short and usually lasts 1–4 days. First symptoms are often elevated temperature, especially in norovirus and rotavirus infections, muscle pain or fatigue. It is related to the activity of proinflammatory cytokines interleukin (IL)-1, -2, -6, and -8 released from macrophages, and interferon gamma (INFγ) released from lymphocytes due to viremia. The lack of appetite, nausea, vomiting, and diarrhea without the presence of blood and painful intestinal cramps occurs during localization of viruses within the gastrointestinal tract. There are also changes in laboratory parameters, for example, lymphopenia or increased number of specific immunoglobulin M (IgM) antibodies. The treatment is only symptomatic. It includes mainly supplementing lost fluids and electrolytes. Convalescence, besides gradual recovery, is accompanied by increasing number of specific IgG antibodies.

13.3 ROTAVIRUS INFECTIONS

Yearly mortality among children due to rotavirus infections reaches 6,00,000, mainly in least developed countries. During 2004–2005, there were studies in Europe carried out within REVEAL program, which determined, among others, the incidence rate in the group of children below the age of 5. The incidence rate was 10.4–36% of tested subjects. The mortality rate was very low (Giaquinto et al. 2007). In the United States, the incidence rate reaches 30–70% of hospitalizations and yearly treatment costs 1 billion per year (Bernstein 2009). Rotavirus infections, due to prodromal symptoms, are often called in Poland the "intestinal flu." They usually start with incidental sicknesses. Infants and small children are most often affected—breast feeding prevents from the infection (high concentration of IgA in mother's milk, especially in first 5 days of infant's life). Incubation period lasts 1–3 days. The infection results in diarrhea lasting 5–8 days, rapidly leading to dehydration.

Rotavirus (Latin: rota—wheel) belongs to the family Reoviridae. Its genome is formed of dsRNA. It has icosahedral symmetry. The genome consists of 11 segments of dsRNA and is surrounded by a three-layered capsid. RNA segments encode six structural and five nonstructural proteins. The proteins possess antigenic properties, thus a serological identification can be performed and seven main species of this virus were determined—from A to G. Some of the proteins form the inner core layer of the virion, and some form the outer layer. The proteins present on the surface—VP4 and VP7—show different resistance on enzymatic proteolysis, hence further division of the virus into strains (serotypes). Protein VP4 defines 23 strains P having the possibility to stimulate antigens production (serological properties). Various serotypes, with differing frequency, caused infections in different continents or countries (Lin et al. 2014). The knowledge of rotavirus serotypes is used for production of polyvalent vaccines containing viral proteins characteristic for the infections in a given area. There was a monovalent vaccine produced in China, but due to improper control research it is not recommended (Lin et al. 2014).

Species A, B, and C are infectious for humans and animals. Species A is the most common and causes 90% of all rotavirus infections in people. The infections primarily occur in winter months. The viruses are resistant to physical factors, temperatures below −20°C, and numerous freezing and thawing. They are also not destroyed by incubation in 56°C or by UV. Thus, the transmission is not only possible via the fecal—oral route but also through objects, hence the infections in hospitals in neonatal units reported in Poland and throughout the world. Viruses do not possess lipid envelope. They are sensitive to disinfectants, for example, alcohol or halogenated compounds. Rotaviruses are destroyed at the temperature above 60°C after 30 min. The disease is most common among children between 4th and 36th month of age. Until the age of 5 almost, 100% children go through rotavirus infections. Yearly in the world 138 million children are infected, 6,00,000 of those die, mainly from Sub-Saharan Africa and South Asia. It was shown that rotaviruses are capable of producing nonstructural NSP4 protein, which is regarded as the first viral endotoxin defined. It is a 22-amino acid peptide increasing the influx of Ca ions to a cell, which results in a higher secretion of chlorine ions to the intestines and diarrhea (Lee et al. 2000). Passing through the infection leaves short-term immunity; so, multiple infections are possible. The only successful form of prevention is using a vaccine containing live attenuated viruses, administered to infants orally. Vaccines used in the United States and popular in the whole world are polyvalent vaccines, for example, *Rotarix* (GlaxoSmithKline) and RotaTeq (Merck and Company). Last year, Rotarix was used in more than 90 countries. These vaccines are given orally from the 6th week of life, in two doses in 4-week intervals to children until the 24th month of life. In studies carried out in Latin America and in Africa, at least 2-year effectiveness of the vaccines was confirmed, in the sense of reducing the prevalence of the disease in vaccinated groups in comparison to unvaccinated ones and significantly milder course of the disease (Gentsch et al. 2005).

13.4 NOROVIRUS INFECTIONS

Norovirus infections are the second most common infections in the world. According to US Centers for Disease Control and Prevention (CDC) estimates, the virus affects 21 million people in the United States each year, which amounts to 60% of gastroenteritis cases. Noroviruses, previously called Norwalk-like viruses, are nonenveloped viruses containing ssRNA. They belong to Caliciviridae family, comprising various types of viruses: Noroviruses, Sapoviruses, which cause diarrhea in children and adults, and Lagovirus, Nebovirus and Vesivirus, infecting animals like cattle, amphibians, reptiles, sea mammals (dolphins), birds (chickens), dogs, and cats (Feline calicivirus). These are small viruses (27–40 nm), icosahedral with 32 bowl-shaped sinuses, nonenveloped, with positive-sense RNA genome. Noroviruses can be divided into six genogroups and more than 40 genotypes, being the reason of its high variation (Robilotti et al. 2015). The genotypes GGII—GGIV were the cause of worldwide pandemic. Infections caused by those genotypes were noted from the 90s in the United States, Japan, Taiwan, New Zealand, and Australia (Chen et al. 2009). The routes of transmission vary via contaminated potable water and in swimming pools, naturally fertilized vegetables, including frozen ones, improperly washed fruits, fecal contaminated objects (viruses can survive up to 7 days), or food not subjected to heat treatment. People are infected directly (person to person) via the aerosol surrounding vomiting person. Transmission from animals is problematic, but it has been proved possible to get infected from a sick person having no symptoms and shedding viruses in feces. Numerous strains belong to noroviruses: Norwalk, Lordsdale, Toronto, Southampton, Hawaii, or Mexico. Epidemics caused by noroviruses occur during the whole year and encompass all age groups; they are, however, more frequent in children. Viruses replicate in intestinal epithelium. The course of infection is characteristic to intestinal viral infections. The consumption of oysters, mussels or other seafood, ready-to-eat foods touched by infected food workers (salads, sandwiches, ice, cookies, fruit), or any other foods contaminated with vomit or feces from an infected person may be a source of infection, especially in institutional feeding or catering points (www.Foodsafety.gov). Drinking stream water or from reservoirs where sewage is released or using such water for cleaning kitchenware or fruits or vegetables (parsley, raspberries) not subjected to heat treatment can also be the source of infection.

Mass outbreaks were noted in enclosed environments: barracks, boarding houses, schools, ship crews, and often in winter season. The cause of the symptoms is gastroenteritis. The dominating symptoms are vomiting, diarrhea, dehydration, and electrolyte imbalance. Self-recovery occurs in most cases after 2–3 days of the illness. After the infection, one gains 2–4 year immunity. People with weakened immune system are especially prone to infection. In a group aged above 85 a severe, long-term (several weeks) illness was observed; however, no deaths were noted, similarly in case of people after marrow and organ transplants (Robilotti et al. 2015).

13.5 SAPOVIRUS INFECTIONS

Sapoviruses, until recently called Sapporo-like viruses, belong to Caliciviridae family. Approximately 23% of patients with diarrhea were infected with Sapoviruses. The majority of infections developed in winter. The structure of Sapoviruses is characteristic to Caliciviridae. Thus, they are ssRNA with icosahedral geometry. Sapoviruses are classified into genogroups from GI to GV, whereas GIII infects pigs and others infect humans. Differentiating Sapoviruses from other Caliciviruses using electron microscope (EM) proved to be very challenging. Due to that serological diagnosis was used, by immunizing guinea pigs and obtaining specific antibodies, which were used in enzyme-linked immunosorbent assay (ELISA) test, which in turn was problematic due to the necessity of collecting stool from 2 days. Better, more precise, and cheaper methods turned out to be nested polymerase chain reaction (PCR) and reverse transcription (RT) PCR, and in interspecies determination Taq-Man RT-PCR.

Sapoviruses were reported in 88% of children below the age of 5, and in only 8% of tested subjects above the age of 10. The infections affect children in concentrations such as kindergartens or schools and are transmitted via fecal—oral route and through the objects: door-handles, phone receivers, and taps. The course of the infection is milder than in case of rota- or noro-virus infections.

Studies concerning the presence of viruses in water revealed that the viruses were found in dirty reservoirs but absent in shallow rivers. No viruses were present in seawater; however, they were observed in seafood, excluding oysters. The studies were limited to Japan (Hansman et al. 2007). It is estimated that in Europe the number of Sapovirus infections is growing.

13.6 ASTROVIRUS INFECTIONS

Astroviruses belong to small viruses whose genome is composed of ssRNA. The viruses replicate in the cytoplasm of infected cells. Astroviruses form the family Astroviridae, which is divided into two genera: “Mamastroviruses” and

"Avastroviruses." Human astrovirus that infects people belongs to Mamastroviruses. They divide into five genotypes, with one being the most common. Depending on the antigenic properties, we can distinguish eight serotypes, with one to five having the highest importance. Besides humans, the viruses also infect animals. Animal astroviruses infect kittens, piglets, puppies, cattle (types 1 and 2), sheep, deer, and mink kittens. *Avastrovirus* includes duck AstV, turkey AstVs (types 1 and 2), and avian nephritis virus of chickens (types 1 and 2). Astroviruses are divided into species, depending on the type of infected animal. The viruses exhibit high genetic variation, thus adjusting themselves to infect new animal species. They are transmitted by contaminated water and food; therefore, it is crucial to provide animals with water free from viruses. Not only domestic but also farming animals can be infected. Astroviruses cause changes in central nervous system of minks, leading to apoptosis of infected cells (shaking mink syndrome) (Gliński and Kostro 2012).

The majority of infections in people were noted between October and January. It is a winter season in China. In seven provinces in China, during 7 years (1998–2005) the average percentage of infected people amounted to 5.5%. Children between 9th and 11th month of age were most frequently affected—7.4%, next—children between 12th and 17th month of age—6.1%. Interestingly, the percentage of infected children between 0 and 2 months of age was 5.6%. The incidence of astrovirus infections in Korea noted during 5 years was 0.6–2.4%. In Spain, a peak of incidence was between 2nd and 4th year of age and 80% of children were affected below the age of three. In Vietnam, children were infected mainly from the end of May to August, or November, that is, during the rainy season. In the United States, France and Finland the prevalence was higher in winter and spring months.

Astroviruses are the cause of mild gastroenteritis. They are resistant to low pH of gastric acid, so they affect the intestines. They were localized in both M cells and in enterocytes in top and side parts of intestinal villi. The incidence of astrovirus infection was observed in all age groups, but children below 2nd year of age were most prone to the infection. The dominating symptoms are vomiting (20–62% sick people), diarrhea (on average 3 days with 4 stools daily), elevated body temperature, sometimes up to 39°C, in 25% of sick people.

More than 70% of adults and 95% of children have specific antibodies against astroviruses. The infections are especially frequent in closed communities or concentrations such as dormitories, nurseries, and kindergartens. More severe course of the infection was observed in those suffering from AIDS (Jeong et al. 2012). Astroviruses are inactivated at 50–60°C for 30 min, stable at low temperatures, resistant to chloroform, and ether; they are destroyed during disinfection with chlorine compounds and glutaraldehyde.

13.7 ADENOVIRUS INFECTIONS

Adenoviruses (90–100 nm) are a large group of ubiquitous viruses. Their genome is linear dsDNA forming eight domains. About 252 capsomeres form a protein capsid with icosahedral geometry. A complete virion resembles a satellite, as it is formed from 20 sides and 12 apexes from which thin peptides protrude. It contains early- and late-structural proteins and maturates in cell nucleus.

Adenoviridae family contains the genera Mastadenovirus, which infects mammals, and Aviadenovirus, infecting birds. Birds infections are very severe and cause losses of body weight. The viruses affect broilers, ducks, geese, and pigeons. The infection causes hepatitis cholangitis and pancreatitis, soft eggs shells, and the lack of proper embryo development. Infections also concern reptiles. Human adenoviruses are classified into A—F species, and then into 51 serotypes with different pathogenicity. Generally, adenoviruses may infect gastrointestinal system, respiratory system, central nervous system, urinary system, and eyes, causing conjunctivitis or keratoconjunctivitis. The viruses are transmitted by the fecal—oral route, by air, or by contact with objects. Incubation period lasts 10 days. Transmission of viruses to eyes happens by improperly washed and disinfected hands or by old type of tonometers measuring the intraocular pressure with contact method. These can be hospital infections, but they can be also related to the occupation and injuries, called "shipbuilder's eye."

Children are affected with the viruses in early childhood. The majority of infections are related to upper respiratory tract, with rhinitis, stomatitis, and pharyngitis. Passing through the infection results in a carrier state for several months. Adenoviruses can also cause intussusception in neonates, necrotic inflammation of small intestine, meningitis and encephalitis, and rarely—urinary tract infections (hemorrhagic cystitis).

Teenagers are affected usually during summer time. Water in swimming pools becomes the source of contamination. The infections are associated with eyes and upper respiratory tract. The disease also more often affects children and teenagers accommodated in dorms, attending schools or summer camps.

In case of adults, the infections develop mainly in people under strain, gathered in barracks. There are often cases of bronchopneumonia. Adenovirus infections can also spread among hospitalized patients, senior centers, generally among people with weakened immune system, especially during chemotherapy, cancer, HTLV3 infection, or marrow transplant.

"Adenovirus" infections are very common. They may be responsible for 13% of all viral infections and thus are placed as second after *Herpesviridae* infections. Gastrointestinal system is mainly affected by type A adenoviruses. They are present in dirty water and sewage, swimming pools, seawater, and drinking water (Mena and Gerba 2009). These are usually viruses of species A, serotypes 40 and 41. The concentration of viral particles in water necessary for an infection to occur is disputable. Water recommended for drinking should not be the cause of more than one infection per 10,000 consumers per year. Water in swimming pools should be biologically as pure as potable water, assuming that inexperienced swimmer drinks approximately 30 mL a day. Two samples of river water and potable water in South Africa contained 1.40 and 2.45 adenoviruses per 10,000 L, respectively (van Heerden et al. 2005a). Nowadays, due to chlorination there are 0.5 adenoviruses per 100 L in surface waters, which indicates the effectiveness of the preventive measures against adenoviruses infections (Mena and Gerba 2009). However, it is crucial to monitor the concentration of viruses in potable water in some parts of South Africa, as well as the efficiency of water treatment processes (van Heerden et al. 2005b). Similar problem occurs in south-eastern Poland, where seasonally waste water is disposed to some rivers (Kozyra et al. 2011).

The presence of adenoviruses in food was mainly related to drinking raw, unprocessed milk. After the introduction of pasteurization the problem was solved. Seafood could be another food carrier. Adenoviruses serotypes 40 and 41 do not multiply in cell cultures. Diagnosis is made by subjecting the feces to EM, latex agglutination, or monoclonal antibody based immune EM examination.

An interesting observation is a potential connection between adenovirus infection and the development of obesity. It was noted that the frequency of the presence of antibodies against adenoviruses is six times higher in obese people than in healthy population. It is assumed that adenovirus AD 36 and avian SMAM 1 affect ventromedial nucleus and paraventricular nucleus of hypothalamus, leading to increased appetite. This hypothesis needs further studies (Dhurandhar et al. 2000), especially in the context of possible spread of the disease through food.

13.8 HEPATITIS INFECTIONS

13.8.1 Introduction

Hepatitis viruses type A and E (HAV and HEV) present in water contaminated with feces, in food (during flood) or in raw seafood in tropical countries, can cause viral hepatitis with comparatively mild symptoms. The illness is characteristic for viral infections. Early stage, lasting several days, called prodromal period (viremia) is similar to flu infection. The dominating symptoms are elevated temperature, fatigue, lack of appetite, nausea, pain in the area of liver, and possibly diarrhea.

In the second stage, liver symptoms occur. It becomes a phase of organ localized infection, occurring approximately 4–6 weeks after the initial infection. The symptoms include jaundice, dark amber color of urine, light colored feces, and skin itching. The symptoms affect only one-third of infected people. The disease is accompanied by enlarged liver, sometimes also spleen and lymph nodes. Mainly small children and teenagers become infected. Antibodies, indicating the contact with the virus, are present in only 30% people in Poland. After the HAV infection one usually recovers completely, there is neither carrier state nor chronic hepatitis. Passing through the infection results in lifelong immunity. The immunity ensures high number of specific IgG antibodies.

HEV infections transmitted via fecal—oral route are present mainly in Asia, Africa, and Central America. The main source of the infection is contaminated water. The course of the infection is usually mild and the recovery complete. Unfortunately, a less favorable prognosis is during pregnancy, when the mortality can reach 10–40% (CDC 2004).

13.8.2 HAV Infection

HAV is a self-limiting inflammatory disease affecting liver parenchyma. People are the reservoir of the virus and the disease spreads via fecal—oral route, by transferring virions to water or food. Viruses can survive for a long time in waste water, ground water, warm shelf waters (up to 10 months), and in food products. The source of the infection could be, for example, shellfish, various types salads containing tomatoes, spring onions, iceberg lettuce, fennel, carrots, raspberries, and even ice cubes added to drinks. In countries with limited access to clean water, it was observed that 90% of the population possessed antibodies, which indicated contact with the virus, most commonly after asymptomatic infection. Therefore, the disease among the youth and adults, after the consumption of contaminated food, are rare (Fiore 2004). In Europe, where the chances of acquiring the disease are lower, there is a tendency for cyclic outbreaks, recurring every 20 years. This is caused by the appearance of next, susceptible generations (cyclic epidemic). Nowadays in the United States, Israel, Italy, and Spain, where vaccination is compulsory, most often against HAV and HBV (Twinrix vaccine) this is less visible; however, the outbreaks cycles appear every decade (CDC 2004).

According to CDC, globally there are approximately 1.5 million symptomatic cases of hepatitis A occurring each year, mainly in the Third World countries. In Poland, the incidence rate amounts to 15/1,00,000 people. People taking part in family events, for example, weddings, baptism, or eating in mass feeding or catering points, such as canteens or cafeterias, are especially at risk of acquiring infection. Thus, schoolchildren, kindergarten children, people living in dorms, and pensioners are most often infected, but so are active homosexuals, people addicted to drugs, people engaged in medical care and close to a patient (need for preventive administration of γ-globulin or a vaccine in advance), and sewage workers (Zuckerman 1996). The majority of outbreaks occur in spring or autumn, which can be related to people returning from trips to regions with higher incidence rate. Those regions are Mediterranean countries, Eastern Europe, Central and Eastern Asia, South America, and Africa. Infectious period in humans lasts from 2 weeks before the symptoms appear to one week after the symptoms occur. A patient, unaware of the infection, poses a threat to those around, especially if working in contact with food or in bottling plant (CDC Advisory Committee on Immunization Practices 1999).

HAV belongs to Picornaviridae family. The size of the virion is 27 nm, and the genome consists of a positive-sense ssRNA. As much as 7500 nucleotides form a capsid, which is serologically one serotype. The virus sustains low pH of gastric acid. It is also resistant to low temperatures (−80°C). Because it does not possess an envelope, it is resistant to detergents and also to chlorine at low concentrations.

Incubation period ranges from 2 weeks to 2 months. After unspecific prodromal symptoms (3–10 days), similar to those mentioned earlier for other viral infections, a second acute phase of the infection begins, characterized by jaundice, the presence of dark amber color of urine, light, clay-colored feces, pains under right costal arch, skin itchiness, lack of appetite, reflux, vomiting, changes in laboratory parameters. The third phase is convalescence. The infection normally ends with spontaneous full recovery usually providing lifelong immunity, without turning into a carrier state. Asymptomatic course or hepatitis without jaundice is also possible. In some patients, the infection develops into acute liver failure, being more common in patients above the age of 50 (Zuckerman 1996).

The prevention of HAV infections is a serious problem. As stressed by Fiore, the infectious dose for hepatitis A is unknown. The infection is spread by fecal—oral route and viruses are transmitted by hands to unprocessed food. Workers having contact with food should undergo preventive vaccination against HAV. Proper sanitary standards, including washing and disinfecting hands after leaving a toilet, are crucial. Using disposable gloves for preparation and handling food should be considered; however, it is not a substitute for hands washing and disinfection. Fresh components of vegetable salads, such as lettuce, require washing under pressure with clean water. Such process leads to 10–100-fold reduction in viruses number, not removing them entirely. Another problem is posed by shellfish—for example, mussels, which are thrown into boiling water for up to 2 min, what does not guarantee their sterility, because the concentration of viruses in cockles is 100 times higher. The number of viruses can be lowered by keeping the shellfish for a week in clean exchanged water to reduce the concentration of hepatovirus A in gastrointestinal tract of the shellfish. Unfortunately, it is not an ideal solution. Only the direct treatment of the product with temperature exceeding 85°C for longer than one minute kills the viruses. The use of gamma globulin in people having contact with food contaminated with hepatovirus A is often stressed as necessary (Fiore 2004).

13.8.3 HEV Infection

HEV is described as an acute, necrotic self-limiting infection of liver parenchyma. It is caused by viruses belonging to Hepeviridae family, with diameter approximately 30 nm, ssRNA genome, 1 and 2 genotypes, capsomeres of spherical geometry, and proteins forming one serotype. The virus does not possess an envelope. People are the reservoir, but HEV strains were reported among wild and domestic pigs, and the presence of IgG antibodies was observed in pigs and cattle. Besides that it has been recognized in almost all domestic animals, as well as in rodents and wildlife species (e.g., deer, boars, and rabbits.) (Christou and Kosmidou 2013). It is known that animal virus species are infectious to humans—genotypes 3 and 4 (Lee et al. 2013). Undoubtedly, the infection is transmitted from person to person by water contaminated with feces. Thus, the infections are noted in hot countries during rainy season, when waste water enters ground waters and drinking water reservoirs. According to WHO, the infections affect Central and Southeast Asia and Northeast Africa. Person to person transmissions affecting people close to the sick person are uncommon, unlike in case of HAV. The number of infections every year is estimated to be 20 million confirmed infections, 3 million presumptive cases and 56,000 deaths due to HEV-fulminant hepatitis (acute liver failure). Besides the transmission of viruses by water and food, another possibility is a vertical transfer from a mother to a child. In pregnant women, especially those in the third trimester, infected by 1 and 2 HEV genotypes, the disease is especially severe (eclampsia, hemorrhage, miscarriage, with or without liver damage) (WHO 2016).

HEV infection is a disease of war, conflicts, and natural disasters. Men between 15 and 30 years of age are most commonly affected. Until recently it was claimed that it is a rare disease throughout EU countries, not exceeding 1% of cases of infectious hepatitis, carried by people returning from endemic regions. Thanks to the research carried out in UK it was proved that approximately 3% of affected people with jaundice in the course of drug poisoning are infected with animal genotype 3 of HEV virus. Thus, shortly cooked pork can be a source of HEV. It was also determined that alcoholism is a factor worsening the prognosis of the disease due to progressing liver damage.

The course of HEV is the following: incubation period, lasting on average 40 days; early period, prodromal, with uncharacteristic flu—like symptoms together with nausea, anorexia and vomiting—lasts several days; acute phase, with symptoms characteristic to previously mentioned hepatitis infections—lasts several weeks; final recovery phase. Recently it has been observed that recovery phase can be preceded by chronic hepatitis E.

In southeast France, an increase in liver enzymes concentration in blood was observed in patients with hematological malignancies or HIV, after transplants, taking Tacrolimus, without jaundice. In as much as 60% of people being at risk of contact with HEV in the period above half a year, a chronic HEV form was observed, confirmed by positive PCR results, leading to cirrhosis in 10% of them. In other regions, the incidence of complications in patients with blood conditions and with HIV did not exceed 1% (Scobie and Dalton 2013).

Another forms of chronic HEV are numerous neurological complications caused by genotype 3 in Europe, and genotype 1 in Asia, with unknown pathogenesis (Scobie and Dalton 2013). The authors stress the necessity to:

1. Use safe water;
2. Consume seafood (oysters) caught in safe reservoirs; in South Korea it was shown that oysters can carry genotype 3 of HAV coming from local pigs;
3. Cook pork thoroughly or deep fry it, resign from grilling or barbecuing, avoid a specific barbecue restaurant; in Japan the presence of ssRNA was determined in 2% of pigs' livers, in the United States—in 11%, in Germany—in 4%;
4. Adhere to hand hygiene regimens;
5. Carry out proper and safe water and sewage management (Christou and Kosmidou 2013).

Due to the presence of HEV among rodents, also the necessity to protect farming animals and human dwellings against rodents could be added to the above, to prevent the spread of the infection.

It is known that the most important means of prevention are vaccinations. A hepatitis E vaccine was developed in China. However, "due to the lack of sufficient information on safety, immunogenicity and efficacy in the following population subgroups, WHO does not recommend routine use of the vaccine in children aged <16 years, pregnant women, chronic liver disease patients, and patients on organ transplant waiting lists, and travelers" (WHO 2015).

13.9 ENTEROVIRUS INFECTIONS: POLIO, COXSACKIE A, B AND ECHO

Enteroviruses belong to Picornaviridae. The genus "Enterovirus" contains Polio viruses, Coxsackie A and B, and ECHO. Enteroviruses are characterized by a positive-strand ssRNA. A virion is 18–30 nm in diameter, and its capsid has icosahedral geometry. The viruses exhibit various cytopathic effects in cell cultures; they also have different affinity to tissues. Those factors lead to classification of the viruses into 68 types: poliovirus contains three serotypes, Coxsackie A—23 serotypes,

Coxsackie B—6, ECHO—28 serotypes, and 5 other types of viruses. Based on the genome structure, the viruses were divided into five groups: polio, human enterovirus A (HEV A), human enterovirus B (HEV B), human enterovirus C (HEV C), and human enterovirus D (HEV D). All five viruses are infectious to humans. Animals are affected by them as well. The infections were observed in farming and wild animals. The disease is present in pigs, calves, dogs, foxes, rabbits, squirrels, monkeys, and enteroviruses were also found in oysters and mussels. Usually humans are the source of the infection. Transmission occurs by fecal—oral route or can be airborne in case of upper respiratory tract infection, or in the presence of the aerosol surrounding vomiting person. The disease can be also transmitted by carriers such as flies or insects. It has been shown that the highest risk is posed by water contaminated with faces, swimming pools, and beach resorts. Children are most commonly affected, especially in countries with low socioeconomic standards. In summer, during heat waves, there are numerous worldwide outbreaks caused by enteroviruses other than polio.

According to WHO 2015 "Polio cases have decreased by over 99% since 1988, from an estimated 3,50,000 cases then, to 359 reported cases in 2014. The reduction is the result of the global effort to eradicate the disease." Polio outbreaks occur mainly in Pakistan and Afghanistan, whereas in other parts of the world there are less than ten cases reported every year. Due to preventive measures taken since 1988 by the Global Polio Eradication Initiative (GPEI), spearheaded by national governments, WHO, Rotary International, the CDC, UNICEF, and supported by key partners including the Bill and Melinda Gates Foundation, a total eradication of the infections with wild and vaccine virus is assumed within the program for the years 2013–2018 (WHO 2015b).

The global interest in polio virus eradication was led by the consequences of this disease. Clinical image of polio may vary—from asymptomatic cases, through meningitis symptoms to acute flaccid paralysis, including death. A person undergoing asymptomatic or mildly symptomatic infection could be a reservoir of the virus. Faces or secretion from upper respiratory tract are the contagious materials. Viruses are shed in the faces after 72 h from the contact with a virus, and when transmitted by insects they contaminate food. The viruses are present in upper respiratory tract after 36 h. The spread of the infection is thus possible by contaminated objects. Polio viruses carried to potable water and beach resorts can infect people. The incubation period lasts up to 2 weeks. After that period, the viruses reach lymphoid tissue of gastrointestinal and respiratory systems, and then are carried via blood to central nervous system. The consequence of the infection is the development of nonparalytic aseptic meningitis, or acute flaccid paralysis due to the damage of anterior horn cells of the spinal cord (paralytic poliomyelitis), leading to permanent disability. The life-threatening forms of the disease are spinal, bulbospinal, bulbar, and progressive bulbar palsy. There is no cure for polio; the only available treatment provides relief of symptoms.

Good effects were obtained by prophylactic, mass, obligatory vaccination: attenuated vaccine containing live polio viruses OPV (oral poliomyelitis vaccine), used in countries where wild polio viruses occur, and IPV (inactivated poliomyelitis vaccine), used in countries where wild polio viruses are not present.

Other infections caused by Enteroviruses, as well as Coxsackie A and B, within the gastrointestinal tract, cause acute gastroenteritis, abdominal pains, constipation, mesenteric lymphadenitis, appendicitis, intussusception, hepatitis, Reye's syndrome, and type I diabetes (mimicry theory assumes antigenic compatibility between β cells in the pancreatic isles and Coxsackie B types 1–5). It is estimated that in the United States approximately 10 million enterovirus infections occur each year. The infections more often affect small children (boys) and infants. One-fourth of those are Coxsackie infections, usually due to type B1. Among neonates also Coxsackie viruses are responsible for approximately 25% of the infections; however, the dominating type of the virus is B4 (Muller et al. 2015).

13.10 DIAGNOSTIC TESTS OF VIRAL CONTAMINATION IN DIFFERENT KIND OF FOOD AND WATER

Potential contamination of water with viruses present in humans' and animals' digestive tracts poses a significant problem. There are two aspects to be considered:

1. Determining the presence of viruses and their numbers,
2. Effective prevention of the contamination and constant monitoring.

The presence of viruses in water and food can be determined by standard methods established long time ago; however, they are unpractical because it takes too long to obtain results and high costs are involved. Such methods include: determination of cytopathic effect in cell cultures, finding viruses in a sample using EM, showing the ability to inhibit the passive hemagglutination reaction if specific sera against targeted viruses are available (SPACE test—solid phase agglutination with coupled erythrocytes).

Other methods practically used nowadays include indirect and direct ELISA and PCR methods: multiplex PCR, nested PCR—when searching for various viruses in food homogenate or in water, or real-time PCR, enabling to determine the amount of genetic material in tested product. These methods require dedicated equipment and proper knowledge on how to use it.

Determination of potential viruses counts on the basis of *Escherichia coli* and coliforms counts does not work, because viruses are much more resistant than bacteria to environmental factors. They also sustain wider pH range (from 3 to 10). Water treatment process has two stages. Basic treatment involves the removal of contaminants and impurities. The efficiency of water purification using different processes was assessed in percentages. The most effective were membrane processes, which enable to remove 90–100% of contaminants due to reverse osmosis. Ultrafiltration and electrodialysis allow for the removal of 60–90–100% of contaminants. Coagulation with sedimentation and filtration is also effective, enabling to remove 60–100% of impurities, similarly as with calcium treatment. It seems that the entire removal of viruses is practically impossible. The second stage of water treatment relies on chlorination with free chlorine or chlorine dioxide. Bacteria are killed by 20-fold lower concentrations than viruses. However, high concentrations of chlorine give the water a specific smell and lead to the formation of toxic compounds, chlorites and chlorates. The viruses exhibiting especially high resistance against lower concentration of chlorine are Coxsackie and ECHO (Kowal and Świderska-Bróż 2007).

13.11 PREVENTION OF FOODBORNE CONTAMINATION AND VIRAL INFECTION IN PATIENTS

Prevention of viral infections on a mass scale is a great challenge, taking into consideration the facts that the majority of viruses present in water or food infect humans at low infectious doses (10–100 virions), they are highly resistant to environmental factors and tolerate wide range of pH, are resistant to low temperatures and to several disinfectants, and they are also able to survive in water for a long time (approximately a year). It is emphasized that the following factors are the causes of the majority of infections:

1. Transmission of viruses by the hands of the personnel, when the reservoir of the infection is either a sick person—worker of the food processing plant, or contaminated raw material, a product or a meal not subjected to heat treatment, or the thermal treatment was too short.
2. Seafood caught in waters contaminated with viruses.
3. Watering or sprinkling the fruits intended for consumption with contaminated water (raspberries in Denmark).
4. Insufficiently heated pork, grilled steaks.
5. Lack of biological treatment of wastewater, disposal of wastewater to rivers or sea.
6. Ineffective prevention against insects' access to food and water (transmission of the infection by flues, cockroaches, Pharaoh ants).
7. Potential contamination of food and water by rodents—mice and rats.
8. Lack of obligatory, preventive use of vaccines against rotaviruses, HAV and polio by the personnel working in contact with food; in case of polio at least some of the infections could be effectively limited in this way.

The problem of viral infections becomes more and more serious in case of people. The reason for that is the growing number of people with weakened immune system or deliberately deprived of the immune response. The first group includes growing older population in developed countries and malnourished children in underdeveloped ones. The second group comprises growing number of patients after organs or marrow transplants, treated with chemotherapeutic agents, those subjected to radiotherapy or treated with biopharmaceuticals in case of autoaggressive diseases.

The issues concerning hand washing and disinfection, and then using protective gloves in contact with food, changing clothes and gloves with the change of food product range, proper procedures regarding handling the equipment and machinery used in food processing, are covered by Good Hygienic Practice, Good Manufacturing Practice, and HACCP.

Research, however, is directed at proper handling of seafood to avoid contamination. It is widely known that high temperature treatment would sterilize a product, but this method cannot be fully applied. On one hand, the viruses are resistant to short thermal treatment, and on the other hand, with longer thermal treatment the product subjected to such treatment has lower sensory properties (becomes rubbery). Thus, the remaining solution is to use preventive measures. They were divided into those used before the catch and during processing.

Preventive measures used before catching seafood include water microbial quality testing, and even though it is known that the number of *E. coli* and coliforms does not correspond to viral contamination, it is still a marker of fecal contamination of water. It was proposed to include the determination of bacteriophages, especially F-specific coliphages, somatic coliphages, and phages of *Bacteroides fragilis* to the monitoring of viral water quality. The hypothesis was attractive, because it allowed to test for one type of bacteriophages, and not particular types of viruses. Because phages are less sensitive to changing environmental factors than viruses contaminating water and food, the research is still ongoing.

Another approach was to test previously caught seafood, especially oysters, for the presence of viruses, after several days of self-purification in clean water, or with the addition of disinfectants: chlorine, ozone, and after UV treatment. The methods are commonly used, but even though they give good results in case of pathogenic bacteria decontamination, they are ineffective in case of contamination of seafood with HAV.

Enteropathogenic viruses survive well during storage at low temperatures in fridges and freezers. However, their life span shortens to several weeks at positive temperatures. It has been shown that subjecting seafood to the temperature above 85°C for one minute eliminates the infectiousness of hepatitis A virus; however, other authors claim that the product becomes safe only after 2 min of heat treatment at the temperature above 90°C.

Using microwaves also does not guarantee the elimination of viruses. The treatment with ionizing radiation at the dose of 3 Gy reduces the number of HAV by 95%, whereas in case of 2 Gy—below 95%. It has been suggested to use a combined approach, that is, depuration with radiation doses 2 Gy, to keep sensory values. The opponents of such a solution point at high costs of the method.

Another means of HAV elimination could be the use of high pressure of 450 MPa for 5 min and 275 MPa for 5 min. For polio viruses the parameters should be changed— 600 MPa for 15 min; however, longer treatment did not improve the outcome.

A challenging task is to reduce the number of viruses on leafy vegetables or small fruits. A commonly used method is to rinse under a strong stream of water containing chlorine compounds (200 mg/L) or organic acids. The addition of ozone did not work, especially in case of slightly damaged produce, as oxidation causes discoloring and aroma loss. The temperature of utilized water was also modified to 22–43°C, which lead to a further reduction in the number of viruses. The addition of washing liquids such as Fit (Proctor and Gamble) and automatic dishwashing detergent (ADWD, 0.05%), 10% vinegar or 2% kitchen salt leads to the reduction in viruses by 95–99%.

Avoiding further contamination of food products is possible with meticulous adherence to hand washing and disinfection recommendations. Noroviruses can survive on the surface of hands for up to an hour. Microbiologically dirty hands pose a major threat in case of ready to eat food. Prevention of food poisoning during food processing relies on maintaining proper hand hygiene, especially before commencing the work. It is crucial to prepare hands for the work, that is, maintain skin integrity, keep short nails, lack of nail enamel or tips. Besides washing hands in warm water with liquid soaps (they can contain disinfectants), there should be a place for hands disinfection with dedicated alcohol-based sanitizers.

Places used for serving food should have the surfaces washed with detergents, especially in hotels, where there is a risk of surface contamination with vomit. Lesser threat is posed by carpets or soft floor-coverings that are cleaned and hovered in a standard way.

It is beneficial for the employers to preventively vaccinate their workers against previously discussed viruses causing food poisoning (Papafragkou et al. 2006).

REFERENCES

Bernstein, D.I. 2009. Rotavirus overview. *Pediatr Infect Dis J* 28(3): S50–S53.

CDC. 1999. Prevention of hepatitis A through active or passive immunization: Recommendations of the Advisory Committee on Immunization Practices (ACIP). *MMWR Recomm Rep* 48(RR-12): 1–37.

Centers for Disease Control and Prevention. 2004. Disease burden from hepatitis A, B, and C in the United States. Available at: http://www.cdc.gov/ncidod/diseases/hepatitis/resource/

Chen, S.Y., C.N. Tsai, M.W. Lai, C.Y. Chen, K.L. Lin, T.Y. Lin, and C.H. Chiu. 2009. Norovirus infection as a cause of diarrhea-associated benign infantile seizures. *Clin Infect Dis* 48(7): 849–855.

Christou, L., and M. Kosmidou. 2013. Hepatitis E virus in the Western world—a pork-related zoonosis. *Clin Microbiol Infect* 19(7): 600–604.

Dhurandhar, N.V., B.A. Israel, I.M. Kolesar, G.F. Mayhew, M.E. Cook, and R.L. Atkinson. 2000. Increased adiposity in animals due to human virus. *Int J Obes Relat Metab Disord* 24: 989–996.

Fiore, E.A. 2004. Hepatitis A transmitted by food. *CliniInfecti Dise* 38: 705–715.

Gentsch, J.R., A.R. Laird, B. Bielfelt, D.D. Griffin, K. Banyai, M. Ramachandran, V. Jain, N.A. Cunliffe, O. Nakagomi, C.D. Kirkwood, T.K. Fischer, U.D. Parashar, J.S. Bresee, B. Jiang, and R.I. Glass. 2005. Serotype diversity and reassortment between human and animal rotavirus strains implications for rotavirus vaccine programs. *J Infect* 192: S146–S159.

Giaquinto, C., P. Van Damme, F. Huet, L. Gothefors, M. Maxwell, P. Todd, and L. da Dalt. 2007. Clinical consequences of rotavirus acute gastroenteritis in Europe, 2004–2005: The REVEAL study. *J Infect Dis* 1(195): 26–35.

Gliński, Z., and K. Kostro. 2012. Astrowiroza norek—obserwacje wstępne. *Życie Weterynaryjne* 7(11): 922–924.

Hansman, G.S., T. Oka, K. Katayama, and N. Takeda. 2007. Human sapoviruses: Genetic diversity, recombination, and classification. *Rev Med Virol* 17(2): 133–141.

Kowal, A., and M. Świderska-Bróż. 2007. *Oczyszczanie wody. Podstawy teoretyczne i technologiczne, procesy i urządzenia.* Wydawnictwo Naukowe PWN: Warszawa, Poland, pp. 85–110.

Kozyra, I., A. Kaupke, and A. Rzeżutka. 2011. Seasonal occurrence of human enteric viruses in river water samples collected from rural areas of South-East Poland. *Food Environ Virol* 3 (3): 115–120.

Leclerc, L., L. Schwartzbrod, and E. Dei-Cas. 2002. Microbial agents associated with waterborne diseases. *Crit Rev Microbiol* 28(4): 371–409.

Lee, C.N., Y.L. Wang, C.L. Kao, C.L. Zao, C.Y. Lee, and H.N. Chen. 2000. NSP4 gene analysis of rotaviruses recovered from infected children with and without diarrhea. *J Clin Microbiol* 38(12): 4471–4477.

Lee, J.T., P.L. Shao, L.Y. Chang, N.S. Xia, P.J. Chen, C.Y. Lu, and L.M. Huang. 2013. Seroprevalence of Hepatitis E virus infection among swine farmers and the general population in rural Tajwan. *PLoS One* 8(6): e67180.

Lee, L.E., E.A. Cebelinski, C. Fuller, W.E. Keene, K. Smith, J. Vinjé, and J.M. Besser. 2012. Sapovirus outbreaks in long-term care facilities, Oregon and Minnesota, 2002–2009. *Emerg Infect Dis* 18: 873–876.

Jeong, H.S., A. Jeong, and D.S. Cheon. 2012. Epidemiology of astrovirus infection in children. *Korean J Pediatr* 55(3): 77–82.

Lin, C.L., S.C. Chen, S.Y. Liu, and K.T. Chen. 2014. Disease caused by rotavirus infection. *Open Virol J* 8: 14–19.

Mena, K.D., and C.P. Gerba. 2009. Waterborne adenovirus. *Rev Environ Contam Toxicol* 198: 133–167.

Muller, M. 2016. Coxsackieviruses. *Medscape.*

Robilotti, E., S. Deresinski, and B.A. Pinsky. 2015. Norovirus. *Clin Microbiol Rev* 28(1): 134–164.

Papafragkou, E., H.D. D'Souza, L.A. Jaykus. 2006. Food-borne viruses: Prevention and control. In *Viruses in Foods*, ed. S.M. Goyal. Minnesota, Minnesota-Saint Paul: Springer.

Rossmann, M.G. 2013. Structure of viruses: A short history. *Q Rev Biophys* 46(2): 133–180.

Scobie, L., and H.R. Dalton. 2013. Hepatitis E: Source and route of infection, clinical manifestations and new developments. *J Viral Hepat* 20(1): 1–11.

van Heerden, J., M.M. Ehlers, and W.O. Grabow. 2005a. Detection and risk assessment of adenoviruses in swimming pool water. *J Appl Microbiol* 99(5): 1256–1264.

van Heerden, J., M.M. Ehlers, J.C. Vivier, and W.O. Grabow. 2005b. Risk assessment of adenoviruses detected in treated drinking water and recreational water. *J Appl Microbiol* 99(4): 926–933.

WHO (World Health Organization). 2015. Poliomyelitis *Fact sheet* N°114.

WHO (World Health Organization). 2016. Hepatitis E. *Fact sheet* N°280.

Zuckerman, A.J. 1996. Hepatitis viruses. Chap. 70 in *Medical Microbiology*. 4th ed. Galveston, Texas. ISBN-10:0-9631172-1-1.

14 Possible Adverse Effects of Food Additives

Shilpi Gupta Dixit

CONTENTS

14.1 INTRODUCTION

Since time immemorial, ingredients have been added for improving various features of food to make it more palatable and reliable. It all started with preservation of food by additives like salt. In ancient times, cloves were added to food to prevent bacterial growth. The Egyptian Era saw the use of food colors, seasoning, spices, and flavors. The spices were worth sometimes more than human lives during Middle Ages. Columbus also discovered America when he explored the world through sea route in search of spices of India.

"Assize of Bread" was the first food regulatory law passed by the King of England in the early thirteenth century. Even in the United States, food regulatory laws also date back to early colonial lives.

In 1960, the first "Food and Drugs Act" was passed that prohibited interstate commerce in misbranded and adulterated foods, drinks, and drugs followed by the "Meat Inspection Act" again in the same year.

"Federal Food Drug and Cosmetic (FDA) Act" was passed in 1938 that set safe tolerance limits for unavoidable poisonous substances, authorization of food inspections, and maintenance of standards of identification and quality of foods.

In 1949, FDA published guidelines for the industry first time called "Procedures for the Appraisal of the Toxicity of Chemicals in Food" (Aka black book).

This was followed by "Oleomargarine Act" in 1950, "Food Additives Amendment" in 1958, "Consumer bill of Rights" in 1962, "Fair Packaging and Labeling Act" in 1965, "Infant Formula Act," and 1980 "Dietary Guidelines for Americans."

In 1982, FDA published "Toxicological principles for the safety assessment of direct food additives and color additives used in food." In 1990, "Nutritional Labeling and Education Act (NLEA)" was passed that required all packaged food to bear nutrition labeling and all health claims for foods to be consistent with terms defined by Secretary of Health and Human Services.

The twenty-first century marked many such regulations and bills passed by regulatory authorities of various countries, the most important ones being "Food Allergy Labeling and Consumer Protection Act" (FDA, USDA, AHA, Company and Organization Websites).

From 1948 to 1994, successive rounds of multilateral negotiation under the General Agreement on Tariffs and Trade (GATT) established the governing international rules for trade between states. Although the first negotiations focused on lowering tariffs on imported goods, later negotiations also covered nontariff barriers. The latest and largest negotiation round was the Uruguay Round of Multilateral Trade Negotiations from 1986 to 1994, which led to the creation of the World Trade Organization (WTO) on January 1, 1995. The Uruguay Round included not only goods but also services and intellectual property, and for the first time brought agricultural products under the discipline of international trade rules. With the progress of twentieth century, public demands of foods of high quality and convenience could be met by reasonably priced and packaged food. Advances in technology have made it possible to meet the demands of variability, accessibility, freshness, palatability, and uniformity that simply did not exist hundreds of years ago. In modern lifestyle, pursuit of happiness through enjoying of food have been made possible due to thousands of highly specialized ingredients known as food additives that contribute to increase in taste, textures, freshness, safety, eye appeal, and nutritional value of food.

The latest concept of labeling all food products is by putting labels like

100 % Natural
No added preservatives
No artificial products added

followed by a list of contents of food products in small print, which says "Added for colors and flavor." In modern times, you might not find even one food product in the market that does not contain at least one food additive. Even organic and the so-called 100% natural products also contain them for manufacturing and you avoid them only if you drink nothing but water.

14.2 WHAT ARE FOOD ADDITIVES?

In the broadest sense, a food additive is any substance added to food.

According to the EC Regulation 1333/2008 Article 3, a food additive is defined as

> Any substance not normally consumed as a food in itself and not normally used as a characteristic ingredient of food whether or not it has nutritive value, the intentional addition of which to food for a technological purpose in the manufacture, processing, preparation, treatment, packaging, transport or storage of such food results, or may be reasonably expected to result, in it or its by-products becoming directly or indirectly a component of such foods. (Guidance on Food Additives, 2010)

14.3 REASONS FOR USING FOOD ADDITIVES

Broadly food additives are mainly ingredients used for four major purposes:

1. Preservation of food and maintenance of product quality: Food additives like ascorbic acid in packaged fruit slices, propionates in bakery products significantly delay the deterioration, and prevent spoilage caused by growth of microorganisms as well as by oxidation.
2. To aid in the processing and preparation of foods that will impact certain desired qualities to them. Examples are emulsifiers such as lecithin used in ice-cream, cake mixes, stabilizers and thickeners like lecithin in ice cream, cake mixes, and leaveners like sorbitol.
3. Enhancement/maintenance of appearance and flavor like flavoring agents, coloring agents, and sweeteners.
4. Nutritional implements either to maintain or improve nutritional quality of food. Examples are addition of iodine to salt to reduce incidence of goiter, vitamin D to milk, and other dairy products, for the elimination of rickets, niacin in bread, and cereals. These additives are basically responsible for fortification in the diet to prevent diseases caused due to deficiencies.

Table 14.1 is showing the classification of food additives.

14.4 NATIONAL AND INTERNATIONAL REGULATIONS REGARDING THE USE OF ADDITIVES IN FOOD PRODUCTION

With the advancement of technology and an ever increasing portion of our population being employed in the working world, the food industry has to satisfy consumer demands of high quality and readily available foods. With the increase in the use of processed food, there has been a great increase in the use of food additives of varying levels of safety. This has led to legislations in many countries regulating their use.

Thousands of ingredients are being used to make foods that are commercially available in the world markets. However, food additives used for whatsoever purpose are ultimately composed of chemicals. Today, these are strictly studied, regulated, and maintained. Federal authorities and various international organizations are now

TABLE 14.1
Classification of Food Additives

Type of Food Additive	Action	Uses	Additives
Preservatives	Substances that prolong the shelf-life of foods by protecting them against deterioration caused by micro-organisms and/or against growth of pathogenic micro-organisms Prevent changes in color, flavor, or texture and delay rancidity	Fruit sauces and jellies, beverages, baked goods, cured meats, oils and margarines, cereals, dressings, snack foods, fruits and vegetables	Ascorbic acid, citric acid, sodium benzoate, calcium propionate, sodium erythorbate, sodium nitrate(III), calcium sorbate, potassium sorbate, BHA, BHT, EDTA, tocopherols (Vitamin E)
Emulsifiers	Substances that make it possible to form or maintain a homogenous mixture of two or more immiscible phases such as oil and water in a foodstuff. control stickiness and crystallization	Salad dressings, peanut butter, chocolate, margarine, frozen desserts	Soy lecithin, mono- and diacylglycerols, egg yolks, polysorbates, sorbitan monostearate sodium phosphate
Stabilizers binders, texturizers	Give foods a firmer texture, and help to stabilize emulsions: substances that make it possible to maintain the physicochemical state of a foodstuff	Frozen desserts, dairy products, cakes, pudding and gelatin mixes, dressings, jams and jellies, sauces	Pectin and agar, ammonium alginate, carragenin
Thickeners	Substances that increase the viscosity of a foodstuff without substantially modifying other properties	Frozen desserts, dairy products, cakes, pudding and gelatin mixes, dressings, jams and jellies, sauces	Agar, acid treated starch, acetylated distarch adipate, acetylated distarch phosphate, acetylated oxidized starch, xanthan gum
pH Control agents and acids	Control acidity and alkalinity, prevent spoilage Added to make flavors "sharper," and also act as preservatives and antioxidants	Beverages, frozen desserts, chocolate, low acid canned foods, baking powder	Lactic acid, citric acid, ammonium hydroxide, sodium carbonate
Leavening agents	Promote rising of baked goods	Breads and other baked goods	Baking soda, monocalcium phosphate, calcium carbonate
Anti-caking agents	Keep powdered foods free-flowing, prevent moisture absorption	Salt, baking powder, confectioner's sugar	Calcium silicate, iron ammonium citrate, silicon dioxide, ammonium silicate

(Continued)

TABLE 14.1 (*Continued*)
Classification of Food Additives

Type of Food Additive	Action	Uses	Additives
Humectants	Retain moisture, prevent foods from drying up	Shredded coconut, marshmallows, soft candies, confections	Glycerin, sorbitol
Enzyme preparations	Modify proteins, polysaccharides and fats	Cheese, dairy products, meat	Enzymes, lactase, papain, rennet, chymosin
Dough strengtheners and conditioners	Produce more stable dough	Breads and other baked goods	Ammonium sulfate, azodicarbonamide, L-cysteine
Firming agents	Maintain crispness and firmness	Processed fruits and vegetables	Calcium chloride, calcium lactate, Epsom Salts, magnesium sulfate
Gases	Serve as propellant, aerate, or create carbonation	Oil cooking spray, whipped cream, carbonated beverages	Carbon dioxide, nitrous oxide
Sweeteners	Add sweetness with or without the extra calories	Beverages, baked goods, confections, table-top sugar, substitutes, many processed foods	Sucrose, glucose, fructose, sorbitol, mannitol, corn syrup, high fructose corn syrup, saccharin, aspartame, sucralose, acesulfame potassium (acesulfame-K), neotame
Color additives	Natural or artificial offset color loss due to exposure to light, air, temperature extremes, moisture and storage conditions; correct natural variations in color; enhance colors that occur naturally; provide color to colorless and "fun" foods	Candies, snack foods margarine, cheese, soft drinks, jams/jellies, gelatins, pudding and pie fillings	FD&C Blue 1 and 2, FD&C Green 3, FD&C Red 3 and 40, FD&C Yellow. 5 and 6, Orange B, Citrus Red 2, annatto extract, beta-carotene, grape skin extract, cochineal extract or carmine, paprika oleoresin, caramel color, fruit and vegetable juices, saffron
Flavors and spices	Add specific flavors (natural and synthetic)	Pudding and pie fillings, gelatin dessert mixes, cake mixes, salad dressings, candies, soft drinks, ice cream, BBQ sauce	Natural flavoring, artificial flavor, and spices

(*Continued*)

TABLE 14.1 (*Continued*)
Classification of Food Additives

Type of Food Additive	Action	Uses	Additives
Flavor enhancers	Enhance flavors already present in foods (without providing their own separate flavor)	Many processed foods	Monosodium glutamate (MSG), hydrolyzed soy protein, autolyzed yeast extract, disodium guanylate or inosinate
Fat replacers (and components of formulations used to replace fats)	Provide expected texture and a creamy "mouth-feel" in reduced-fat foods	Baked goods, dressings, frozen desserts, confections, cake and dessert mixes, dairy products	Olestra, cellulose gel, carrageenan, polydextrose, modified food starch, microparticulated egg white protein, guar gum, xanthan gum, whey protein concentrate
Nutrients	Replace vitamins and minerals lost in processing (enrichment), add nutrients that may be lacking in the diet (fortification)	Flour, breads, cereals, rice, macaroni, margarine, salt, milk, fruit beverages, energy bars, instant breakfast drinks	Thiamine hydrochloride, riboflavin niacin, niacinamide, folate or folic acid, beta carotene, potassium iodide, iron or ferrous sulfate, alpha tocopherols, ascorbic acid, Vitamin D, amino acids (L-tryptophan, L-lysine, L-leucine, L-methionine)
Yeast nutrients	Promote growth of yeast	Breads and other baked goods	Calcium sulfate, ammonium phosphate
Bulking agents	Additives that increase the bulk of a food without affecting its nutritional value		Modified food starch or modified corn starch
Glazing agents	Provide a shiny appearance or protective coating to foods		Beeswax, Candelilla wax, Carnauba wax, paraffin wax, refined microcrystalline wax

carefully regulating all of these food additives so that the consumers are ensured of the safety and accurate labeling of the foods they are eating.

Expansion of food trade, both within countries and in between the nations, needs regulation not only at national but also at international level to ensure that the desirable characteristics of food are retained during various stages of production, handling, processing, packaging, distribution, and preparation for meals. With the increase in consumer rights, the state should ensure good quality and safe food supply that will promote healthy diets, reduce economic losses, and encourage domestic and international trade of food.

Various nations along with international food control organizations have introduced various food laws and regulations. A food law is generally based on scientific studies. Harmonization of food law on international level is a worldwide trend from late twentieth century.

Generally the structure of a food laws consists of two parts:

1. Basic food act that contains broad principles of food standards, hygienic provisions, food additives. It includes definition of basic concepts, enforcement of law by inspections and analytical procedures, penalties of defaulters, and also procedures for amendments in regulations if and when necessary.
2. Regulations that contain detailed specifications governing food processing packaging, labeling, food standards, additives, advertising hygienic practices, and pesticides. Revisions in regulations are necessary and should be prompt because of advent of new findings in science and food processing technology or in case of emergencies that require instant action to protect consumer's health (Vapnek and Spreij, 2005).

Following various initial laws mentioned in the introduction a number of regulation agencies have been formed in various countries.

1. One of the major ones is US Food and Drug Administration (FDA) that has the legal responsibility of protecting public health by assuring the safety, cleanliness, security and efficacy of food products, human and veterinary drugs, biological products, medical electives, cosmetics, and also those products that emit radiation. It includes:
   EAFUS—everything added to food in United States, food ingredients, packaging and labeling, GRAS.
2. European Commission (EC) is responsible for defending general interest of all European countries and implementing various common policies and managing European Unions (EU's) budget and programs.
   The European Food Safety Authority (EFSA) is the keystone of EU risk assessment regarding food and feed safety.
3. Food Standards Australia, New Zealand, Food Additives give information pertinent to reading food labels, including names of food additives associated with code numbers, functional classes/uses, and information on food intolerance.

4. Health Canada gives general information on food additives, including regulations and other Canadian resources (Final Report to Canadians Reducing Food Safety Risks, 2016).
5. Japan Ministry of Health, Labour & Welfare, Food Additives gives regulatory information, including lists of additives designated as approved, substances being evaluated for authorization, lists of substances exempted from the "designation system," Japan's specifications and standards for use of food additives, and guidance for the designation of food additives and revision of standards for use.

Other agreements/associations and organizations international acclaimed include:

1. SPS Agreement (Application of Sanitary and Phytosanitary Measures) defines rights and responsibilities of WTO members and can apply measures to protect human and animal life and health sanitary measures and plant life and health (phytosanitary measures). SPS Agreement also requires that the member states should take into account the special needs of developing countries, in particular the least developed countries that are granted longer time frames for compliance with the agreement.
2. TBT Agreement ensure that technical regulations and standards including packaging, marketing, and labeling requirements as well as testing and certification procedures do not create unnecessary obstacles for the international trade. It covers all technical standards not covered by SPS Agreement and applies to all food products including agricultural products (Food Standards Agency, 2002).

Several other international technical organizations that have joined the food safety initiative and that have expertise in SPS issues include Codex Alimentarius that is a UN international body and jointly funded by WHO and FAO. This body is concerned with the setting and implementation of international standards and protecting the health of consumers. Then there is other like International Food Information Council (IFIC) that is responsible for communication of science-based information about food safety standards to health professionals, governments, educators, journalists, as well as consumers. Others include International Food Additives Council (IFAC), Food Chemicals Codex (FCC), and Joint FAO/WHO Expert Committee on Food Additives (JECFA) (WHO Technical Report Series, 1987).

14.5 SAFETY GUIDELINES TO CONTROL RISK OF USING OVERDOSE OR BANDED ADDITIVES

The decision of whether an additive (either natural or manmade) can be permitted for its use in food depending on its safety.

Every additive no matter what its source or intended purpose is composed of chemicals. Universal food safety requirements state that food is considered as unsafe if it is potentiality "injurious to health, unfit for human consumption or contaminated keeping into consideration both short- and long-term effects, its effects on subsequent generations or effect on specific sensitive categories of consumers that are pregnant women, diabetics, infants or old people where the foods are intended to be used.

The words "toxic" "harmful," and "safe" should be used carefully as every substance has potential to be harmful either due its chemical composition, due to quantity in which it is being used, route, conditions of exposure, or susceptibility of organisms exposed to those substances (Toxic substances strategy committee 1980 Report).

Food safety testing has progressed a long way since early 1900s to twenty-first century. Both industry and government evaluate safety through comprehensive testing and accepted scientific procedures. The process of introducing a new food additive is quite rigorous and time consuming.

The evaluation of a food additive is done by examining its chemical structure and physical characteristics, its specifications, impurities, and the potential breakdown products in its intended use. For direct additives, the first step is to conduct a battery of tests with its chemical analyses to determine that a substance does what it is intended to do, and that it can be measured accurately in minute quantities. These tests assure that the usage can be checked, and that unwanted manufacturing by-products are adequately removed. Animal testing is carried out using higher doses of the additive than would be used in food for humans. Since no animal is a perfect model, a number of tests in different laboratory conditions and doses should be carried out and totality of scientific evidence must be evaluated and cautiously interpreted before being extrapolated to man. Large doses over extended periods are administered to determine whether an additive may be harmful over a lifetime of use. Human studies if adequate and when available are most significant. Studies on metabolism, genetic toxicity, carcinogenicity, and reproduction are among those required.

Various tests have now been developed to detect even miniscule quantities of indirect food additives (with accuracy of detection 1 part per billion or 1 part per trillion) as it helps in determine the margins of safety. It is well known that potential toxic effects of any food substance/additive are dose dependent.

Few terms generally used during the safety testing and approval of new food additives are:

1. ADI (Acceptable Daily Intake)—It is defined as "an estimate of the amount of food additive, expressed on a body weight basis, that can be ingested daily over a lifetime without appreciable health risk" and is used extensively by regulatory and advisory bodies throughout the world. It is expressed on a milligram per kilogram body weight per day basis (mg/kg bw/day). Various toxicological studies are used to identify the dose levels at which the additive causes toxic effects on the health of test animals (usually rats or mice).
2. NOAEL (No-observed-adverse-effect-level)—It is defined as the highest level at which no toxic effect is observed on the health of animals. An ADI is derived by dividing the NOAEL obtained from these studies, by an appropriate "uncertainty" factor, which is intended to take account the differences between animals on which the additive was tested, and humans, in order to further reduce the possibility of risk to humans.
3. Uncertainty factor—It is commonly 100 (assuming that human beings are 10 times more sensitive than test animals and that the different levels of

sensitivity within the human population is in a 10-fold range), but may be as much as 1,000 (if the toxic effect in animals is particularly severe) or as low as 10 (humans less likely to be effected than animals based on actual human studies).
4. E number—It is a unique number assigned to all additives to regulate their use and to provide correct information to consumers. This has been extended by Codex Alimentarius Commission and widely accepted internationally across many countries to identify all additives. E numbers are used in Europe; other countries use only the number without the prefix of "E" although the number is the same.

Any new food additive when brought to FDA for approval, all the testing mentioned above is done for the evaluation of its safety (the chemical composition and physical properties of the substance, the amount that would generally be consumed, immediate and long-term health effects, and various other safety factors). FDA determines the "reasonable certainty of no harm" for the additive proposed to be used and generally approves quite lower levels for use than the quantity that is tested for harmful effects (Rees and Watson, 2000).

Following the initial laws for food safety, a number of amendments have been made due to advances in scientific evaluation. The Food Additives Amendment of 1958 (including the Delaney Clause) and the Color Additives Amendment of 1960 created three legal categories of additives:

1. Group 1—Those approved by the government prior to 1958 ("prior-sanctioned" substances): Examples are sodium nitrate (III) and potassium nitrate (III) used to preserve luncheon meats.
2. Those not requiring government approval (GRAS—substances). Those that are generally recognized by experts as safe, based on their extensive history of use in food before 1958 or based on published scientific evidence. Among the several hundred GRAS substances are salt, sugar, spices, vitamins, and monosodium glutamate (MSG).
3. Those requiring governmental approval in order to be used ("food additives" and "color additives").

Each direct and indirect additive is classified into one of these legal categories.

The Delaney Clause states:

> That no additive shall be deemed to be safe if it is found to induce cancer when ingested by man or animal, or if it is found, after tests which are appropriate for the evaluation of the safety of food additives, to induce cancer in man or animal.

Regulatory agencies of various countries also impose penalties defined in the food laws for various offenses including deliberate adulteration of food products, production or marketing of prohibited or unauthorized food products or additives, unhygienic conditions, mislabeling, fraudulent use of trademarks, or failure in compliance with the food safety requirements.

14.5.1 Labeling

Federal government regulations generally require that all food ingredients, including direct additives, be listed on the package label by their common names in order of weight. Manufacturers of food products have to list all ingredients in the food on the label. On the label, the ingredients used in the greatest amount are listed first, followed in descending order by those in smaller amounts.

The label must list the names of any FDA-certified color additives (e.g., FD&C Blue No. 1 or the abbreviated name, Blue 1).

Some ingredients can be listed collectively as "flavors," "spices," "artificial flavoring," or in the case of color additives exempt from certification, "artificial colors," without naming each one. Declaration of an allergenic ingredient in a collective or single color, flavor, or spice could be accomplished by simply naming the allergenic ingredient in the ingredient list.

Nutrition information is also required. The Nutrition Facts Panel on the food label includes content information on calories, fat, sodium, carbohydrates, protein, vitamins, and minerals, while the ingredient statement lists the product's ingredients in order of predominance by weight.

14.5.2 Side Effects

Food along with additives can also be responsible for side effects, both immediate and long term. Immediate side effects include most commonly allergies like dermatitis, pruritus, angioedema, urticaria and gastroenteritis, headache, alteration in concentration levels, or behavior or immune response. Then there can be other contaminants of food like bacteria, parasites, and toxic residues from pesticides. For example, butylated hydroxytoluene (BHT), butylated hydroxyanisole (BHA) and tertiary butylhydroquinone (TBHQ) that are added to foods containing fat are said to cause ADHD (attention deficit hyperactivity disorder) in children and young adults.

Long-term side effects include risk of cancer, cardiovascular diseases, or other degenerative conditions. For example, sodium nitrate(III) and nitrate(V) that are added to cured meats and fish to preserve their color and flavor may cause thyroid cancer.

14.6 RESEARCH AND PROCEDURES LEADING TO INCREASED SAFETY OF FOOD ADDITIVES

Many new techniques are being researched upon that will allow the production of additives in various ways that were not possible in previous times. One approach is the use of biotechnology, which can use simple organisms to produce food additives. These additives are the same as food components found in nature. In 1990, FDA approved the first bioengineered enzyme, rennin, which traditionally had been extracted from calves' stomachs for use in making cheese. Other measures used are like monitoring and food inspections; environmental monitoring is done to ensure that harmful bacteria are not present in the food-processing environment. This involves the sampling (swabbing) and testing of facility surfaces and areas.

Pesticide residues are controlled through a system of statutory maximum residue levels (MRLs). The MRL is the maximum amount of residue likely to remain in food products when a pesticide has been used correctly. It is expressed as milligrams of residue per kilogram of food product.

Monitoring is done to check that:

- No unexpected residues occur in crops
- Human dietary intakes of residues in foods are within acceptable levels
- Pesticide residues do not exceed the statutory MRL (Vapnek and Spreij, 2005)

The consumer demands placed on technology have resulted in the development of additives that afford us abundant, convenient, nutritious, appetizing, and economical foods. While the levels of use of food additives compared to our total diet are minor, their contributions have proven to be major.

To conclude, food additives are essential ingredients added to food products to maintain their palatability and freshness, enhancement of color and nutritional value as well as to improve their sustainability. Strict guidelines have been laid down by various agencies for maintaining the food quality both at national and international level. Therefore, the consumers are advised to read the instructions on the food labels before buying as well as consuming the food products.

REFERENCES

Action on Weatherill Report Recommendations to Strengthen the Food Safety System: Final Report to Canadians Reducing Food Safety Risks on 25th March, 2016.

Evaluation of certain food additives and contaminants. Thirteenth Report of the Joint FAO/WHO Expert Committee on Food Additives. WHO Technical Report Series, 1987.

Food Standards Agency. Producing and distributing food—guidance chemicals in food: Safety controls. In: *Food Labelling and Safety and Producing and Distributing Food*, Aviation House, 125 Kingsway, London, UK, 2002.

Guidance on Food Additives. *Food Safety Authority of Ireland.* Abbey court, Dublin, Ireland, 2010.

Rees, N. and D. Watson. *International Standards for Food Safety*. Aspen Publishers, Maryland, ISBN-0-8342-1768-6, 2000.

Toxic substances strategy committee 1980 Report.

Vapnek, J. and M. Spreij. *Perspectives and Guidelines on Food Legislation, with a New Model Food Law*. Food and Agriculture Organization of the United Nations: Rome, Italy, 2005.

15 Food Allergens

Elżbieta Kucharska and Barbara Wróblewska

CONTENTS

15.1 WHAT IS AN ALLERGY? INFLUENCE OF GENETIC AND ENVIRONMENTAL FACTORS

15.1.1 Introduction

Approximately a hundred years ago, in 1906, a Viennese pediatrician Pirquet introduced the concept of "allergy," being a synonym of modified reaction of an organism at the contact with triggering substances—allergens. The allergens were supposed to trigger the formation of ergins. The coupling of allergens with ergins was, according to Pirquet, the cause of allergic symptoms. Nowadays, due to the development of molecular methods, biochemistry and immunology, the structure of allergens has been shown, and numerous allergens have been obtained *in vitro*. Also, at least some of the mechanisms responsible for allergic reactions have been recognized.

The incidence of allergies varies in different geographic regions. Despite significant progress in research, prevention and treatment are still the matter of studies performed in the majority of countries in the world. The growth in the number of cases in the last 40 years is attributed to the changes in lifestyle, and also, paradoxically, to better access to health care in developed regions, limiting the natural selection of biologically weaker individuals. The incidence of allergies varies depending on age and sex. The condition most often affects children until the age of 5 and boys (Pawankar et al. 2013).

According to WAO (World Allergy Organization), allergic disorders affect 30%–40% of the world population. In 2020, every second person can suffer from an allergy (EAACI, 2011 Marshall 2004) in Europe. It is hard to estimate and give a precise incidence rate in the view of insufficient health care, even in economically developed countries. The dominating disorders are atopic. In Europe, the incidence rate is estimated to be 35%. Allergic conditions can affect one system or more, which also makes the estimation difficult.

Hundreds of thousands of people suffer from allergic rhinitis, and approximately 300 million from allergic asthma. Ignoring the fact that the symptoms can be seasonal, the two conditions can be present together, or allergic rhinitis can precede asthma. Combining those with allergic conjunctivitis or symptoms from the skin or digestive tract makes the qualification of the patients difficult. Asthma was noted in 29%–76% of patients with food allergy. The accompanying symptoms were bronchoconstriction—sometimes life-threatening, rash, swelling of throat (laryngeal edema), and allergy to pollen (Summers 2008; Branum and Lukacs 2009; McGowan et al. 2015).

Food allergy is a common condition with atopic background. The incidence of this disease in Europe was estimated to be 0.1%–6% on the basis of the data collected from four electronic databases gathering results of studies obtained during 10 years. The most common cause of the allergy was cow's milk and eggs in the group of youngest children. Older children were allergic to wheat, soy, peanuts, tree nuts, fish, and shellfish. The incidence rate was higher among children from northeastern Europe than those from the southern part (Pawankar et al. 2013). The risk of the occurrence of irreversible anaphylactic shock in the course of food allergy was less common than death for other reasons; however, it significantly increased in case of allergy to peanuts and nuts (Umasunthar et al. 2013).

Allergic diseases occur in majority of cases in first months or years of human life. However, it is possible to be affected at every age. It is disputable which allergens, and when administered to a pregnant mother, can induce tolerance in a child after birth. Based on the results of the research, it seems that allergens of peanuts and tree nuts act as tolerogens if children in third trimester of fetal life have a contact with them (Maslova et al. 2012). Thus early exposure to some allergens during pregnancy does not induce allergy in a child, acting in an opposite, protective way. However, high consumption of citruses and celery during pregnancy correlates with an allergy to inhalant allergens (Nwaru et al. 2010).

Next stage in human life—neonatal period and infancy—is associated with the possibility to acquire allergies due to the penetration of immature mucosa barriers by inhalant and food allergens. Even in case of breastfeeding it is possible that the allergens of cow's milk, beef, eggs and then fish, shellfish, and soy sensitize children when traversing gastrointestinal mucosa. Bacterial and viral infections and inflammations of respiratory tract and gastrointestinal system, anatomic defects and primary immunological deficiencies facilitate the development of allergies. Too early introduction of solid foods, cow's milk, or gluten can often lead to the development of an allergy localized in various systems. Rashes, atopic dermatitis, running nose, wheezing, conjunctivitis, allergic sinusitis and otitis, bronchospasm, diarrhea, and abdominal pains are often observed. Early childhood (until 5 years of age) is the period of the greatest manifestation of the symptoms. Approximately, 30% of children seasonally develop allergic symptoms; however, the majority of symptoms pass with age.

In adults, food allergy concerns 2%–3% people (White allergy paper 2004; Nwaru et al. 2014). Nowadays, the number of people suffering from food allergy is estimated to be 22–250 mln (Pawankar et al. 2013). It is also assumed that the percentage of people with allergic asthma reaches 30%, similarly as in the case of allergic dermatitis. These are often accompanied by allergies to drugs, insects, allergic conjunctivitis, and other inflammations. Allergic diseases are thus defined as a major global health issue (Pawankar et al. 2011, 2013).

15.1.2 What Is an Allergy?

An allergy is the response of the body's immune system to normally harmless substances, such as pollens, foods, and house dust mite. While in most people these substances (allergens) pose no problem, in allergic individuals their immune system identifies them as a "threat" and produces an inappropriate response. The most severe and life-threatening form of allergy is anaphylaxis.

> "Anaphylaxis is a hypersensitivity reaction to foreign substances such as foods, medications, and insect bites or stings. Anaphylaxis is a serious, life-threatening generalized or systemic hypersensitivity reaction and a serious allergic reaction that is rapid in onset and can be fatal. Symptoms may be throat swelling, itchy rash, and low blood pressure." (Johansson et al. 2004, pp. 832–836)

Risk factors for allergy can be sought in patient's genotype, environmental factors, including climate change, change in lifestyle, changes in microbiome, successive colonization of the gastrointestinal tract by bacteria, infections, especially during childhood, and used medications.

15.1.3 Genetic Determinants of Atopic Diseases

Allergy has a polygenic character, thus by analyzing the genotype it will be possible to predict the risk of allergy development in the future. Despite many years of research, all polymorphisms and possible mutations have not been recognized yet. Moreover, the knowledge on genotype does not provide certain diagnosis, because genes undergo post-translational modifications: methylation, acetylation, and therefore can be silenced, that is, the transcription into mRNA will not occur.

Familial predisposition to allergy is called an atopy. The concept of atopy is connected with excessive immunoglobulin E (IgE) reaction. If one of the parents suffers from an allergy, then the probability of passing the genes to a child reaches 40%; if both parents are affected, then the risk increases to 60%. The predisposition to allergy is mainly inherited on mother's side. Boys have a 1.5 times higher risk of developing allergies than girls (Pawankar et al. 2011–2012).

Allergy symptoms are conditioned not only by genes responsible for producing antibodies, but also those related to simulation and inhibition of patient's immune response and those controlling the structure of certain proteins. A good example is

1q21 gene determining proper synthesis of filaggrin responsible for physiological functionality of the epidermis. Gene polymorphisms can lead to functional disorders, that is, the disruption of the balance between the release of proinflammatory and anti-inflammatory cytokines, for example, a variant of the gene for Il 13 +2044GA is related to excessive release of IgE and often to atopic diseases. Polymorphism in promoter region *IL13*(−1055)C>T (in other works also described as (−1111), (−1112), (−1124), rs1800925) is responsible for the development of allergies in ethnically different populations, for example, Russian, Dutch, Danish (Dmitrieva-Zdorova et al. 2010). Eosinophils are the cells directly involved in allergic processes. They release numerous compounds that escalate allergic reaction, including eosinophil peroxidase. It was shown that the polymorphism in gene P358L, which corresponds to the presence of leucine 358, is often present in people with hay fever allergic to pollen of Japanese red-cedar (Nakamura et al. 2007).

The genes determining the profile of immune response and the function of Th2 lymphocytes are on the chromosome 5q31-34 containing genes of interleukin (IL)4 complex (IL4, IRF1—interferon regulatory factor 1, IL3, IL13, IL5, CD25C—cell division cycle 25 protein), granulocyte-macrophage colony-stimulating factor (GM-CSF), IL9, EGR (early grown response 1) and CD14. The production of interferon gamma (INFγ) and protein for T helper-2 (Th2) lymphocytes signal transducer and activator of transcription (STAT) 6 is regulated by the genes present on chromosome 12. These are 14.3-q24.1, and for IL10 1q32; also 13q14 is a gene for cysteinyl-leukotriene long terminal repeat (Cys LTR), and 16p12 for IL4 receptor (Ober and Yao 2011).

Most commonly recognized genetic mutations are single mutations, so called SNPs (single nucleotide polymorphisms). They can also concern IgE receptors on mast cells and basophils. Therefore, the mutations in the promoter region Fce R1 (−109)T>C and a point mutation in intron 2 of Fce RI b gene are related to atopy and increased concentration of IgE, which results in increased release of histamine and cytokines from mast cells (Imada et al. 2009; Kim et al. 2009). Second receptor for IgE, Fcε RII, has a secondary importance for the development of an allergy. It is estimated that approximately 79 genes are involved in the development of an atopy or asthma, and further 30 wait for confirmation (Ober and Hoffjan 2006).

Many researchers point at the fact of single mutations in the genes encoding for IL 13 linked to point mutation in gene IL 18. With too little concentration of such ILs as 15, 23, and mainly IL 12 in stroma, there occurs an increase in the concentration of IL4 and IL13, what, in consequence, leads to the polarization of lymphocytes toward Th2. It was shown that basophils and mast cells originating from bone marrow may release IL-4, IL-13, and histamine without the stimulation of FceRI receptor with specific IgE. This process occurs after the stimulation of IL-8 together with IL-3 released by lymphocytes with cytokine profile common for Th1 and Th2. Administration of IL 12 does not inhibits the atopic reaction (Nakanishi et al. 2001). As a result, the developing cellular infiltration, which is characteristic for cellular allergy response, is accompanied by the early allergic symptoms without increased concentration of IgE, which indicates pleiotropic activity of IL 8.

Single mutations in genes encoding for cytokines responsible for the inhibition of immune response were noted in chromosome 1q32 for IL 10 and within the receptors for transforming growth factor β receptor (TGFβR) 1 and TGFβR 2, as well as for TGFβ itself, which led to vast inflammatory allergic reactions within many systems: respiratory—asthma, rhinitis, digestive—eosinophil infiltration in stomach and intestines, and skin—eczema (Frischmeyer-Guerrerio et al. 2013).

Fox p3 protein is a characteristic marker for TCD 4 CD25 lymphocytes, that is, Treg, taking part in immunosuppression by inhibiting the release of proinflammatory cytokines. Seven point mutations were reported in gene *FoxJ1*, which could probably attribute to higher risk of the development of pollinosis. The most commonly observed mutations in people suffering from pollinosis were (−460)C>.T,1805G>.T, 3375G.>C (Li et al. 2006).

Lack claims that genetic predispositions for food allergy are identical as in the case of other atopic conditions. Moreover, some genes can be linked to allergies to specific food ingredients. If parents or siblings are allergic to peanuts, then a child is at seven times higher risk of having an allergy to peanuts in case of allergic parents and 64% in case of allergic siblings (Lack 2008).

Other factors, such as the polymorphism in the antigens of the major histocompatibility complex (MHC) system (HLA—human leukocyte antigen), or mutations in genes encoding for IL4 and IL13, are also reported (Lack 2008). Eczema can be a first symptom of food allergy, and if it occurs in the first 6 months of life, then the risk of food allergy to milk, eggs, or peanuts is twice as high as in the case when eczema appears in the next 6 months or later (Hill et al. 2008).

Polygenic character of allergy makes it impossible, with the current knowledge, to develop a genetic vaccine applicable for all, in all the types of the disease.

15.1.4 Environmental Factors

Environmental factors can affect the human body in various ways:

- Enabling the penetration of antigens through damaging some natural immunity mechanisms, for example, bronchial ciliary apparatus, change in composition of proteoglycans, reduced release of sIgA coating mucous membranes of respiratory, digestive and genitourinary systems.
- Unsealing mucous barrier, enabling the penetration of not only haptens, but also oligopeptides, and even peptides in inflammatory states.
- Modifying immune response toward inflammation by disrupting the balance between pro- and anti-inflammatory cytokines, either directly or by an adjuvant effect.
- Strengthening allergic reactions and expression of the symptoms of the disease.
- Modifying the immunity in early childhood by blocking the domination of Th2 and Th1 lymphocytes, which leads to the development of an allergy.

Environmental factors can damage skin and mucous membranes by increasing environmental pollution in some countries. The contributing factors are gases and dust, and this theory is confirmed by higher occurrence of allergy among the people living in the cities, as compared to those living in the country. Such emissions as sulfur dioxide, nitrogen dioxide, ozone or compounds formed during combustion in a diesel engine can damage natural protective barriers and enable the penetration of pollen to upper respiratory tract, and also the penetration of pollen fragments of less than 5 μm in size, released after pollen grains burst after rain, into lower respiratory tract.

It was observed that due to global warming—early spring, long and hot summer, and autumn—there is earlier pollination and the presence of higher concentration of pollen in the air. Larger number of storms and hurricanes contribute to the migration of pollen over longer distances with air currents. Thus, the allergies to pollen occur earlier and the symptoms become more severe. Allergy symptoms affecting respiratory tract can occur in new areas and last longer in comparison to similar periods in the previous years (Pinkerton and Rom 2014).

In the cities, Diesel exhaust particles (DEPs) contain aromatic hydrocarbons, formaldehyde, carbon oxide, and sulfur dioxide. Their concentration can accumulate in windless periods. Exhaust emissions not only irritate and damage the mucous membranes but can also affect cell biology by increasing proliferation, having adjuvant effect or be carcinogenic. It was reported that they induce the release of IL8, GM CSF, and soluble intercellular adhesion molecule 1 (sICAM1) in the bronchial tree (D'Amato et al. 2015). Adjuvant effect manifests by several-fold increase in IgE levels in patients' blood, if inhalant allergens reach respiratory tract together with DEPs (Trasande and Thurston 2005).

Ozone also has a proallergenic properties, and by damaging mucous membranes via free radicals, it can facilitate the development of bacterial, viral, and allergic inflammatory reactions due to increased release of IL 1, 6, 8, PAF (D'Amato et al. 2015) and IL13, which escalates the formation of free radicals in respiratory tract cells, leading to increased inflammatory reaction and tissue damage. Moreover, the chances of acquiring allergy to own, physiological bacterial flora or molds in the form of spores, and their enzymes released by vegetative forms, also increase (Williams et al. 2008).

In recent years, several aspects of "the hygiene hypothesis" for allergy have been questioned. "The hygiene hypothesis" states that increased incidence rate of allergy observed in western countries results from too high standards of microbial and parasitic cleanliness of children's environment. The lack of exposure to a large panel of microorganisms, especially those containing lipopolysaccharide, and parasites, suppresses the natural development of the immune response from the domination of Th2 lymphocytes to Th1. It seems that the hypothesis has certain limitations resulting from the following observations: spending time in the country reduces the incidence rate of both atopic and nonatopic asthma; people living in the Central America live in the conditions entirely different from those in the western countries but suffer from asthma as often as people in the developed countries. Thus is seems that "the hygiene hypothesis" concerns only people in early stages of life, that is, fetal period and early childhood. Exposure to certain microorganisms leads to Th2 suppression. This thesis needs further confirmation (Brooks et al. 2013).

It was, however, reported that pregnant women spending time in the country reduce the incidence rate of allergic conditions in their children. This refers to asthma, hay fever, and eczema. Child exposure during fetal period and just after birth (i.e., in the period of immune system development) to fur of farming animals and their bacterial flora, especially to lipopolysaccharide in gram-negative rods, leads to stimulation of toll-like receptor (TLR)2, TLR4, and CD 14 receptors and retunes the immune response from Th2 to Th1 lymphocytes (Douwes et al. 2008). There were trials to give pregnant women fresh, unprocessed milk, but there was no effect in allergy prevention (Perkin and Strachan 2006). Contradictory results were reported by Douwes for unpasteurized milk. Therefore, it was shown that for pregnant women a continuous contact with potential environmental country allergens is necessary to possibly develop immune tolerance by their children (Douwes et al. 2006).

Change in lifestyle is also regarded as a cause of allergy. This involves: different diets of pregnant women, decreased size of families, lower exposure to contagions, higher usage of antibiotics and paracetamol. According to Pearce and Douwes, this is a "package" that leads to the increased risk of developing asthma (Pearce and Douwes 2013).

Contacts between children and animals were also the subject of research. It was noted that early (up to the age of 4) contact with cats increased the risk of sensitization to cat allergens but decreased the risk of an allergy to other inhalant allergens, whereas contacts with dogs lowered the chance of sensitization to inhalant allergens and the risk to develop asthma (Almqvist et al. 2003).

Smoking or passive smoking during pregnancy increases the risk of asthma in children (Bousquet et al. 2007). Similarly, the risk is higher among the youth, with even higher in nonallergic than allergic teenagers, so smoking can disclose new cases of allergic rhinitis or asthma (Polosa et al. 2008).

Obesity is regarded as a plague of the twenty-first century. It was observed that excessive body weight (body mass index, BMI, higher than 30 kg/m^2) favors the development of an allergy (Netting 2014), especially in women (Chen et al. 2002). The same dependency was reported for kindergarten and school children, regardless of sex (Gilliland et al. 2013).

Consumption of too high amounts of n–6 *polyunsaturated fatty acid* (PUFA) with relation to n–3 PUFA is also considered as an environmental risk factor for food allergy (Netting 2014). The deficiency in eicosapentaenoic acid (EPA) is especially stressed, and results in increased production of prostaglandins by cyclooxygenase, including PGE2, which in turn leads to decreased release of INFγ, the dominance of Th2, and the increase in IgE. Regular consumption of fish by children lowered the concentration of IgE directed against various allergens, even though the presence of specific IgE does not directly correspond to an allergy, but may be the sign of an allergy in the future. It was reported that the number of allergy conditions decreased in children below the age of 4 (Kull et al. 2006).

Another factor contributing to the development of food allergy may be the deficiency of antioxidants, such as vitamins A, C, and E, and bioflavonoids and carotenoids, in total food ratios. It was shown that adhering to Mediterranean Diet, rich in these compounds, decreased the risk of food allergy through overall anti-inflammatory effect (Lack 2008).

An environmental factor modifying incidence rate of allergies, including food allergy, is the supply of vitamin D. It seems that both excessive supply of vitamin D (inhibition of Th1 lymphocytes proliferation, decrease in IL2, IL12, and INFγ release) and its deficiency (western lifestyle, staying at home, and not in the sun, as children in the country) can increase the risk of allergy. Physiologically, vitamin D promotes the proliferation of Treg lymphocytes, and thus has anti-inflammatory and anti-allergenic properties (Cantorna et al. 2008).

The incidence of food allergy is also facilitated by Cesarean birth. The lack of early colonization of a neonate by mother's flora leads to microbiome disorders and improper colonization of the intestines by microorganisms. It is not certain whether and which probiotics can replace the physiological flora.

Another issue is the development of atopic dermatitis (eczema) followed by food allergy. There is a hypothesis that the penetration of food allergens, for example, peanuts by disrupted skin barrier (mutations in filaggrin gene) leads to the presentation of allergens by Langerhans cells to Th2 lymphocytes and to altered, proallergic immune response (Strid et al. 2004).

Strong allergens delivered via a healthy gastrointestinal tract with properly formed microflora develop immune tolerance. This hypothesis is confirmed by the low number of peanut allergies in countries with high consumption, for example, Israel or the Philippines. It seems that proper development of bacteria flora has a significant effect. Allergy can develop with the absence of microbiome ("germ-free" mice) or after microbial selection due to antibiotic therapy (Sudo et al. 1997).

Therefore, diet recommendations for healthy, nonallergic pregnant women have been modified. Instead of avoiding strong allergens, it is proposed to introduce them in large amounts via digestive tract to make use of the tolerance phenomenon. Thus peanuts should not be avoided during pregnancy, provided that the mother is not allergic to them. The recommendations also concern the timeframe for the introduction of gluten from grains into infant's diet. A child should be given grains between 4th and 6th months of life, especially it is fed naturally (breastfed—5th month, if not—6th month). It was observed that later administration of gluten poses a risk of IgE-dependent food allergy (Pool et al. 2006).

15.2 FOOD ALLERGENS, OCCURRENCE IN DIFFERENT FOOD RAW MATERIALS AND PRODUCTS. PATOMECHANISM OF FOOD ALLERGY AND SYMPTOMS

15.2.1 Cow's Milk Allergy

15.2.1.1 Introduction

Cow's milk is the most common food allergen in case of small children and affects 0.25%–4.9% or more children according to WAO 2011 (Pawankar et al. 2011). Cow's milk allergy more often affects children partly fed with milk than those who were breastfed, if mothers drank milk or consumed dairy products. Milk allergens include casein fractions: α-s1, α-s2, β, κ (known under a common name as Bos 8 allergen), α-lactalbumin (α-la), β-lactoglobulin (β-lg), transferrin, lactoferrin, bovine serum albumin (BSA), and immunoglobulins.

15.2.1.2 α-s1-Casein

α-s1-casein is a protein with a molecular mass of 27–32 Da, containing peptides with similar amino acid structure forming hydrophilic and hydrophobic domains bound by α-helix segment (Kumosinski et al. 1991) complexing calcium phosphate. Several casein epitopes and specific IgE were recognized. Most children "grow out" of cow's milk allergy before the age of 5. It was determined that IgE specificity for casein epitopes localized between AAs 69–78 (EEIVPNSVEQ) and AAs 123–132 (MKEGIHAQQK) in children above the age of 8 is characteristic for persistent allergy (Beyer et al. 2005; Lisson and Erhardt 2016).

15.2.1.3 α-s2-Casein

α-s2 casein is built from larger and smaller components. Ten regions binding-specific IgE were determined by using synthetic decapeptides. Persistent allergy is mainly connected to IgE for α-s2-casein, AAs 33–42 (ENLCSTFCKE) and AAs 171–180 (YQKFALPQYL) (Beyer et al. 2005). The degree of phosphorylation of the components may decide on the persistence of the allergy (Bernard et al. 2000).

15.2.1.4 β-Casein

β-casein breaks down into three subunits when attacked by proteases. It is less phosphorylated than α-caseins. It binds calcium ions, forming nanoclusters. The sequences of amino acids responsible for persistent allergies have been recognized. It has been confirmed that nonphosphorylated epitops have weaker allergenic properties than native ones. Persistent allergy was observed in case of the presence of IgE specific for AA: 1–16, 45–54, 55–70, 83–92, 107–120, 135–144, 149–164, 167–184, and 185–208 (Chatchatee et al. 2001).

15.2.1.5 κ-Casein

κ-casein has numerous disulfide bridges spatially connecting dimers and octamers. It is sensitive to proteolysis, but during thermal treatment it does not lose its allergenic properties. During proteolysis it breaks down into para κ-casein and casein macropeptides. Persistent allergy is caused by the following decapeptide: AAs 155–164 (SPPEINTVQV) (Beyer et al. 2005).

15.2.1.6 Whey Proteins: α-Lactalbumin (Bos d4)

Despite being hydrolyzed by pepsin at pH2 it is a strong allergen. It is built of two domains: larger with α-helix structure and smaller forming β-sheet structure. It denatures at temperature above 95°C, linearly unwinding folded structure (the concentrations of IgE against those fragments exceed 100U/l). At lower temperatures, it forms large aggregates due to changes in disulfide bridges (Chang, 2004). Besides antigenic properties, the whole particle and its components have antibacterial properties.

15.2.1.7 Whey Proteins: β-Lactoglobulin (Bos d5)

It binds retinol, β-carotene, *unsaturated fatty acid* (UFA) and PUFA. It comprises 50% of whey proteins. It is a mixture of mono- and dimers and has crab-like shape with crooked "arms." In the secondary structure of β-lg, the α-helix makes up 1.5% of the structure, beta sheet—ca. 43% and random coil—ca. 47% (Darewicz and Dziuba 2005). It aggregates and denatures irreversibly at pH above 7.5. No structural changes, besides higher number of monomers, were noted at the temperature up to 70°C. Heating to 90°C reduces its allergenic properties but does not eliminate them entirely. It breaks down to oligopeptides at pH lower than 6 (Kuriyan and Eisenberg 2007). β-lg is a strong allergen as it is not present in human milk.

When analyzing persistent allergy to milk with respect to comparable features of the epitopes, it was determined that persistent allergy is mainly caused by antibodies against epitopes with linear structure, present in caseins and α-la, but absent in β-lg (Järvinen et al. 2001). This lead to a hypothesis that persistent allergy to β-lg would be mainly dependent on the formation of IgG4 antibodies. It is debatable, because IgG4 are generated by vaccines during desensitization. However, the development of the tolerance, both in IgE-dependent and IgE-independent allergy, was conditioned by the growth of specific IgA (Sletten et al. 2006). Sensitizing properties were also tested for the mixture of β-lg and glycomacropeptides in various ranges of pH. It was observed that at pH 3.5 the digestion is so effective that the products of enzymatic hydrolysis do not bind to sera from children suffering from allergy to milk. This effect was not obtained at pH 7 (Martinez et al. 2016). Lowering the concentrations of IgE specific for Bos d4 and Bos d 5.0102 allergens and for κappa-casein and αs1-casein gives positive prognosis for obtaining immune tolerance to milk allergens (Ahrens et al. 2012).

15.2.1.8 Lactoferrin

Lactoferrin binds Fe ions and has bacteriostatic properties (AA 265–284). Specific antibodies against lactoferrin were reported in 50% of children allergic to cow's milk (4–14 months of life) (Natale et al. 2004).

15.2.1.9 Bovine Serum Albumin

Bovine serum albumin is similar to human with respect to its structure and functionality. It is present in both milk and beef. It contains allergens with linear and conformational epitopes. IgE antibodies are directed against conformational epitopes, so some technological processes, such as homogenization and lyophilization, can significantly lower the allergenic properties. BSA structure is well known. It has three domains folded into nine coils linked with 17 disulfide bridges. The reduction of disulfide bridges lowers the ability to bind specific IgE, but it does not entirely eliminate allergenic properties, which are also dependent on linear epitopes (Restani et al. 2004). Allergy to BSA is airborne through inhalation of albumin present in epithelia of domestic, laboratory or farming animals, containing conservative fragment of albumins. Another route is oral—allergy symptoms after eating cooked meat, but also goat's cheeses. Therefore, BSA is regarded as a panallergen. The symptoms of allergic response usually correspond to the way of allergen penetration. A case of anaphylactic shock was described after giving a sick person cells multiplied in liquid culture with BSA. The preparation serum albumin peptide—ABBOS was claimed responsible for autoimmune reaction against pancreatic islands and further development of diabetes. This opinion is controversial. Some vaccines obtained from cell cultures, where culture medium was supplemented with albumin, can be dangerous for allergic people (Chruszcz et al. 2013).

15.2.1.10 Bos d7 IgG

Bos d7 IgG are antibodies directed against environmental microorganisms present in milk, which give immunity when fed to a calf. These are tetramers linked by disulfide bridges. Bos d7 IgG are panallergens, similarly as albumins. Sensitization begins by oral route in first months of child's life, when cow's milk is introduced to a diet. Later in life, due to the presence of Ig in such meats like beef or veal, it is possible that reaction becomes more severe due to further immunization via gastrointestinal route. It was observed that IgG present in pork or chicken meat do not stimulate the production of IgE, so they should be used in everyday diet. The possibility of cross—reactions between antigens similar to bovine albumins, present in hair and fur of other animals: cats, dogs, and farming animals, is still being studied. High chemical similarity between bovine IgG and allergen present in dust mites—Der pl—is also taken into consideration. These are amino acids 81–94 and 101–111 building flexible coil connecting two domains. Allergy to IgG present in milk precedes the allergy to beef (Ayuso et al. 2000).

15.2.2 Hypoallergenic Products as an Alternative to Cow's Milk

15.2.2.1 Introduction

Alternative products to cow's milk in Poland are hypoallergenic products. In the United States, South Africa and southern Europe people sometimes use goat's or ewes' milk (25% of children allergic to cow's milk do not react to these types of milk). In Asia, Africa and southern Europe (Italy) people sometimes use donkey's milk but also camel's and horse milk. Official standpoint of the societies European Society for Paediatric Gastroenterology, Hepatology and Nutrition and European Society for Paediatric Allergology and Clinical Immunology and Food and Drug Administration (FDA) is that other types of milk than cow's milk are not approved for the production of hypoallergenic products for children suffering from allergy to cow's milk. There were trials to perform desensitization of children allergic to cow's, ewe's and goat's milk with cow's milk oral immunotherapy. Positive results were not obtained for other allergens (sheep's and goat's) (Rodríguez del Río et al. 2012).

15.2.2.2 Goat's Milk

Allergic reactions to goat's milk among adults become more and more frequent, due to higher consumption of goat's cheeses. The most sensitizing fraction, with similar structure as in cow's milk, is caseins, which are the main allergen of goat's milk. Small amounts of α-la, which remain in cheeses, are the cause of food allergy. Despite undisputable benefits of goat's milk, for example, better digestibility and slightly higher vitamins content, goat's milk cannot be a substitute in case of allergy to cow's and ewe's milk, and also sheep milk cheese (Tavares et al. 2007).

15.2.2.3 Donkey's Milk

Human adaptation to donkey's milk is better than to cow's milk, because it is similar to human milk in terms of protein composition, the contents of linoleic and linolenic acids and bioelements, the content of lactose stimulating intestines to Ca absorption, and Ca(calcium):P(phosphorus) ratio (1,48:1,0). It contains low number of bacteria due to high content of lysozyme (LYS). Similar content of protein and bioelements as in human milk protects infants' kidneys. No cross-reactive allergens were found between donkey's and cow's milk, and no allergy symptoms were observed in people allergic to cow's milk (Monti 2007). In case of 83% of short stature children allergic to cow's milk, it was possible to increase their height after the diets supplementation with donkey's milk. Because of the farms in central Italy, France, and Switzerland, donkey's milk is easier to obtain than horse milk, and even if not as tasty as cow's (less sweet) it is a good therapeutic alternative (Monti et al. 2007). In Asia (China) it is treated as a drink that elongates older people's life.

15.2.2.4 Camel's Milk

Camel's milk is the closest in composition to human milk and does not contain cross-reactive β-casein and β-lg—main allergens of cow's milk. Immunoglobulins are identical as in human milk. Camel's milk contains 2% of homogenized fat in the form of PUFA. Lactose content amounts to 4.8%, so it is more digestible by people with lactase deficiency. It is rich in Ca, Fe, and vitamin C (camel does not belong to ruminants but Tylopoda) (Shabo et al. 2005). It can very rarely cause an allergic reaction. A case of anaphylactic shock was described after drinking heated but uncooked camel's milk by a 6-year-old child without an allergy to cow's milk (Al-Hammadi et al. 2010).

15.2.2.5 Mare's Milk

Mare's milk is similar to camel's and donkey's milk and is treated as an alternative in diets of atopic children. The composition of the milk is similar to human milk, but mare's milk contains twice less fat and, whey and casein proteins do not contain allergens cross-reacting with cow's, ewe's, or goat's milk. There are twice as much *N* caseins in horse than in human milk, but the content of lactose and bioelements is similar (Potočnik et al. 2011). Allergies to mare's milk are rarely reported. The cause may be previous allergy on horse epithelium or other inhalant allergens, for example, hamster fur.

15.2.3 Allergy to Egg Proteins

15.2.3.1 Introduction

It is a common condition among children until the age of 5, affecting 1.8%–2% of children, especially those living in highly developed countries (Japan, Spain, France). The symptoms pass away during puberty or in young adults during studies. Twenty allergens have been recognized (Urisu et al. 2015). It is known that proteins contained in egg yolk are weaker allergens than those in egg white. Eliminating diets are very difficult to adhere to because eggs are added to many meals. Allergy to eggs can be an occupational disease for people involved in processing of this food ingredient. An allergy can be acquired by ingestion or by exposure to inhalation, when egg powder is added to cakes, icings, or bakery wares. Another problem is the presence of egg proteins in cell cultures used for production of vaccines, for example, flu vaccines or MMR (mumps, measles, rubella), with the possibility of advanced allergic reactions to occur within skin, increased bronchial hyper-reactivity or anaphylactic shock. Aminoglycosides, which ensure the sterility of the vaccine, can also cause allergic reaction. The four major allergens in egg white are: ovalbumin (OVA; Gal d 2, 54% of the total protein content), ovotransferrin (OVT; conalbumin, Gal d 3, 12%), ovomucoid (OVM; Gal d 1, 11%), and LYS (Gal d 4, 3.5%). Two yolk proteins have been identified: α-livetin (chicken serum albumin, Gal d 5) and lipoprotein YGP42 (Gal d 6) (Martos et al. 2013b). Due to the importance of the problem, for many years particular proteins were isolated and the levels of specific IgE were measured. The decrease in IgE, but also in IgG levels were observed after subjecting egg proteins to various technological processes (Martos et al. 2013a). Also single allergens were used in desensitizing vaccines. Dhanapala et al. (2015) developed a genetic vaccine containing four recombined antigens for egg proteins, introduced on plasmids to *E.coli*, and then isolated and compared to natural ones with respect to purity of the product, compatibility with natural proteins and immunogenicity in vitro, that is, ability to bind specific IgE. In the nearest future, it is planned to administer the vaccine sublingually to allergic children and use it for laboratory studies (Dhanapala et al. 2015). Child's diet should be enriched by introducing egg yolk prior to egg white.

A protein present in egg yolk is α-livetin, which is regarded as a weak allergen. It can sensitize by exposure to inhalation, it is identical with chicken serum albumin and cross-reactive with bird allergens causing bird-egg syndrome. Similarly, apo-livetins are weak allergens.

Egg proteins trigger IgE-dependent, IgE-independent, or mixed reactions. The conditions described included: eosinophilic esophagitis, eosinophilic allergenic gastroenteritis, and proctocolitis. It is debatable what is the threshold level of IgE, and against which egg allergens, that enables to predict the representation of clinical symptoms. The symptoms include: rash, vomiting, abdominal pain, and diarrhea. It is difficult because IgE levels change with children's age. Most of allergens are thermolabile and are digested by enzymes. The strongest allergen is OVM, which is not digested in alimentary tract and can present linear epitopes. High levels of IgE directed against OVM, main egg protein allergen, which is resistant to high temperatures, in majority of cases do not allow "to grow out" of allergy. Fragments of OVM partly digested by pepsin were found in IgE idiotopes in children with persistent allergy (Urisu et al. 2015). However, the consumption of muffins showed the lack of allergic properties of such processed allergen. It is justified by the formation of indigested complexes between gluten present in flour and OVM during baking (Urisu et al. 2015).

15.2.3.2 Ovalbumin

Ovalbumin contains four sulfhydryl groups with single disulfide bridges. It is a glycoprotein belonging to serpin family. Active center has α-helix structure. Usually, 100% of patients allergic to egg show positive allergic reaction to the presence of OVA. It is sensitive to proteases and high temperature, thus eggs cooked for a long time often do not cause any symptoms in children allergic to raw eggs (Verhoeckx et al. 2015). In case of cooking for 10 minutes the allergic properties decrease by 75% and even more after frying or baking (Fu et al. 2010). This could be caused by increased digestibility of thermolabile egg allergens and lower the stimulation of T lymphocytes and basophils present in intestinal submucosa (Martos et al. 2013a).

15.2.3.3 Ovotransferrin

Ovotransferrin called conalbumin, Gal d 3, with a molecular mass of 77 kDa and built of 686 AA, is a common allergen sensitive to changes in temperature in the range 60°C–82°C, generating the formation of isoforms (Tong et al. 2012). It has antibacterial properties, as it is able to bind iron. Approximately 50% of people allergic to egg proteins have specific IgE. OVT from chicken eggs is compatible with that of duck and goose.

15.2.3.4 Lysozyme

Lysozyme (Gal d 4) is built by 129 AA (14.3 kDa). It is formed by a single polypeptide chain linked by four disulfide bridges. Antigenic properties, comparable with Gal d3, are reduced during heating. There is a cross-reactivity between LYS from chicken and other birds. It is sometimes used as a preservative in some medicaments, causing allergic reaction in sensitive people, for example, in eye drops (Urisu et al. 2015).

15.2.3.5 Alpha-Livetin

Alpha-livetin, Gal d 5, present in egg yolk is similar to chicken serum albumin and is a protein with a molecular mass of 65–70 kDa. It can cause egg-bird syndrome by ingestion or by exposure to inhalation through a contact with meat, serum, chicken albumin, feathers, or egg yolks. Alpha-livetin allergy can be an occupational disease of pigeon fanciers, ornamental bird breeders, or farm workers. The symptoms of allergy response by inhalation are allergic rhinitis and conjunctivitis and symptoms of asthma. The symptoms of allergy occurring after the consumption of egg yolks or homemade mayonnaise, the oral allergy syndrome (OAS), include swelling of lips, itching, and swelling of tongue and mucous membrane of the oral cavity. Heating of chicken albumin at 90°C for 30 minutes reduces its allergenic properties by 88% (Quirce et al. 2001).

15.2.4 Fish Allergens

The incidence rate of allergy to fish in the whole population is estimated to 0.1%–0.4%. Parvalbumin is a panallergen. It is present in the muscles of cod and also in wide range of commonly consumed species such as salmon, carp, mackerel, tuna, and pilchard.

Only micro amounts of the allergen are required for allergic reaction to occur (facial urticaria and angioedema), as it was in the case of a kiss in a cheek given to a child allergic to many allergens (including fish) by a grandfather, who ate fish 2 hours earlier (Monti et al. 2003). The inhalation of allergens during cooking or frying of fish, as well as during fish preparation, could be the cause of allergy symptoms. Reactions localized in alimentary tract, skin, and respiratory system caused by consumption of fish are the effect of contact with both the raw and thermally processed product. Parvalbumin is thermally stable. Therefore, such symptoms as nausea, vomiting, stomach ache, diarrhea, hives (also called urticaria or nettle rash), swelling under the skin (also called angioedema), itching and reddening of the skin, worsening of eczema, asthma (wheezing, breathlessness, coughing), hay fever (itchy nose and eyes, sneezing/runny nose), swelling of the airways, and sometimes fatal episodes of allergic shock can occur individually or together.

Allergy to fish occurs more often in Norway and Japan, but allergy sufferers from EU countries are "catching up." The main allergen is Cod M, the name was changed into Gad c1 (2001). It is parvalbumin with a molecular weight of 12.3 kDa. It is built from 113 amino acids and one molecule of glucose. Tertiary structure has three domains: AB, CD, and EF, and the latter two are responsible for the transfer of calcium ions in a cell. Dark meat of mackerel or tuna contains hundredth parts of mg of Gad c1. It is one order of magnitude less than in white fish meat. Gad c1 is present in sea and freshwater fish. Approximately 50% of people are allergic to all fish species. Due to high rate of consumption a recombined carp parvalbumin was developed (Swoboda et al. 2002). It is possible to get rid of fish allergens by canning—a total loss of allergenic activity is obtained due to the pressure and temperature (Elsayed and Jaran 1983). Besides parvalbumin, which is present in several dozen isoforms displaying cross-reactivity, various enzymes were also isolated from different fish species. Potential allergens of known identity were found in cod (aldehyde phosphate isomerase), salmon (triose-phosphate isomerase, fructose-bis-phosphate isomerase, serum albumin), and tuna (creatine kinase, beta-enolase). Most commonly present allergens are enolases, aldolases, and fish gelatine, which seems to be a weak allergen. Specific IgE for parvalbumin were reported in 72.6% of examined people, IgE for enolase—in 62.9% of people allergic to other allergens than to parvalbumin, for aldolase—in 50%, and for fish gelatine—in 19.3%. Tropomyosin, found not only in tilapia, was also indicated, as in humans it can provoke autoaggressive disease—colitis ulcerosa. Parvalbumin has two phylogenetic lineages—alpha and beta lineage. Generally, IgE antibodies were observed only against beta form; however, in frog meat alpha form is the main allergen (Kuehn et al. 2014).

15.2.5 Crustaceans Allergens

15.2.5.1 Introduction

The consumption of crustaceans in Poland is limited to special occasions and is not popular. In the world, however, it is a serious issue and crustaceans were placed on the "Big 8" food allergens list. In the United States, there are approximately 30 edible crustaceans distinguished.

15.2.5.2 Shrimp Allergens

Major shrimp allergen is a coiled-coil dimer with molecular weight of 45 kDa, built of 189 amino acids, and 0.5% of carbohydrates. It was first isolated from raw shrimps and carapace extracts and then also from cooked *Penaeus aztecus* and *Penaeus indicus*. The comparison between the amino acid composition of the allergens proved their similarity, and the protein was named shrimp tropomyosin. It was shown that it is a glycoprotein soluble in water, resistant to heat and digestive enzymes. The consumption of 1–2 average size shrimps can induce anaphylactic reaction.

The reaction to crab allergens was mainly observed in environments with occupational exposure due to crab meat processing. IgE-dependent reactions are mainly related to extracts obtained during cooking of crabs, but no to direct contact with raw produce.

Tropomyosin was also determined as an allergen of Chinese spiny lobster (*Panulirus stimpsoni*) and American lobster (*Homarus americanus*). Both proteins were cloned and their sequences analyzed. It was reported that they are homologous to Pen a1 shrimp allergen and, moreover, are compatible with a protein isolated from a nematode *Anisakis simplex* infesting fish, and tropomyosin from mites, cockroaches, moths, and other invertebrates found in food. It was thus concluded that "tropomyosins are the major allergens in invertebrates such as crustaceans (shrimp, crab, lobster), arachnids (dust mites), insects (cockroaches, midges), and mollusks (squid, snail, and oyster)" (Rees et al. 1999).

For a long time it was not understood why crustacean tropomyosin was allergic, whereas that present in vertebrates was not. After subjecting crustacean tropomyosin to pepsin A digestion, Mikita and Padlan found undigested tropomyosin fragments originating from different invertebrates. Those compounds also penetrated through intestine wall into the bloodstream, because numerous specific IgE were found. They observed that those fragments could even sensitize people who were not suffering from allergy. Such compounds were not present in mammalian skeletal muscles (Mikita and Padlan 2007).

15.2.5.3 Another Issue Concerning Products Obtained from Crustaceans

Another issue concerned products obtained from crustaceans: chitin, chitosan, and glucosamine present in cosmetics and food. The opinions on potential allergenic characters of these compounds were divided. In 2010, Muzzarelli summarized previous studies on their potential allergenic properties and pointed out all the mistakes. He observed that, irrespective of the origins of the products, they did not contain proteins, carbohydrates, or fats. Therefore, they should be regarded as chemically pure, nonsensitizing substances (due to the lack of observed allergy symptoms in recipients) and not as potential allergens (Muzzarelli 2010).

15.2.6 Plant Allergens

Plant allergens are commonly present in various plant species. Diagnosis of the cause of the symptoms can be difficult, because even within one species plants can vary with respect to their allergenic properties. Therefore, "prick-to-prick" tests, that is, skin prick testing performed by pricking the skin with a needle containing juice of a tested plant, reported as potential allergen by a patient, are reliable diagnostic methods. It is generally regarded that the diagnosis can be made after performing a double-blind test, and the gold standard is a provocation allergy testing, involving the direct administration of the allergen to gastric mucosa. Moreover, the elevated level of specific IgE can also be a good marker of the disease. The increase in antibodies alone, without the symptoms of the condition, can only be a signal preceding the development of the allergy in the future.

Such procedure allows to differentiate food hypersensitivity from allergy.

In recent years, a lot of controversial articles have been published about gluten.

15.2.6.1 Gluten

Gluten is a protein found in wheat and related grains, containing gliadin and gluteine. It belongs to prolamins. Prolamins present in wheat—gliadin, barley—hordein, rye—secalin, and oats—avenin cause several diseases, which in 2012 were classified by a panel of 15 experts as gluten-related disorders (Sapone et al. 2012). Among these are autoimmune disorders, which include celiac disease, Duhring's disease (dermatitis herpetiformis) and gluten ataxia. Nonautoimmune and nonallergic diseases include nonceliac gluten sensitivity (NCGS), and allergic disease—IgE-dependent and IgE-independent food allergy, wheat-dependent exercise-induced anaphylaxis (WDEIA), baker's asthma, and contact dermatitis.

Celiac disease is an autoimmune disorder developing in people possessing one of two types of the MHC class II alleles: HLA-DQ2 (DQA1*05 and DQB1*02) and HLA-DQ8 (DQA1*03 and DQB1*0302). HLA-DQB1*02 homozygotes are in a greater risk of disease development. The incidence rate in Poland reaches from 1:300 to 1:100. As much as 95% of celiac patients have HLA DQ2 variant on the surface of their immunocompetent cells, whereas the remaining 5%—DQ8. Mc Mowat claims that gluten is broken down in alimentary tract into polypeptides rich in proline and glutamine, which are resistant to digestion and penetrate through the wall of small intestine, possibly unsealed by inflammatory process (e.g., rotavirus infection). In submucous layer, the polypeptides undergo deamidation by transglutaminase and strongly immunogenic (AA p57–73) deamidated peptides (DPG) containing glutamic acid are formed (Mc Mowat 2003).

Transpeptidase itself becomes autoantigen (due to viral infections) capable to cross-link actins. It was reported that Epstein–Barr virus (EBV) or Coxsackie infections lead to modifications within domain 8 of transpeptidase. Antibodies released against transpeptidase are not only markers for celiac disease, but also for some infections (Ferrara et al. 2010). Moreover, gluten peptides p31–43/49 can directly induce the production of IL 15, released by dendritic cells and macrophages after gluten phagocytosis, which activates intestinal intraepithelial T cells—IELs. Transglutaminase also leads to the increase in the number of T CD8+ lymphocytes and induces overproduction of MIC A ligand on intestinal villi and NKG2D receptor on the surface of cytotoxic cells. MIC A is a ligand for lectin-like receptor NKG2D found on the surface of cytotoxic lymphocytes and responsible for the recognition of foreign proteins, for example, DPG present on the cells.

The DPG in the context of HLA class II antigens DQ2 and DQ8, to which they strongly bind, are presented to TCD 4, T CD8, TCRαβ+ and TCRγδ+ lymphocytes, and NK cells. Increased release of interferon (IFN)γ and TNFα, triggered by IL 15 and DPG presentation, increases the cytotoxicity of T lymphocytes and NK cells. This results in tissue damage, gradual villous atrophy, and further loss of intestinal barrier capacity leading to condition called "leaky gut syndrome."

Stimulation of Th lymphocytes, and then B lymphocytes, activates the production of antibodies directed against: gliadin, transglutaminase, endomysium, and DPG, which increases the damage done to the intestine by the antibody-dependent cell-mediated cytotoxicity (ADCC). The best markers for the disease are antiendomysium p-c Ig A, IgG against tissue transglutaminase, and also anti-DPG IgG. Pathology changes of celiac disease in the small intestine are categorized as III and IV in a 4-stage Marsh classification.

According to Fasano, the cause for the "leaky gut syndrome" is a direct activity of gluten containing peptides AA 110–130 and AA 151–170, increasing the production of zonulin. It is a protein that modulates the permeability of tight junctions between enterocytes. The possibility of gluten polypeptides to penetrate this way can be the cause of a strong primary immune response, which is marked by increased levels of zonulin (haptoglobin) in blood and next by a secondary cytotoxic immune response. Gluten itself, having polypeptide AA 30–43, can have a cytotoxic effect in a nonallergic way.

Fasano indicates that impairment of intestinal barrier, as the reason for various allergens penetration, can lead to the development of type I diabetes, asthma, some autoaggression disorders such as rheumatoid arthritis and autoimmune cholangitis, and due to the disruption of blood–brain barrier—the development of schizophrenia and glioma (Fasano 2011).

Celiac disease symptoms may come from the gastrointestinal system and outside of it. These include abdominal pain, diarrhea, vomiting, recurring aphthous stomatitis and dental erosion, symptoms of progressing hypochromic anemia, vitamins and bioelement deficiencies, reduced release of disaccharidases (milk intolerance), growth inhibition in children, and body weight loss.

Dermatitis herpetiformis is an autoimmune disease in which the precipitations of IgA and IgA together with skin transglutaminase are deposited in skin blisters causing polymorphic, intensely itchy papulovesicular eruptions occurring symmetrically on various body parts. The most common sites of involvement are the sacral region, buttocks, scapulae, nape, elbows, knees, face, and scalp. After gluten consumption, the skin symptoms proceed from sharply separated red bumps, through papules or vesicles to blisters. Skin itching is the dominating symptom, which leads to numerous scratches and scabs. The disease is caused by gluten deamidation. IgA antibodies against endomysium are a serological marker. Damages to small intestine are less severe than in case of the celiac disease, but despite that, the deficiencies in iron, magnesium, calcium, B-group vitamins, and fat soluble vitamins, including vitamin D3, can occur. If the disorders occur during childhood, the patient may not build her/his peak bone mass, which may lead to the development of osteopenia or osteoporosis. Similarly as in the celiac disease, the recurring aphthous stomatitis was observed. Diarrheas did not occur; however, moderate villous atrophy was also diagnosed. Gluten-free diet introduced at early stages lead to significant improvement (Żebrowska and Waszczykowska 2007).

Gluten ataxia is the next condition belonging to autoimmune disorders. It is caused by cross-reactivity between antigens in Purkinje cells located in the cerebellum, the stem and the pons, and gluten epitopes after deamidation. Antitransglutaminase antibodies were detected in clusters surrounding brain vessels. Approximately 10% of patients exhibited changes in intestinal villi, confirmed by biopsy. The symptoms of ataxia include difficulties with maintaining balance and coordinated walking (walking on a widened base), trembling limbs, intention tremor, writing abnormalities, inability to perform precise movements, muscle spasms, nystagmus, and slow, often slurred speech (Fasano 2011).

The NCGS is a syndrome classified from 2012 as a nonautoaggressive disorder. It is the most commonly occurring form of nonallergic sensitivity to gluten in which the introduction of gluten-free diet leads to entire regression of the symptoms. Half of the affected people possess HLA DQ2 and DQ8, whereas both antigens are present in 30% of healthy people. It was noted that diarrheas are more frequent in people having HLA DQ2 than in those having DQ8. Other symptoms include: headache, joint and muscle pain, muscle cramps, leg or arm numbness, anemia, "foggy mind," depression, abdominal pain, fatigue, but also constipation or body weight loss. Histopathologic examination of the gastrointestinal tract did not reveal any manifestations in duodenum, except slightly increased infiltration of intraepithelial lymphocytes T. Damages to the small intestine were assessed as mild and categorized as I or II in Marsh classification. In 50% of the affected the antibodies against transglutaminase and endomysium were not present. Antigliadin antibodies are also not an ideal marker because they are also present in gluten ataxia, Duhring's disease, Sjögren's syndrome, sarcoidosis, and SLE—systemic lupus erythematosus. Eosinophil infiltrations have been recently reported within lamina propria, and the symptoms of the disease appeared after several hours or days after gluten consumption, for example, in provocation allergy testing (in celiac disease—after 2 hours) (Czaja-Bulsa 2015). It is assumed that NCGS is caused by overexpression of innate immunity. The condition was not accompanied by the "leaky gut syndrome," but higher expression of TLR 1, 2, and 4 was observed, as well as proper expression of claudin-1 and zonulin, but increased expression of CLDN-4 gene encoding for claudin, and decreased concentration of TGF-beta 1 and FOXP3 marker of Treg lymphocytes below the level present in healthy people. Temporary increase of IFNγ and intraepithelial T CD3 concentrations in blood were also reported.

Allergic diseases related to gluten consumption include IgE-dependent and IgE-independent food allergy, WDEIA, baker's asthma, and contact dermatitis. Common feature of these conditions, except IgE-independent food allergy, is that they have an atopic background. Specific IgE occur against α-, β-, γ-, and ω-gliadin. In patients there are neither symptoms of the "leaky gut syndrome" nor antibodies against endomysium or transglutaminase. However, the course of the diseases is different. The reason for the disorders is immune hypersensitivity. Early symptoms of gluten allergy result from the activity of biogenic amines and other compounds found in preformed granules, or eicosanoids formed from the degradation of arachidonic acid, found in generated granules. In case of food allergy, besides the symptoms from gastrointestinal tract, a bronchial spasm, asthma symptoms or rash can occur. Additional testing shows increased level of IgE, slight damage of duodenal mucous membrane, and positive result of provocation test after gluten contact with gastric mucosa.

Wheat-dependent exercise-induced anaphylaxis is characterized by food allergy symptoms enhanced by physical activity. Physical activity can also accelerate and pronounce the symptoms from bronchial tree, up to, and including anaphylactic shock. These symptoms are accompanied by diffuse urticaria and angioedema. The main allergen is ω5-gliadin, and sever other epitopes were also found.

Baker's asthma involves bronchospasms and acute dyspnea after the contact with flours—wheat, barley, or rye, containing, besides gluten, α-amylase, peroxidase and nonspecific lipid transfer proteins (LTPs), water-soluble albumin, and α-amylase inhibitor, all identified as allergens. Skin symptoms may include both hives and contact dermatitis. Although early respiratory symptoms, usually induced in alimentary tract, occur after several minutes (baker's asthma) or several hours (food allergy), in case of contact dermatitis the symptoms appear after a day or two from the contact of the skin with gluten. The pathogenesis of contact dermatitis is different than in case of hives. It is a type IV allergy mechanism according to Gell and Coomb's classification, involving activation of Th lymphocytes and increased levels of IL 1, 2, 6, 12, IFNγ, and TNF, but without the activation of IgE. The symptoms include intense itching, characteristic skin bumps and redness, and vesicles. The skin is thickened with marked furrows, dry, and cracks easily. To make a diagnosis patch tests are performed and read out after 24–48 hours. The treatment is based on entire elimination of gluten from a diet and patient's surroundings (Czaja-Bulsa 2015).

15.2.6.2 Profilins

Profilins are proteins found in animal and plant cells. In animals they are present in almost all the tissues and are bound to actin. They are a group of panallergens also found in pollen, fruits, vegetables, and latex. They sensitize by inhalation. Consumption of products containing these compounds usually cause moderate allergy symptoms localized in oral cavity (Fernández Rivas 2003). They include itchiness, redness, edema, and wheals, which disappear after 30 minutes without trace. Profilins are proteins having low molecular weight of 15–30 Da.

Profilins are divided into pollen and food profilin allergens. Pollen profilin allergens include birch (Bet v2), hazel tree (Cor b2), olive tree (Ole e2), plane tree (Pla a), European ash (Fra e2), and profilins of grasses: timothy grass (Phl p12), *Ambrosia* (ragweed) (Amb a), *Artemisia* (Artemisia v4), latex (Hev b8), ryegrass (Lol p12), and many more. Food profilins include: celery (Api g4), carrot (Dau c4), soybean (Gly m3), tomato (Lyc e1), apple (Mal d4), pear (Pyr c4), peach (Pru p4), peanut (Ara h5), hazelnut (Cor a2), rapeseed (Bra n), and many more. They can be responsible for up to 43% of allergies in people affected by pollen or food allergy, due to having cross-reactive allergens in pollen, fruits, and vegetables (Valenta et al. 1991). It was observed that allergy to birch pollen is often accompanied by allergy to some fresh fruits and vegetables.

15.2.6.3 Bet v-1 Allergen from Pollen of Birch

Bet v-1 allergen from pollen of birch (*Betula verrucosa*) is cross-reactive with allergens of many fruits, but not all people allergic to Betv-1 develop allergic reactions. This may be attributed to the fact that warty (silver) birch is common in Scandinavia. Birch trees pollinating in our country release pollen having slightly different expression of determinants. Moreover, there are several different varieties of apples, pears, and other fruits. Allergy symptoms are often triggered by specific variety of apples, hence the necessity to perform prick-to-prick testing.

Pollen homologues of Bet v1 are: hazel tree (Cor a1), oak (Que a1), alder (Aln g1), and hornbeam (Car b1). The cross-reacting allergens of vegetables and fruits are the following: peanuts (Ara h8), hazelnut (Cor a1), celery (Api g1), carrot (Dau c1), soybean (Gly m4), pear (Pyr c1), sweet cherry (Pru av1), apricot (Pru a1), potato (Sol t1), strawberry (Fra a1), and mung bean (Virg r1).

15.2.6.4 Proteins Resistant to Pathogens

Proteins resistant to pathogens form 14 groups but not all of them are allergenic. The most commonly allergenic are given as follows.

15.2.6.4.1 Lipid Transfer Proteins

LTPs are responsible for intracellular membrane transport, contribute to plants resistance to infections, and are found in fruit cuticles. They are resistant to pepsin digestion at the pH of gastric juice and are thermostable. Their concentration increases with fruit ripening (Yeats and Rose 2008).

The LTP present in pollen include *Artemisia* (Art v3), latex (Hev b3), olive tree (Ole e7), Ambrosia (ragweed) (Amb a6), and those present in food are hazelnut (Cor a8), walnut (Jug r3), cabbage (Bra o3), tomato (Lyc e3), apricot (Pru ar3), orange (Cit s3) and plants of the rose family (*Rosaceae*), and many more (Hauser et al. 2010). Similarly as in the case of other plant allergens, they commonly induce medium OAS, or gastrointestinal allergy symptoms and rashes.

15.2.6.4.2 Chitinases

Chitinases are a group of allergens found in many fruits. Chitinase-induced IgE cross react with latex Hev b 11 and Hev b 6 and fruit allergens (from papaya, avocado, banana, chestnut, passion fruit, fig, melon, mango, kiwi, pineapple, peach, tomato, and green beans). They are also formed during fruit ripening in ethylene oxide. The allergens are responsible for latex-fruit syndrome. They are thermolabile, so cross-reactions do not occur between IgE specific for latex and cooked green beans (Sánchez-Monge et al. 2000). Chitinases are a group of enzymes hydrolyzing chitin found in cell walls of fungi.

15.2.6.4.3 Thaumatin-Like Proteins

Thaumatin-like proteins show antifungal activity. They belong to proteins induced by biotic and abiotic stress. They are thermoresistant. They are found in strawberries, apples, cherries, bell peppers, corn, cocoa, papaya fruits, and even in tobacco plants (osmotin) and cannabis, causing "cannabis-fruits/vegetables" syndrome. IgE are cross reacting with plant-food-derived alcoholic beverages, tobacco, and latex (Decuyper et al. 2015).

15.2.6.4.4 Glucanases

Glucanases are a group of enzymes hydrolyzing β-glucans, being the polymers of 1–3 and 1–6 glucose, produced by *Saccharomyces cerevisiae* and present in many food products, as well as in edible mushrooms and algae. Specific antiglucanase IgE cross react with latex, tomato, potato, and banana allergens (Hoffmann-Sommergruber 2000). Plant panallergens also include polcalcin Phl p7 engaged in growth of grasses, found, for example, in timothy grass (*Phleum pratense*), and trypsin inhibitors present in olive tree pollen.

15.2.6.5 Enolases

Enolases are panallergens of yeast-like fungi and molds such as: *Candida albicans, Penicillium citrinum, Fusarium solani, Aspergillus fumigatus, Rhodotorula mucilaginosa*, and also *Cladosporium* spp. and *Alternaria alternata*, which can grow in long or improperly stored food. In 60% they are compatible with latex allergens (Hev b9) (Ferreira et al. 2004).

15.2.7 Nuts Allergens

Nuts (tree nuts) often cause cross-reactions with other antigens. This group comprises of several species, not always related. Most frequently consumed are hazelnuts, walnuts, pistachios, Brazil nuts, coconuts, almonds, cashews, and chestnuts. Main allergens of hazelnuts include Cor a 1, which belongs to RP (pathogenesis—related) proteins (its release is induced by viral, viroidal, or fungal infection and by salicylic acid) and is homologous to Bet v 1, Cor a 2, belonging to profilins, and Cor a 8, being an LPT. Walnut contains: Jug r 1 of 2S albumins family, which is a storage protein, thermostable vicilin Jug r 2 and also thermostable Jug r 3 belonging to LTP. The danger of accidental consumption of nuts proteins by allergic people is high, because nuts are often a component of sweets, Asian meals, and can also contaminate production lines. Thus they are regarded as hidden allergens, not always disclosed on food product labels.

15.2.8 Peanuts

Peanuts are a no lesser threat. They are classified as grain legumes. Peanuts contain three thermostable proteins: Ara h1—vicilin, Ara h2—conglutinin, and Ara h3 being a legumin, and roasting increases the allergenic properties. Moreover, in peanuts we can also find: Ara h4—a legumin (a group of proteins present in legumes), Ara h5—a profilin, Ara h6—a homologue of conglutinin, similarly as Ara h7. Ara h8 is a thermolabile homologue of Bet v1, and Ara h9 is a protein belonging to LTP group. Strong cross-reactivity is observed with other legumes. It is stressed that only 20% of children grow out of allergy, so allergy symptoms persist for the whole life.

Allergen Nomenclature Sub-Committee of the International Union of Immunological Societies systematized the nomenclature and determined the structure of several hundreds of cloned and sequenced allergens, which are put on the website (www. allergen.org). It was impossible to discuss all of them so only selected were presented (Radauer et al. 2014).

15.3 INFLUENCE OF SOME TECHNOLOGICAL PROCESSES ON FOOD ALLERGENS

15.3.1 Introduction

The common food processes involved in the technological treatment of raw material are thermal processing (heating), hydrolysis (acid and enzymatic), physical treatment (high pressure, extrusion, microwave ultrasounds, γ-radiation), and bioconversion as a result of bacterial fermentation with the use of endogenous enzymes. Food processing changes the structural and chemical properties of proteins, activates the nonspecific interactions between proteins, protein–carbohydrate, and protein–fat. Proteins denature, aggregate, bind to lipid structures, and undergo glycosylation and/or glycation (Maillard reaction). These changes have the potential to influence the allergenicity of food (Wróblewska et al. 2007).

Microbial fermentation and enzymatic or acid hydrolysis may have the potential to reduce the allergenic integrity and allergenicity to such an extent that reactions will not be elicited. The combination of heat processing and the aforementioned methods may improve this hypoallergenic potency of a food product. Other processing methods, such as high pressure treatment, gamma radiation, and chemical modification, demonstrate promising results. Moreover, processing may also create new epitopes that may have the potential to induce sensitization and food allergy.

In addition, processing may influence, but not abolish, the allergenic potential of proteins at all. All these processes exert an impact on the potential allergenicity of food matrix and binding the specific IgE antibodies.

Food processing may affect the allergenicity of proteins in two aspects.

- The impact on the integrity of epitopes recognized by IgG or IgE antibodies. It influences the ability of antibodies to bind to the modified protein. During the IgE antibody binding this may result in an altered capacity to elicit an allergic reaction.
- It remains unsolved whether food processing has an impact on the capacity of a protein to stimulate the production of the IgE antibody (Verhoeckx et al. 2015).

The impact of food processing on the allergenicity of the most well-known sources of food allergens are summarized below.

15.3.2 Milk

Thermal processes, for example, pasteurization, increase the allergenicity of milk possibly due to aggregation, enhanced binding of proteins to the IgE and activation of mast cells in organisms by denatured proteins. Denaturation and Maillard reaction as a consequence of sterilization, trigger a decrease in the IgE- and IgG-binding capacity of existing epitopes of both β-lg and α-la. The condition of denaturation and nonenzymatic glycation leads to a destruction of already existing epitopes or renders them inaccessible. Up to date, there is not enough data concerning the ultra high temperature (UHT) processing, vacuum condensing, and spray drying on the allergenicity of milk. Fermentation of milk with lactic acid bacteria leads to the reduction of the allergenicity due to proteolytic activity of enzymes of bacteria (Wróblewska et al. 2011). Hydrolysis, used during baby formulae's production, usually allows to obtained low-antigenic products. However, there are also some data on enhanced allergenicity, being the effect of the specificity of the enzymes used.

15.3.3 Egg

Cooking and extensive heating diminishes the allergenicity of egg white proteins. Glycation by Millard reaction increased the IgE binding. Physical treatment methods, for example, irradiation, may modulate the allergenic properties of eggs.

15.3.4 Tree Nuts (Hazelnut, Almond, Cashew Nut, Brazil Nut, Walnut, Pistachio, Pecan Nut)

Heat processing exerts mainly a destructive effect on the allergenicity of proteins related to Bet v 1 (PR-10 and profilins) from tree nuts (hazelnut, almond, cashew nut, Brazil nut, walnut, pistachio, pecan nut). The binding of IgE was reduced. There are no data on the allergenicity of the homologs of the seed storage protein and LTP family.

Dry roasting of English walnuts (*Juglans regia*) at a temperature of 132°C or 180°C for 5, 10, or 20 minutes showed that both the soluble and insoluble protein fractions remained IgG and IgE immunoreactive. Consequently, this proved that walnut proteins are relatively stable under certain thermal processing conditions (Downs et al. 2016).

15.3.5 Peanut

The allergenic properties of peanut proteins may be altered by cooking and processing conditions, including temperature level, time of boiling, and hydration. The reduction of peanuts allergenicity during boiling results from denaturation of allergenic proteins and transferring water-soluble low molecular weight mass (<30 kDa) fraction of proteins into cooking water (Bennett and Lee 2016). Roasting of dry peanuts is one of the processes that may enhance the allergenicity due to oxidation-driven generation of advanced glycation end products (AGEs) from the Maillard reaction of peanut proteins with either exogenous simple sugars or glucose and fructose under a high temperature of process. Frying did not reduce the IgE-binding capacity.

15.3.6 Soybean

There are some studies concerning the reduction of soy allergenicity by food processing. Up to date, one-step processing may not fully abolish soy allergenicity. However, highly refined soybean oil and a few soybean products demonstrate the reduction of allergenicity below clinically relevant levels.

15.3.7 Wheat

Before consumption, wheat is subjected to various technological processes: baking, extrusion, and cooking, which may affect the digestibility of wheat proteins. Heating at high temperature in the presence of carbohydrates may induce the formation of protein aggregates with allergenic potential that are resistant to digestibility. Acid-hydrolyzed wheat gluten may also induce the allergenicity of traditional wheat products. It was noticed that proteolytic properties of enzymes are useful to lower the allergenicity of wheat. It was also proved that pH, temperature, and shear cause considerable conformational changes in the antigenicity of gluten. At pH 3, up to 90°C, the antigenicity was reduced by 30% in comparison to the control sample. Further heating to 100°C revealed new epitopes and enhanced antigenicity. High shearing rate (1,000 or 1,500/s) with high temperature (100°C) and pH 7 synergistically increased the antigenicity (Rahaman et al. 2016).

15.3.8 Mustard

The best method to reduce the allergenicity of mustard is to apply a combination of physical and thermal treatment (e.g., extrusion). The process of extraction of the potential allergens from mustard oil may suppress the allergenicity. Edible oils that are bleached and deodorized are devoid of any allergenicity.

Allergies to the oils of seeds remain controversial. The source of the allergenic proteins in the oil is not clear: they may be native proteins or may have been modified by the industrial process. The severity of the clinical reactions induced by the

DBPCFC conducted using a few milliliters of oil (corresponding to a few micrograms of protein) suggest that an adjuvant effect may be involved (Fremont et al. 2002).

15.4 CONCLUDING REMARKS

Summarizing, food allergens are relatively stable proteins, resistant to proteolysis in a simulated gastric fluid containing pepsin. It is possible that processing, as well as the food matrix, may have a significant impact on the digestibility of proteins by altering the susceptibility to gastrointestinal enzymes. For this reason, a combination of processing and digestion shall be taken into account in the assessment of allergenicity. Solubility of proteins after processing may undergo changes, improving after heat processing in some cases, yet decreasing in other, affecting the allergenicity.

REFERENCES

Ahrens, B., L.C. Lopes de Oliveira Grabenhenrich, G. Schulz, B. Niggemann, U. Wahn, and K. Beyer. 2012. Individual cow's milk allergens as prognostic markers for tolerance development? *Clin. Exp. Allergy* 42(11): 1630–1637.

Al-Hammadi, S., T. El-Hassan, and L. Al-Reyam. 2010. Anaphylaxis to camel milk in an atopic child. *Allergy* 65(12): 1623–1625.

Almqvist, C., A.C. Egmar, G. Hedlin, M. Lundqvist, S.L. Nordvall, G. Pershagen, et al. 2003. Direct and indirect exposure to pets—risk of sensitization and asthma at 4 years in a birth cohort. *Clin. Exp. Allergy* 33(9): 1190–1197.

Ayuso, R., S.B. Lehrer, M. Lopez, G. Reese, M.D. Ibañez, M. Esteban, et al. 2000. Identification of bovine IgG as a major cross-reactive vertebrate meat allergen. *Allergy* 55(4): 348–354.

Bennett, L., and A. Lee. 2016. Extractable low mass proteins <30 kDa from peanut display elevated antigenicity (IgG-binding) and allergenicity (IgE-binding) in vitro and are attenuated by thermal reactivity with non-peanut food ingredients. *Food Chem.* 194: 811–819.

Bernard, H., C. Creminon, M. Yvon, and J.M. Wal. 2000. Specificity of the human IgE response to the different purified caseins in allergy to cow's milk proteins. *Int. Arch. Allergy Immunol.* 115(3): 235–244.

Beyer, K., K.M. Jarvinen, L. Bardina, M. Mishoe, K. Turjanmaa, B. Niggemann, et al. 2005. IgE-binding peptides coupled to a commercial matrix as a diagnostic instrument for persistent cow's milk allergy. *J. Allergy Clin. Immunol.* 116(3): 704–705.

Bousquet, J., R. Dahl, and N. Khaltaev. 2007. Global alliance against chronic respiratory diseases. Allergy 62(3): 216–223.

Branum, A.M., and S.L. Lukacs. 2009. Food allergy among children in the United States. *Pediatrics* 124(6): 1549–1555.

Brooks, C., N. Pearce, and J. Douwes. 2013. The hygiene hypothesis in allergy and asthma: An update. *Curr. Opin. Allergy Clin. Immunol.* 13(1): 70–77.

Cantorna, M.T., Y. Zhu, M. Froicu, and A. Wittke. 2008. Vitamin D status, 1,25-dihydroxyvitamin D3, and the immune system. *Am. J. Clin. Nutr.* 80(6): 1717S–1720S.

Chang, J.Y. 2004. Evidence for the underlying cause of diversity of the disulfide folding pathway. *Biochemistry* 43(15): 4522–4529.

Chatchatee, P., K.M. Jarvinen, L. Bardina, L. Vila, K. Beyer, and H.A. Sampson. 2001. Identification of IgE and IgG binding epitopes on beta- and kappa-casein in cow's milk allergic patients. *Clin. Exp. Allergy* 31(8): 1256–1262.

Chen, Y., R. Dales, M. Tang, and D. Krewski. 2002. Obesity may increase the incidence of asthma in women but not in men: Longitudinal observations from the Canadian National Population Health Surveys. *Am. J. Epidemiol.* 155(3): 191–197.

Chruszcz, M., K. Mikolajczak, N. Mank, K.A. Majorek, P.J. Porebski, and W. Minor. 2013. Serum albumins—unusual allergens. *Biochim. Biophys. Acta.* 1830(12): 5375–5381.

Czaja-Bulsa, G. 2015. Non coeliac gluten sensitivity—A new disease with gluten intolerance. *Clin. Nutr.* 34(2): 189–194.

Darewicz, M., and J. Dziuba. 2005. Struktura a właściwości funkcjonalne białek mleka. *Żywność: nauka - technologia - jakośćZNTJ* 2(43): 47–60.

Decuyper, I., H. Ryckebosch, A.L. Van Gasse, V. Sabato, M. Faber, C.H. Bridts, et al. 2015. Cannabis allergy: What do we know Anno 2015. *Arch. Immunol. Ther. Exp. (Warsz)* 63(5): 327–332.

Dhanapala, P., T. Doran, M.L. Tang, and C. Suphioglu. 2015. Production and immunological analysis of IgE reactive recombinant egg white allergens expressed in Escherichia coli. *Mol. Immunol.* 65(1): 104–112.

Dmitrieva-Zdorova, E., O. Voronko, M. Aksenova, and N.V. Bodoev. 2010. Association of interleukin-13 gene polymorphisms with atopic bronchial asthma. *Russ. J. Gen.* 46(1): 99–104.

Douwes, J, R. van Strien, G. Doekes, J. Smit, M. Kerkhof, J. Gerritsen et al. 2006. Does early indoor microbial exposure reduce the risk of asthma? The Prevention and Incidence of Asthma and Mite Allergy birth cohort study. J Allergy Clin Immunol 117: 1067–1073.

Douwes, J., S. Cheng, N. Travier, C. Cohet, A. Niesink, J. McKenzie, et al. 2008. Farm exposure *in utero* may protect against asthma, hay fever and eczema. *Eur. Respir. J.* 32(3): 603–611.

Downs, M.L., A. Simpson, A. Custovic, A. Semic-Jusufagic, J. Bartra, M. Fernandez-Rivas, et al. 2016. Insoluble and soluble roasted walnut proteins retain antibody reactivity. *Food Chem.* 194: 1013–1021.

D'Amato, G., S.T. Holgate, R. Pawankar, D.K. Ledford, L. Cecchi, M. Al-Ahmad, et al. 2015. Meteorological conditions, climate change, new emerging factors, and asthma and related allergic disorders. A statement of the World Allergy Organization. *World Allergy Organ. J.* 8(1): 25.

EAACI-the European Academy of Allergy and Clinical Immunology. 2011. A European Declaration on Immunotherapy. Combating allergy beyond symptoms. Zurich, Switzerland.

Elsayed, S., and A. Jaran. 1983. Immunochemical analysis of cod fish allergen M: Locations of the immunoglobulin binding sites as demonstrated by the native and synthetic peptides. *Allergy* 38(7): 449–459.

Fasano, A. 2011. Zonulin and Iits regulation of intestinal barrier function: The biological door to inflammation, autoimmunity, and cancer. *Physiol. Rev.* 91(1): 151–175.

Fernández Rivas, M. 2003. Cross-reactivity between fruit and vegetables. *Allergol. Immunopathol. (Madr)* 31(3): 141–146.

Ferrara, F., S. Quaglia, I. Caputo, C. Esposito, M. Lepretti, S. Pastore, et al. 2010. Anti-transglutaminase antibodies in non-coeliac children suffering from infectious diseases. *Clin. Exp. Immunol.* 159(2): 217–223.

Ferreira, F., T. Hawranek, P. Gruber, N. Wopfner, and A. Mari. 2004. Allergic cross-reactivity: From gene to the clinic. *Allergy* 59(3): 243–267.

Frischmeyer-Guerrerio, P.A., A.L. Guerrerio, G. Oswald, K. Chichester, L. Myers, M.K. Halushka, et al. 2013. TGFβ receptor mutations impose a strong predisposition for human allergic disease. *Sci. Transl. Med.* 5(195): 195ra94.

Frémont, S., Y. Errahali, M. Bignol, I. Montagnon, M. Metche, J.P. Nicolas. 2002. What about the Allergenicity of Vegetable Oils? Internet Symposium on Food Allergens 4(2): 111–118.

Fu, T.J., N. Maks, and K. Banaszewski. 2010. Effect of heat treatment on the quantitative detection of egg protein residues by commercial enzyme-linked immunosorbent assay test kits. *J. Agric. Food Chem.* 58(8): 4831–4838.

Gilliland, F.D., K. Berhane, T. Islam, R. McConnell, W.J. Gauderman, S.S. Gilliland, et al. 2013. Obesity and the risk of newly diagnosed asthma in school-age children. *Am. J. Epidemiol.* 158(5): 406–415.

Hauser, M., A. Roulias, F. Ferreira, and M. Egger. 2010. Panallergens and their impact on the allergic patient. *Allergy Asthma Clin. Immunol.* 6(1): 1.

Hill, D.J., C.S. Hosking, F.M. de Benedictis, A.P. Oranje, T.L. Diepge, V. Bauchau, and EPAAC Study Group. 2008. Confirmation of the association between high levels of immunoglobulin E food sensitization and eczema in infancy: An international study. *Clin. Exp. Allergy* 38(1): 161–168.

Hoffmann-Sommergruber, K. 2000. Plant allergens and pathogenesis-related proteins. What do they have in common? *Int. Arch. Allergy Immunol.* 122(3): 155–166.

Imada, Y., M. Fujimoto, K. Hirata, T. Hirota, Y. Suzuki, H. Saito, et al. 2009. Large scale genotyping study for asthma in the Japanese population. *BMC Res. Notes* 2: 54.

Järvinen, K.M., P. Chatchatee, L. Bardina, K. Beyer, and H.A. Sampson. 2001. IgE and IgG binding epitopes on α-lactalbumin and β-lactoglobulin in cow's milk allergy. *Int. Arch. Allergy Immunol.* 126(2): 111–118.

Johansson, S.G., T. Bieber, R. Dahl, P.S. Friedman, B.Q. Lanier, R.F. Lockey, et al. 2004. Revised nomenclature for allergy for global use: Report of the Nomenclature Review. *J Allergy Clin Immunol.* 113(5): 832–836.

Kim, E.S., S.H. Kim, K.W. Kim, H.S. Park, E.S. Shin, J.E. Lee, et al. 2009. Involvement of FcεR1β gene polymorphisms in susceptibility to atopy in Korean children with asthma. *Eur. J. Pediatr.* 168: 1483–1490.

Kuehn, A., I. Swoboda, K. Arumugam, C. Hilger, and F. Hentges. 2014. Fish allergens at a glance: Variable allergenicity of parvalbumins, the major fish allergens. *Front. Immunol.* 22(5): 179.

Kull, I., A. Bergstrom, G. Lilja, G. Pershagen, and M. Wickman. 2006. Fish consumption during the first year of life and development of allergic diseases during childhood. *Allergy* 61(8): 1009–1015.

Kumosinski, T.F., E.M. Brown, and H.M. Farrell. 1991. Three-dimensional molecular modeling of Bovine Caseins: αs1-Casein. *J. Dairy Sci.* 74(9): 2889–2895.

Kuriyan, J., and D. Eisenberg. 2007. The origin of protein interactions and allostery in colocalization. *Nature* 450(7172): 983–990.

Lack, G. 2008. Epidemiologic risks for food allergy. *J. Allergy Clin. Immunol.* 121(6): 1331–1336.

Li, C.S., S.C. Chae, J.H. Lee, Q. Zhang, and H.T. Chung. 2006. Identification of single nucleotide polymorphism in FOXJ1 and their association with allergic rhinitis. *J. Hum. Genet.* 51(4): 292–297.

Lisson, M., and G. Erhardt. 2016. Mapping of epitopes occurring in bovine α_{s1}-casein variants by peptide microarray immunoassay. *Methods Mol. Biol.* 1352: 279–296.

Marshall, J.B. 2004. European Allergy White Paper. Allergic diseases as a public health problem in Europe. The UCB Institute of Allergy.

Martinez, M., G. Martos, E. Molina, and A.M.R. Pilosof. 2016. Reduced β-lactoglobulin IgE binding upon *in vitro* digestion as a result of the interaction of the protein with casein glycomacropeptide. *Food Chem.* 192(1): 943–949.

Martos, G., I. Lopez-Exposito, R. Bencharitiwong, M.C. Berin, and A. Nowak-Węgrzyn. 2013a. Mechanisms underlying differential food allergy response to heated egg. *J. Allergy Clin. Immunol.* 127(4): 990–997.

Martos, G., R. López-Fandiño, and E. Molina. 2013b. Immunoreactivity of hen egg allergens: Influence on in vitro gastrointestinal digestion of the presence of other egg white proteins and of egg yolk. *Food Chem.* 136(2): 775–781.

Maslova, E., C. Granström, S. Hansen, S.B. Petersen, M. Strøm, W.C. Willett, et al. 2012. Peanut and tree nut consumption during pregnancy and allergic disease in children. *J. Allergy Clin. Immunol.* 130(3): 724–732.

McGowan, E.C., G.R. Bloomberg, P.J. Gergen, C.M. Visness, K.F. Jaffee, M, et al. 2015. Influence of early-life exposures on food sensitization and food allergy in an inner-city birth cohort. *J. Allergy Clin. Immunol.* 135(1): 171–178.

Mc Mowat, A. 2003. Coeliac disease—a meeting point for genetics, immunology, and protein chemistry. *Lancet* 361(9365): 1290–1292.

Mikita, C.P., and E.A. Padlan. 2007. Why is there a greater incidence of allergy to the tropomyosin of certain animals than to that of others? *Med. Hypotheses* 69(5): 1070–1073.

Monti, G., E. Bertino, M.C. Muratore, A. Coscia, F. Cresi, L. Silvestro, et al. 2007. Efficacy of donkey's milk in treating highly problematic cow's milk allergic children: An *in vivo* and *in vitro* study. *Pediatr. Allergy Immunol.* 18(3): 258–264.

Monti, G., G. Bonfante, M.C. Muratore, A. Peltran, R. Oggero, L. Silvestro, et al. 2003. Kiss-induced facial urticaria and angioedema in a child allergic to fish. *Allergy* 58(7): 684–685.

Muzzarelli, R.A.A. 2010. Chitins and chitosans as immunoadjuvants and non-allergenic drug carriers. *Mar. Drugs* 8(2): 292–312.

Nakamura, H., F. Higashikawa, Y. Nobukuni, K. Miyagawa, T. Endo, T. Imai, et al. 2007. Genotypes and haplotypes of CCR2 and CCR3 genes in Japanese cedar pollinosis. *Int. Arch. Allergy Immunol.* 142(4): 329–334.

Nakanishi, K., T. Yoshimoto, H. Tsutsui, and H. Okamura. 2001. Interleukin-18 is a unique cytokine that stimulates both Th1 and Th2 responses depending on its cytokine milieu. *Cytokine Growth Factor Rev.* 12(1): 53–72.

Natale, M., C. Bisson, G. Monti, A. Peltran, L.P. Garoffo, S. Valentini, C, et al. 2004. Cow's milk allergens identification by two-dimensional immunoblotting and mass spectrometry. *Mol. Nutr. Food Res.* 48(5): 363–369.

Netting, M.J., P.F. Middleton, and M. Makrides. 2014. Does maternal diet during pregnancy and lactation affect outcomes in offspring? A systematic review of food-based approaches. *Nutrition* 30(11–12): 1225–1241.

Nwaru, B.I., L. Hickstein, S.S. Panesar, G. Roberts, A. Muraro, A. Sheikh, and EAACI Food Allergy and Anaphylaxis Guidelines Group. 2014. Prevalence of common food allergies in Europe: A systematic review and meta-analysis. *Allergy* 69(8): 992–1007.

Nwaru, B.I., S. Ahonen, M. Kaila, M. Erkkola, A.M. Haapala, C. Kronberg-Kippilä, et al. 2010. Maternal diet during pregnancy and allergic sensitization in the offspring by 5 yrs of age: A prospective cohort study. *Pediatr. Allergy Immunol.* 21(1 Pt. 1): 29–37.

Ober, C., and S. Hoffjan. 2006. Asthma genetics 2006: The long and winding road to gene discovery. *Genes Immun.* 7(2): 95–100.

Ober, C., and T.C. Yao. 2011. The genetics of asthma and allergic disease: A 21st century perspective. *Immunol. Rev.* 242(1): 10–30.

Pawankar, M.R., G.W. Canonica, S.T. Holgate, and R.F. Lockey. 2011. *Allergic Diseases as a Global Public Health Issue in White Book on Allergy*. By World Allergy Organization copyright 2011.

Pawankar, M.R., G.W. Canonica, S.T. Holgate, and R.F. Lockey. 2011–2012. *Biała Księga Alergii Światowej Organizacji Alergii*. Streszczenie wykonawcze. By World Allergy Organization copyright 2011.

Pawankar, M.R., G.W. Canonica, S.T. Holgate, R.F. Lockey, and M.S. Blaiss. 2013. *Allergic Diseases as a Global Public Health Issue in White Book on Allergy*. By World Allergy Organization copyright 2013.

Pearce, N., and J. Douwes. 2013. Lifestyle changes and childhood asthma. Symposium on Chronic Noncommunicable Diseases and Children. *Indian J. Pediatr.* 80(1): 95–99.

Perkin, M.R., and D.P. Strachan. 2006. Which aspects of the farming lifestyle explain the inverse association with childhood allergy? *J. Allergy Clin. Immunol.* 117(6): 1374–1381.

Pinkerton, K.E., and W.N. Rom. 2014. *Global Climate Change and Public Health.*: New York: Springer Science + Business Media.

Polosa, R., J.D. Knoke, C. Russo, G. Piccillo, P. Caponnetto, M. Sarvà, et al. 2008. Cigarette smoking is associated with a greater risk of incident asthma in allergic rhinitis. *J. Allergy. Clin. Immunol.* 121(6): 1428–1434.

Poole, J.A., K. Barriga, D.Y. Leung, M. Hoffman, G.S. Eisenbarth, M. Rewers, et al. 2006. Timing of initial exposure to cereal grains and the risk of wheat allergy. *Pediatrics* 117(6): 2175–2182.

Potočnik, K., V. Gantner, K. Kuterovac, and A. Cividini. 2011. Mare's milk: Composition and protein fraction in comparison with different milk species. *Mljekarstvo* 61(2): 107–113.

Quirce, S., F. Maranon, A. Umpierrez, M. de las Heras, E. Fernandez-Caldas, and J. Sastre. 2001. Chicken serum albumin (Gal d 5*) is a partially heat-labile inhalant and food allergen implicated in the bird-egg syndrome. *Allergy* 56(8): 754–762.

Radauer, C., A. Nandy, F. Ferreira, R.E. Goodman, J.N. Larsen, J. Lidholm, et al. 2014. Update of the WHO/IUIS Allergen Nomenclature Database based on analysis of allergen sequences. *Allergy* 69(4): 413–419.

Rahaman, T., T. Vasiljevic, and L. Ramchandran. 2016. Shear, heat and pH induced conformational changes of wheat gluten—Impact on antigenicity. *Food Chem.* 196: 180–188.

Reese, G., R. Ayuso, and S.B. Lehrer. 1999. Tropomyosin: An invertebrate pan–allergen. *Int. Arch. Allergy Immunol.* 119(4): 247–258.

Restani, P., C. Ballabio, A. Cattaneo, P. Isoardi, L. Terracciano, and A. Fiocchi. 2004. Characterization of bovine serum albumin epitopes and their role in allergic reactions. *Allergy* 59(78): 21–24.

Rodríguez del Río, P., S. Sánchez-García, C. Escudero, C. Pastor-Vargas, J.J. Sánchez Hernández, I. Pérez-Rangel, et al. 2012. Allergy to goat's and sheep's milk in a population of cow's milk-allergic children treated with oral immunotherapy. *Pediatr. Allergy Immunol.* 23(2): 128–132.

Sánchez-Monge, R., C. Blanco, A.D. Perales, C. Collada, T. Carrillo, C. Aragoncillo, et al. 2000. Class I chitinases, the panallergens responsible for the latex-fruit syndrome, are induced by ethylene treatment and inactivated by heating. *J. Allergy Clin. Immunol.* 106(1 Pt. 1): 190–195.

Sapone, A., J.C. Bai, C. Ciacci, J. Dolinsek, P.H. Green, M. Hadjivassiliou, et al. 2012. Spectrum of gluten-related disorders: Consensus on new nomenclature and classification. *BMC Med.* 10: 13.

Shabo, Y., R. Barzel, M. Margoulis, and R. Yagil. 2005. Camel milk for food allergies in children. *Isr. Med. Assoc. J.* 7(12): 796–798.

Sletten, G.B., R. Halvorsen, E. Egaas, and T.S. Halstensen. 2006. Changes in humoral responses to beta-lactoglobulin in tolerant patients suggest a particular role for IgG(4) in delayed, non-IgE-mediated cow's milk allergy. *Pediatr. Allergy Immunol.* 17(6): 435–443.

Strid, J., J. Hourihane, I. Kimber, R. Callard, and S. Strobel. 2004. Disruption of the stratum corneum allows potent epicutaneous immunization with protein antigens resulting in a dominant systemic Th2 response. *Eur. J. Immunol.* 34(8): 2100–2109.

Sudo, N., S. Sawamura, K. Tanaka, Y. Aiba, C. Kubo, and Y. Koga. 1997. The requirement of intestinal bacterial flora for the development of an IgE production system fully susceptible to oral tolerance induction. *J. Immunol.* 159(4): 1739–1745.

Summers, C.W., R.S. Pumphrey, C.N. Woods, G. McDowell, P.W. Pemberton, and P.D. Arkwright. 2008. Factors predicting anaphylaxis to peanuts and tree nuts in patients referred to a specialist center. *J. Allergy Clin. Immunol.* 121(3): 632–638.

Swoboda, I., A. Bugajska-Schretter, R. Valenta, and S. Spitzauer. 2002. Recombinant fish parvalbumins: Candidates for diagnosis and treatment of fish allergy. *Allergy* 57(72): 94–96.

Tavares, B., C. Pereira, F. Rodrigues, G. Loureiro, and C. Chieira. 2007. Goat's milk allergy. *Allergol Immunopathol (Madr)* 35(3): 113–116.

The UCB Institute of Allergy. 2004. *European Allergy White Paper—Summary.*

Tong, P., J. Gao, H. Chen, X.M. Li, Y. Zhang, and S. Jian. 2012. Effect of heat treatment on the potential allergenicity and conformational structure of egg allergen ovotransferrin. *Food Chem.* 132(2): 603–610.

Trasande, L., and G.D. Thurston. 2005. The role of air pollution in asthma and other pediatric morbidities. *J. Allergy Clin. Immunol.* 115(4): 689–699.

Umasunthar, T., J. Leonardi-Bee, M. Hodes, P.J. Turner, C. Gore, P. Habibi, et al. 2013. Incidence of fatal food anaphylaxis in people with food allergy: A systematic review and meta-analysis. *Clin. Exp. Allergy* 43(12): 1333–1341.

Urisu, A., Y. Kondo, and I. Tsuge. 2015. Hen's egg allergy. In: Ebisawa, M., B.K. Ballmer-Weber, S. Vieths, and R.A. Wood (eds): *Food Allergy: Molecular Basis and Clinical Practice.* (*Chem Immunol Allergy*), vol. 101. Basel, Switzerland: Karger, pp. 124–130.

Valenta, R., M. Duchêne, K. Pettenburger, C. Sillaber, P. Valent, P. Bettelheim, et al. 1991. Identification of profilin as a novel pollen allergen: IgE autoreactivity in sensitized individuals. *Science* 253(5019): 557–560.

Verhoeckx, K.C.M., Y.M. Vissersb, J.L. Baumertc, R. Faludid, M. Feyse, S. Flanaganf, et al. 2015. Food processing and allergenicity. *Food Chem. Toxicol.* 80: 223–240.

Williams, A.S., P. Nath, S.Y. Leung, N. Khorasani, A.N. McKenzie, I.M. Adcock, et al. 2008. Modulation of ozone-induced airway hyperresponsiveness and inflammation by interleukin-13. *Eur. Respir. J.* 32(3): 571–578.

Wróblewska, B., A. Kaliszewska, P. Kołakowski, K. Pawlikowska, and A. Troszyńska. 2011. Impact of transglutaminase reaction on the immunoreactive and sensory quality of yoghurt starter. *World J. Microbiol. Biotechnol.* 27: 215–227.

Wróblewska, B., A. Szymkiewicz, and L. Jedrychowski. 2007. Wpływ procesów technologicznych na zmiany alergenności żywności. *Żywność. Nauka. Technologia. Jakość. ZNTJ* 6(55): 7–19.

Yeats, T.H., and J.K.C. Rose. 2008. The biochemistry and biology of extracellular plant lipid-transfer proteins (LTPs). *Protein Sci.* 17(2): 191–198.

Żebrowska, A., and E. Waszczykowska. 2007. Clinical research Osteopenia and osteoporosis in patients with dermatitis herpetiformis: Effect of gluten-free diet. *Arch. Med. Sci.* 3(3): 252–258.

16 The Effect of Processing on the Safety and Nutritional Value of Food

Zdzisław E. Sikorski and Hanna Staroszczyk

CONTENTS

16.1 INTRODUCTION

Agricultural crops as well as animal food raw materials are usually somehow processed before being used by humans. Processing should make them more useful, increase their safety and nutritional value, extend the shelf life, and modify the sensory properties. As stressed by Damazy Jerzy Tilgner, the cofounder of the International Union of Food Science and Technology, "Man does not 'take nourishments,' he rather wants to eat various tasty dishes, because eating must provide consumer's satisfaction. Thus, the flavor, color, shape, texture, and taste of food are equally important as the contents of nutrients." However, the opinion, expressed even by some food professionals and journalists that only unprocessed foods are healthy, is at least misleading.

Processing, depending on its parameters and the properties of the commodity, may improve or decrease the nutritional value and safety of foods. This could be illustrated by numerous examples. Various enzymatic reactions improve the functional and nutritive value of lipids. Transesterification in presence of regiospecific or selective lipases makes it possible to produce fats containing nutritionally desirable fatty acid (FA) residues and concentrates of eicosapentaenoic acids (EPA) and docosahexaenoic acids (DHA). Hydrogenation turns liquid oils into plastic fats and protects them against oxidation, but this may generate nutritionally undesirable *trans*-FA. Smoking contributes to the formation of delicious properties and extension of the shelf life of meat and fish products. In improper conditions, however, it may contaminate the products with carcinogenic hydrocarbons. Nitrate(III) used in curing meat serves to develop the desirable heat-stable pink color of nitrosyl hemochrome and inhibits the growth of *Clostridium botulinum.* However, if applied in excessive amounts, it leads to the formation of toxic *N*-nitroso compounds.

Numerous toxins and other harmful components, present in the raw materials naturally or due to contamination, can be eliminated by physical separation, as well as destroyed in enzyme catalyzed reactions or by heating. Detailed information on the specific treatments applied in the food chain to minimize the human health hazards has been presented in several chapters of this book. However, changes and interactions of various compounds in the conditions of processing may generate products toxic or otherwise unsafe for the human organism. The food industry endeavors to find and apply processes that do not adversely affect the desirable properties of the products. The aim of the processor or cook is to maximize the beneficial and minimize the undesirable effects. Disseminating knowledge on the occurrence and properties of the harmful compound in foods may help in achieving this goal.

16.2 INCREASING FOOD SAFETY

16.2.1 Physical Elimination of Harmful Compounds

Knowing the localization and form of distribution of the undesirable compounds it is possible to physically remove them from the raw materials. This is routinely made both in the food industry and in the kitchen. Some representative examples are presented below.

The first step is the prevention of entering of raw materials, containing harmful compounds, into the food chain. The means of achieving this depend on the commodity and are different in various regions. They include:

- Good agricultural practice and traceability in plant production, animal husbandry, and fisheries
- Visual and laboratory examination of the feedstock
- Prevention of the use of materials not allowed as human food
- Implementation of adequate legislation
- Education of the population in recognizing toxic plants and animal sources

Different parts of the plants of the *Solanaceae* family contain the toxic glycoalkaloid solanine in various concentrations. In potato tubers its content may be high enough to cause in humans various gastrointestinal malfunctions and neurological disorders. The tubers contain usually less solanine than 0.2 mg/g of, but potatoes of some varieties much more. The glycoalkaloid is mainly in the skin and in a thin layer beneath. Its content is especially high in sprouted tubers or those which were stored unprotected from light. Green color of the surface of such potatoes may indicate that they contain even five times more solanine than the unchanged tubers. The best way of preventing poisoning is not eating green potatoes. The alkaloid is water soluble and thus gets extracted during cooking. However, unpeeled boiled, especially baked green potatoes may cause various health troubles, since in some circles the skin of baked potatoes is also consumed.

Severe human health hazards may be caused by mycotoxins present in grains, corn, pulses, nuts, and fruits harvested and/or stored in adverse conditions (see Chapter 6). Most effective in preventing such hazards is applying conditions inhibiting the proliferation of the toxin producing organisms. They include mainly low water activity in the crop and low air humidity during storage, as well as strict professional control of the commodities entering the food chain. Mechanical cleaning of crops infested by molds does not eliminate the health hazards, because the toxins accumulate in the molded tissues.

In Poland, where wild mushroom hunting in the forests is a very popular summer and autumn outdoor activity, up to hundreds cases of mushroom poisoning occur annually. Severe intoxications may be even fatal. To minimize this hazard several educational programs on recognizing poisonous species are run. Furthermore, regulations have been set safeguarding the food chain from being entered by wild, poisonous mushrooms difficult to be recognized as such by untrained people. They require certification by qualified inspectors of all mushrooms offered on the market. An official list of species allowed to be sold in Poland has been published. Various techniques of soaking and cooking aimed at decreasing the toxicity, popular among the population, have been practiced and described. The only foolproof approach, however, is to refrain from eating unknown, possibly poisonous mushrooms. The subject of mushroom toxins has been described in Chapter 3 of this volume.

Fish of several species may contain toxins causing severe health hazards, like tetrodotoxin and ciguatoxin. Eating shellfish may be seasonally dangerous because of the paralytic, diarrheic, amnesic, neurotoxic, or azaspiracid poisons (see Chapter 4). Shellfish toxins are generally heat resistant, thus normal cooking does not inactivate them. To prevent polluted shellfish from being harvested, various microbiological and chemical surveys of seawater are carried out to determine the sanitary standard of the fishing grounds. Depending on the results of the surveys, the harvesting areas are classified accordingly, from approved to prohibited. The detailed conditions of the surveys and the resulting regulations are different in various countries, although all of them aim at preventing poisoning of the consumers. Actual information regarding the harvesting areas and shellfish species is being published by the responsible authorities. However, recreational harvesters not observing the official warnings run a great risk caused by seasonally poisonous shellfish. Thus, the most reasonable decision, just like that regarding wild mushrooms, is to refrain from eating shellfish other than purchased from a source that sells only tested ware. In the fisheries industry a standard procedure is depuration of the live animals to minimize the hazards induced by eating polluted bivalve molluscs. Live oysters are kept for up to a few days in sterilized water to remove from their intestines fecal pathogenic microorganisms of several species.

As regards the toxic puffer fish, containing tetrodotoxin, the safest approach is not to catch them. However, since there are consumers who value the exquisite sensory properties of *Tetraodontidae* and the thrill connected with having a puffer fish for dinner, there are numerous chefs qualified to safely prepare these dishes. They skillfully remove the parts of the body known to contain the highest amounts of the deadly tetrodotoxin, especially the ovaries, liver, intestines, and skin.

Eating fish of several species rich in dark meat, especially tuna, mackerel, mahi-mahi, sardine, anchovy, herring, bluefish, amberjack, and marlin may cause light to severe symptoms of intolerance or intoxication known as scombroid or histamine poisoning. The responsible factor may be not only histamine but also a group of other biogenic amines (Figure 16.1) (Flick and Granata 2005; Visciano et al. 2014). Scombroid poisoning may cause gastrointestinal, circulatory, and cutaneous disturbances. The effect depends significantly on the individual susceptibility of the consumer involved, the contents of various biogenic amines in the diet, and the presence of other food components. Heat processing applied normally to foods does not destroy the toxic compounds.

Histamine and the other amines in fish muscles are products of decarboxylation of amino acids by bacterial enzymes (Figure 16.2). Their accumulation in fish can be inhibited by rapid chilling of the catch on board vessel and storage at a temperature

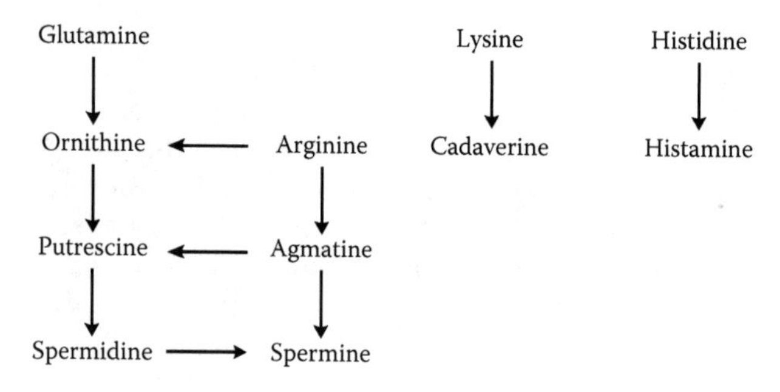

FIGURE 16.1 Biogenic amines.

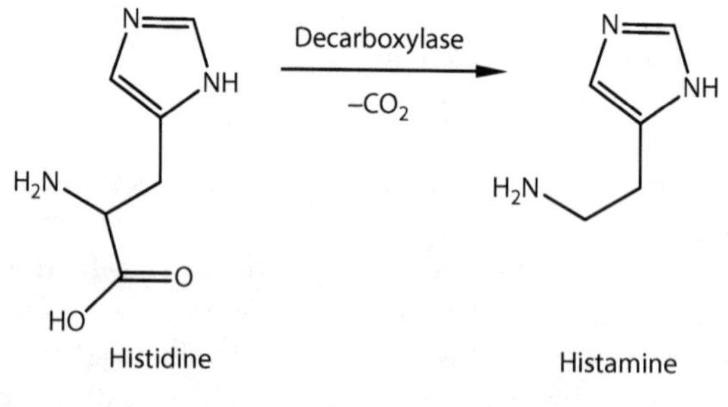

FIGURE 16.2 Decarboxylation of histidine.

close to 0°C or freezing. The bacterial decarboxylase accumulated prior to freezing can be activated after thawing; therefore, cold storage is required also for defrosted fish. Limits for the content of histamine in fish and fishery products have been set to prevent scombroid poisoning. In the European Union, the limit is 400-μg histamine/g of products made by enzyme maturation in brine of fishes of the families *Scombridae*, *Clupeidae*, *Engraulidae*, *Coryferridae*, *Pomatomidae*, and *Scombresosidae* (Commission Regulation (EC) No 2073/2005, Commission Regulation (EU) No 1019/2013).

Biogenic amines occur not only in fishery products but also in small amount in various fresh vegetables and fruits, as well as in fermented commodities (Malinowska-Pańczyk 2015). Cheeses contain predominantly tryptamine, tyramine, cadaverine, putrescine, and histamine in total concentration up to 300 μg/g, depending on the conditions of ripening. The subject of biogenic amines has been expertly treated in Chapter 5 of this book.

Of deep-water fish, orange roughy, highly valued for the superb sensory properties of its fillets, the nutritionally undesirable element is the under skin lipid layer rich in high-molecular wax. The lipids of the fish *Hoplostethus atlanticus* and *Pseudocyttus maculatus* may contain up to 95% waxes. Deep skinning of the fillets effectively removes the wax layer.

To prevent poisoning by mercury accumulated in large specimen of predatory fish from several polluted fishing grounds upper size limits for setting ashore such catch are obligatory, or else fishing in some lakes is prohibited. Toxic microelements in foods have been described in Chapter 9 of this book.

The hazards caused by pesticide residues and environmental pollutants in fishery products are being limited by restricting the fishery in certain aquae or advising the removal of some parts of the fish body, for example, the livers. The hazards caused by pesticide residues in foods have been discussed in Chapter 8.

Since the end of the twentieth century, the meat industry has to cope with the bovine spongiform encephalopathy (BSE). This disease is caused by prions, extremely heat-resistant proteins, which cannot be denatured/destroyed during heat sterilization. They are concentrated in BSE infected cattle in the tissues of the central nervous system, but they have not been detected in the muscle meat. Therefore, the BSE specified risk material, that is, the skull, brain, tonsils, trigeminal ganglia, eyes, spinal cord, distal ileum, and dorsal root ganglia must be removed at slaughter/deboning and splitting of the cattle carcasses. This material is not allowed to enter the food and fodder chain. The requirements regarding the age of the slaughtered cattle to be thus treated are somewhat different in various countries.

Soaking in water or in appropriate solutions is applied to extract and remove different harmful components from some agricultural crops. Soaking decreases the content of phytic acid (inositol polyphosphate) in legumes and cereals. Phytic acid binds mineral components of the diet, especially Ca, Mg, Fe, Cu, and Zn and complexes the basic groups of amino acid residues in proteins, thus their absorption in the digestive tract of human consumers is impaired. The efficiency of removal of phytic acid can be increased by lowering the pH of the soaking medium. Fermentation, as in the sour dough in manufacturing rye bread, decreases the contents of phytic acid due to the hydrolyzing activity of endogenous and bacterial phytase (Lopez et al. 2003). In kidney beans soaking lowers also the contents of phytohemagglutinins—proteins, which agglutinate erythrocytes and leucocytes.

Various treatments are necessary to prevent the toxic effects caused by changes of the cyanogenic glucosides, linamarin and lotaustralin, present in cassava roots, one of the major staple foods for millions of people. The enzymes of the roots catalyze the hydrolysis of the glucosides and liberate the toxic hydrogen cyanide (HCN) (Figure 16.3). The amount of HCN generated in the bitter variety may reach 1-μg/g fresh tuber. Cooking may eliminate the risk of toxicity of cassava that contains much less glucosides. The tubers rich in linamarin and lotaustralin have to be peeled, ground, soaked in water, pressed, and toasted. Alternatively, the roots may be soaked for several days and fermented prior to cooking.

Unrefined, crude cottonseed oil is red or brown since it contains several pigments, including gossypol, a polyphenolic aldehyde, which serves in the seed as a natural insecticide. Gossypol is toxic for monogastric animals, but the microflora of the rumen is able to utilize it. The cottonseed oil used extensively in producing numerous processed foods and snacks is free of gossypol, since alkaline refining removes this pigment effectively.

To the category of physical elimination of harmful compounds belongs also the sanitization of food plants to control the spoilage and pathogenic microflora in the processing environment (Table 16.1).

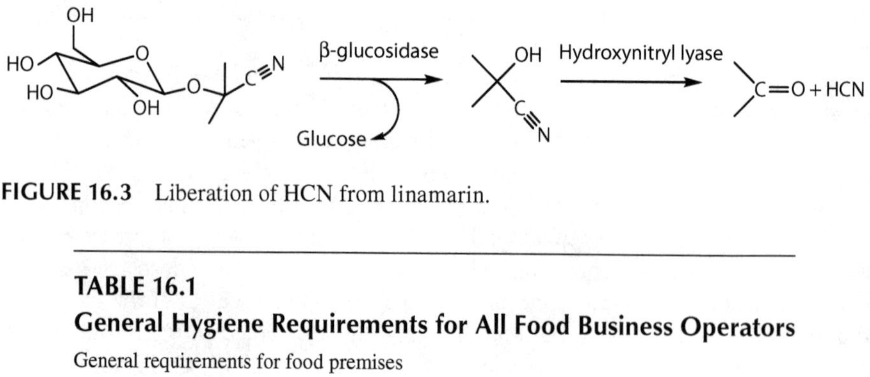

FIGURE 16.3 Liberation of HCN from linamarin.

TABLE 16.1
General Hygiene Requirements for All Food Business Operators

General requirements for food premises
Requirements in rooms where foodstuffs are prepared, treated/processed
Requirements for movable and/or temporary premises
Transport
Equipment requirements
Food waste
Water supply
Personal hygiene
Provisions applicable to foodstuffs
Provisions applicable to the wrapping and packaging of foodstuffs
Water treatment
Training

Source: Regulation (EC) No 852/2004 of the European Parliament and of the Council of 29 April 2004 on the hygiene of foodstuffs. Annex II.

16.2.2 Preventing Health Hazards to Nutritionally Compromised Persons

Some food components perfectly safe for the majority of the consumers may cause severe health hazards for other people. Industrial processing as well as home preparation of foods may in numerous cases prevent these undesirable health effects to such persons.

A large number of plants and foods of animal origin contain various allergens. The health hazards involved, and the treatments applied in the food industry to inactivate the allergens have been expertly presented in Chapter 15.

Gluten, the valuable component of wheat flour, responsibles for the desirable texture of bread, contains gliadin, the cause of the gluten-sensitive enteropathy or celiac disease in genetically susceptible persons. To avoid the dangerous health consequences, the food consumed by such individuals must be completely free of gluten proteins. That means that all products and dishes containing gluten proteins of wheat, barley, rye, and triticale should be excluded from the diet of such persons. Ordinary bread and cakes cannot be produced without using wheat or rye flour. However, equally tasty and nourishing bread and other products can be baked using flour made of other grains, for example, buckwheat, rice, or millet. The food industry helps the people suffering from the celiac disease by manufacturing a large variety of gluten-free products.

A great percentage of the adult humans in the world does not tolerate lactose in the diet because of lack in their digestive tract of β-galactosidase necessary to hydrolyze this disaccharide to galactose and glucose. The lactose not hydrolyzed in the small intestine cannot be absorbed there, but it is metabolized by the colon microflora. The gaseous products of fermentation induce various gastrointestinal disorders, including abdominal cramps, vomiting, and diarrhea. Lactose is present mainly in milk (in cow's milk about 4.7%) and in unfermented dairy products, but it is also used as an ingredient in a number of other commodities. The simplest way to avoid the harmful health effects is to refrain from consuming lactose-containing foods. Proper information on the labels of packaged commodities regarding the contents of lactose is required. Separation of sweet whey removes most of the disaccharide from the casein curd, since lactose is water soluble. In fermented dairy products the contents of lactose may be substantially decreased by bacteria converting it into lactic and/or propionic acid. By using β-galactosidase of bacterial origin, often immobilized, the dairy industry manufactures lactose-free milk. Commercial preparations of β-galactosidase are also offered for home use.

Persons with phenylalanine hydroxylase deficiency must avoid foods rich in proteins containing much phenylalanine. For such consumers various modified protein preparations with less or no phenylalanine are manufactured, for example, the glycomacropeptide separated from casein. Protein hydrolysates can be modified enzymatically to remove phenylalanine and produce phenylalanine-free polypeptides (plasteins).

16.2.3 Control of Infestation by Parasites

Numerous food raw materials are infested with various parasites. Roundworms live on vegetables grown on sewage-contaminated soil, *Trichinella spiralis* in the muscles of pigs and game, mainly boars, *Toxoplasma gondii* in meat, tapeworms in meat animals and fish, and *Anisakid nematodes* and protozoans in fish.

In the pork industry, the first sanitary inspection is carried out prior to slaughter to prevent diseased animals to enter the processing line. Later, the diaphragm, cheek muscle, or tongue of the carcasses is examined visually on the slaughter line by veterinary inspectors, and samples taken here are analyzed in the laboratory to eliminate the parasitized bodies. The carcasses and entrails are tagged to allow for their later identification. The pig carcasses containing *Trichinella spiralis* are removed and undergo adequate procedures inactivating the parasites, for example, freezing to −35°C or cooking to internal temperature of 70°C.

The number of parasites living on or in fish may be larger than that of the animals caught for human consumption. It is not possible to examine individually the vast number of small fish landed by the industrial fishing vessels and small craft. Some parasites are harmful for the human consumer (see Sobecka and Piasecki 2011), other have to be avoided due to aesthetic reasons or because their activity decreases the sensory properties and technological value of the meat. The parasite *Capillaria philippinensis* causes severe gastrointestinal disorders in countries where raw fish are eaten habitually. The muscles of hake and blue whiting heavily infested by the microscopic *Myxosporidia* of the *Kudoa* sp. turn gray, watery, and gel-like due to the activity of the proteinases of the parasites. The infestation of some fish in certain areas and seasons is very high, thus the fishery refrains from exploitation of such waters. In the case of large fish, for example, large cod, removing of the belly flaps from the fillets, the parts of the carcasses predominantly infested, followed by candling to check for remaining *Anisakis* is done routinely on the industrial filleting lines. To kill the larvae at least 1 minute heating at 60°C is required. Generally, effective treatment against parasites in uncooked fishery products is freezing and storage for at least 3 days at −20°C.

16.2.4 Treatments against Food Poisoning Microorganisms

Various methods of food preservation are used to inhibit the growth or kill the spoilage and pathogenic microorganisms. The bacteria in foods differ in their sensitivity toward temperature, oxygen, water activity, pH, nutrient availability, ionizing radiation, and chemical preservatives, as well as in their ability to produce spores (Table 16.2). Predictive microbiology equations relate the growth rate of microorganisms to temperature, atmosphere composition, water activity, pH, and concentration of preservatives. This makes it possible to quantify the hazards caused in every step of food handling, processing, and storage (McMeekin et al. 1993).

Inhibition of the growth of the undesirable microflora can be achieved in conditions which decrease the rate or stop the metabolism of the microbial cells—low temperature, absence of water available for the biological processes, restricted access of oxygen, low pH, or chemical changes in the enzyme systems (Table 16.3). Thus, harmful microflora can be inhibited by chilling, freezing, modifying the atmosphere, drying/lyophilization, smoking, salting, curing, other means of decreasing the water activity, acidifying, fermentation, adding various preservatives and by combined action of several factors—the hurdle technology. Harsh parameters, that

TABLE 16.2
Growth Conditions of *Listeria monocytogenes*

Temperature: 0°C–45°C
Generation time: at 1°C–3 days; at 5°C–1 day
pH: 4.3 to 9.6, depending on the growth medium and temperature
NaCl: up to 10%
Water activity: above 0.92
Oxygen requirements: aerobic environment or restricted oxygen supply
Thermal resistance: survives high-temperature short-time (HTST) pasteurization (71.7°C, 15 sec) in milk if present at 1.000 to 10.000 cells/cm^3

TABLE 16.3
Minimum Water Activity (a_w) and Temperature Tolerated by Bacteria

Bacteria	a_w	°C
Campylobacter jejuni	0.99	30–45
Clostridium botulinum type E	0.97	3.3–45
Escherichia coli O157:H7	0.95	6.5–49
Clostridium perfringens	0.93	10–52
Yersinia enterocolitica	0.95	−1.3–42
Vibrio parahaemolyticus	0.94	5–45
Salmonella spp.	0.94	5–46
Listeria monocytogenes	0.92	−0.4–45
Staphylococcus aureus	0.83	7–50

is, drying to very low water content, acidifying to very low pH or heavy salting, increase the shelf life of the products but may degrade the sensory properties of the food. Mild processing, like salting of tender fish with small amounts of salt, leads to high-quality products, as has been noted by Biegler (1960):

> "Auf 100 kg Herringe rechnet man 12 bis 15 kg Salz. Gerade die milde Salzung verhalf diesem Salzherringsprodukt zu seinem delikaten Charakter. Ein mild gesalzener Schinken, oder mild gesalzener Kaviar oder mild gesalzener Lachs dürften schon den Göttern gut gemundet haben."

To effectively extend the shelf life of such commodities, however, additional treatments, mainly refrigerated storage and approved preservatives should be applied.

In eliminating the health hazards created by pathogenic microflora the quality management system HACCP has high priority. An example of its application is presented in (Table 16.4). One of the crucial points in this system is the flow sheet, which visualizes the unit operations and processes in which food safety hazards may occur.

TABLE 16.4
Hazard Analysis in Hot Smoking of Baltic Sprats

Unit Operation/Process	Potential Hazard	Source of Hazard	Degree of Risk	Preventive Action	Control Point/Critical Control Point
Inspection of raw material	Low freshness, initial signs of spoilage, high number of pathogenic bacteria	High initial number of bacteria, too long storage at too high temperature	High	Refuse to accept, strict freshness control at inspection point, change of supplier	CCP
Storage	Loss of freshness, high growth of microorganisms	Too high temperature, too long time of storage	Low	Decrease the storage temperature, increase the flow rate of the process	CP
Brining	Growth of *Clostridium. botulinum* and *Listeria monocytogenes*	Too low concentration of NaCl in the brine, differences in contact fish/brine	High	Increase the time of brining and/or concentration of NaCl, control the brine temperature, improve mixing of the fish in the brine	CCP
Smoking	Survival of vegetative forms of pathogens	Too low temperature and time of smoking	High	Increase the temperature and time of smoking, control the yield of smoked fish	CCP
Chilling	Growth of bacteria and recontamination	Too low chilling rate, contaminated air	Low	Decrease the air temperature, improve air circulation, control air cleaning	CP
Packaging	Recontamination with pathogens	Low hygiene standard, bad organization of work	High	Comply with general hygiene requirements Regulation (EC) No 852/2004	CCP
Storage	Growth of putrefactive and pathogenic microorganisms	Too high temperature and storage time	Low	Decrease temperature, shorten the time from producer to retailer	CP

Destruction of the microbial population can be achieved by heat pasteurization or sterilization and by ionizing radiation. The antimicrobial effects and the sensory quality of the products caused by such treatments depend upon the properties of the food and the conditions of processing. The parameters of the treatment are selected so as to achieve the highest or just sufficient preservative/bactericidal effect at minimal loss of the sensory and nutritional value of the products. One of such approaches is the HTST thermal processing. A typical example of the application of heat treatment to destroy most of the vegetative forms of spoilage microorganisms and of common pathogenic bacteria is pasteurization which, if properly carried out, eliminates the risk of diseases caused by contaminated, untreated milk. The risk and benefit considerations show that the loss of nutritional value due to thermal destruction of some vitamins is negligible as compared to the increase in safety of the product.

The death of bacteria in heated wet foods proceeds generally in a logarithmic order. The time required to reduce by 90% the original number of microorganisms at any given temperature is known as the D-value. For the spores of any given bacterial species, the D-value decreases as the temperature increases. The number of °C to cause a 10-fold reduction of the D-value is called the z-value. The time required to destroy a spore in a specific medium at 121°C, the F-value can be calculated as:

$$F = D\,(\log N_0 - \log N_f) \tag{16.1}$$

where:

N_0 = maximum initial number of bacteria per container
N_f = acceptable number of surviving bacteria per container

Inactivation of the vegetative forms and spores of bacteria can be also achieved by ionizing radiation at room temperature or in the frozen state. The dose of radiation necessary for sterilization is 25–35 kGy. It depends on the initial number of bacteria, their radiation sensitivity, as well as on the conditions of the treatment, including temperature, access of oxygen, contents of water and of reducing compounds.

The preservation methods applied in food processing are expected not only to prevent spoilage of the products, but they should also safeguard the consumer against microbial food poisoning. Microbial foodborne diseases include:

- Infections caused by bacteria present in the food or water that grow in the consumer's organism
- Intoxications caused by toxins accumulated in the eaten food, products of the metabolism of the microorganisms

The resistance of microbial toxins to the lethal conditions of heat pasteurization or sterilization differs substantially. In some cases, the time–temperature regimes lethal to the vegetative cells do not inactivate the toxin, whereas microorganisms of other species produce spores that are much more heat stable than their toxins. This can be illustrated as below. *Staphylococcus aureus*, a nonspore forming bacteria, is inactivated by heat pasteurization, but its enterotoxins can withstand sterilization.

The vegetative form of *Clostridium botulinum* can be destroyed in a few minutes at 60°C, the spores are heat resistant, their *D*-value at 121.1°C is 1–2 minutes, depending on the properties of the medium, but the toxins can be inactivated by pasteurization, in about 3 minutes at 74°C. Thus, the resistance of the microbial toxins to heating should be regarded as a crucial factor in securing food safety. The human health hazards caused by bacterial toxins have been very thoroughly discussed in Chapter 7 of this book.

16.2.5 Inactivating of Some Antinutrients

Different antinutritive constituents occur in various food raw materials. They serve special physiological purposes in the plant or animal. When consumed, however, they adversely affect the digestive processes or impair the utilization of nutrients in humans.

One group of such compounds is the proteinaceous inhibitors of proteolytic enzymes. They form enzymatically inactive complexes with various proteinases. Their physiological role is to protect the plants against the attack of invaders. However, when consumed they impair digestion in the human organism. Protein inhibitors are in grains, potatoes, beans, *Cruciferae*, and in high concentration up to 20 mg/g in soybeans. They can be extracted by soaking and inactivated by cooking, for example, 5-min boiling decreases in about 80% the inhibitory activity of common beans. In soybean processing, the inhibitors are denatured by toasting and extrusion.

The biological value of pulses may be decreased by the activity of endogenous lipoxygenase, which catalyzes the oxidation of linoleic and linolenic acids. Oxidation decreases the biological value of soybeans and generates secondary products, which impart to some commodities, for example, soy milk, the unpleasant beany flavor. The development of the beany flavor may be prevented by inactivation of the enzyme by 10 minutes of blanching at 100°C.

Soybeans, faba beans, peas, peanuts, cereal grains, nuts, potato tubers, and many other agricultural crops contain also various lectins in different concentration. Lectins are predominantly glycoproteins, which may contain up to 10% of saccharide moieties. They can bind different saccharides and thus display hemagglutinating activity. Being fairly resistant to the digestive enzymes they may cause gastrointestinal disturbances and nutritional deficiencies. Some lectins are heat resistant, thus only prolonged cooking of various plant foods inactivates them.

Some plants used for food contain water-soluble α-galactooligosaccharides, soybeans even as much as 4% dry matter. These oligosaccharides are indigestible, because humans do not synthesize α-galactosidase necessary to hydrolyze them in the digestive tract. They are easily metabolized by bacteria in the colon and turn into short chain FA, CO_2, CH_4, and H_2. These changes may decrease the absorption of some nutrients and cause uncomfortable flatulence. However, α-galactooligosaccharides may also be regarded as prebiotics, facilitating the growth of the beneficial bifidobacteria. Various treatments can decrease the content of these saccharides in soybeans intended for human consumption, predominantly soaking, enzyme treatment, and fermentation as practiced in manufacturing of the traditional Asian soy products—tempeh, soy sauce, and miso (Figure 16.4). Soy protein isolates

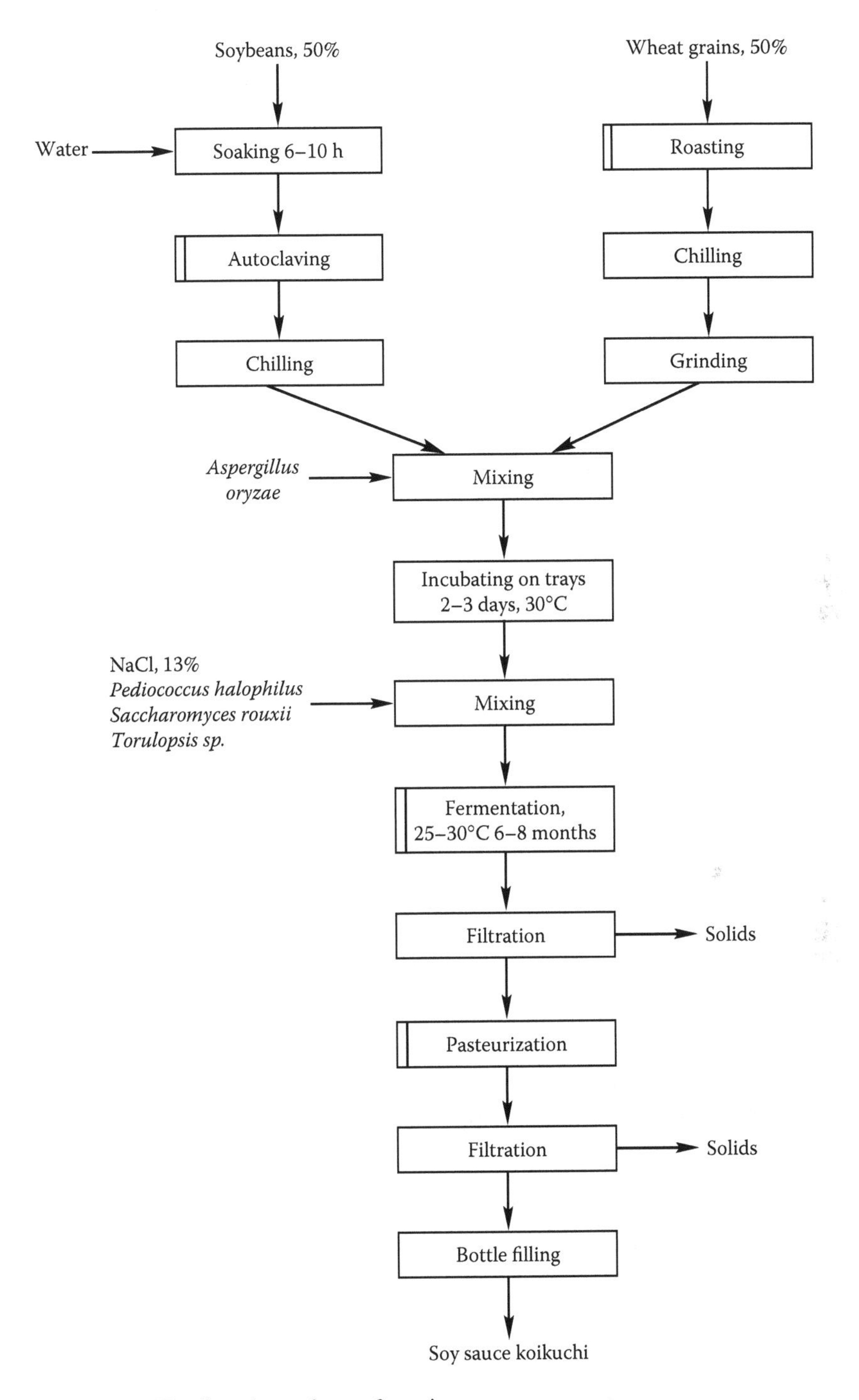

FIGURE 16.4 The flow sheet of manufacturing soy sauce.

are also free of α-galactooligosaccharides, since nonprotein components of the soybeans are removed in the manufacturing process.

Egg white contains avidin—a biotin-binding protein. It is a glycoprotein composed of four subunits. Each of these subunits can form a stable complex with one molecule of biotin, resistant to several proteolytic enzymes, thus making the vitamin unavailable for the consumer of raw eggs. The biotin-binding activity of avidin is destroyed to different degrees in preparing egg dishes; total inactivation occurs after 4 minutes of boiling.

16.3 LOSS OF SAFETY AND NUTRITIONAL VALUE OF FOODS

16.3.1 Introduction

Leaching, mechanical separation, as well as several biochemical and chemical reactions during storage and/or processing of foods generally do not yield toxic or otherwise harmful compounds. However, they may decrease the biological value of the dishes by removing or destroying some nutritionally valuable components or making them unavailable to the human organism. Examples of such undesirable changes include:

- Loss of mineral components and vitamins due to leaching and cooking drip
- Loss of mineral components and vitamins in the fractions separated during grain milling
- Loss of some calcium from the milk curd that is transferred into the acid whey
- Thermal changes of some heat-labile proteins, lipids, and vitamins
- Oxidation of various food components
- Loss of nutritionally valuable EPA and DHA by hydrogenation of oils

16.3.2 Effects of Oxidation

Autoxidation of lipids is initiated by an attack of any free radical (R•) on a C–H bond in the FA chain (LH), yielding an alkyl radical (L•), that in the propagation step forms with oxygen a lipid peroxide radical (LOO•). Reacting with a next unsaturated FA residue this radical turns into a hydroperoxide (LOOH) and generates again an L• (Figure 16.5). Furthermore, lipoxygenases may catalyze the stereo- and regio-specific oxidation of polyenoic FA with the formation of respective LOOH (Bartosz and Kołakowska 2011). Decomposing of the unstable LOOH leads to LO• and HO•. Repeating this sequence keeps the chain reaction running. In photosensitized oxidation initiated by a singlet oxygen molecule ($^1O_2$), the LOOH is formed directly, omitting the LOO• (Figure 16.6). Decomposition of LOOH, accelerated by high temperature, radiation, and cations yields alkoxy radicals and a large number of various low-molecular secondary products, including aldehydes, ketones, epoxy compounds, alcohols, and hydroxy acids. In the third stage, the accumulated radical secondary products of autoxidation react to form various lipid–lipid and lipid–protein polymers, thus terminating the chain reaction (Kołakowska and Bartosz 2014) (Figure 16.7).

$$LH + R^{\bullet} \longrightarrow L^{\bullet} + RH$$

$$L^{\bullet} + O_2 \longrightarrow LOO^{\bullet}$$

$$LOO^{\bullet} + LH \longrightarrow LOOH + L^{\bullet}$$

FIGURE 16.5 Formation of lipid hydroperoxides.

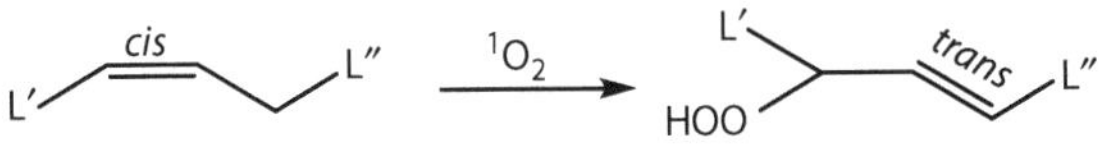

FIGURE 16.6 Photosensitized oxidation.

$$L^{\bullet} + LOO^{\bullet} \longrightarrow LOOL \qquad L^{\bullet} + L^{\bullet} \longrightarrow LL$$

$$L^{\bullet} + P^{\bullet} \longrightarrow LP \qquad LOO^{\bullet} + P^{\bullet} \longrightarrow LOOP$$

FIGURE 16.7 Termination of the chain reaction.

Oxidation of food lipids has a deleterious effect on the human organism. It destroys the nutritionally valuable EPA and DHA, as well as essential amino acids that react with the products of decomposition of LOOH. Among the secondary products are several dialdehydes and other reactive, toxic compounds that may increase the oxidative stress in the consumer's organism and impair vascular function. They activate inflammatory reactions that may affect the digestive tract, the circulatory system, and several other organs, as well as possibly participate in carcinogenesis. Oxidative stress is one of the important causes of a score of human diseases. The formation of polymers in the termination stage decreases the digestibility of fats. To prevent lipid oxidation in foods the temperature of heating should be as low as possible, transition metals, oxygen, and light should be excluded, and appropriate antioxidants purposely selected for the specific products may be effective. In long-term stored unprotected foods oxidation of lipids proceeds even at freezing temperature.

Protein oxidation is caused mainly by reactive oxygen species present in foods and radicals formed as secondary products of lipid oxidation, as well as by the activity of peroxidase, lipoxygenase, polyphenol oxidase, oxygen, metal ions, photosensitizers, and exposure to light and elevated temperature. An attack of a radical may abstract a hydrogen at the α-carbon atom in the polypeptide chain or involve the functional groups of the amino acid residues–arginine, cysteine, methionine, histidine, lysine, and tryptophan. Abstraction of a hydrogen from the cysteine residue generates a cysteinyl radical that participates in the formation of intra- and intermolecular –S–S– cross-links in proteins. The amino acid residues may also react with low-molecular secondary products of lipid oxidation, thus decreasing the biological value of proteins (Figure 16.8). The loss of essential amino acids in foods stored and processed in controlled, rational conditions is generally low, but may reach about 10% in over sterilized meat or fish and in the outer layers of products fried in oxidized oil. The polyphenol oxidase catalyzes the oxidation of tyrosine and formation of brown polymers, thus

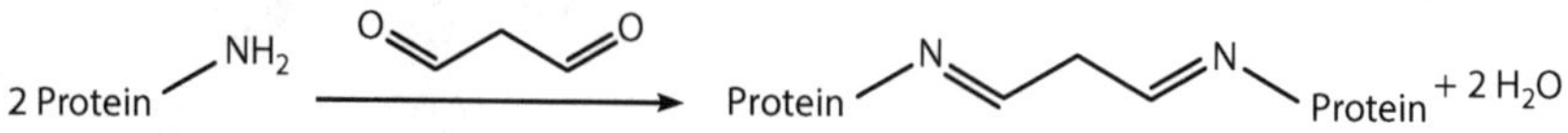

2 Protein–NH_2 + malonaldehyde → Protein–N=CH–CH₂–CH=N–Protein + $2\ H_2O$

FIGURE 16.8 Cross-linking of proteins in the reaction of malonaldehyde with a lysine residue.

Tyrosine —(PPO + O)→ DOPA colorless —(PPO + O)→ o-Quinone colored —(Amino acids + O)→ Melanins brown and black

PPO = polyphenoloxidase
DOPA = dihydroxyphenylalanine

Protective measures

Enzyme inhibitors, reducing compounds, chelating agents, citric or phosphoric(V) acid, enzymes

FIGURE 16.9 Enzymatic browning.

deteriorating not only the color of fruits and shellfish but also causing loss of essential amino acids (Figure 16.9). Polyphenols present naturally in foods or used as additives are easily oxidized and may form cross-links with proteins. These reactions decrease the biological value of the proteins.

16.3.3 Safety Aspects of Smoking and Grilling

Smoking serves to develop desirable sensory properties and increases the shelf life of foods. This is caused by a multitude of smoke components, partial loss of water, added salt, and enzymatic or thermal changes of proteins. Smoking and grilling in uncontrolled conditions, however, may contaminate foods with polycyclic aromatic hydrocarbons (PAHs), nitropolycyclic aromatic hydrocarbons (nitro-PAHs), *N*-nitroso compounds, and heterocyclic aromatic amines.

Several hundred PAHs are generated naturally in forest fires and volcano eruptions, as well as in various combustion and pyrolysis processes carried out in the industry. Therefore, their mixtures are present, generally in minute concentration, in the air, seawater, soil, agricultural crops, and food raw materials. The movement of PAHs in the environment and their natural degradation processes, as well as concentration in various food products, has been described by Alexander et al. (2008). Processing like smoking, grilling, roasting, and drying may increase the contamination of foods with PAHs to levels that may constitute a health hazard for the consumers.

Wood smoke contains a large number of PAHs, including those of molecular weight higher than 216 Da, known to be genotoxic or carcinogenic. In the human organism, they are metabolized by various enzymes to form promutagenic and carcinogenic DNA adducts. These changes are affected by the chemical structure of the compounds. Therefore, the carcinogenicity of the various members of the group of 15 potentially harmful PAHs is different. Actually, according to the Commission Regulation (EU) of 2011, a realistic representative of the carcinogenicity of foods is the content

TABLE 16.5
Maximum Allowable Content of PAHs in Foods

	Maximum Content of PAHs (ng/g)	
Food Product	**Benzo(a) pyrene (BaP)**	**Polycyclic aromatic hydrocarbon (PAH4)**
Smoked meat and meat products, meat of smoked fish and fish products	2	12
Smoked sprats and canned smoked sprats	5	30
Smoked bivalves	6	35

Source: Commission Regulation (EU) of 6 May 2011 amending Regulation (EC) No 1881/2006.

of benzo(a)pyrene (BaP) + benz(a)anthracene + benzo(b)fluoranthene + chrysene (known as the PAH4), or that of PAH4 + benzo(k)fluoranthene + benzo(g,h,i)perylene + dibenzo(a,h)anthracene + indeno(1,2,3-cd)pirene (PAH8). The maximum allowable level of PAHs in smoked foods has been set as shown in Table 16.5. In traditional old-type kilns it is hardly possible to produce smoked foods with a PAHs content not higher than these limits. Such kilns are heated and supplied with smoke by burning wood and smoldering sawdust, with the fish or meat placed on meshes or hanging directly above the firebed. In such products the concentration of PAHs may exceed even 50 times the acceptable limits. However, food smoked in modern smokehouses equipped with heaters and supplied by smoke produced in a separate generator by smoldering wood logs, shavings, chips, or sawdust of standard quality at controlled air access at a temperature not exceeding 400°C does not contain excessive amounts of PAHs (Sikorski 2016).

Also grilled foods contain some PAHs, generated due to pyrolysis of fat at the high temperature of the flame and as products of incomplete combustion of the fuel. Just as in the case of smoked products the pollution of grilled foods depends on the conditions of processing, that is, the construction of the grill and the temperature of the surface of the meat or fish.

Smoked foods may be also contaminated with trace amounts of nitro-PAHs, including 1-nitropyrene, 2-nitronaphtalene, and 2-nitrofluorene, present in urban air and in many agricultural crops. The total contents of different nitro-PAHs, in ng/g, is about 1.5 in olive oil, 3 in grilled meats, 15 in smoked meats, 30 in smoked sausages, and 35 in roasted coffee beans. In 1 g of tea leaves of different brands 10 to several hundreds ng of nitro-PAHs were found.

Some wood smoke components, particularly aldehydes and nitrogen oxide, may react with meat and fish constituents to generate various *N*-nitroso compounds. Among the products of such reactions *N*-nitrosothiazolidine, *N*-nitrosothiazolidine-4-carboxylic acid, 2-(hydroxymethyl)-*N*-nitrosothiazolidine and 2-(hydroxymethyl)-*N*-nitrosothiazolidine-4-carboxylic acid were detected. The concentration of *N*-nitroso compounds in different smoked meat products and fish may reach from a few to hundreds ng/g. Heavy smoking leads to accumulation of larger amounts of these compounds than mild processing.

Heterocyclic aromatic amines have been detected in various smoked foods in minute concentrations, of the order of 1 ng/g or lower. Generally smoking in mild conditions, at low temperature, does not favor the formations of these amines in foods (see Section 16.4.3).

16.3.4 Safety Aspects of Food Additives

Hundreds of natural products and synthetic compounds have been used in foods as additives to prevent spoilage, inhibit the growth of pathogenic microflora, change or improve the sensory properties, as well as facilitate processing and decrease its cost. In the past, many of them were abused intentionally in the food industry to achieve unethical financial gain, or applied although at that time their toxicological effects were unknown.

To prevent consumer's health hazards the national and international bodies responsible for the safety of foods have introduced regulations regarding the use of additives. These regulations are based on the results of sound, unbiased scientific investigations. Actually, the food additives have internationally recognized numbers. In the European Union, the additives permitted to be used in foods are marked by the letter E, followed by the identifying number, for example, E 320 butylated hydroxyanisole (BHA) or E 250 sodium nitrate(III). The additives are permitted to be added in strictly limited quantities to specified categories of food products or, if there are no set limits, only in minimum concentration required to achieve the intended effect (*quantum satis*).

According to the requirements of the EU law a food additive may be placed on the positive register only, if

- It does not constitute a human health hazard when used in the allowed concentration in strictly defined product categories
- There is no other technologically or economically justified treatment available to achieve the intended result
- Its use does not mislead the food consumer

The list of allowed food additives is being revised as the accumulating results of toxicological investigations bring new evidence regarding the safety or harmful effects of various compounds. Thus, some additives may be deleted from the list, while other ones after year-long tests may be added. There are still published opinions raising the question of some possible toxic effects of interactions of various additives. According to the present state of knowledge, however, the use of approved additives in accordance with the law requirements poses no health hazard to the consumer. Thus, only the application of additives not respecting the law requirements may be dangerous (Dąbrowski and Rutkowski 2015), but here the ethics of the food processor is involved. However, lack of knowledge among the population regarding the above presented rules may add to the mistrust of the consumers toward foods containing any additives. Avoiding generally the consumption of foods containing any additives is not justified.

16.4 GENERATION OF HARMFUL COMPOUNDS

16.4.1 Introduction

A vast number of chemical compounds build the structure of plant and animal tissues, as well as participate in the physiological reactions in the living organisms. These are predominantly proteins, saccharides, lipids, numerous low-molecular organic compounds, various mineral components, and water (Yannai 2013). They appear in different structures bound by physical and chemical forces, like protein bodies and fibers, starch granules, lipid crystals and globules, as well as lipid and protein micelles and membranes. They are in contact with true and colloidal solutions of various compounds, in purposely organized cells and tissues. Most of these chemicals are biochemically and chemically active due to their reactive groups (Table 16.6).

In the living plants and animal organisms, their interactions are controlled by biochemical mechanisms. After harvesting, as a result of uncontrolled catabolic effects, microbiological activity, and processing, the compartmentalization is disturbed or damaged. In consequence, the chemical components of the tissues may participate in various uncontrolled, haphazard reactions due to their increased mobility. Some products of these reactions may be harmful to the human organism. Their real effect depends on their properties and concentration and may not always be a reason for concern.

The kinetics of the reactions of the components in the conditions of food storage and processing depend on:

- State of the structure of the tissues
- Temperature, pH, water activity, and pressure
- Activity of enzymes and enzyme inhibitors
- Ionizing radiation, light, radicals, and active oxygen species
- Activity of sensitizers and antioxidants
- Composition of the surrounding atmosphere
- Ionic strength and availability of polyvalent cations

One of the major factors affecting the changes of food components during processing is heating. Its role is to cause changes in the physical state and rheological properties

TABLE 16.6
Reactive Groups of Food Components

Reactive Group	Typical Food Components
$-SH$, $-S-S-$, $-NH_2$, $-MH-C(=NH)NH_2$, $-CONH_2$	Proteins, amino acids
$-OH$, $-CHO$, $R_2C=O$, $-COOH$, $-OSO_3H$, $-O-P_3H_2$	Saccharides
$^1O_2$, $^{\bullet}O_2-$, $^{\bullet}OH$, H_2O_2, $RO^{\bullet}$, $ROO^{\bullet}$, ROOH, $ArO^{\bullet}$, $ArOO^{\bullet}$	Oxidation products
$-CH=CH-$, $-CH=CH-CH_2-CH=CH-$	Lipids
$CH_3-(CH_2)_n-CH_2-$ and other hydrophobic groups	Lipids
Inorganic anions and cations	Proteins, tissue fluids

of foods, destruction of pathogenic microflora, parasites, and toxic or other harmful compounds, creation of optimal parameters for intended unit operations and enzymatic or chemical processes, increase in the digestibility and availability of various nutrients, and separation of various fractions of the raw materials. It serves to accelerate the removal of fat, water, and volatile compounds, the extraction of many components, including sugar and lipids, as well as develop the desirable sensory properties. However, harsh heating parameters, that is, too long time or excessively high temperature decrease of the nutritional value and safety of food due to partial loss of vitamins (Seidler 2015), undesirable changes in proteins or lipids, and generation of toxic products of chemical reactions. Generally, these undesirable effects are negligible if mild processing conditions are applied, and the parameters of heating are well under control (Sikorski 2005).

The toxic or otherwise harmful compounds generated in foods due to storage and processing may result from the activity of microorganisms or are caused by oxidation, hydrogenation, or other chemical reactions, often affected by heating. The harmful products of microbiological metabolism have been described in Chapter 7 of this volume, whereas other categories are presented below.

16.4.2 Reactions of Lipids

Fats and oils heated to about 180°C in absence of air may change due to thermal decomposition. The sensitivity of different lipids to heating depends on the number and distribution of double bonds and on the chain length of their FA residues. Homolytic cleavage of the C–C bonds adjacent to the double bond yields various radicals, which participate in further reactions (Figure 16.10). Among the reaction products are short chain FA, dicarboxylic acids, dimers of FA and acylglycerols, cyclic compounds, and various *trans*-FA. There is also the irritant, toxic acrolein (Stevens and Maier 2008). Although acrolein is ubiquitous since it is a product of thermal decomposition of different materials and occurs in polluted air, its content in various foods is generally not higher than 1 μg/g. This is well below the provisional tolerable concentration for ingestion (Gomes et al. 2002). Thermal reactions

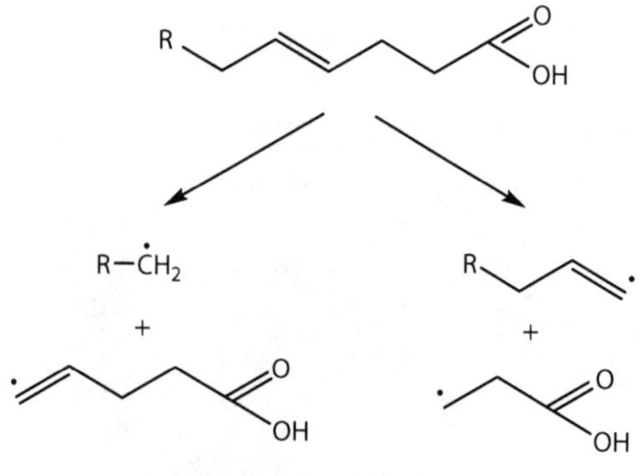

FIGURE 16.10 Homolytic cleavage of the C–C bond.

of the unsaturated acylglycerols result in the formation of various cyclic compounds, dimers, oligomers, and polymers. Cyclization of monoenoic FA residues in acylglycerols yields saturated fats, whereas in polyenoic acids one double bond in the hydrocarbon chain gets lost.

Unsaturated lipids can be protected against oxidation, and the melting point of oils can be increased by hydrogenation of the double bonds in the FA chains. This turns the fluid oils into fats that are plastic at room temperature and more resistant to oxidation. The commercial process of hydrogenation involves reactions of gaseous hydrogen with the double bonds under a pressure of about 10^5 Pa at 120°C–220°C in the presence of catalyzers containing Ni, Pt, Pd, Cu, or Co. In the first stage, hydrogen and the unsaturated acyls are activated on the surface of the catalyst and half hydrogenated labile intermediates are formed. At locally low concentration of hydrogen the intermediates may decompose with regeneration of unsaturated acyls. However, the regenerated double bonds may have either a *cis* or *trans* configuration. Furthermore, positional isomers may be formed (Figure 16.11) (Stołyhwo 2007).

Hydrogenation destroys in food lipids the polyenoic FA, including EPA and DHA, and increases the proportion of saturated residues, which is nutritionally disadvantageous. The *trans*-FA generated during partial hydrogenation present in foods are regarded as severe health hazard for the consumers. There are indications that they can contribute to obesity and high blood pressure. They also increase the risk of coronary heart disease by unfavorably changing the concentration of various lipids

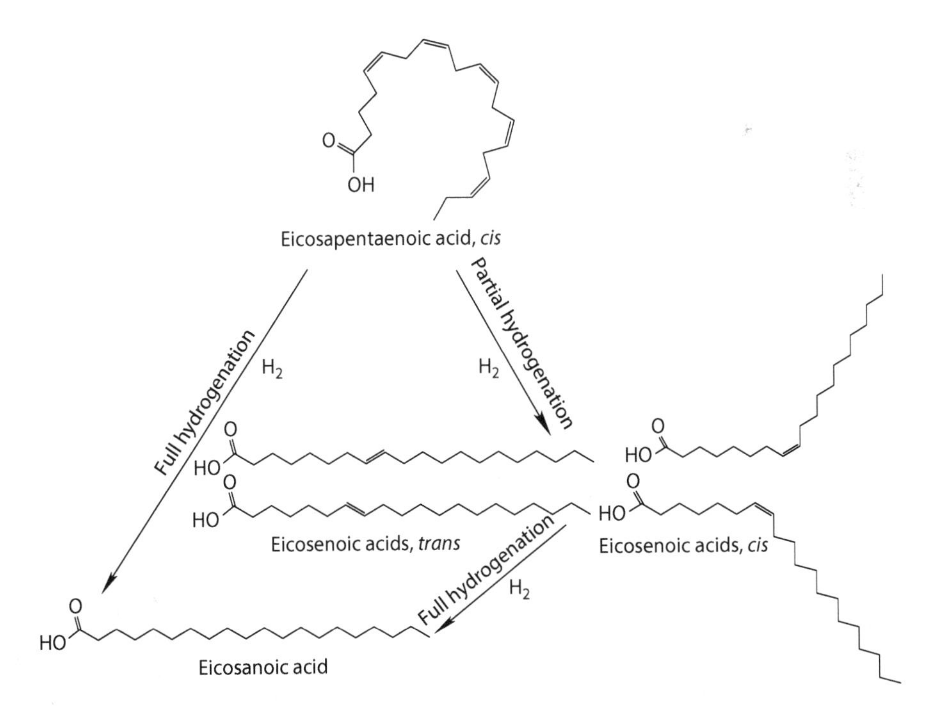

FIGURE 16.11 Hydrogenation and formation of *trans*-fatty acids.

in the human blood (Forycki 2011). Since the risks caused by *trans*-FA of the diet are generally recognized by nutritionists and health authorities, there is a consent that their content in foods should be as low as possible and at least declared on the labels. Different actions regarding limiting the presence of "*trans*-fats" in foods are in progress in various countries. These include such decisions as establishing a highest acceptable level of 2% of "*trans*-fats" in fats and oils or treating "*trans*-fats" as not Generally Recognized as Safe (GRAS) in human food.

Trans-FA occur also in small amount as natural components of beef and milk fat. They are the products of biohydrogenation in the rumen and differ from those generated by industrial hydrogenation of oils. The predominant component of the *trans*-fraction in beef, up to 80%, is *trans*-vaccenic acid ($C_{18:1}$ trans 11), which by desaturation in the human organism turns into conjugated linoleic acid (CLA). This, a mixture of geometric and positional isomers of linoleic acid, is claimed to have various beneficial health effects.

To avoid the nutritionally bad consequences of hydrogenation of oil the food industry endeavors to decrease the generation of *trans*-FA by improving the distribution of hydrogen in the reactor, optimizing other process parameters, and introducing new selective catalyzers. There is also a trend to replace hydrogenation by chemical or enzymatic transesterification.

Heating of fat-containing foods may lead to the formation of the possibly carcinogenic 3-monochloropropane-1,2-diol (3-MCPD) as a result of a reaction of triacylglycerols, phospholipids or glycerol and hydrochloric acid. During production of hydrolyzed vegetable protein (HVP), chloropropanols and chloroesters can be formed in a reaction of glycerol with hydrochloric acid or sodium chloride in the presence of other acids, for example, citric and acetic acids at high temperature. The chloropropanols found in HVP are 3-MCPD, 1,3-dichloropropan-2-ol (1,3-DCP), 2-chloropropane-1,3-diol (2-MCPD), 2,3-dichloropropan-1-ol (2,3-DCP), and 3-chloropropan-1-ol. FA esters of 3-MCPD and 1,3-DCP can also be formed in acid HVP, but the majority of them are removed during filtration of the hydrolysates. Chloropropanols occur also in ready-to-eat processed foods, including soy and oyster sauces, food ingredients such as processed garlic, and related food products such as cereal-based products, soups, meat, cheese, and cooked fish. In 11 food groups, 3-MCPD was found in concentrations from not detectable to several hundred ng/g: in herbs, spices and condiments 6–12 ng/g, in grains and grain-based products 26–39 ng/g, in smoked fish meat 36–37 ng/g, and in margarine 1480–1530 ng/g (European Food Safety Authority 2013). Its maximum permitted level in HVP has been set in the Commission Regulation (EC) No 1881/2006 as 20 ng/g.

3-MCPD and 1,3-DCP show clear carcinogenic effects in rats and mice. Although no epidemiological or clinical studies on humans have been reported concerning 3-MCPD, a provisional maximum tolerable daily intake of up to 2 μg/kg body weight has been established on the basis of the lowest observed effect level. Regarding 1,3-DCP and 2,3-DCP, it has been concluded that their exposures are of low concern for human health. An adequate risk assessment for 2-MCPD cannot be performed due to limited data on its toxicology and occurrence in food.

16.4.3 Reactions of Proteins

Most foods are heated at neutral or slightly acidic pH, but in several cases also in alkaline conditions, for example, for extraction and separation of proteins from various raw materials or for inactivation of proteinase inhibitors and mycotoxins. Heating at high pH may cause hydrolysis of amides and of some peptide bonds in proteins, as well as β-elimination in amino acid residues. This generates carbanions and dehydroalanine residues (Figure 16.12). By recombination of the carbanions with protons the L and D amino acids are formed. The rate of racemization depends on the properties of the proteins and the amino acid residues. The dehydroalanine residue participates in intra- and intermolecular cross-linking of proteins and formation of modified amino acids (Figure 16.13). These reactions decrease the biological utilization of proteins due to D-isomers of amino acids, lower digestibility caused by cross-linking, inhibition of proteolytic enzymes, as well as loss of lysine, threonine, cysteine, and arginine. They may also cause kidney damage by lysinoalanine. The extent of the modification of amino acid residues in heated foods depends on the pH of the product, properties of the proteins, and temperature. Very small amounts of the modified amino acids occur in foods heated at neutral and slightly acidic pH, but at alkaline pH their concentration may reach several μg/g. Cooked, baked, or fried proteinaceous products contain lysinoalanine in amounts from about 50 to 500 μg/g. According to Gilani, Xiao, and Cockell (2012) its no-effect level in liquid infant formulae has been suggested as 0,5–1 μg/g.

Heating of proteinaceous foods may lead to formation of small amounts of mutagenic or carcinogenic heterocyclic amines. They are generated mainly in the surface parts of grilled, roasted, baked, or fried products as well as in gravies and pan residues exposed to high temperature for long time. The concentration of these compounds in such heat processed foods is generally several ng/g. A more detailed presentation of this subject has been published earlier (Sikorski 2005).

The health hazards caused by the presence of small amounts of *N*-nitrosamines in foods have also been described earlier (Sikorski 2005) and discussed thoroughly in Chapter 5 of this book.

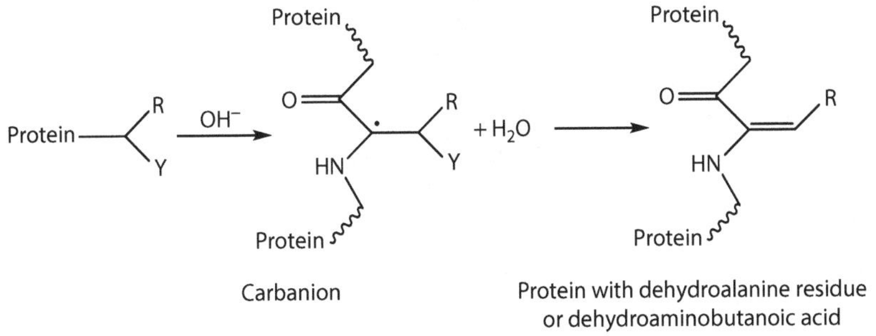

Carbanion

Protein with dehydroalanine residue or dehydroaminobutanoic acid

where: R = H, CH_3; Y = H, OH, OPO_3H_2, SH, SR^+, OR, $N(R)_3$ or SSR

FIGURE 16.12 Formation of carbanions and dehydroalanine.

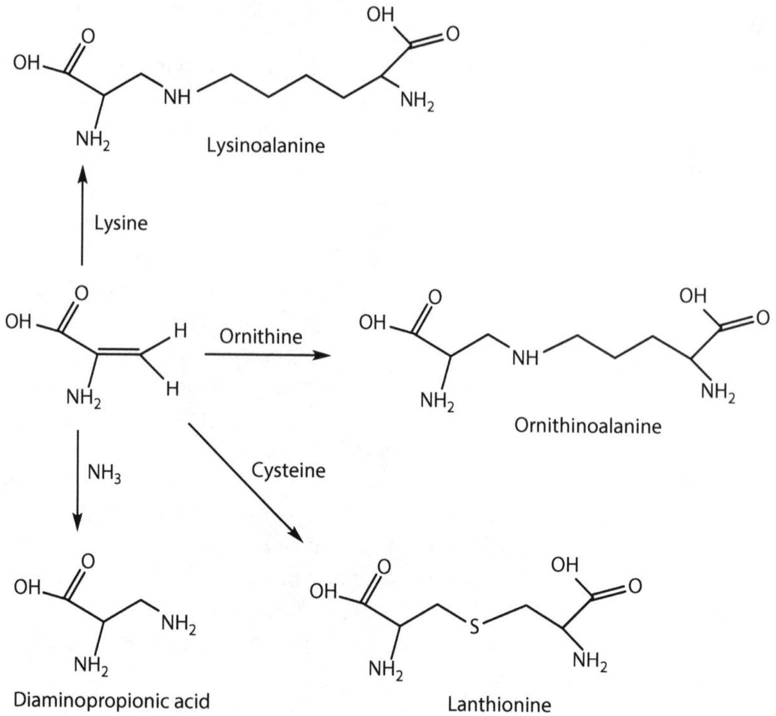

FIGURE 16.13 Generation of modified amino acids by reaction with dehydroalanine.

Several nutritionally objectionable compounds are generated also in the reactions of amino acid residues with reducing saccharides. These reactions have been presented in section 16.4.4.

Generally various procedures of heating applied in the industry and in the kitchen do not generate objectionably high amounts of nutritionally harmful protein degradation products, simply because high sensory quality of foods can be guaranteed only by not too harsh conditions. The temperature of the internal part of a chicken or turkey roasted at 200°C in the oven or of a fish fillet deep-fat fried in oil at 180°C is usually about 70°C. A much higher temperature, above 100°C, is only in the thin, dehydrated surface layer, which is necessary for developing the desirable color and flavor of the product. Even sterilization at 130°C does not generate significant amounts of harmful compounds in the cans, because such high core temperature is there not longer than about 1 minute.

16.4.4 Reactions of Saccharides

Whenever saccharide-rich foods are heat processed, a series of chemical reactions, summarized as Maillard reaction and/or caramelization, follow one another resulting in formation of compounds that contribute to desired color and flavor. However, these processes, for example, frying, baking, roasting, and dry heating, should be controlled, as they can also be implicated in the formation of compounds with toxicological potential, including acrylamide (AA), furan, 5-hydroxymethylfurfural (5-hydroxymethyl-2-furaldehyde, HMF), and 4-methylimidazole with its tautomer 5-methylimidazole (4(5)-MEI).

The major pathway for AA formation in food during heating at temperatures above 120°C and low moisture is the Maillard reaction, which involves reducing saccharides and amino acid residues, especially free L-asparagine, as main precursors (Figure 16.14). L-Asparagine can thermally decompose by deamination and decarboxylation, but when a carbonyl source is present, the yield of AA from L-asparagine is much higher. Other reaction routes for AA formation in food have been postulated to originate from acrolein (Stevens and Maier 2008), which might be derived from lipids, amino acids, or saccharides, from wheat gluten (Claus et al. 2006), and by deamination of 3-aminopropionamide (Zamora et al. 2009), which is formed as an intermediate in the Maillard reaction.

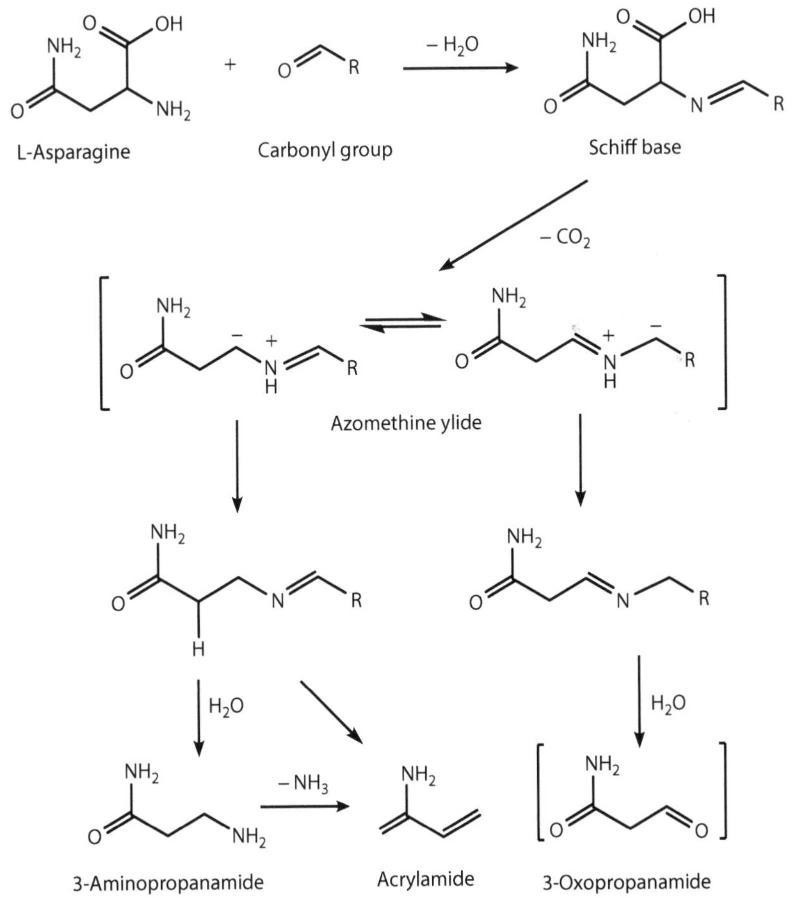

FIGURE 16.14 Formation of acrylamide in food.

TABLE 16.7
Acrylamide Level (ng/g) in Different Food Products vs. Indicative Acrylamide Value

Food Products	Acrylamide		Number of Samples
	Middle Bound	Indicative Value[a]	
Coffee roasted bean	522	450	17
Gingerbread	407	1000	na
Potato crisp and snacks	389	1000	47
Potato fried products	308	600	33
Biscuits, crackers, crisp bread, and similar	265	500	73
items	161	400	41
Breakfast cereals	73	50	53
Processed cereal-based baby foods	42	150	31
Soft bread	24	80	32

Source: *EFSA J.* 13, 1–321, 2015.
na: not analyzed.
[a] Indicative values for AA in food products according to Commission Recommendation 2013/647/EU.

Acrylamide is present in a wide range of everyday foods. The most important food groups contributing to AA exposure are coffee, fried potato products, especially potato chips and French fries, and also foods made from grains, such as cookies, crisp bread, soft bread, and breakfast cereals (Table 16.7).

In dairy, meat, and seafood products, AA does not form, or forms at very low levels. How to reduce the level of AA in coffee is not known yet, although it is clear that it occurs when coffee beans are roasted, and not when coffee is brewed. To limit the AA content in processed potatoes and cereals, the factors that affect reducing saccharide levels in the former and asparagine concentration in the latter case should be controlled, as in potatoes reducing saccharides are present in excess in relation to asparagine, and in cereals conversely. Since the AA level in food is temperature and time dependent, raw plant-based foods or foods cooked by steaming, boiling, or microwaving are safer than fried, baked, or roasted.

Unlike AA, the furan formation in food is not well understood. Five routes of its formation have been proposed. Apart from the Maillard reaction/thermal degradation of reducing saccharides in the presence or absence of amino acids, there are thermal oxidation of polyenoic FA and thermal decomposition of ascorbic acid and carotenoids (Figure 16.15) (Perez and Yaylayan 2004).

Furan and its derivatives naturally occur in many foods. They are found in coffee and various products that have been subjected during processing to heat treatment at temperatures above 200°C (Table 16.8). The amount of furan formed in coffee beans varies according to the level of roasting. Grinding may reduce furan levels by up to 60%. Further decreases occur in the production of instant coffee powder and in the brewing process. Since furan is highly volatile, it may evaporate from processed

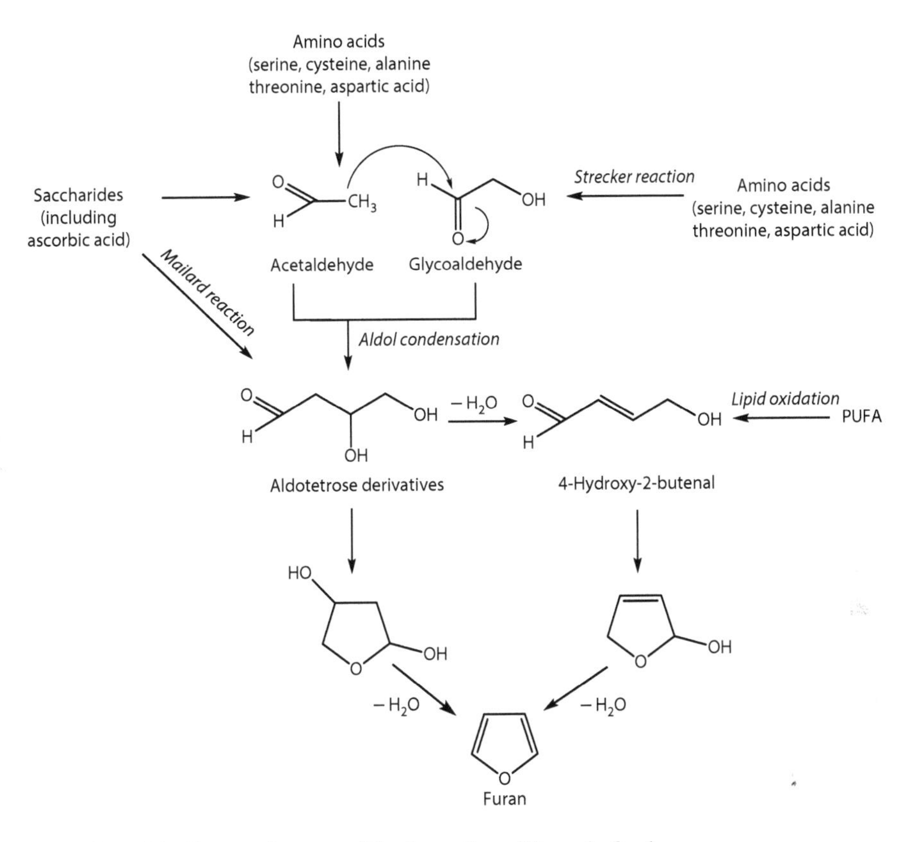

FIGURE 16.15 Proposed routes of the formation of furan in food.

TABLE 16.8
Furan Level (ng/g) in Different Food Products

Food Products	Furan	Number of Samples
Coffee roasted bean	3660	30
Coffee brew	42–45	89
Baby foods other than cereal based	31–32	1617
Soy sauce	27	94
Soups	23–24	270
Cereal products	15–18	190
Fish	17	47
Meat products	13–17	174
Cocoa	9–10	14

Source: EFSA *J.* 9, 1–33, 2011.

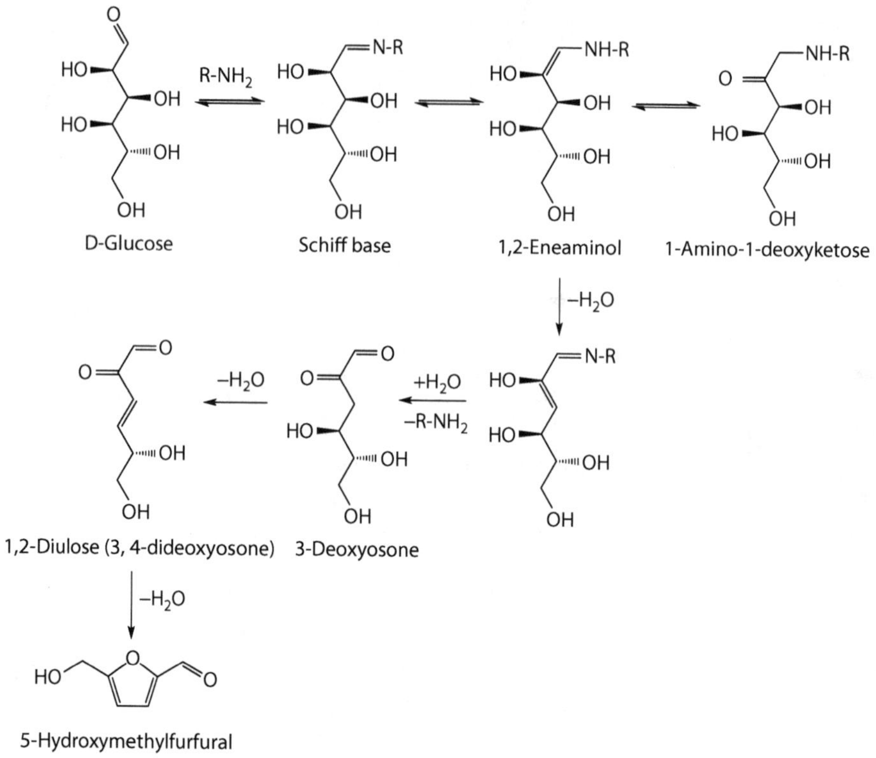

D-Glucose $\xrightleftharpoons{R\text{-}NH_2}$ Schiff base $\rightleftharpoons$ 1,2-Eneaminol $\rightleftharpoons$ 1-Amino-1-deoxyketose

1,2-Eneaminol $\xrightarrow{-H_2O}$ $\xrightarrow[-R\text{-}NH_2]{+H_2O}$ 3-Deoxyosone $\xrightarrow{-H_2O}$ 1,2-Diulose (3, 4-dideoxyosone) $\xrightarrow{-H_2O}$ 5-Hydroxymethylfurfural

FIGURE 16.16 Formation of 5-hydroxymethylfurfural in food.

food contained in an airtight sealed pack when the container is opened. Hence, the amount of furan lost depends on the conditions of food storage.

The HMF is formed naturally as an intermediate in the Maillard reaction and by direct dehydration of hexoses under mild acidic conditions (caramelization) (Figure 16.16). The activation energy for HMF formation is higher than that for HMF degradation, hence its concentration increases with increasing temperature. The rate of formation of HMF in food also depends on the type of sugar, pH, and water activity.

The HMF is not present in fresh or untreated food, but it collects rapidly during heat treatment and storage of saccharide-rich products. HMF occurs in honey, coffee, fruit juices, tomato paste, and heat-treated dairy products, where it is generated as a result of overheating and/or improper storage conditions, and is recognized as a marker of quality deterioration. HMF also occurs in cereal products such as pasta, cookies, bread, extruded baby cereals, breakfast cereals, and toasted bread, where it is used for monitoring the heating process applied. Another source of HMF in food is alcoholic beverages, in which the presence of HMF can be related to ingredients used in product formulation, for example, the addition of caramel solutions.

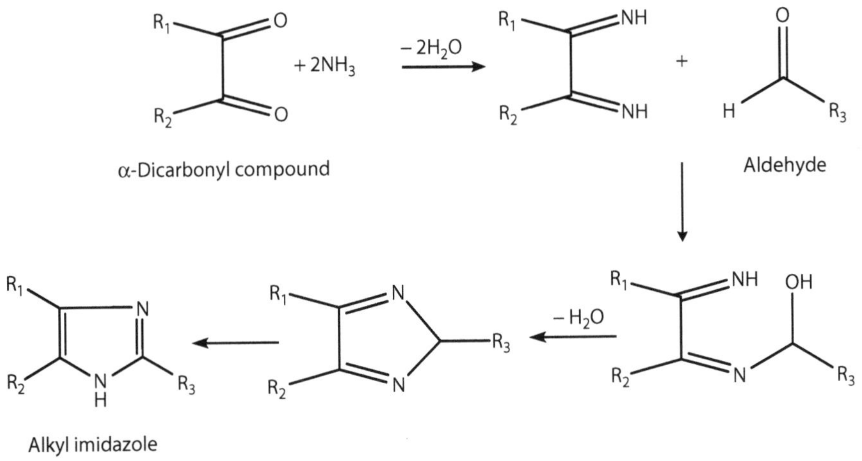

FIGURE 16.17 Formation of imidazole.

Imidazoles, including 4(5)-MEI, are also formed in the Maillard reaction. During thermal treatment of foods and beverages, saccharides degrade into alkyl dicarbonyls and alkyl ketones, and amino acids form ammonia and alkyl carbonyls via the Strecker degradation. 4(5)-MEI occurs as a result of the interaction between the products of these reactions (Figure 16.17).

Higher concentrations of saccharide and ammonia, higher temperatures, higher water activity, and longer reaction times increase the amount of 4(5)-MEI.

4(5)-MEI has been identified in roasted foods, grilled meats, coffee, and in various commercial caramel colors used for food and beverage coloring. In particular, high 4(5)-MEI levels have been found in class III and IV caramel colorings, which are created by heating saccharides with ammonium compound, in the absence and presence of sulfate(IV)-containing compounds, respectively. The amounts of 4(5)-MEI, in dark beers range from 0 to 424 mg/dm^3, is about one thousand times lower in common brands of cola drinks, and in coffee these may reach levels of up to 2 mg/dm^3 (Hengel and Shibamoto 2013).

Although there have been many reports on heat-induced toxic products of the Maillard reaction, these compounds are generally found only at trace levels. The average daily AA consumption for the general population, and for consumers with high dietary exposure, has been estimated as 1 and 4 μg/kg body weight, respectively, and the values of 1 and 2 μg/kg body weight were taken to represent mean and high dietary intake of furan (EFSA 2015). Thus, AA and furan are present in foods at levels that are far below those which would significantly raise health risks. Nevertheless, both compounds are considered by the International Agency for Research on Cancer (IARC) as probable or potentially carcinogenic to humans, or might be metabolized by humans to potentially carcinogenic compounds. In turn, the daily dietary intake of HMF has been estimated as 1600 μg/person (EFSA 2005). This means that it is by several orders of magnitude higher than that reported for AA or furan, and according to IARC criteria, the evidence for carcinogenicity of HMF appears to be inadequate. The IARC does not mention 4(5)-MI at all, but in 2011, the State of California added this compound to the list of probable carcinogens and stipulated 29 μg/day as the "No Significant Risk Level" intake (Hengel and Shibamoto 2013). Long-term dietary exposure to caramels among children aged 1–10 years, estimated based on analytical data in 11 European countries (EFSA 2010), have shown that the median daily exposure ranges from 4.3 to 41 mg/kg body weight for ammonia-sulfate(IV) caramels (class IV) and from 32 to 105 mg/kg body weight for ammonia caramels (class III).

In 2007, the European Union project Heat-Induced Food Toxicants, Identification, Characterization and Risk Minimization (HEATOX) compiled a database including around 800 compounds generated as a result of the Maillard reaction and lipid oxidation. This database contains compounds that belong to different chemical classes, including alcohols, aldehydes, hydrocarbons, furans, ketones, pyrazines, pyridines, pyrroles, thiazoles, and thiophenes, as well as a variety of S-, N-, and O-containing compounds. Information on toxicity of these compounds is scarce; therefore, a molecular modeling approach has been employed to assess the potential toxicity of each compound. From this *in silico* evaluation, 53 compounds were identified as potentially harmful. These include, for example, 5-propionyl-2,3-dihydro-1,4-thiazine and 2-propionyl-1,4,5,6- tetrahydropyridine.

16.5 CONCLUDING REMARKS

The thought that in the industrialized world of the twenty-first century the billions of its population, especially those living in urbanized areas, could sustain without contemporary preservation and processing of food resources is beyond human imagination. Processing of food raw materials is ages old and a must. Opinions that only unprocessed foods are healthy mislead the consumers and undermine the trust to the food industry. Processing serves *inter alia* the purpose of eliminating natural harmful components and pollutants from the raw materials and, if carried out in rational conditions, should improve the sensory properties of foods, not decreasing the nutritive value nor generating toxic compounds. However, in handling foods, the risk and benefit principle should be observed just like in almost every human activity.

The international bodies responsible for the safety of food have established rules and requirements regarding the parameters of storage and processing. These regulations aim at achieving the intended benefit, that is, high sensory quality and shelf life at minimum risk of impairing the nutritional value and safety of the products. They are based on the results of unbiased research showing the effects of the conditions of producing and handling foods on the contents of harmful compounds in various commodities. Observing these rules brings to a minimum the health hazards caused by unsafe foods. A very important factor in eliminating these hazards is full implementation of the quality management system HACCP and traceability in agriculture, fisheries, and food industry. In controlling the safety of foods modern analytical techniques make it possible to determine even trace amounts of harmful compounds at the level of a few pg/g (Plutowska and Jeleń 2015). However, regardless all systematic arrangements and sound professional knowledge, one of the decisive factors is the ethics of the personnel in all segments of the food economy.

REFERENCES

Alexander, J., D. Benford, A. Cockburn, J.-P Cravedi, E. Dogliotti, A.D. Domenico 2008. Scientific opinion of the panel on contaminants in the food chain on a request from the European commission on polycyclic aromatic hydrocarbons in food. *EFSA J.* 724: 1–114.

Bartosz, G., and A. Kołakowska. 2011. Lipid oxidation in food systems. In: Sikorski Z.E., and A. Kołakowska (eds) *Chemical, Biological, and Functional Properties of Food Lipids*, 2nd edn. Boca Raton, FL: CRC Press, pp. 163–184.

Biegler, P. 1960. Fischwaren-Technologie. Theorie und Praxis der Fabrikationsmethoden zur Konservierung von Fischen. In: *Der Fisch. Band V.* Verlag Der Fisch. Clara Bader, Lübeck.

Claus, A., G.M. Weisz, A. Schieber, and R. Carle. 2006. Pyrolytic acrylamide formation from purified wheat gluten and gluten-supplemented wheat bread rolls. *Mol. Nutr. Food Res.* 50: 87–93.

Commission Recommendation of 8 November 2013 on investigation into the levels of acrylamide in food. *OJ. L* 301: 15–17.

Commission Regulation (EC) No 2073/2005. Microbiological criteria for foodstuffs *OJ. L* 338 1–26.

Commission Regulation (EU) of 6 May 2011 amending Regulation (EC) No 1881/2006.

Commission Regulation (EU) No 1019/2013 amending Annex I to Regulation (EC) No 2073/2005 as regards histamine in fishery products.

Dąbrowski, K., and A. Rutkowski. 2015. Food additives—Properties, role and rules of application. In: Sikorski, Z.E., and H. Staroszczyk (eds) *Food Chemistry*, vol. 2. Warszawa, MO: Wydawnictwo WNT (in Polish), pp. 215–252.

EFSA. 2005. Opinion of the Scientific Panel on Food Additives, Flavourings, Processing Aids and Materials in contact with Food (AFC) on a request from the Commission related to Flavouring group evaluation 13: Furfuryl and furan derivatives with and without additional side-chain substituents and heteroatoms from chemical group 14. *EFSA J.*, 215: 1–73.

EFSA. 2010. Long-term dietary exposure to different food colours in young children living in different European countries. EXPOCHI Scientific report submitted to EFSA. EFSA-Q-2010–00787 7(5): 1–27.

EFSA. 2011. Update on furan levels in food from monitoring years 2004–2010 and exposure assessment. *EFSA J.* 9(9)2347: 1–33.

European Food Safety Authority. 2013. Analysis of occurrence of 3-monochloropropane-1,2-diol (3-MCPD) in food in Europe in the years 2009–2011 and preliminary exposure assessment. *EFSA J.* 11(9): 3381–3426.

EFSA. 2015. Scientific opinion on acrylamide in food. EFSA panel on contaminants in the food chain (CONTAM). *EFSA J.* 13(6): 4104: 1–321.

Flick, G.J., and L.A. Granata. 2005. Biogenic amines in foods. In: Dąbrowski, W.M., and Z.E. Sikorski (eds) *Toxins in Food.* Boca Raton, FL: CRC Press, pp. 121–154.

Forycki, Z.F. 2011. Dietary lipids and coronary heart disease. In: Sikorski Z.E, and A. Kołakowska, (eds) *Chemical, Biological, and Functional Properties of Food Lipids*, 2nd edn, Boca Raton, FL: CRC Press, pp. 211–226.

Gilani, G.S., Ch. W. Xiao, and K.A. Cockell. 2012. Impact of antinutritional factors in food proteins on the digestibility of protein and the bioavailability of amino acids and on protein quality. *Brit. J. Nutr.* 108: 315–333.

Gomes, R., M.E. Meek, and M. Eggleton. 2002. *Acrolein. Concise International Chemical Assessment Document 43*. Geneva: World Health Organization.

Hengel, M., and T. Shibamoto. 2013. Carcinogenic 4(5)-methylimidazole found in beverages, sauces, and caramel colors: Chemical properties, analysis, and biological activities. *J. Agr. Food Chem.* 61: 780–789.

Kołakowska, A., and G. Bartosz. 2014. Oxidation of food components. An introduction. In: Bartosz, G. (ed) *Food Oxidants and Antooxidants. Chemical, Biological, and Functional Properties*, Boca Raton, FL: CRC Press, pp. 1–20.

Lopez, H.W., F. Leenhardt, C. Coudray, and C. Remesy. 2003. Minerals and phytic acid interactions: Is it a real problem for human nutrition? *Int. J. Food Sci. Tech.* 37: 727–739.

Malinowska-Pańczyk, E. 2015. Nonprotein nitrogenous compounds. In: Sikorski, Z.E., and H. Staroszczyk (eds) *Food Chemistry*, vol. 1, Warszawa: Wydawnictwo WNT (in Polish), pp. 240–262.

McMeekin, T.A., J.N. Olley, T. Ross, and D.A. Ratkovsky. 1993. *Predictive Microbiology. Theory and Practice*. New York: John Wiley & Sons.

Perez, L.C., and V.A. Yaylayan. 2004. Origin and mechanistic pathways of formation of the parent furan—A food toxicant. *J. Agric. Food Chem.* 52: 6830–6836.

Plutowska, B., and H. Jeleń. 2015. Food analysis. In: Sikorski, Z.E., and H. Staroszczyk (eds) *Food Chemistry*, vol. 2. Warszawa: Wydawnictwo WNT (in Polish). pp. 279–316.

Regulation (EC) No 852/2004 of the European Parliament and of the Council of 29 April 2004 on the hygiene of foodstuffs. Annex II.

Seidler, T. 2015. Vitamins. In: Sikorski Z.E., and H. Staroszczyk (eds) *Food Chemistry*, vol. 1. Warszawa: Wydawnictwo WNT (in Polish), pp. 265–294.

Sikorski, Z.E. 2005. The effect of processing on the nutritional value and toxicity of foods. In: Dąbrowski, W.M., and Z.E. Sikorski (eds) *Toxins in Food*. Boca Raton, FL: CRC Press, pp. 285–312.

Sikorski, Z.E. 2016. Smoked foods: Principles and production. In: *The Encyclopedia of Food and Health*, eds. B. Caballero, P. Finglas, and F. Toldrá, vol. 5, 1–5. Oxford: Academic Press.

Sobecka, E., and W. Piasecki. 2011. Fish and shellfish diseases and seafood quality. In: Daczkowska-Kozon, E.g., and B. Sun Pan (eds) *Environmental Effects on Seafood Availability, Safety, and Quality*, 1st edn, Boca Raton, FL: CRC Press, pp. 245–259.

Stevens, J.F., and C.S. Maier. 2008. Acrolein. Sources, metabolism, and biomolecular interactions relevant to human health and disease. *Mol. Nutr. Food Res.* 52: 7–25.

Stołyhwo, A. 2007. Lipids and food quality. In: Sikorski, Z.E. (ed) *Chemical and Functional Properties of Food Components,* 3rd edn, Boca Raton, FL: CRC Press, pp. 177–207.

Visciano, P., M. Schirone, R. Tofalo, and G. Suzzi. 2014. Histamine poisoning and control measures in fish and fishery products. *Front. Microbiol.* 5: 500.

Yannai, S. 2013. *Dictionary of Food Compounds with CD-Rom*, 2nd edn. Boca Raton, FL: CRC Press.

Zamora R., R.M. Delgado, and F.J. Hidalgo. 2009. Conversion of 3-aminopropionamide and 3-alkylaminop, ropionamides into acrylamide in model systems. *Mol. Nutr. Food Res.* 53: 1512–1520.

17 Toxic Components of Food Packaging Materials

Lidia Wolska and Maciej Tankiewicz

CONTENTS

17.1 INTRODUCTION

In the beginning, food was consumed where it was found. Then, if transportation of food was necessary, man began to use various forms of food packaging. Initially, they were obtained directly from the environment, such as leaves, tree bark, or seashell. Afterward, the earthenware vessels appeared, and from 1500 BC to 500 AD ceramic vessels and amphoras were used. Glass was first industrialized in Egypt in 1500 BC. In ancient age, paper appeared (Egypt, China) and metal production process was discovered (silver, gold, bronze, iron, lead). Lead has been used for at least 5,000 years and early applications included pigments for glazing ceramics, pipes for water supply, and sweetener for wine (lead acetate). It is speculated that in ancient Rome, the consumption of lead by some Romans was at the level of 1 gram per day (Järup 2003).

Our ancestors also used for packaging naturally sourced cellulose, cotton, and flax. Plastic packaging appeared together with the synthesis of polymers in the early nineteenth century (Raheem 2012).

Packaging of food provides unquestionable benefits. It enables and increases logistics and transportation processes, preservation and storage of food products, marketing, and consumer information. Essentially, the packaging protects food from the environment and from chemical and physical agents, thus playing a crucial role in the protection of quality and safety of food products. It also provides biological protection against microorganisms, insects, rodents, and other pests. Food packaging constitutes part of human history and is still evolving and developing (Conti 2007; EFSA n.d.).

Traditionally used packaging materials include glass, metals (aluminum foils and laminates, tinplate, and tin-free steel), paper and paperboards, ceramics, and plastics. They are applied because they do not influence the taste and flavor of the packed food. Recently, a wider variety of plastics has been introduced in both rigid and flexible forms. Nowadays, packages often combine several materials to exploit each material's functional or aesthetic properties. As research to improve food packaging continues, advances in the field may affect the environmental impact of packaging. Initially, the materials and the method of packaging of food did not constitute a burden for the environment and did not generate any threat to humans. Over time, it has been noted that the production processes of packaging and the subsequent fate of the disposal materials (storage, recycling, waste) constitute a growing hazard (Montanari 2015).

Presently, we have access to a new generation of packaging materials, such as intelligent packaging (IP), active packaging (AP), modified atmosphere packaging (MAP), and the use of antimicrobial agents to extend the shelf life of foods under storage and distribution conditions.

Modern food packagings are controlled in terms of their impact on the food quality, especially those that are in direct contact with food. Packaging may be also potential sources of chemical contamination of food and the relevance of these sources is often underestimated. Some of them are toxic and constitute an increasingly scientifically documented threat to human health. The transfer process of chemicals from the packaging to the food is known as migration.

17.2 MIGRATION PROCESS

The qualitative and quantitative analysis of migrants from food packaging materials can be achieved by different means. Regulation of chemicals that can be used for food packaging materials is managed on a substance-by-substance approach with generic or specific thresholds for different contaminants. Quantifying the exposure of the general population to substances from food packaging materials relies on estimation of food consumption and leaching into the food. The migration process can be divided into three phases (Figure 17.1; Mattsson and Sonesson 2003):

(a) Diffusion within the polymer
(b) Solvatation at the polymer–food interface
(c) Dispersion into food

In general, any migration of chemical substances from packaging to food is the result of a series of diffusion processes subjected to both thermodynamic and kinetic control. The following factors are crucial on the process: the physicochemical properties of migrant (size below 1,000 Da), the packaging material, and the food matrices (e.g., fat and salt content, the pH value); temperature; storage time;

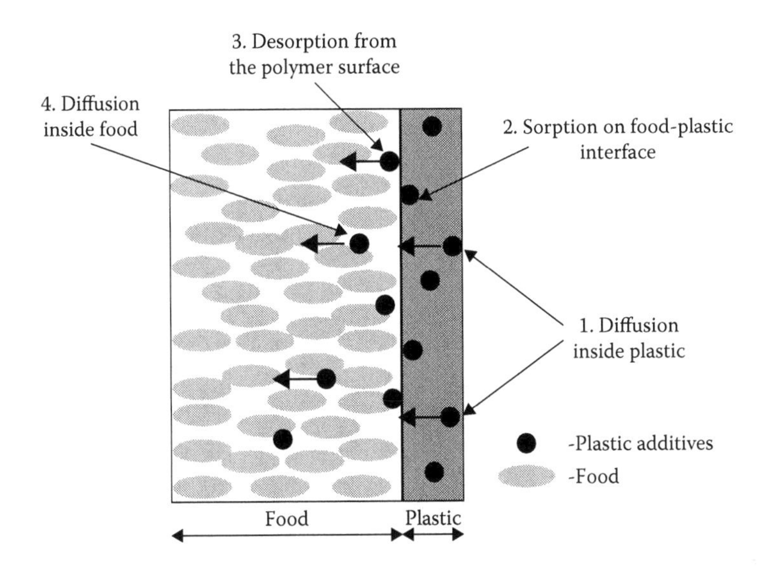

FIGURE 17.1 Phases of migration process.

and size of packaging in proportion to food volume (smaller size packaging has a larger surface-to-volume ratio). The types of chemicals that can migrate are highly diverse and depend on the type of packaging material.

Different mathematical models derived from the Fick's laws can describe the migration process (Crank 1975). For example, the Crank's mathematical model was applied to evaluate the migration of butylated hydroxytoluene from polypropylene film (Rubino and Xia 2016).

17.3 REGULATORY CONTROL

The regulations concerning food and food contact materials are well developed and established (see Chapter 19). In Europe, the community level legislations and national legislations continue to coexist (Schaefer 2010), whereas in the United States the Food and Drug Administration (FDA) exercises control on the food safety (Baughan and Attwood 2010).

EU legislation sets the acceptable limits for migration of substances from packaging to food. For all substances that can migrate from plastic to food, the Overall Migration Limit—OML—is designated and for individual substances the Specific Migration Limit—SML. In 2011, the European Commission has updated and consolidated the regulations related to plastics in contact with food. In accordance with this legal regulation only substances included in the EU list may be intentionally used in the manufacture of plastic layers in plastic materials and articles (European Commission 2011a, 2015).

Generally, regulations are divided into two different series: one refers to generic requirements on all food packaging materials and another to specific rules with relation to individual materials, such as ceramics, epoxy resins, regenerated cellulose film, recycled plastic material, active and IP, and plastics (Council of Europe 2002;

European Parliament and the Council 2004). At present, there are no harmonized documents related to the use of stainless steel.

17.4 METALS AND NONORGANIC CONTAMINANTS

Metals and alloys are widely applied as food contact materials, for example, as process equipment in the food industry, household utensils, and as food packagings (Table 17.1; Muncke 2014).

Some packaging materials are metallic or may be naturally present in raw materials used in the preparation of preserved foods. In other situations (plastics, glass, ceramic), metals are only one of the components with a specific role. Therefore, they are a potential source of food contamination. Metal contamination can take place during the handling and processing of foods, from the farm to the point of consumption. The presence of some heavy metals such as arsenic, cadmium, lead, mercury, and zinc in foods have been reported as a result of environmental pollution from soil, water, and plants (fruits and vegetables) utilized during production (Cederberg et al. 2015). The main sources of these elements in the environment are natural or as a consequence of human activity from industrial processes, agricultural facilities, and traffic. Finally, metals can get into the food from the packaging by a variety of processes. Migration must not occur in amounts that endanger human health. Relevant for food contact materials made from metals and alloys are the migration (release) of metals, both the main components and foreseen impurities. As a conclusion, the study of metals migration and their concentrations in food is important due to their negative effects (Mayfield et al. 2015).

TABLE 17.1
Application of Metals in the Modern Industry of Food Packaging Materials

General Function or Uses	Industrial Applications
Structural material (metals, alloys)	Aluminum
	Tinplate
	Foils and laminates
	Tin-free steel
	Electro-coated chromium steel
Additives and processing aids (paper, ceramic, glass, textile, plastic)	Fillers
	Stabilizers
	Colorants (pigments and dyes)
	Ceramic glazes
Active and intelligent packaging materials	Antimicrobic agents
	Antioxidants
	Oxygen scavengers
	Gas barrier agents
	Microwave susceptors
Nanomaterials	Nanocompounds (Ti, Ag, Zn)

Metals readily form cations, oxides, hydroxides, and binary metal hydrides. Moreover, they can react with nonmetals forming ionic compounds and with other metals giving metallic compounds. These metallic compounds composed of several metals might be referred to as alloys. Stainless steel is the most widely used alloy. Metalloids can be divided into two categories, because they possess metallic and nonmetallic properties. Examples of these are antimony and arsenic. Furthermore, the speciation of metals is of great importance for toxicology. For example, Cr(III) is the most stable state and is an essential element for humans. Cr(VI) is highly toxic, including effects such as genotoxicity (Marsh and Bugusu 2007).

In addition, a number of metals that play important roles in biological functions (essential for good health), at appropriate concentrations, may be potentially toxic. For example, iron is an integral fragment of many proteins and enzymes and is crucial for the production of hemoglobin. Its deficiency is a generally acknowledged problem and in some countries wheat flour is fortified with iron to provide the necessary amount of iron in the diet. Cobalt is a necessary component of vitamin B_{12} (cyanocobalamin) and is required for the production of red blood cells. This element accumulated in large amounts is toxic. It increases the activity of the thyroid gland and bone marrow. Copper is an important component of several enzymes and participates in the utilization of iron. Manganese is an essential element for humans. In case of occupational exposure, deleterious effects on the central nervous system and neurological effects have been observed. Zinc is a cofactor for more than 200 enzymes (Lemos et al. 2008; Saçmacı et al. 2012).

Nonessential metals are those that have no beneficial role in biological functions, for example, beryllium, thallium, and titanium. Especially, heavy metals, such as cadmium, lead, and mercury, have shown harmful and toxic properties and constitute a serious public health concern. These elements may be very deleterious even at low concentration levels when ingested over a long time. Cadmium and lead have no known physiological functions and may cause adverse health effects. Cadmium accumulates in kidneys and can cause kidney damage, including cancer, whereas lead influences the nervous system. Especially, children are affected as their developing nervous system is sensitive. It affects the intelligence and the ability to learn (Ibrahim et al. 2006).

The main application examples of 14 popularly used metals for food packaging materials with their risk characterization are presented in Table 17.2 (European Commission 2007, 2011b, 2011c, 2012, 2014; EFSA 2009).

Paper and its derivatives are among the primary food packaging materials all over the world. They are inexpensive and have high quality standards of safety of use. Paper packagings are composed of pulp from different vegetable sources and are most often used in contact with dry foods. Metals used in this type of material have the function of additives, which include fillers, starch and derivatives, wet strength sizing agents, retention aids, biocides, fluorescent whitening, and grease-proofing agents. For production processes, different compounds are used; for example, oxides and hydroxides of aluminum, calcium, magnesium, silicon, and metal silicates or hydrated silicates (European Commission 2002). Recycled fiber is considered a major source of migrants. The de-inking process is very often used to enhance the quality of the recycled paper. The inks may contain heavy metals, such as cadmium, chromium, and lead (Hauder et al. 2013).

TABLE 17.2
Examples of Application and General Toxic Effects of Selected Metals

Metal	Food Contact Materials	Toxic Effects	Tolerable Daily Intake (mg/kg of Body Weight)	Specific Release Limits (mg/kg)	Recommendations
Aluminum (Al)	Food-trays, cans, can ends and closures, packaging foil, coating or lamination of carton packages, aluminum powder in pigments and paints; aluminum alloys for food contact materials may contain magnesium, silicone, iron, manganese, copper, and zinc	There have been no adverse health effects caused by released aluminum from packaging material	1.0 (weekly intake)	5.0	Storage of acidic (fruit juices), alkaline, or salty food, especially as liquids, in uncoated aluminum should be avoided (to minimize migration)
Antimony (Sb)	Used in the production of lead, tin, and copper alloys; pigment in paint; fire-proofing agent in textiles and plastic; opacifying agent in glass, ceramic, and enamels	Causes reduced body weight gain; long-term exposure can lead to increased blood cholesterol and decreased blood sugar	0.0060	0.040	Concentration in plastic food contact materials (used as catalyst) should be evaluated and be lower than limit
Chromium (Cr)	Component of alloys, certain cans; used as a coating to protect other metals from corrosion (in cans it serves to passivate the tinplate surface); used in dyes	Lung cancer ($Cr^{6}+$); respiratory effects; allergic dermatitis	0.30 ($Cr^{3}+$)	0.25	Acidic foodstuffs (e.g., fruit juices) in non-lacquered cans may be significantly higher in chromium than fresh foodstuffs
Cadmium (Cd)	Used as pigments and stabilizers in plastics; pigments in certain enamels; present in pewter can	Kidney damage; lung cancer; bone disorders	0.0025 (weekly intake)	0.005	Pewter should not be used for acidic or salty food; cadmium in zinc sulphate used as a food supplement or for feed can be a problem

(Continued)

TABLE 17.2 (*Continued*)
Examples of Application and General Toxic Effects of Selected Metals

Metal	Food Contact Materials	Toxic Effects	Tolerable Daily Intake (mg/kg of Body Weight)	Specific Release Limits (mg/kg)	Recommendations
Cobalt (Co)	Used as a blue color in glass, enamels and ceramics, to neutralize the yellow tint from iron in glass; used in enamel coatings on steel to improve the adherence of the enamel to the metal	Heart problems; abdominal pain; difficulties with breathing	0.0014	0.020	Correct use in alloys, glass, and glazing pottery only do not raise any problem
Lead (Pb)	Pigment in ceramic glazes; used in printing inks; present in crystal glass	Neurological and reproductive effects; hematopoietic system damage	0.025 (weekly intake)	0.010	Due to the low safety factor, use of lead in food contact materials should be abandoned or avoided; storage of acidic food (e.g., wine) in crystal glass should be avoided (increase the release of lead); glaze on ceramics may contain lead or cadmium, which can migrate into the food
Manganese (Mn)	Used in the production of steel; in the manufacture of glass to bleach the color of any iron present; used in pigments and glazes	Central nervous system effects	9.0 mg/day (based on neurological effects)	1.8	Specific migration of manganese from plastic food contact materials should be lower than 0.60 mg/kg

(Continued)

TABLE 17.2 (*Continued*)
Examples of Application and General Toxic Effects of Selected Metals

Metal	Food Contact Materials	Toxic Effects	Tolerable Daily Intake (mg/kg of Body Weight)	Specific Release Limits (mg/kg)	Recommendations
Nickel (Ni)	Used in coloring ceramics and in glazes; used in manufacture of glass and the corrosion resistant alloys (cookware, materials for food transportation, e.g., milk and wine tanks, for processing equipment, e.g., in chocolate industry and processing of fruit such as apples, grapes, oranges, and tomatoes)	Allergic dermatitis; there is evidence that nickel is carcinogenic by inhalation	0.012	0.14	Nickel-plated food contact materials should not be used
Silver (Ag)	Used as coloring agent for decorations in confectionery, in alcoholic beverages, and as food additive (E174); alloyed with 7.5% of copper is known as sterling silver; used in the production of cutlery and tableware	Long-term exposure may result in anemia, cardiac enlargement, growth retardation, and liver damage	1.29	0.08	Silver used in nanomaterials has not been considered and must be evaluated separately on a case by case basis
Thallium (Tl)	Used in glass manufacture	Vomiting, diarrhea, temporary hair loss, and effects on the nervous system, lungs, heart, liver, and kidneys	0.010	0.00010	Content in food contact materials should be lower than 0.050%

(*Continued*)

TABLE 17.2 (*Continued*)
Examples of Application and General Toxic Effects of Selected Metals

Metal	Food Contact Materials	Toxic Effects	Tolerable Daily Intake (mg/kg of Body Weight)	Specific Release Limits (mg/kg)	Recommendations
Tin (Sn)	Tinplate is used in steel cans, for foods with a light color, for example asparagus and pineapple; it acts as an antioxidant; used in cans, can ends, and closures mainly for glass bottles and jars; used in alloys, for example with copper for conversion into bronze and with zinc for galvanization	Inorganic tin is relatively nontoxic; organic compounds—neurological effects, diarrhea, and vomiting	14 (weekly intake)	100	Food contact with tin materials should be avoided at low pH and high temperatures other than for food packaged in tin plated cans; do not store food in open cans because opening the can will break the lacquer sealing, which allows direct contact between food and metals
Titanium (Ti)	Present up to 1% in stainless steel cans; used in white pigments in, for example paints, lacquers, enamels, paper coatings, and plastics; used as a food additive and catalysts in the manufacture of plastics	Practically inert (pass through the human body)	0.30–1.0 mg/person/day (dietary intake)	no limit	It is estimated that 0.80 mg/day is absorbed
Vanadium (V)	Used in ceramics and glass pigments with blue and green colors	Effects on kidneys, spleen, lungs, and blood pressure	0.010–0.030	0.010	The level in food contact materials is not considered to be harmful
Zinc (Zn)	Used in silos for storing food (galvanized steel); used for paints and ceramics; may contain small amounts of cadmium and lead as impurities	Nausea, vomiting, epigastric pain, abdominal cramps, and diarrhea	25 for adults, 7.0 for children aged 1–3 years	5.0	Do not use galvanized iron for contact with liquid (moist) and acidic foodstuffs

A study concerning heavy metals migration from packaging paper boards to food was performed (Conti 1997). Pb and Cd were detected in the range of 0.41–2.37 μg/g for Pb and 0.08–0.1 μg/g for Cd respectively from pizza packaging made from 100% virgin cellulose fibers.

Both stainless steels and glass for food packaging material production contain heavy metals, such as nickel, cadmium, chromium, and lead. Thus, all these elements can migrate into foods (FSA 2002). Most metal cans are made from tinplate (steel coated with tin), tin-free steel (steel coated with chromium and chromium oxides), or aluminum. Tinplate is the most popular for food cans and aluminum for beverage cans. Most cans are internally coated with a polymeric layer (mostly a polymerized resin), and thus the layer of food contact is not the metal but the lacquer. In case of acid beverages, several tests should be performed to evaluate the risk of contaminant migration (Dionisi and Oldring 2002). Metals are readily solubilized in acidic medium; thus, they may easily migrate. Moreover, a high storage temperatures and salt concentrations (over 3.5% of sodium chloride) can also increase metal migration from packaging materials. The substances used in can production are therefore not only the metals involved, but also components migrating from the coatings, such as starting substances and their potential derivatives (Francisco et al. 2015). For ceramic glazes, lead and cadmium pigments have been often used. The most popularly used pigment is white lead. Moreover, colorants used in glaze paints can contain pigments with lead, cadmium, zinc, and other heavy metals (Lu et al. 2014). Nowadays, leaching of these elements from ceramic materials is strictly regulated due to their high toxicity.

There are many substances of toxicological interest, restricted for plastic materials and articles that may come into contact with foodstuffs. For the production of thermoplastic polymers, such as polyethylene, polystyrene, polyethylene terephthalate, and polyamide, different catalysts are used, which may contain heavy metals. Lead and cadmium are sometimes detected in plastic packaging materials. The sources of these elements are impurities from inorganic pigments and stabilizers. Additives that may migrate from plastic materials include antioxidants, antistatics, antifogging agents, slip additives, plasticizers, heat stabilizers, dyes, and pigments. Antioxidants can contain nickel, while thermal stabilizers nickel, lead, and antimony (Montanari 2015). In the production process of polyvinyl chloride some metallic compounds are used as stabilizers, which may contain tin, cadmium, and zinc. The calcium/zinc stearates and carboxylates stabilizer systems are often used for manufacture of nontoxic articles. Also, lead compounds may be applied as stabilizers. For example, the Sb contamination of soft drinks and waters bottled in plastic (polyethylene terephthalate—PET) was examined (Shotyk et al. 2006; Shotyk and Krachler 2007). Sb_2O_3 is used in the manufacturing of PET as a catalyst. The concentration of Sb observed from PET resin ranged from 6.08 mg/kg to 216.49 mg/kg, while the range of Sb in bottled solutions was from 0.26 μg/dm^3 to 1.55 μg/dm^3.

Colorants, including pigments, dyes, and inks, used for plastic packaging material production or surface coatings can also contain metals, such as antimony, arsenic, barium, cadmium, chromium, and lead. Several types of inorganic pigments containing cadmium and lead have been banned due to restrictions on the use of heavy metals. All the application of chromium(VI) pigments for food packaging use is discouraged because of carcinogenic properties. For example, the migration of metals from wrappers with colorfully printed outer covers used in packages of candy products in South Korea was examined (Kim et al. 2008). Pb and Cr(VI) were detected at high concentrations in a part of candy packages. Pb was detected from about 110 mg/kg to 6,394 mg/kg in 10 of 92 candy packages, whereas Cr concentrations ranged from about 137 mg/kg to 1,429 mg/kg in 7 of the 92 candy packages. The outer cover of these candy packages was green or yellow. These results indicate that heavy metals could migrate from the printed outer packages to food.

Recently, the development of active and IP has dominated the market. Metals are also used in this field and have diverse functions, such as clays as oxygen scavengers and humidity absorbers, titanium dioxide as antimicrobic agent, or ferric carbonate with metal as carbon dioxide emitters. Transition metal salts, such as iron, are also used as oxo-biodegradation promoter (Martirosyan and Schneider 2014).

17.5 ORGANIC CONTAMINANTS

17.5.1 Introduction

The main sources of contamination of food with organic compounds are nowadays primarily polymeric packaging. There are hundreds of plastics, but only very few are utilized in food packaging. The most common are polyolefin, copolymers of ethylene, substituted olefins, polyesters, polycarbonate, and polyamide (nylon). Silicones, due to their versatile properties, are a class of polymers broadly used in food contact materials too. The market of polymeric packaging is growing rapidly, and is driven by new developments in plastics and bio-plastics area (inter alia to reduce the bulk and weight of metal and glass containers; Ozen and Floros 2001; Mattsson and Sonesson 2003; Raheem 2012).

Low-molecular-weight chemical compounds are incorporated into plastics to improve their functional properties (primarily physical and chemical).

Additives are not chemically bonded in the plastics; therefore, they may leach into the food. Research studies show that chemical substances with a molecular weight smaller than 600 g/mol will have high tendency to migrate from polymer to food.

Possible chemical migrants include additives like plasticizers, antioxidants, light and thermal stabilizers, slip compounds, antistatic agents, lubricants but also monomers, residual solvents, and degradation products.

The potential influence of these substances on product safety and quality remains in question when the amount of these migrating compounds in food exceeds their specified limits.

17.5.2 Sources of Low-Molecular-Weight Chemical Compounds Migrating from Packaging Materials

Until 2004, the state of the art on the toxic components of food packaging materials was summed up by Piotrowska (Dąbrowski and Sikorski 2004), who focused on plastics as packaging materials and additives as toxic compounds migrating from packaging to food.

A brief description of the components used in plastics production like additives and monomers is given below.

Plasticizers. Plasticizers are the group of compounds used to improve flexibility, workability, and stretchability of polymeric films. The most commonly used plasticizers in certain plastics are given in Table 17.3.

The quantities of plasticizers added, for example, to the PVC polymer vary between 15% and 60%, with typical ranges for most flexible applications around 35–40% (Krupa et al. 2011).

Antioxidants. Antioxidants are added to plastics to reduce or prevent oxidative degradation of polymer structure caused by UV light. Arylamines (diphenylamine), phenolics (butylated hydroxytoluene (BHT), 2- and 3-*t*-butyl-4-hydroxyanisole (BHA), tetrakismethylene-(3,5-di-*t*-butyl-4-hydroxyhydrocinnamate) methane (Irganox 1010), and bisphenolics such as Cyanox 2246 and 425, and bisphenol A), and organophosphate (tris-nonylphenyl phosphite—TNPP, tris (2,4-di-*tert*-butylphenyl) phosphite, also known as Irgafos 168) are common antioxidants used in plastic food packaging. Oxidation processes significantly increase at high

TABLE 17.3
Plasticizers Commonly Used in Certain Plastics

Plasticizers (Used in Plastic Formulation)	Plastics			
	PVC	PE	PVDC	Other Plastics
Diethyl phthalates (DEP),		✓		
Diisobutylphthalate (DiBP),		✓		
Di-*n*-butyl phthalate (DBP)		✓		✓
Dipentyl phthalate (DPP),		✓		
Dicyclohexyl phthalate (DCHP),				✓
Di-2-ethylhexyl phthalate (DEHP)	✓			✓
Butyl benzyl phthalate (BBP),				✓
Diheptyl adipate (DHA),				✓
Heptyl adipate (HAD),				✓
Heptyl octyl adipate (HOA)				✓
Di-(2-ethylhexyl) adipate (DEHA),		✓		
Di-octyladipate (DOA),		✓		
Acetyltributyl citrate (ATBC)			✓	

Source: Bhunia et al. *Compr. Rev. Food Sci. F,* 12, 523–545, 2013.

temperatures or exposure to infrared heating, retort processing, and, potentially, microwave heating.

Heat stabilizers. Heat stabilizers prevent thermal degradation of resins. There are three major types of primary heat stabilizers: mixed metal salt blends, organotin compounds (they have been found to be effective in the control of many fungi and bacteria), and lead compounds; and three secondary heat stabilizers such as beta diketones, alkyl organophosphites, and epoxy compounds (Piver 1973; Bhunia et al. 2013).

Slip agents. Slip compounds have many functions in the plastics (impart lower surface resistivity, reduce melt viscosity, better mold release, and antisticking properties) but the main function is to reduce the coefficient of friction of the surface of a polymer.

Common slip compounds are fatty acid amides (primary erucamide and oleamide), fatty acid esters, metallic stearates (e.g., zinc stearate), and waxes (Bhunia et al. 2013).

Monomers and oligomers. Small molecules like ethene, propene, vinyl chloride, styrene, acrylonitrile, tetrafluoroethane, and others, which build blocks of polymers are called monomers. During the polymerization process not all molecules of the monomers are bonded chemically with the chain of polymer. That's why plastics may be a source of migration of toxic compounds to food.

The report, prepared by COWI and Danish Technological Institute, summarizes very useful information on the most used plastic types and their characteristics and uses, as well as hazardous substances used in plastics and present on the priority list of hazardous substances (Hansen et al. 2013).

Silicones due to their versatile properties are also often used as additives. Applications include lubricants, adhesives, films and barriers, as well as process additives like surfactants or plasticizers.

Although plastic packagings are major sources of food contamination by organic compounds (relatively well documented), other packaging materials like paper, wood, or ceramic can be also sources of organic toxins in food.

Food packaging materials are still in a development stage. Today, nanomaterials (materials in the size range of up to about 100 nm in one or more dimensions) are incorporated to packaging materials and perform the following tasks (Bradley et al. 2011). They improve:

- Physical performance, durability, and barrier properties (either at the inside or the outside surface, or sandwiched as a layer in a laminate).
- Antimicrobial properties acting on the packaging surface (chemicals such as nano silver, zinc oxide, or magnesium oxide may have an effective action as a surface biocide in food contact plastics, rubber, or silicones).
- Antimicrobial or other properties (e.g., antioxidant) with intentional release into, and consequent effect on, the packaged food.
- Food quality and freshness by monitoring of condition of the food storage and transport with new generation of nanosensors.

Among nanomaterials are metals (silver, gold, copper), metal oxides (nano-zinc oxide, ZnO, and titanium), carbon nanotubes, carbon black particles, and also organic compounds such as cellulose or polylactic acid (PLA; Jamshidian et al. 2010; Tantra 2016).

17.5.3 Levels of Certain Contaminants in Food

The migration process is modified by common-use stresses like temperature, moist heat via boiling or dishwashing, microwaving, ultraviolet radiation, or autoclaving (Alin 2012). With time the concentration of the migrating substances decreases in the packaging.

To protect the quality and safety of food, many organizations and governments agree that the amount of these migrating compounds in food mustn't exceed the specified limits.

The number of low-molecular-weight compounds, which could migrate from polymeric food packaging, is now estimated as higher than 100 (Iwanowicz et al. 2016).

Information concerning the level of migration of these compounds to food can be found in the literature, but most of them are focused on phthalate, adipate, and bisphenol A (BPA; Fasano et al. 2012). Definitely less data are available for the other low-molecular-weight compounds (Gao et al. 2011) and other packaging materials like paper, wood, or ceramic.

Paper and paperboard are sheet materials made from an interlaced network of cellulose fibers derived from wood by using sulfate(VI) and sulfate(IV). During the paper production, the fibers are pulped and/or bleached and treated with chemicals. Paper packaging materials are often coated with waxes, polymeric materials, or aluminum to improve their poor barrier properties.

In such materials like paper and wood (e.g., wood barrels for wine, packaging for fresh fruit and vegetables, boxes for tea), decorated and/or printed ceramic dioxins can be found including pentachlorophenol, polychlorinated biphenyl (whitening process; Makuch and Wolska 2000), trace amounts of pesticides (biocides; Rosero-Moreano et al. 2014), volatile organic compounds, and benzophenone (ink components; Huang 2015).

In Table 17.4 are gathered examples of food concentration of contaminants, which migrated from packaging materials.

In 2012, Fasano and co-workers published results of their extensive research on migration of phthalates (DMP, DBP, DEHP, BBP), alkylphenols (OP, NP), bisphenol A (BPA), and DEHA from the different food packaging items into appropriated simulants (Fasano et al. 2012). Packaging items with highest migration of polymer additives are given in Table 17.5.

The values obtained by Fasano and co-workers are generally higher than those presented in Table 17.4. However, the real migration from packaging into food differs from migration process to simulants (under controlled conditions) and depends on real storage conditions and sometimes analytical problems (see Chapter 18).

17.5.4 Toxicity of Compounds, Which Migrate from Packaging Materials to Food

The toxic effects of many compounds have been known for years and well documented. The big problem is to prove the occurrence of certain health effects with long-term (chronic) exposure of humans to low concentrations of specific compounds. Unfortunately, the situation is complicated by the fact that compounds

TABLE 17.4
Level of Food Contaminants Concentration, Which Migrated from Packaging Materials (Mainly from Plastics)

Food or Food Simulants	Migrating Substances	Concentration in Food	Reference
Water (plastic bottle)	Styrene	0.04–0.73 mg/cm^3	Oi-Wah and Siu-Kay (2000)
Yogurt (plastic pot)	Styrene	0.2–0.5 mg/g	Oi-Wah and Siu-Kay (2000)
Soft drinks[a]	DMP	60–760 µg/dm^3	Bośnir et al. (2007)
	DEP	0–17 µg/dm^3	
	DBP	12–26 µg/dm^3	
	DEHP	15–37 µg/dm^3	
	BBP	0–5 µg/dm^3	
Mineral water (plastic bottle)	DMP	ND	Bośnir et al. (2007)
	DEP	0.1 µg/dm^3	
	DBP	11 µg/dm^3	
	DEHP	9 µg/dm^3	
	BBP	ND	
Mineral water (plastic bottle)	DBP	26 µg/dm^3	Czernych (2016)
	DEHP	18 µg/dm^3	
Tea (plastic box)	DBP	26 µg/g	Czernych (2016)
	DEHP	46 µg/g	
dried plum (plastic vessel)	DBP	5 µg/g	Czernych (2016)
	DEHP	2 µg/g	
Frozen broccoli	DBP	9 µg/g	Czernych (2016)
	DEHP	9 µg/g	
Fresh cucumber (greenhouse)	DBP	30 µg/g	Czernych (2016)
	DEHP	14 µg/g	
Fresh cucumber (ground)	DBP	ND	Czernych (2016)
	DEHP	ND	
Cheese	DEHP	310 µg/g	Page and Lacroix (1995)
Bread	DEHP	314.0 ng/g ww	Cirillo et al. (2011)
	DBP	101.0 ng/g ww	
Fish	DEHP	136.5 ng/g ww	Cirillo et al. (2011)
	DBP	60.4 ng/g ww	
Water-food simulants (cartoon)	PCB	0.53 µg/g	Makuch and Wolska (2000)
Water-food stimulants (PCV films)	Bisphenol A (BPA)	12 µg/dm^3	Lopez-Cervantes and Paseiro-Losada (2003)
Olive oil-food stimulants (PCV films)	Bisphenol A (BPA)	31 µg/dm^3	Lopez-Cervantes and Paseiro-Losada (2003)
Milk (commercial canned)	Bisphenol A (BPA)	1.7–15.2 ng/g	Taskeen and Naeem (2009)
Palm oil	DBP	0.63 mg/dm^3	Nazarudin et al. (2014)
	BBP	0.19 mg/dm^3	

(*Continued*)

TABLE 17.4 (*Continued*)
Level of Food Contaminants Concentration, Which Migrated from Packaging Materials (Mainly from Plastics)

Food or Food Simulants	Migrating Substances	Concentration in Food	Reference
Cheese (PVC films)	Nonylphenol (NP)	0.2 to 0.8 mg/kg	FSA (2009)
Cake (PVC films)	Nonylphenol (NP)	0.3 to 0.6 mg/kg	FSA (2009)
Carbonate water	Total cyclosiloxanes	0.05 mg/dm^3	Forrest (2006)
Oil	Total cyclosiloxanes	0.43 mg/dm^3	Forrest (2006)
Food	Organotin	0.01 mg to 0.24 mg organotin/kg of food	Mercer (1990)
Mineral water (PCV bottle)	Organotin	0.01 mg/dm^3	Piver (1973)
Milk (PCV bottle)		0.126 mg/dm^3	
Apple juice (PCV bottle)		0.126 mg/dm^3	
Vegetable oil (PCV bottle)		0.063 mg/dm^3	
Water simulants (gamma-irradiated PVC) water simulants (electron-irradiated PVC)	Organotin	73–422 g/dm^3 296–513 g/dm^3	Zygoura et al. (2011)
Water (migration from PCV pipe)	Organotin	<100 ng/dm^3 (depends on conditions)	Richardson and Edwards (2009)

ND: Non–detected.

[a] According to type of preservative and pH of the drink.

as a complex mixture give often toxicological interactions. It is well known that a mixture may produce a toxic effect that is either additive, antagonistic, or synergistic (Groten et al. 2001; Danish Veterinary and Food Administration 2003).

The plastic polymers are generally not regarded as toxic, but low-molecular-weight additives and monomers can lead often to serious health problems for human and animals such as neurological problems, impaired immune function, hormone disruption, cancer, and birth defects.

Since the early 1980s, endocrine disruption in humans, fish, and wild life has been recognized as a global environmental concern (Mercer 1990). Many studies have reported skewed sex ratios and reproductive failure in resident fish species (Iwanowicz et al. 2016).

Substances having estrogenic activity can produce many human health-related problems too, such as early puberty in females, reduced sperm counts, altered functions of reproductive organs, obesity, altered sex-specific behaviors, and increased rates of some breast, ovarian, testicular, and prostate cancers (Diamanti-Kandarakis et al. 2009; Yang et al. 2011).

TABLE 17.5
Range of Concentration of Polymer Additives Migrated to the Simulants

Migrant	Packaging Items	Food Simulant	Range of Concentration [ng/dm³]
DMP	Marmalade cap	Distilled water	271–421
	Plastic wine top	Ethanol 15%	155–375
DBP	Plastic wine top	Ethanol 15%	1,389–1,948
	Baby's bottle	Distilled water	96–159
BBP	Marmalade cap	Distilled water	210–344
	Plastic wine top	Ethanol 15%	151–355
DEHP	Plastic wine top	Ethanol 15%	10,999–17,694
	Marmalade cap	Distilled water	7,141–8,609
	Oil tuna can	Acetic acid 3%	1,986–3,027
OP	Plastic wine top	Ethanol 15%	25,676–27,956
	Bread bag	Distilled water	18–512
NP	Natural tuna can	Distilled water	3,382–4,185
	Plastic wine top	Ethanol 15%	415–1,368
	Bread bag	Distilled water	123–376
BPA	Natural tuna can	Distilled water	677–973
	Baby's bottle	Distilled water	345–480
DEHA	Yogurt packaging	Acetic acid 3%	1,876–2,902
	Plastic wine top	Ethanol 15%	780–1,470

Source: Fasano et al., *Food Control* 27, 132–138, 2012.

With the reference to the position statements of the Endocrine Society, the Pediatric Endocrine Society, and the European Society of Pediatric Endocrinology, the Polish Society of Endocrinology points out the adverse health effects caused by endocrine disrupting chemicals (EDCs) commonly used in daily life as components of plastics, food containers, pharmaceuticals, and cosmetics (Rutkowska et al. 2015b).

The group of these compounds includes many substances that migrate from plastics as monomers (styrene), plasticizers (phthalate esters, alkylphenols: APs, and di(2-ethylhexyl)adipate: DEHA), antioxidants (2,2-bis(4-hydroxyphenyl)propane: bisphenol A, BPA), heat stabilizers (organotin compounds), and substances migrated from paper and wood such as pesticides or dioxins and dioxin-like polychlorinated biphenyls (Diamanti-Kandarakis et al. 2009; Fasano et al. 2012).

Epidemiological studies on human exposure to phthalates from different countries have shown that increased phthalate exposure might have associations with potential health risks to children involving allergic diseases such as asthma and eczema, attention-deficit/hyperactivity disorder (ADHD), high blood pressure, and increasing body mass index (BMI), waist circumference (WC; Baol et al. 2015), and, importantly, generate some endocrine health problems.

Fetal, newborn, and juvenile mammals are especially sensitive to very low (sometimes picomolar to nanomolar) doses of substances having estrogenic activity (Yang et al. 2011).

Higher serum concentrations of some EDCs in women with PCOS and their impact on the hormonal profile suggest their potentially negative role in this endocrinopathy (Rachoń et al. 2015; Rutkowska et al. 2015a).

Below there are given examples of well-known substances whose toxic effects on humans have been documented scientifically:

- Vinyl chloride (monomer) is carcinogenic to humans and it is classified by the International Agency for Research on Cancer (IARC) to Group 1 (IARC 2011)
- Styrene (monomer) is possibly carcinogenic to humans and it is classified by IARC to Group 2B, and additionally styrene is shown to cause mammary gland tumors in animal studies (IARC 2011)
- Di(2-ethylhexyl) phthalate (plasticizers) causes liver cancer and develops damaged kidneys (Rusyn et al. 2006; Myers and Spoolman 2014)
- Bisphenol-A (antioxidants) disrupts the endocrine system by mimicking the female hormone estrogen (vom Saal and Hughes 2005; Rochester 2013; Acconcia et al. 2015)

A relatively new issue is the question about the effects of nanostructures on human health. Scientists initially struggled with the development of analytical methods for determination of nanostructures. Foods contain many nanostructures; some of them are natural as proteins, saccharides, and fats, but others, as engineered nanomaterials (ENMs), are produced to a particular usage. The distinction between them is not always clear. Silvestre and co-authors sum up that there is limited scientific data about migration of most types of nanoparticles from packaging to food, but it is reasonable to assume that migration may occur (Silvestre et al. 2011).

In 2007, Handy and Shaw concluded that toxicology studies on animals, and cells *in vitro*, raise the possibility of adverse effects on the immune system, oxidative stress related disorders, lung disease, and inflammation. However, the doses needed to produce these effects are generally high (Handy and Shaw 2007).

The European Food Safety Authority (EFSA) published guidance document on the Risk Assessment of Engineered Nanomaterials (ENM), which provides directions on how to determine the chemical composition of an ENM, its physico-chemical properties, *in vitro* and *in vivo* interactions with tissues, and potential exposure levels (Sauer 2011).

Unfortunately, up to now there is still limited data on exposure to specific ENMs and any consequent toxicity (Reidy et al. 2013; Smolkova et al. 2015). Potential applications of nanomaterials in food packaging will need to be evaluated for their potential risks and benefits.

17.6 CONCLUSIONS

The concepts of precaution and prevention have always been at the heart of public health practice. That's why substances for which there is insufficient knowledge of toxicology should not be allowed in food. Packaging is one of the possible sources of contamination of food with toxic substances. Nowadays, three main ways of development of packaging are observed. All of them take into account the complete life cycle of the packaging (from raw material selection, through production, analysis of interaction with food, use, and final disposal) to consider both health and environment.

The first way is connected with continuation and improvement of packaging materials and functions that they perform. These materials may include MAP, AP, IP, the use of antimicrobial agents to extend the shelf life of foods under storage and distribution conditions, and bio-based polymers.

The second way is a return to bio-derived materials (e.g., starch, cellulose, chitosan, proteins, and polymers produced on bio-based monomer as lactic acid) to build "greener" packaging (recyclable and biodegradable materials, reusable with reduced weight packaging). The future of these two kinds of packaging materials in the food industries is related to continued research on migration and the impact of packaging on human health and the environment.

The third way is also connected with using Life Cycle Assessment but the emphasis is on the reduction of the distance between the consumer and the producer of food.

Transportation of food needs time, appropriate packaging, and transport conditions. In the United States, food travels 1,500 miles on average from farm to consumer. Academic and marketing literature often cites environmental benefits of purchasing local foods that include reduced transportation, less processing and packaging, and farmland preservation. Which way will dominate in the future depends on public decisions, which will be a consequence of public engagement and awareness, but, above all, sufficient scientific evidence.

REFERENCES

Acconcia, F., V. Pallottini, and M. Marino. 2015. Molecular mechanisms of action of BPA. *Dose-Response: An Int. J.* 13(4): 1–9.

Alin, J. 2012. *Migration from Plastic Food Packaging during Microwave Heating* (TRITA-CHE-Report 2012:25). Stockholm: KTH Royal Institute of Technology.

Baol, J., X.W. Zeng, X.D. Qin, Y.L. Lee, X. Chen, Y.H. Jin, N.J. Tan, and G.H. Dong. 2015. Phthalate metabolites in urine samples from school children in Taipei, Taiwan. *Arch. Environ. Contam. Toxicol.* 69: 202–207.

Baughan, J.S., and D. Attwood. 2010. Food packaging law in the United States. In: *Global Legislation for Food Packaging Materials*, eds. R. Rijk and R. Veraart, pp. 223–239. Weinheim: Wiley-VCH.

Bhunia, K., S.S. Sablani, J. Tang, and B. Rasco. 2013. Migration of chemical compounds from packaging polymers during microwave, conventional heat treatment, and storage. *Compr. Rev. Food Sci. F.* 12: 523–545.

Bośnir, J., D. Puntraić, A. Galić, I. Škes, T. Dijanić, M. Klarić, M. Grgić, M. Čurković, and Z. Šmit. 2007. Migration of phthalates from containers into drinks. *Food Technol. Biotechnol.* 45(1): 91–95.

Bradley, E.L., L. Castle, and Q. Chaudhry. 2011. Applications of nanomaterials in food packaging with a consideration of opportunities for developing countries. *Trends Food Sci. Tech.* 22: 604–610.

Cederberg, D.L., M. Christiansen, S. Ekroth, et al. 2015. *Food Contact Materials—Metals and Alloys. Nordic Guidance for Authorities, Industry and Trade.* Copenhagen: Nordic Council of Ministers. TemaNord 2015:522.

Cirillo, T., E. Fasano, E. Castaldi, P. Montuori, and R.A. Cocchieri. 2011. Children's exposure to di(2-ethylhexyl)phthalate and dibutylphthalate plasticizers from school meals. *J. Agric. Food Chem.* 59: 10532–10538.

Conti, M.E. 1997. The content of heavy metals in food packaging paper boards: An atomic absorption spectroscopy investigation. *Food Res. Int.* 30: 343–348.

Conti, M.E. 2007. Heavy metals in food packagings. In: *Mineral Components in Food*, eds. J. Nriagu and P. Szefer, pp. 339–362. Boca Raton, FL: CRC Press/Taylor & Francis Group.

Council of Europe. 2002. *Guidelines on Metals and Alloys Used As Food Contact Materials.* Strasbourg: Social and Public Health Field, Partial Agreement Department, Council of Europe.

Crank, J. 1975. *The Mathematics of Diffusion,* 2nd ed. Oxford: Oxford University Press.

Czernych, R. 2016. Possibilities of using bioassays for estimating health risks in terms of exposure to environmental chemicals emissions. PhD thesis, Medical University of Gdansk, Poland.

Dąbrowski, W., and Z. Sikorski. 2004. *Toxin in Food.* Boca Raton, FL: CRC Press/Taylor & Francis Group.

Danish Veterinary and Food Administration. 2003. *Combined Actions and Interactions of Chemicals in Mixtures. The Toxicological Effects of Exposure to Mixtures of Industrial and Environmental Chemicals* (Report 2003:12). Glostrup: Danish Veterinary and Food Administration.

Diamanti-Kandarakis, E., J.P. Bourguignon, L.C. Giudice, R. Hauser, G.S. Prins, A.M. Soto, R.T. Zoeller, and A.C. Gore. 2009. Endocrine-disrupting chemicals: An endocrine society scientific statement. *Endocrine Rev.* 30(4): 293–342.

Dionisi, G., and P.K.T. Oldring. 2002. Estimates of per capita exposure to substances migrating from canned foods and beverages. *Food Addit. Contam.* 19: 891–903.

EFSA (European Food Safety Authority, European Union Agency). 2009. Panel on contaminants in the food chain (CONTAM); scientific opinion on arsenic in food. *EFSA J.* 7: 1351: 1–199.

EFSA. n.d. Metals as contaminants in food. http://www.efsa.europa.eu/en/topics/topic/metals (accessed March 22, 2016).

European Commission. 2002. *Resolution AP (2002)1 on Paper and Board Materials and Articles Intended to Come in Contact with Foodstuffs.* Strasbourg: Council of Europe, Committee of Ministers on 18 September 2002.

European Commission. 2007. Commission Regulation No. 333/2007 of 28 March 2007 laying down the methods of sampling and analysis for the official control of the levels of lead, cadmium, mercury, inorganic tin, 3-MCPD and benzo(a)pyrene in foodstuffs. *Off. J. Eur. Union L.* 88: 29–38.

European Commission. 2011a. Commission Regulation (EU) No. 10/2011 of 14 January 2011 on plastic materials and articles intended to come into contact with food. *Off. J. Eur. Union L.* 12: 1–89.

European Commission. 2011b. Commission Regulation No. 420/2011 of 29 April 2011 amending Regulation (EC) No. 1881/2006 setting maximum levels for certain contaminants in foodstuffs. *Off. J. Eur. Union L.* 111: 3–6.

European Commission. 2011c. Commission Regulation No. 836/2011 of 19 August 2011 amending Regulation No. 333/2007 laying down the methods of sampling and analysis for the official control of the levels of lead, cadmium, mercury, inorganic tin, 3-MCPD and benzo(a)pyrene in foodstuffs. *Off. J. Eur. Union L.* 215: 9–16.

European Commission. 2012. Commission Regulation No. 380/2012 of 3 May 2012 amending Annex II to Regulation (EC) No. 1333/2008 of the European Parliament and of the Council as regards the conditions of use and the use levels for aluminium-containing food additives. *Off. J. Eur. Union L.* 119: 14–38.

European Commission. 2014. Commission Regulation No. 488/2014 of 12 May 2014 amending Regulation (EC) No. 1881/2006 as regards maximum levels of cadmium in foodstuffs. *Off. J. Eur. Union L.* 138: 75–79.

European Commission. 2015. Commission Regulation (EU) 2015/174 of 5 February 2015 amending and correcting Regulation (EU) No. 10/2011 on plastic materials and articles intended to come into contact with food. *Off. J. Eur. Union L.* 30: 2–9.

European Parliament and the Council. 2004. Regulation (EU) No. 1935/2004 of 27 October 2004 on materials and articles intended to come into contact with food and repealing Directives 80/590/EEC and 89/109/EEC. *Off. J. Eur. Union L.* 338: 4–17.

Fasano, E., F. Bono-Blay, T. Cirillo, P. Montuori, and S. Lacorte. 2012. Migration of phthalates, alkylphenols, bisphenol A and di(2-ethylhexyl)adipate from food packaging. *Food Control* 27: 132–138.

Forrest, M.J. 2006. *Food Contact Rubbers 2: Products, Migration and Regulation* (Rapra Review Report, Vol. 16, No. 2). Shawbury/Shrewsbury, UK: Rapra Technology Limited.

Francisco, B.B.A., D.M. Brum, and R.J. Cassella. 2015. Determination of metals in soft drinks packed in different materials by ETAAS. *Food Chem.* 185: 488–494.

FSA (Food Standards Agency). 2002. *Investigation of the Significant Factors in Elemental Migration from Glass in Contact with Food.* Final Report Project Code A03029. London: Food Standards Agency.

FSA. 2009. *Nonylphenol in Food Contact Plastics and Migration into Foods.* Report FD 09/05. FSA PROJECT A03057. London: Food Standards Agency.

Gao, Y., Y. Gu, and Y. Wei. 2011. Determination of polymer compounds—antioxidants and ultraviolet (UV) absorbers by high-performance liquid chromatography coupled with UV photodiode array detection in food simulants. *J. Agric. Food Chem.* 59: 12982–12989.

Groten, J.P., V.J. Feron, and J. Sühnel. 2001. Toxicology of simple and complex mixtures. *Trends Pharmacol. Sci.* 22(6): 316–322.

Handy, R.D., and B.J. Shaw. 2007. Toxic effects of nanoparticles and nanomaterials: Implications for public health, risk assessment and the public perception of nanotechnology. *Health Risk Soc.* 9(2): 125–144.

Hansen, E., N.H. Nilsson, D. Lithner, and C. Lassen. 2013. *Hazardous Substances in Plastic Materials* (Report). Vejle: COWI and Danish Technological Institute.

Hauder, J., H. Benz, M. Rűter, and O.G. Piringer. 2013. The specific diffusion behavior in paper and migration modelling from recycled paper and board into dry foodstuffs. *Food Addit. Contam.* 30: 599–611.

Huang, W.W. 2015. Analysis on the industrial design of food package and the component of hazardous substance in the packaging material. *Adv. J. Food Sci. Technol.* 9(1): 44–47.

IARC (International Agency for the Research on Cancer). 2011. *Agents Classified by the IARC Monographs.* Lyon, France: World Health Organization. http://monographs.iarc.fr/ENG/Classification/ClassificationsAlphaOrder.pdf (accessed March 30, 2016).

Ibrahim D., B. Froberg, A. Wolf, and D.E. Rusyniak. 2006. Heavy metal poisoning: Clinical presentations and pathophysiology. *Clin. Lab. Med.* 26: 67–97.

Iwanowicz, L.R., V.S. Blazer, A.E. Pinkney, et al. 2016. Evidence of estrogenic endocrine disruption in small mouth and largemouth bass inhabiting Northeast U.S. national wild life refuge waters: A reconnaissance study. *Ecotox. Environ. Safe.* 124: 50–59.

Jamshidian, M., E.A. Tehrany, M. Imran, M. Jacquot, and S. Desobry. 2010. Poly-lactic acid: Production, applications, nanocomposites, and release studies. *Compr. Rev. Food Sci. F.* 9: 552–571.

Järup, L. 2003. Hazards of heavy metal contamination. *Brit. Med. Bull.* 68: 167–182.

Kim, K.Ch., Y.B. Park, M.J. Lee, J.B. Kim, J.W. Huh, D.H. Kim, J.B. Lee, and J.C. Kim. 2008. Levels of heavy metals in candy packages and candies likely to be consumed by small children. *Food Res. Int.* 41: 411–418.

Krupa, K.H., A. Wolny, and G. Dziubanek. 2011. The health risks associated with exposure to phthalates—how to effectively protect children from phthalates? In: *Health Risks Among Children and Youth*, eds. M. Seń and G. Dębska, pp. 115–122. Kraków: Krakowskie Towarzystwo Edukacyjne - Oficyna Wydawnicza AFM.

Lemos, V.A., M.S. Santos, G.T. David, M.V. Maciel, and M. Almeida Bezerra. 2008. Development of a cloud-point extraction method for copper and nickel determination in food samples. *J. Hazard. Mater.* 159: 245–251.

Lopez-Cervantes, J., and P. Paseiro-Losada. 2003. Determination of bisphenol A in, and its migration from, PVC stretch film used for food packaging. *Food Addit. Contam.* 20(6): 596–606.

Lu, L., Z. Dong, Z. Liu, T. Yali, and J. Wang. 2014. Migration of toxic metals from ceramic food packaging materials into acid food simulants. *Math. Probl. Eng.* 2014: 1–7.

Makuch, B., and L. Wolska. 2000. Modern analytical methods in studies of specific migration and toxic substances in packaging. *Opakowanie* 6: 34–37.

Marsh, K., and B. Bugusu. 2007. Food packaging—roles, materials, and environmental issues. *J. Food Sci.* 72: R39–R55.

Martirosyan, A., and Y.J. Schneider. 2014. Engineered nanomaterials in food: Implications for food safety and consumer health. *Int. J. Environ. Res. Public Health* 11: 5720–5750.

Mattsson, B., and U. Sonesson. 2003. *Environmentally-Friendly Food Processing*. Cambridge, MA: Woodhead.

Mayfield, D.B., A.S. Lewis, L.A. Bailey, and B.D. Beck. 2015. Properties and effects of metals. In: *Principles of Toxicology: Environmental and Industrial Applications,* eds. S.M. Roberts, R.C. James, and P.L. Williams, pp. 283–307. Hoboken, NJ: John Wiley.

Mercer, A. 1990. Migration studies of plasticizers from PVC film into food. PhD thesis, Leicester Polytechnic, Leicester, UK.

Montanari, A. 2015. Inorganic contaminants of food as a function of packaging features. In: *Food Packaging Hygiene*, eds. C. Barone, L. Bolzoni, G. Caruso, et al., pp. 17–41. Basel: Springer.

Muncke, J. 2014. Hazards of food contact material: Food packaging contaminants. In: *Encyclopedia of Food Safety*, eds. Y. Motarjemi, G. Moy, and E. Todd, pp. 430–437. Cambridge, MA: Academic Press.

Myers, N., and S.E. Spoolman. 2014. *Environmental Issues and Solutions: A Modular Approach.* Pacific Grove, CA: Brooks/Cole, Cengage Learning.

Nazarudin, I., O. Rozita, A. Azmui, and S. Norashikin. 2014. Determination of phthalate plasticisers in palm oil using online solid phase extraction-liquid chromatography (SPE-LC). *J. Chem.* ID 682975. doi:10.1155/2014/682975.

Oi-Wah, L., and W. Siu-Kay. 2000. Contamination in food from packaging material. *J. Chromatogr.* A882: 255–270.

Ozen, B., and J.D. Floros. 2001. Effects of emerging food processing techniques on the packaging materials. *Trends Food Sci. Tech.* 12: 60–67.

Page, B.D., and G.M. Lacroix. 1995. The occurrence of phthalate ester and di-2-ethylhexyladipate plasticizers in Canadian packaging and food sampled in 1985–1989: A survey. *Food Addit. Contam.* 12(1): 129–151.

Piver, W.T. 1973. Organotin compounds: Industrial applications and biological investigation. *Environ. Health Persp.* 4: 61–79.

Rachoń, D., A. Rutkowska, R. Czernych, A. Kowalewska-Włas, and L. Wolska. 2015. Serum phthalates concentrations correlate with serum testosterone levels in women with polycystic ovary syndrome (PCOS), paper presented at the 13th Annual Meeting of Androgen Excess and PCOS Society, Siracusa, SR.

Raheem, D. 2012. Application of plastics and paper as food packaging materials—An overview. *Emir. J. Food Agric.* 25(3): 177–188.

Reidy, B., A. Haase, A. Luch, K.A. Dawson, and I. Lynch. 2013. Mechanisms of silver nanoparticle release, transformation and toxicity: A critical review of current knowledge and recommendations for future studies and applications. *Materials* 6: 2295–2350.

Richardson, R., and M. Edwards. 2009. *Vinyl Chloride and Organotin Stabilizers in Water Contacting New and Aged PVC Pipes*. Web Report. Denver, CO: Water Research Foundation.

Rochester, J.R. 2013. Bisphenol A and human health: A review of the literature. *Reprod. Toxicol.* 42: 132–155.

Rosero-Moreano, M., E. Canellas, and C. Nerin. 2014. Three-phase hollow-fiber liquid-phase microextraction combined with HPLC-UV for the determination of isothiazolinone biocides in adhesives used for food packaging materials. *J. Sep. Sci.* 37: 272–280.

Rubino, M., and Y. Xia. 2016. Effect of cut edge area on the migration of BHT from polypropylene film into a food simulant. *Polym. Test.* 51: 190–194.

Rusyn, I., J.M. Peters, and M.L. Cunningham. 2006. Effects of DEHP in the liver: Modes of action and species-specific differences. *Crit. Rev. Toxicol.* 36(5): 459–479.

Rutkowska, A., A. Konieczna, K. Wilczewska, et al. 2015a. The commonly used plasticizers (bisphenols and phtalates) as endocrine disrupting chemicals in healthy women and women with polycystic ovary syndrome (PCOS), in Proceedings of the 17th European Congress of Endocrinology 2015, Dublin, Ireland, 16–20 May 2015, http://www.endocrine-abstracts.org/ea/0037/ECE2015AbstractBook.pdf. (accessed June 8, 2015).

Rutkowska, A., D. Rachoń, A. Milewicz, et al. 2015b. Polish Society of Endocrinology Position statement on endocrine disrupting chemicals (EDCs). *Endokrynologia Polska* 66: 276–280. DOI: 10.5603/EP.2015.0035.

Saçmacı, S., S. Kartal, Y. Yılmaz, M. Saçmacı, and C. Soykan. 2012. A new chelating resin: Synthesis, characterization and application for speciation of chromium (III)/(VI) species. *Chem. Eng. J.* 181–182: 746–753.

Sauer, U.G. 2011. Eating nanomaterials: Cruelty-free and safe? The EFSA guidance on risk assessment of nanomaterials in food and feed. *ATLA-Altern. Lab Anim.* 39: 567–575.

Schaefer, A. 2010. EU legislation. In: *Global Legislation for Food Packaging Materials*, eds. R. Rijk and R. Veraart, pp. 1–25. Weinheim: Wiley-VCH.

Shotyk, W., and M. Krachler. 2007. Contamination of bottled waters with antimony leaching from polyethylene terephthalate (PET) increases upon storage. *Environ. Sci. Technol.* 41: 1560–1563.

Shotyk, W., M. Krachler, and B. Chen. 2006. Contamination of Canadian and European bottled waters with antimony leaching from PET containers. *J. Environ. Monitor.* 8: 288–292.

Silvestre, C., D. Duraccio, and S. Cimmino. 2011. Food packaging based on polymer nanomaterials. *Prog. Polym. Sci.* 36: 1766–1782.

Smolkova, B., N.E. Yamani, A.R. Collins, A.C. Gutleb, and M. Dusinska. 2015. Nanoparticles in food. Epigenetic changes induced by nanomaterials and possible impact on health. *Food Chem. Toxicol.* 77: 64–73.

Tantra, R. 2016. *Nanomaterial Characterization: An Introduction*. Hoboken, NJ: John Wiley.

Taskeen, A., and I. Naeem. 2009. Bisphenol A toxicity in milk: A review. *Nat. Sci.* 7(8): 83–85.

vom Saal, F.S., and C. Hughes. 2005. An extensive new literature concerning low-dose effects of bisphenol A shows the need for a new risk assessment. *Environ. Health Perspect.* 113(8): 926–933.

Yang, Ch. Z., S.I. Yaniger, V.C. Jordan, D.J. Klein, and G.D. Bittner. 2011. Most plastic products release estrogenic chemicals: A potential health problem that can be solved. *Environ. Health Perspect.* 119: 989–996.

Zygoura, P., E. Paleologos, and M. Kontominas. 2011. Effect of ionizing radiation treatment on the specific migration characteristics of packaging-food simulant combinations: Effect of type and dose of radiation. *Food Addit. Contam.* 28(5): 686–694.

18 Detection of Harmful Compounds in Food

Grażyna Gałęzowska and Lidia Wolska

CONTENTS

18.1 INTRODUCTION

Numerous compounds found in small amounts in food products have been indicated to influence substantially the state of human health. The detection of harmful compounds in food plays an important role in the food industry. The determination of toxicity of these substances enables to establish the potential adverse effects on heath and consumer safety. At the turn of many years, the food industry has changed in terms of number of compounds used for production and as a consequence quality of products. Foods used at early times were mostly without additives, hence they also had a short period for consumption. Nowadays, food without additives is virtually nonexistent. It is extremely important to increase the nutritional value of foods (vitamins, mineral compounds, amino acids, and their derivatives), the sensory properties (pigments, flavoring components, or flavor enhancers), and the shelf life of foods (antimicrobial additives and buffer additives). Additives or their degradation products generally remain in food. Although, in some cases, they can be removed during processing it is generally assumed that applied doses of food additives and their degradation products should be nontoxic. This also applies to both acute and chronic toxicity and is extremely important for compounds with teratogenic, mutagenic, or carcinogenic effects.

Consequently, for detection of these harmful substances sensitive and universal methods are required, which allow their determination at low concentration levels, with good repeatability and reproducibility. New procedures, which fulfill to some extent the requirements of the concept of sustainable development expressed by green chemistry and green analytical chemistry, are needed.

Currently, many parameters can be determined in food, from simple physicochemical ones, like the pH up to the concentration of specified analytes, including harmful substances. In the case of food compounds occurring at very low concentration levels, it is necessary to use highly effective and selective analytical techniques.

This chapter establishes evaluation criteria for methods used to detect harmful compounds such as volatile and semivolatile organic compounds, polar compounds, and metals that may be present, or have the potential to be associated with food products. The principles of operation and the range of use of these techniques are explained. Particular attention is paid to the indication of advantages and disadvantages of various techniques used for separation and determination of harmful compounds in food. Due to the multitude of techniques used in food analysis, the chapter will focus on chromatographic techniques, spectroscopic methods, and immunoassay analysis.

18.2 CHROMATOGRAPHIC TECHNIQUES

18.2.1 Introduction

Since the 1950s, a rapid development of the chromatographic techniques has begun. Various separation techniques have been developed for identification and quantification of diverse substances in food. Nowadays, most of the methods used for food analysis are based on chromatography, including: gas chromatography (GC), liquid chromatography (LC), and thin layer chromatography (TLC). In the case of all chromatographic techniques, the determination of harmful compounds in complex matrices, such as food, often requires extensive sample extraction and preparation prior to instrumental analysis. Sample preparation is often the critical step in analysis and there is a need to minimize the number of operation used, to reduce both sources of errors and analysis time. The trends in food analysis focus also on selection of techniques more environmentally friendly, which use less toxic solvents. Optimal sample preparation should reduce analysis time, sources of error, enhance sensitivity, and enable unequivocal identification and quantification of the analytes. The sample preparation procedure for the investigation of food composition includes at least three steps, the first two being always used (for solid and liquid samples), while the third one is common, although not required (often used to isolate and preconcentrate of harmful compounds or even extract clean-up).

18.2.2 Preliminary Sample Preparation

This includes extraction/leaching of soluble components of the examined material with suitable solvents or their mixtures, or a supercritical fluid, and also desorption, hydrolysis, or saponification. When planning extraction/leaching of the food harmful compounds, a fraction of the total amount of the components can be adsorbed to other food components. Each step of a sample preparation procedure can lead to loss of a fraction of analyte. This is especially important when the amounts of isolated substances are very small. Additionally, some samples (animal or fish tissue and similarly moist or wet solids) can cause special problems, for example, reduction of particles penetration by the extraction media as well as problem with drying of the whole sample volume. A solution may be to distribute the sample with additional matrix, such as cleaned sand. However, this requires a large sample size.

Consequently, in order to relate the content of harmful compounds in the final extract to their content in food sample, it is necessary to examine the recovery. The range of extracted components depends on the kind of extrahent and conditions of the extraction process. First of all, solvents and conditions that enable isolation of a wide range of compounds should be used. The extracts will contain other substances that can interfere with the analysis belonging to such groups as lipids, phospholipids, glycosides, saccharides, or peptides. To reduce the errors in recovery determining, for homogenized samples a standard addition is used. However, even this approach may not eliminate the analytical errors completely.

For solid food samples the following extraction techniques can be used: Soxhlet extraction, matrix solid phase dispersion (MSPD), accelerated solvent extraction (ASE®), super-heated water extraction (SHWE), supercritical fluid extraction (SFE), microwave-assisted extraction (MAE), and ultrasonic extraction (USE; Table 18.1). The example food applications for sample preparation techniques were presented by K. Ridgway and co-workers (Ridgway et al. 2007).

Analyte enrichment is practiced for solid and liquid food samples with the simultaneous removal of interferences by techniques, such as traditional, and the most

TABLE 18.1
Advantages and Disadvantages of Sample Preparation Techniques

Technique	Advantages	Disadvantages
Soxhlet extraction	Use for the isolation and enrichment of thermally stable and low volatility components; Can be automated	Preliminary extraction technique; Further clean-up and preconcentration steps are often necessary; Long extraction time; Large consumption of organic solvents, cooling water, and electric energy
MSPD	Good solvent penetration of food matrix; Low solvent consumption; Elimination of the multiple extractions	Not easily automated; Time consuming; Additional clean-up step is often necessary for fatty matrices
ASE	Fast extraction at elevated temperature and pressure; Improves the solubility of analytes; Enhances kinetics of dissolution processes and favors desorption of analytes from the food matrix; Can be performed in both static and dynamic (flow through) mode	Extraction conditions should be optimized; For lipid matrices, clean-up step is often required; High cost of the equipment

(Continued)

TABLE 18.1 (*Continued*)
Advantages and Disadvantages of Sample Preparation Techniques

Technique	Advantages	Disadvantages
SHWE	"Green" solvent (water); Environmentally friendly (fast, cheap, and clean); High selective extraction type; Temperatures and pressures of water are lower than in SFC	Concentration step of diluted extracts is required; Further extraction or clean-up steps are often required (trace analysis); Suitable for thermally stable analytes; Risk of analyte precipitation during cooling process
SFE	An inexpensive, nonflammable and environmentally friendly solvent (carbon dioxide); More selective extraction; Fast reaction kinetics; Salvation power can be changed by controlling pressure and/or temperature and by adding modifiers; Can be automated	Decrease of selectivity by adding of other solvents, for example, methanol; Extraction of wet or liquid samples quite difficult
MAE	Good extraction efficiency; Low solvent consumption; Short extraction time	Analytes should be stable in high temperatures; Further concentration or clean-up step is generally required (trace analysis); Extraction of nonpolar analytes from nonpolar matrices requires the use of solvents with dipole moments greater than zero
USE	Several extractions can be performed simultaneously; Specialized laboratory equipment is not required; Relatively inexpensive	Separation of the extract from the sample after the extraction is necessary; Further concentration or clean-up step is generally required (trace analysis)
SPE	Involves a liquid–solid partition; Availability of wide range of sorbents; Clean-up and concentration of trace analytes from liquid samples; Specific selective sorbents are commercially available; Can be automated	The packing should be uniform to avoid poor efficiency; Sample matrix can affect the ability of the sorbent to "extract" the analyte; Low selectivity and insufficient retention of very polar compounds
SPME	Solvent-free sample preparation technique; Elimination or reduction of solvent consumption during desorption; Good sensitivity coupled with both LC and GC; Relatively low cost; Possibility of extraction from a variety of matrices; Can be automated	An equilibrium technique; Extraction conditions should be optimized; Volume of stationary phase is limited; Batch to batch variation; Weak robustness of fiber coatings; An internal standard should be considered; Direct immersion can be difficult (an alternative is headspace analysis); Proteins can adsorb irreversibly to the fiber

(*Continued*)

TABLE 18.1 (*Continued*)
Advantages and Disadvantages of Sample Preparation Techniques

Technique	Advantages	Disadvantages
SBSE	Large surface area of stationary phase; Better recovery and sample capacity; Good sensitivity coupled with both LC and GC; Can be used for liquid or semisolid complex food matrices	Problems with high recoveries and reproducibility; Low availability of different types of sorptive phases; Applications are limited to nonfatty matrices and nonpolar or semipolar analytes
LPME	Miniaturized version of LLE; Very low organic solvent consumption; Environmentally friendly; Static, dynamic analysis	Applications are limited; Problems with high recoveries and reproducibility; Cannot be automated

common method is liquid/liquid extraction, as well as modern techniques: solid-phase extraction (SPE), selective adsorption, and solid phase micro-extraction (SPME) or solvent (liquid phase) micro-extraction (LPME; Table 18.1).

The emerging issues during liquid/liquid extraction include incomplete separation of the two formed phases or unexpected reduction of the analytes concentration. The formation of two phases during extraction can be cumbersome. To avoid emulsions forming inorganic salt may be added, centrifugation or alternatively an MSPD approach can be used. Therefore, to separate proteins in food samples instead of extraction with chloroform, the sedimentation with lead acetate could be used (Heperkan et al. 2012). The major disadvantage of liquid/liquid extraction is the usage of relatively large volumes of organic solvents, often toxic. Also, due to the limited selectivity, particularly for trace level analysis, there is a need to extract clean-up and concentration steps prior to chromatographic analysis.

Furthermore, the reduction of concentration could be associated with the sample complete evaporation (in rotary evaporator) or high temperature of the solvent evaporation. The filtrate should be evaporated in a rotary evaporator to about 2–3 cm^3 and then the evaporation should be continued with gentle air stream to nearly dryness. The temperature during extraction should be maintained between 25°C and 33°C to obtain high extraction efficiency (Heperkan et al. 2012). Frequently, if the temperature exceeds 35°C, volatile compounds may be lost and labile compounds may decompose.

Recently, the Quick, Easy, Cheap, Effective, Rugged, and Safe (QuEChERS) method was proposed for the safe (also for analysts) and rapid extraction of harmful compounds such as pesticides (from fruits, vegetables, cereals, and honey samples; Anastassiades et al. 2003). The extract is often not much concentrated. For that reason, this method is not applied for the determination of food harmful compounds with low permissible levels, but it has been documented to give a better recovery compared with classical techniques, such as liquid/liquid extraction (Daba et al. 2011).

The QuEChERS method has the following advantages: high recovery, high sample throughput, low solvent and glassware usage (no chlorinated solvents), less labor and bench space, lower reagent costs, ruggedness, and low worker exposure (Mekonen et al. 2014). Nowadays, QuEChERS sample preparation method coupled with a high resolution GC and LC can be used for the determination of pesticides, monomers and plasticizers, antibiotics, β-blockers, and many other substances.

18.2.2.1 Thin Layer Chromatography

TLC is a simple LC technique capable of not only separating compounds but also determining the purity of a substance. A small concentrated spot of solution containing the sample is applied to a strip of chromatography plate with a stationary phase. Because different analytes ascend the TLC plate at different rates (different strength of interactions), the separation is achieved. TLC is without doubt one of the few options for the separation of samples in complex matrices including food. It does not require sample preparation and is limited to one or two steps. TLC is an effective, low cost, and rather simple method used for the analysis of organic compounds in food (Table 18.2).

Apart from the high matrix tolerance for TLC, another huge advantage is the possibility of analyzing many components in a parallel one plate. However, in view of the low resolution factor of TLC plates, the number of components in food sample, which can be detected with a given detection method is limited. Frequently present substances in the sample have the same or very similar retention coefficient. Considering the size of plates used for analysis at best only about 10 spots can be separated.

In cases of overlapping spots, solvent mixtures should be used for more selective separation or combination of solvent system (two-dimensional separation). This provides much more selective and efficient separation of the food compounds. Nevertheless, it could be associated with the increased spreading of the spots after the two-dimensional elution. Finally, the minimum detectable quantities of the analytes would decrease and, thus, frequently limits of detection would be too high for determination of harmful substances.

Another stage, in which it is possible to make mistakes, is the preparation of the chromatographic system for separation. It is important that plates are activated at 105°C for 20–30 min before use to eliminate water content. The activity of the layers, even in the original packing, changes depending on environmental conditions (humidity or temperature). Before analysis the plates can be also prewashed by immersion in appropriate solvents and dried. Therefore, the layers also should be freshly reactivated.

The differences in the activity of the layer and also the saturation of the vapor phase of the developing tank can be the major sources of the variation of the retention coefficients. The vapor phase may be equilibrated by inserting filter paper in the tank and waiting for at least 30 min. The dosage speed of the samples should not be too slow or too fast. Slow dosage leads to a problem with surface penetration (e.g., formation of a shiny layer). Too high speed dosage leads to problems with effective evaporation of solvent and formation of blurry spots.

TABLE 18.2
The Application Examples of TLC for Determination of Harmful Compounds in Food

Sample	Analytes	Stationary Phase	Mobile Phase	Detection	LOQ	References
Helva (traditional Turkish food)	Aflatoxin B-1	TLC plate	Two-step separation: A: anhydrous diethyl ether; B: chloroform/acetone/methanol (87/10/3, v/v/v)	– UV 365 nm	1 μg/kg	Var et al. (2007)
Fish	Biogenic amines: histamine, cadaverine, putrescine, and tyramine	Silica gel G 0.20 mm	Chloroform/benzene/triethylamine (6/4.5/1)	UV 365 nm; densitometry using wavelength 254 nm (sample derivatization to densylamines)	–	Ayesh et al. (2012)
Plant commodities including cabbage, green peas, orange, tomato, maize, rice, and wheat	Pesticides	Silica gel F 0.25 mm or RP-18		UV 254/365 nm, UV scan	–	Ambrus et al. (2005)
Dried figs	Cyclopiazonic acid	Silica gel 60	Ethyl acetate/2-propanol/ammonium hydroxide (40/30/20, v/v/v)	Erlich's reagent; visual comparison with standards	25 μg/kg	Heperkan et al. (2012)
Honey	5-hydroxymethylfurfural	Silica gel 60	Two steps HPTLC: A: ethanol/methanol 9/1 (v/v) B: ethyl acetate	Densitometry using wavelength 290 nm		Hošťálková et al. (2013)

In view of the variability of *Rf* values and the detection procedures, control of the TLC conditions is important for obtaining reliable analytical data. Therefore, on each plate a mixture of analytical standards should be applied. If the marker compounds are well detectable and their *Rf* values are within the expected range, the analyst can be sure that the applied method is correct. The compounds used as markers should be relatively stable, sensitive under the detection conditions, and have reproducible *Rf* values.

The TLC techniques are intended for screening and confirmation of harmful compounds in food for laboratories, when the irregular supply of electricity, lack of service, or the limited budget do not allow a continuous use of more sensitive but more expensive techniques. TLC can be also used as sample preparation method before GC or LC analysis. TLC has a number of advantages, which include: simplicity, cheapness, is certified in many different industries, needs only a small amount of solvents, and many different samples can be applied on one plate. Recently, new adsorbents, plates, and automated sample applicators in TLC analysis have been applied. In contrast, the disadvantages of this technique include the lack of precise, quantitative results and no possibility of automated coupling to other techniques.

TLC is rarely applied, even though it has many advantages. Presently, more sensitive and selective techniques are available, such as GC or LC.

18.2.3 High Performance Liquid Chromatography

High performance liquid chromatography (HPLC) is one of the most dynamically developing techniques, also for determination of harmful compounds in food. The separation process involves interactions between the stationary and the mobile phase, using the affinity of the analytes to both phases. HPLC is used to determine many components in milk, animal tissues, foodstuffs, wines, or oils (Table 18.3).

The food samples must be subjected to a pretreatment prior to HPLC analysis. The steps of sample preparation often take more time than the chromatographic analysis itself. Therefore, it is important to avoid mistakes, which may lead to false or wrong results or even blocking of the chromatographic system. In the case of food compounds hazardous to health, it is especially important, because the administrative decisions are often based on the results of analysis. The pretreatment is based on multistage purification procedures such as liquid/liquid extraction (LLE), solid-phase extraction (SPE), solid phase microextraction (SPME), and TLC. Some food components may precipitate in the vial, hampering the correct injection. Thus, sample filtration prior to injection is very important. In common HPLC use, the sample should be filtered through a 0.45 μm filter. However, in the case of ultra efficient/ultra HPLC, when the diameter of the capillary is very small or when a mass spectrometer is used, the size of the filter should be at most 0.2 μm.

Additionally, the dissolved compounds of the matrix are responsible for the shifted retention times and ion suppression or ion enhancement. Dilution can minimize the matrix effect, but it can result in a reduced analyte detectability. Hence, "dilute-and-shoot"-LC-MS (DS-LC-MS) methods are predominantly available for substances for which the required detection levels are high and which show good ionization efficiency. In other cases, so-called matrix effects for specific food sample should be determined.

TABLE 18.3
The Application Examples of HPLC Analysis in Food Testing

Sample	Analytes	Column	Eluent	Flow	Detection	Detection Limits	References
Wine	Acesulfame, aspartame, benzoic acid, caffeine, saccharin, salicylic acid, and sorbic acid	C18	Isocratic: A: (acetonitrile, 12%) and solvent; B: (10 mM phosphate buffer, pH 5.0, 88%)	1.2 ml/min/25°C/5 µl/25 min	UV-VIS 202 nm (aspartame, saccharin, and salicilic acid), 206 nm (caffeine), 227 nm (acesulfame and benzoil acid), and 256 nm (soric acid)	1.83–3.74 mg/dm^3	Amidžić et al. (2015)
Oil bean curd, yellow croaker, and paprika	Chrysoidine	C18	Isocratic: methanol and ammonium acetate solution (65/35, v/v)	1.0 ml/min/35°C/–/15 min	UV-VIS, 451 nm	6 ng/dm^3	Fang et al. (2014)
Edible oil (sunflower, canola, and blended oil)	Terephthalic acid and isophthalic acid	C18 AQ column (250 mm, 5 µm particle, 4.6 mm diameter)	Gradient elution A: H_2O buffered with 0.1 TFA/ACN (90/10, v/v); B: H_2O buffered with 0.1 TFA/ACN (60/40, v/v) with the following proportions: A–B 90–10, 83–17, 75–25, and 60–40 at 0, 3, 6, and 12 min, respectively	1.0 ml/min/30°C/10 µl/12 min	DAD	6 ng/cm^3	Khaneghah et al. (2014)

(*Continued*)

TABLE 18.3 (*Continued*)
The Application Examples of HPLC Analysis in Food Testing

Sample	Analytes	Column	Eluent	Flow	Detection	Detection Limits	References
Wines (red wine, white wine, and rice wine), yogurt, potato crisps, fried dough sticks, dried shrimps, brined fish, and honey	Formaldehyde, acetaldehyde, propanal, furaldehyde, butanal, pentanal, hexanal, heptanal, octanal, nonaldehyde, decanal	Hypersil BDS-C8	A: 5% of aqueous acetonitrile; B: acetonitrile (100%); 40–55% (B) at10 min; 55%–100% (B) at 15 min	1.0 ml/min/30°C/10 µl/25 min	FLD $\lambda_{ex} = 280$ nm and $\lambda_{em} = 510$ nm	LOQ: Formaldehyde and acetaldehyde- 1.95, propanal- 1.76, furaldehyde- 0.65, butanal- 1.65, pentanal- 1.15, Hexanal- 1.02, heptanal and nonaldehyde- 1.56, octanal- 1.35, decanal- 1.50	Wang et al. (2014)
Milk	Sulfonamides	N/A	N/A	N/A	Amperometric detection	1.2–6.0 ng/cm^3	Bueno et al. (2014)
Animal tissues	Sulfonamides	SB-AQ C18	Methanol/ acetonitrile/1% acetic acid with a gradient system	N/A	UV and MS/MS	3 µg/kg and 10 µg/kg, respectively, for both of the UV and MS/MS detection	Yu et al. (2011)

Many types of detectors can be used for detection of harmful compounds in food, such as UV-VIS, DAD, fluorescence, or even a refractometer. Actually, tandem mass spectrometry or high resolution mass spectrometry (HRMS) became the standard tools for trace analysis. The advantages provided by HRMS over classic unit-mass-resolution tandem mass spectrometry are considerable. They include the collection of full-scan spectra, which provide the ability to assess more fully the composition of a sample. Consequently, the analyst does not have to do the tuning for specific compounds before analysis. It enables retrospective data analysis, and the capability of performing structural elucidations of unknown or suspected compounds. Users should select a precursor and product ion masses (in LC-MS precursor, ion mass often corresponds to the molecular mass of the analyte molecule plus a proton-positive ionization or minus a proton-negative ionization). Within the last few years, LC-HRMS has become increasingly popular in the field of pesticide analysis. The second area of research seems to be the determination of mycotoxins, which should be detected at a very low level. The use of very specific but expensive and time-consuming immunoassay steps can be circumvented by employing LC-MS/MS. However, HRMS is not widely used yet for the analysis of mycotoxins. The limited availability of reference materials for many mycotoxins and the determination of the so-called masked mycotoxins increase HRMS usage. However, a single-stage quadrupole based on LC-MS instrumentation are insufficiently selective and their sensitivity is low. As a consequence, LC-MS/MS would be useful for the determination of many other harmful compounds in food (Kaufmann 2012).

The presented examples are just a small part of the application of HPLC possibilities. HPLC allows the determination of many different compounds. Generally in HPLC, less sample pretreatment is required than in GC. Moreover, this method is very sensitive and selective.

18.2.3.1 Gas Chromatography

GC is a technique that can be used to separate organic volatile and semivolatile compounds. GC analysis of low-volatility polar compounds results in poor sensitivity and in peak tailing; therefore, derivatization has been extensively used to improve the accuracy, reproducibility, and sensitivity of the analyses. GC is used to determine many components in food products such as milk, animal tissues, foodstuffs, wines, or oils (Table 18.4).

In most cases the food samples require pretreatment. It is based on multistage purification procedures such as LLE, SPE, SPME, purge and trap (PT), or headspace (HS), and also HPLC. PT and HS techniques are often used to determine volatile compounds in food samples. However, the conventional HS technique is sensitive enough to determine only part of them like residual solvents (Uematsu et al. 2002), furan (La Pera et al. 2009), trichloroethylene and/or tetrachloroethylene (Boekhold et al. 1989), thiocyanate (Song et al. 2012), or benzene, toluene, ethylbenzene, *o*-, *m*- and *p*-xylenes, and styrene (Gilbert-López et al. 2010). Dynamic sampling methods, such as PT, coupled to GC are particularly suitable for the determination of volatile compounds at low concentration. The other, more sensitive techniques include HS

TABLE 18.4
The Application Examples of GC Analysis in Food Testing

Sample	Analytes	Column	Temperature Program	Flow	Detection	Detection Limit	References
Wine	Methanol, ethanol, ethyl acetate, propan-1-ol, amyl alcohol, and isoamyl alcohol	HP-1 (30 m × 0.32 mm × 0.25 μm)	26°C (7 min)–1°C/min–50°C–15°C/min–200°C (4 min)	1 μl/30 min	FID: 250°C/nitrogen carrier gas 25 ml/min	0.107% vol. (ethanol); 10 mg/dm³ (prop. amyl, iso.); 10 mg/dm³ (ethyl acet.); 20 mg/dm³ (methanol)	Amidžić et al. (2015)
Pork ham	PAHs	Multiresidue-1 (30 m × 0.25 mm × 0.25 μm)	50°C(1 min)–15°C/min–320°C (6 min)	1 μl/25 min	MS	0.00030–0.0030 mg/kg pyrene—benzo[a] anthracene	Surma et al. (2014)
Food packaging	Nonylophenols	ZB-5 MS (60 m × 0.25 mm × 0.25 μm)	65°C (1.1 min)–10°C/min–230°C–6°C/min–270 °C–40°C/min–300°C (1 min)	2 μl/22.5 min	MS/MS	0.1 ng/mm³	Alfirevic et al. (2011)
Dry-cured sausage	N-nitrosamines	Polyethylene glycol (30 m × 0.25 mm × 0.25 μm)	70°C (3 min)–15°C/min–140°C–5°C/min–180°C–20°C/min–250°C (3 min)	1 μl/22 min	MS	0.05–0.2 μg/cm³	Li et al. (2012)
Plant oil (containing olive oil and grape seed oil), chicken eggs, milk powder, beverages (milk, tea, and juice),	Cholesterol, brassicasterol, stigmasterol, b-sitosterol, and campesterol	VF-5 MS (30 m × 0.25 mm × 0.25 μm)	–	–/17 min	MS/MS	2 mg/kg	Chen et al. (2015)
Baby foods	Pesticides	N/A	N/A	N/A	MS/MS	0.003–0.008 mg/kg	Amendola et al. (2015)

coupled with an aqueous drop extraction or SPE and SPME. As shown, GC with mass spectrometry (GC-MS) uses many pretreatment techniques prior to analysis. The choice of a suitable technique depends on the type of substance analyzed.

Some GC methods do not require extraction, but, for example, derivatization and clean-up on the column. In typical derivatization processes, the reaction requires from 30 min up to several hours at elevated temperature. However, the time required can be reduced to a few minutes in microwave-assisted derivatization procedures. Consequently, it can very effectively shorten the overall analysis time.

The analysis of persistent halogenated pesticide residues in food was at first performed with GC and an electron capture detector (ECD). The widening range of compounds included in analysis led to the use of nitrogen- and phosphorous-specific detectors and then to single-stage low-resolution MS. Electron ionization (EI) was and still is the most frequently used type of GC-MS ionization. GC-HRMS was not used to any relevant extent by food analysts; attempts were made to introduce time-of-flight mass spectrometry (TOF spectrometry) in GC. However, TOF spectrometry became more popular in the field of GC because of the fast scan speed rather than the mass resolution. The situation has changed with the very recent commercial introduction of several new types of HRMS based on GC-TOF instrumentation (Kaufman 2012).

The main disadvantages of the GC method are the long time of food sample pretreatment and multistages prior to analysis. This makes the method rather expensive due to the use of large amounts of solvents and specialized instrumentation, for example, columns. However, derivatization allows for analysis of nonvolatile compounds, too. An additional advantage of this method is a small sample volume for analysis and the possibility of identification of a large number of compounds present at very low concentrations in the food.

18.3 SPECTROSCOPIC METHODS

Spectroscopic methods are the main tool of modern chemistry for the identification of molecular structures in food samples. Generally, the spectroscopic methods can be used to determine metals or for identification of organic chemicals structure (Figure 18.1).

The direct determination of compounds in food is difficult if they are present at trace level in a sample containing strongly interfering components. The enrichment of trace elements permits to increase sensitivity, improve precision and accuracy, and reduce the detection limits. There are many methods of preconcentration and/or isolation of trace components from food samples. These include: precipitation, co-precipitation, the use of a chelating resin, LLE, and SPE. The preconcentration of harmful compounds can be done using digestion of food samples with microwaves or ultrasound-assisted digestion with oxidants at room temperature, of which the latter type is carried out in an off-line mode.

Most of all metals can be determined by Atomic Absorption Spectrometry (AAS). The sample components are atomized, their absorbance measured, and their concentration calculated on the basis of standard samples. Depending on the type of metal, its quantification, and detection limits, different types of AAS are used.

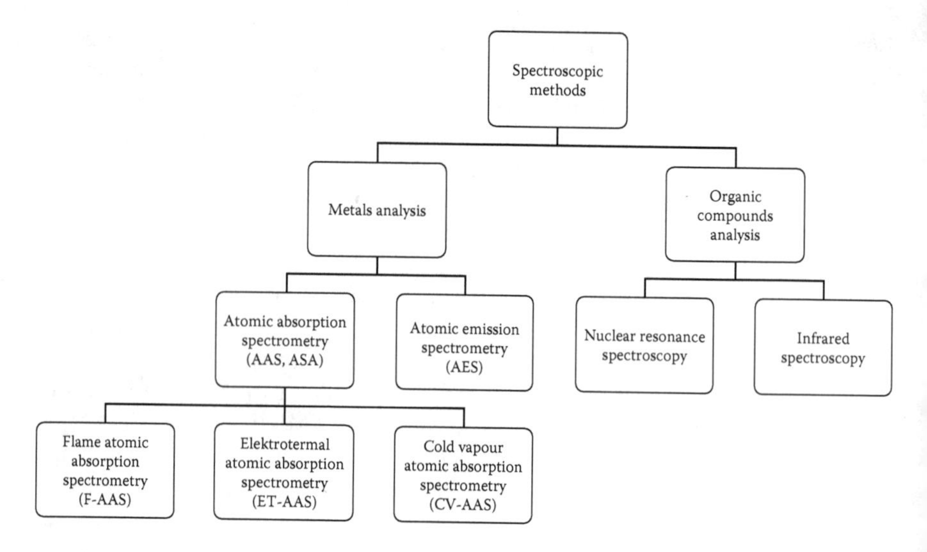

FIGURE 18.1 Classification of spectroscopic methods used for determination of harmful compounds in food.

The Electrothermal Atomic Absorption Spectrometry (ET-AAS) is a type of AAS in which sample modifiers are used, causing the matrix components more volatile and easily removed before atomization or, on the contrary, they bind the analyte to less volatile form. A problem of different atomization yield of an analyte in a sample from that of the same analyte in calibration standards can be resolved by using a reference standard, having a similar matrix to that of the analyzed sample, or by comparing the slopes derived from aqueous standards with those from certified reference materials (Marval-León et al. 2012; Junior et al. 2014; Leite et al. 2015).

For mercury determination, an extremely sensitive method of Cold Vapor Atomic Absorption Spectrometry (CV-AAS) has been developed. The CV-AAS is widely used for mercury tracer analysis because of its simplicity, robustness, and its relative freedom from interferences (Ferreira et al. 2015).

The alternative for AAS is an atomic emission spectrometer (AES), which permits to determine trace elements in a small volume of food materials. AES allows for determination of a few harmful elements in one run: Se, As, Cr, Zn, Cd, Pb, Ni, Mn, and Cu. For AES analysis, the food samples sometimes need a special pretreatment such as SPE (Qin et al. 2015) or after preconcentration with substance immobilized on silica gel and nanometer SiO_2 (Qun et al. 2008).

Some of these elements, for example, Cd, Pb, or Cu, can be determined by both AAS and AES. There are groups of elements, which can be determined by only one method:

- Ni, Cd, Cu, Co, and Pb by F-AAS
- As, Cd, Cu, Hg, and Pb by ET-AAS
- Se, As, Cr, Zn, Cd, Pb, Ni, Mn, and Cu by AES

In methods used for analysis of trace elements in food, it is important to measure many elements at the same time. For example, the inductively coupled plasma mass spectrometry (ICP-MS) is able to determine many elements at high sensitivity and precision in a wide dynamic range. However, in specimens for trace elemental analysis such as food, the concentrations of elements to be analyzed are generally low, while the concentrations of major component elements such as alkali metals, alkaline earth metals, carbon, nitrogen, and chlorine are high. ICP-MS is able to measure rapidly at high sensitivity, but many problems remain to be solved. For example, when samples containing salts at a high concentration are analyzed, the signal intensity of the elements of interest is suppressed, and a correction by the internal standard may not be effective, depending on the concomitant salt concentration (Orecchio et al. 2014; Ohki et al. 2016).

18.4 IMMUNOASSAY ANALYSIS

Recently, analysis including harmful compounds in food was addressed by HPLC or GC with different detection systems. Alternatively, for low cost or rapid applications in samples immunoassay methods can be an attractive strategy. However, it is only for limited number of target harmful analytes. Immunoassays are based on the reaction of an antigen (Ag) with a specific antibody (Ab) to give a product in a predetermined concentration (Ag-Ab complex), which can be measured. The two most commonly used immunoassay tests are plate-based enzyme-linked immunosorbent assays (ELISA) and lateral flow devices (LFD). ELISA can be used as either a qualitative or a quantitative assay but LFDs are designed only for qualitative (yes/no) testing. ELISA methods are used for the determination of many harmful compounds such as thiamphenicol, florfenicol, and chloramphenicol (Guo et al. 2015), residue of trifloxystrobin (Mercader et al. 2014) or antibiotics (Reig and Toldrá 2011), pyrrolizidine alkaloids and their N-oxides (Oplatowska et al. 2014), botulinum (Stanker et al. 2013), or even mercury ion (Wang et al. 2012). Commercially available LFDs for rapid detection are used for determination of peanut (*Arachis hypogaea*) and hazelnut (*Corylus avellana*; Röder et al. 2009), aflatoxins (Anfossi et al. 2013), *Staphylococcal enterotoxin* B (Boyle et al. 2010), ochratoxin (Anfossi et al. 2012), and many other toxins including mycotoxins (Anfossi et al. 2013).

ELISA tests have certain advantages like high sensitivity, strong specificity, or measurement of amount of offending food component (e.g., allergens). An antibody can selectively detect harmful compounds or their marker in food fairly rapidly; equipment needs are minor (plate reader) and require low to medium skill level. However, there are also limitations, such as some training required, adherence to instructions, correct sampling is important, as well as extraction, immunoreactivity and food matrix, polyphenols or oils may interfere, suitable pH and processing are required, etc. Also adverse reactions like cross-reactivity can be observed. It should be understood what does the kit detect—for example, some milk kits detect casein, while other detect whey proteins. The problems are reference materials and validation of ELISA.

The errors at each stage of analysis influence the quality of the results. They can be specified similarly as in the case of parameters regarding other techniques, including:

- Collection of samples (representative amount of samples, prevent cross contamination, label the sample, or record the shelf-life for the sample product),
- Sample preparation.
- Performing of immunoassay.
- Calculation and interpretation of the results.

The sample should be a representative part of the total batch and as homogeneous as possible. The matrix effect should be considered, including high background value and the dilution factor. Turbid sample should be purified or filtered. Do not use kit compounds after the expiry date and do not intermix kit compounds with different lot numbers. The temperature during the performance should be uniform and the edge effect minimized, for example, by placing an empty strip besides the strip containing the standards or samples.

It is important that the coefficient of variability between the duplicates should not be higher than 10–20% depending on the concentration read from the standard curve. When the curve becomes very flat (OD values below 0.8) the interpretation is difficult and the results are not acceptable.

Food samples have a complex composition, contain various levels of target analytes, and their preparation for analysis is very important until their clean up prior to quantitative determination. Numerous improvements have been made to sample preparation methods, most of which have involved miniaturizing the process to reduce the amounts of solvents consumed. Several techniques offer consistently high enrichment factors and consequently higher sensitivity for the analytes, together with a significant reduction of organic solvent consumption as well as extraction time.

The fundamental assumption underlying any methodology for determining harmful compounds is that it should guarantee true and precise results at appropriately low limits of detection for a wide spectrum of analytes in a short period of time.

Methodology also should be environmentally friendly, can be easy to carry out, and applicable with a small amount of solvents and inexpensive reagents, thus limiting the amount of waste generated by the analytical process. Their utility should concern both screening and targeted tests to fulfill legal requirements.

18.5 CONCLUSION

The analysis of harmful compounds in food samples requires method validation, which is a process by which a laboratory confirms by examination of critical parameters, and provides objective evidence, that the particular requirements for specific uses are fulfilled. It serves to demonstrate that the method can detect and identify an analyte or analytes in one or more matrices and in one or more instruments. Any type of analysis should determine sensitivity, specificity, accuracy, trueness, reproducibility, ruggedness, and precision to ensure that the results are appropriate.

In general, sample handling should be minimized to allow cost-effective investigations. Separation using robust LC columns with a long lifetime or high performance thin layer chromatography (HPTLC) plates displaying a high matrix tolerance is desirable. The sample preparation can be as simple as a dissolution step followed by precipitation, filtration, or a multistep SPE procedure. The sample preparation procedures strongly correlate to the subsequent separation experiment.

Although new applications about immunoassay tests appear daily in the literature, little innovation and few real breakthroughs in materials, procedures, or signaling have been described and discussed. The research is application-driven; it is driven by the demand for rapid devices. Therefore, the strategy has been focused on the development of good antibodies. The evaluations of immunoassay methods should include assessment of new kits developed for food samples and examining rapid methods for nontraditional agents for detection of harmful compounds.

REFERENCES

Alfirevic, M.B., E. Krizanec, and D.B. Voncina. 2011. Presence of nonylphenols in plastic films and their migration into food simulants. *Acta Chim. Slovenica* 58: 127–133.

Ambrus, A.M., T. Szathmary, I. Hatfaludi, I. Korsos, and J. Lantos. 2005. Application of TLC for confirmation and screening of pesticide residues in fruits, vegetables, and cereal grains. 2. Repeatability and reproducibility of Rf and MDQ values. *J. Environ. Sci. Health B* 40: 485–511.

Amendola, G., P. Pelosi, and A. Barbini, D. 2015. Determination of pesticide residues in animal origin baby foods by gas chromatography coupled with triple quadrupole mass spectrometry. *J. Environ. Sci. Health B* 50: 109–120.

Amidžić, K.D., I. Klarić, A. Mornar, and B. Nigović. 2015. Evaluation of volatile compound and food additive contents in blackberry wine. *Food Control* 50: 714–721.

Anastassiades, M., S.J. Lehotay, D. Stajnbaher, and F.J. Schenck. 2003. Fast and easy multiresidue method employing acetonitrile extraction/partitioning and "dispersive solid-phase extraction" for the determination of pesticide residues in produce. *J. AOAC Int.* 86: 412–431.

Anfossi, L., C. Baggiani, C. Giovannoli, G. D'Arco, and G. Giraudi. 2013. Lateral-flow immunoassays for mycotoxins and phycotoxins: A review. *Anal. Bioanal. Chem.* 405: 467–480.

Anfossi, L., C. Giovannoli, G. Giraudi, F. Biagioli, C. Passini, and C. Baggiani. 2012. A lateral flow immunoassay for the rapid detection of ochratoxin A in wine and grape must. *J. Agric. Food Chem.* 60: 11491–11497.

Ayesh, A.M., M.N. Ibraheim, A.E. El-Hakim, and E.A.H. Mostafa. 2012. Exploring the contamination level by biogenic amines in fish samples collected from markets in Thuel–Saudi Arabia. *African J. Microbiol. Res.* 6: 1158–1164.

Boekhold, A.J., H.A. van der Schee, and B.H. Kaandorp. 1989. Rapid gas-chromatographic determination of trichloroethylene and/or tetrachloroethylene in lettuce by direct headspace analysis. *Z. Lebensm. Unters. For.* 189: 550–553.

Boyle, T., M. Principato, R.L. Jones, L.J. Robert, and J.M. Njoroge. 2010. Detection of staphylococcal enterotoxin B in milk and milk products using immunodiagnostic lateral FLOW devices. *J. AOAC Intern.* 93: 569–575.

Bueno, A.M., A. Rouos, and A.M. Contento. 2014. Determination of sulfonamides in milk samples by HPLC with amperometric detection using a glassy carbon electrode modified with multiwalled carbon nanotubes. *J. Sep. Sci.* 37: 382–389.

Chen, Y.-Z., S.-Y. Kao, H.-Ch. Jian, Y.-M. Yu, J.-Y. Li, W.-H. Wang, and Ch.-W. Tsai. 2015. Determination of cholesterol and four phytosterols in foods without derivatization by gas chromatography-tandem mass spectrometry. *J. Food Drug Anal.* 23: 636–644.

Daba, D., A. Hymete, A.A. Bekhit, A.M.I. Mohamed, and A.E.D.A. Bekhit. 2011. Multi residue analysis of pesticides in wheat and khat collected from different regions of Ethiopia. *B. Environ. Contam. Tox.* 86: 336–341.

Fang, G., C. Liu, S. Wang, J. Feng, and Y. Yan. 2014. Highly selective determination of chrysoidine in foods through a surface molecularly imprinted sol–gel polymer solid-phase extraction coupled with HPLC. *Food Anal. Meth.* 7: 345–351.

Ferreira, S.L.C., V.A. Lemos, L.O.B. Silva, A.F.S. Queiroz, A.S. Souza, E.G.P. da Silva, W.N.L. dos Santos, and C.F. das Virgens. 2015. Analytical strategies of sample preparation for the determination of mercury in food matrices—a review. *Microchem. J.* 121: 227–236.

Gilbert-López, B., J. Robles-Molina, J.F. García-Reyes, and A. Molina-Díaz. 2010. Rapid determination of BTEXs in olives and olive oil by headspace-gas chromatography/mass spectrometry (HS-GC-MS). *Talanta* 83: 391–399.

Guo, L., S. Song, L. Liu, J. Peng, H. Kuang, and Ch. Xu. 2015. Comparison of an immunochromatographic strip with ELISA for simultaneous detection of thiamphenicol, florfenicol and chloramphenicol in food samples. *Biomed. Chromatogr.* 29: 1432–1439.

Heperkan D., S. Somuncuoglu, F. Karbancioglu-Gűler, and N. Mecik. 2012. Natural contamination of cyclopiazonic acid in dried figs and co-occurrence of aflatoxin. *Food Control.* 23: 82–86.

Hošťálková, A., I. Klingelhöfer, and G. Morlock. 2013. Comparison of an HPTLC method with the Reflectoquant assay for rapid determination of 5-hydroxymethylfurfural in honey. *Anal. Bioanal. Chem.* 405: 9207–9218.

Junior, M.M.S., L.O.B. Silva, D.J. Leao, and S.L.C. Ferreira. 2014. Analytical strategies for determination of cadmium in Brazilian vinegar samples using ET-AAS. *Food Chem.* 160: 209–213.

Kaufmann, A. 2012. The current role of high-resolution mass spectrometry in food analysis. *Anal. Bioanal. Chem.* 403: 1233–1249.

Khaneghah, A.M., S. Mazinani, S. Shoeibi, and S. Limbo. 2014. HPLC study of migration of terephthalic acid and isophthalic acid from PET bottles into edible oils. *J. Sci. Food Agric.* 94: 2205–2209.

La Pera, L., G. Dugo, P. Agozzino, S. Fanara, A. Liberatore, and G. Avellone. 2009. Analysis of furan in coffee of different provenance by head-space solid phase microextraction gas chromatography-mass spectrometry: Effect of brewing procedures. *Food Addit. Contam.* A26: 786–792.

Leite, C.C., A.V. Zmozinski, M.G.R. Vale, and M.M. Silva. 2015. Determination of Fe, Cr and Cu in used lubricating oils by ET-AAS using a microemulsion process for sample preparation. *Anal. Method.* 7: 3363–3371.

Li, L., P. Wang, X.L. Xu, and G.H. Zhou. 2012. Influence of various cooking methods on the concentrations of volatile N-nitrosamines and biogenic amines in dry-cured sausages. *J. Food Sci.* 77: 560–565.

Marval-León, J.R., F. Cámara-Martos, F. Pérez-Rodríguez, M.A. Amaro-López, and R. Moreno-Rojas. 2012. Optimization of selenium determination based on the Hg-ET-AAS method for its application to different food matrices. *Food Anal. Method.* 5: 1054–1061.

Mekonen, S., A. Ambelu, and P. Spanoghe. 2014. Pesticide residue evaluation in major staple food items of Ethiopia using the QuEChERS method: A case study from the Jimma Zone. *Environ. Toxicol. Chem.* 33: 1294–1302.

Mercader, J.V., R. López-Moreno, F.A. Esteve-Turrillas, A. Abad-Somovilla, and A. Abad-Fuentes. 2014. Immunoassays for trifloxystrobin analysis. Part II. Assay development and application to residue determination in food. *Food Chem.* 162: 41–46.

Ohki, A., T. Nakajima, S. Hirakawa, K. Hayashi, and H. Takanashi. 2016. A simple method of the recovery of selenium from food samples for the determination by ICP-MS. *Microchem. J.* 124: 693–698.

Oplatowska, M., C.T. Elliott, A.C. Huet, M. McCarthy, P.P.J. Mulder, C. von Holst, P. Delahaut, H.P. Van Egmond, and K. Campbell. 2014. Development and validation of a rapid multiplex ELISA for pyrrolizidine alkaloids and their N-oxides in honey and feed. *Anal. Bioanal. Chem.* 406: 757–770.

Orecchio, S., D. Amorello, M. Raso, S. Barreca, C. Lino, and F. Di Gaudio. 2014. Determination of trace elements in gluten-free food for celiac people by ICP-MS. *Microchem. J.* 166: 163–172.

Qin, W.X., Q. Gong, M. Li, L.X. Deng, L.S. Mo, and Y.L. Li. 2015. Determination of arsenic in food package aluminum by ultrasound assisted solid phase extraction/ICP-AES. *Spectrosc. Spect. Anal.* 35: 1043–1047.

Qun, H., C. Xijun, H. Xinping, and H. Zheng. 2008. Determination of trace elements in food samples by ICP-AES after preconcentration with p-toluenesulfonylamide immobilized on silica gel and nanometer SiO_2. *Microchim. Acta.* 160: 147–152.

Reig, M., and F. Toldrá. 2011. Patents for ELISA tests to detect antibiotic residues in foods of animal origin. *Recent Pat. Food Nutr. Agric.* 3: 110–114.

Ridgway, K., S.P.D. Lalljie, and R.M. Smith. 2007. Sample preparation techniques for the determination of trace residues and contaminants in foods. *J. Chromatogr.* A1153: 36–53.

Röder, M., S. Vieths, and T. Holzhauser. 2009. Commercial lateral flow devices for rapid detection of peanut (Arachis hypogaea) and hazelnut (Corylus avellana) cross-contamination in the industrial production of cookies. *Anal. Bioanal. Chem.* 395: 103–109.

Song, J., Y. Fu, L. Du, Y. Yao, X. Mu, L. Kang, Y. Zhao, and P. Se. 2012. Determination of thiocyanate in dairy products by headspace gas chromatography. *Chinese J. Chromatogr.* 30: 743–746.

Stanker, L.H., M.C. Scotcher, L. Cheng, K. Ching, J. McGarvey, D. Hodge, and R. Hnasko. 2013. A monoclonal antibody based capture ELISA for botulinum neurotoxin serotype B: Toxin detection in food. *Toxins* 5: 2212–2226.

Surma, M., A. Sadowska-Rociek, and E. Cieślik. 2014. The application of d-SPE in the QuEChERS method for the determination of PAHs in food of animal origin with GC-MS detection. *Europ. Food Res. Technol.* 238: 1029–1036.

Uematsu, Y., K. Hirata, K. Suzuki, K. Iida, and K. Kamata. 2002. Survey of residual solvents in natural food additives by standard addition head-space GC. *Food Addit. Contam.* 19: 335–342.

Var, I., B. Kabak, and F. Go. 2007. Survey of aflatoxin B in helva, a traditional Turkish food, by TLC. *Food Control* 18: 59–62.

Wang, W., G. Li, Z. Ji, N. Hu, and J. You. 2014. A novel method for trace aldehyde determination in foodstuffs based on fluorescence labeling by HPLC with fluorescence detection and mass spectrometric identification. *Food Anal. Method.* 7: 1546–1556.

Wang, Y., H. Yang, M. Pschenitza, R. Niessner, Y. Li, D. Knopp, and A. Deng. 2012. Highly sensitive and specific determination of mercury(II) ion in water, food and cosmetic samples with an ELISA based on a novel monoclonal antibody. *Anal. Bioanal. Chem.* 403: 2519–2528.

Yu, H., Y. Tao, D. Chen, Y. Wang, L. Huang, D. Peng, M. Dai, Z. Liu, X. Wang, and Z. Yuan. 2011. Development of a high performance liquid chromatography method and a liquid chromatography–tandem mass spectrometry method with the pressurized liquid extraction for the quantification and confirmation of sulfonamides in the foods of animal origin. *J. Chromatogr.* B. 879(25): 2653–2662.

19 Regulations Established to Control Harmful Food Contaminations

Stefan S. Smoczyński

CONTENTS

19.1 INTRODUCTION

Hazardous chemicals not occurring normally in food must be controlled in order to ensure food safety. Food safety covers fulfillment of all operations undertaken at all stages of its production, storage, and sale, in order to ensure the health and life of consumers. The primary objective consists in satisfying conditions ensuring the presence in food of those components that are indispensable for the body and a complete absence of hazardous chemicals. The presence of hazardous chemicals in food is practically unavoidable. This results both from the degree of environmental pollution and the technological processes applied. After the existence of a potential threat to consumer health due to hazardous chemicals was confirmed with the results of specialist examinations, controls of substances in food were initiated. In addition, activities were undertaken to establish legal acts concerning the health safety of food. Nowadays, they belong to the most important legislative activities in virtually all countries of the world. The Food and Agriculture Organization (FAO) and the European Union (EU) have been particularly active in this regard, operating under the Codex Alimentarius Commission. With this aim in view, regulations have been introduced to set the maximum acceptable levels of hazardous chemical substances in most types of food products. The current Codex Alimentarius (CA) provides a basis for regulations established in order to control the content of hazardous chemicals in food.

This chapter, after the introduction, presents international regulations concerning food control established in the CA. Additionally, as briefly as it is necessary, it describes the regulations of the EU and other countries of the world concerning food hygiene and control of potentially hazardous components in food. Afterward, regulations established in the EU concerning the content of heavy metals—lead (Pb), cadmium (Cd), and mercury (Hg)—nitrates (V) and (III), polychlorinated biphenyls (PCBs), dioxins, polycyclic aromatic hydrocarbons (PAH), and mycotoxins are presented. The final part describes the requirements set for the sampling method and for determining hazardous chemical compounds in food and presents a summary and conclusions.

19.2 INTERNATIONAL REGULATIONS CONCERNING THE CONTROL OF CHEMICAL HAZARDOUS SUBSTANCES IN FOOD: CA

CA, established in 1963, provides an example of worldwide activity concerning food safety and its control systems, and was developed through international arrangements by the FAO/World Health Organization (WHO) Codex Alimentarius Commission (CAC 2010). The Code is the set of accepted standards, recommendations, and guidelines related to food and nutrition based on the results of worldwide research. The documents established by the Code are used by official food control authorities and research institutions of Member States. The main aim of the Codex Alimentarius is to guarantee the production of safe food with high nutritional value, which meets consumer expectations, as well as to promote fair practices in the international food trade. The is the most important international, intergovernmental organization concerned with food safety and consumer health. The organizational structure of CAC includes 10 General Subject Committees and 11 Commodity Committees under the Executive Committee. The General Subject Committees include the Committee on Contaminants in Food, which monitors the problem of hazardous chemicals in food. Decisions, recommendations, and guidelines included in the CA provide much internationally recognized information to be used by manufacturing plants operating within the food industry. They facilitate the organization of systems for supervising food safety and for improving internal methods for controlling and monitoring the nutritional and health quality of food. The Codex currently includes documents setting the maximum levels of remains of pesticides and chemical contaminants in food. The norms presented in the Codex are not mandatory; they are treated as recommendations and good practice as regards safe food production. By the EU Council Decision No 2003/822/EC of 17 November 2003, the European Community joined the FAO/WHO Codex Alimentarius Commission and has been acting as its member (Council Decision 2003). The Codex Alimentarius Working Party at the EU Council operates as an advisory body. The procedure for elaborating Codex standards is based on eight subsequent steps. It is initiated by a decision made by the Commission to develop a specific standard of the Codex by an appointed committee in order to prepare the draft. Next, the draft is commented upon through the Secretariat of the Commission by Member States and cooperating international expert organizations. After taking into account any comments and amendments made, the Secretariat presents the draft standard to the Commission to be approved as the final one. Any proposals of amendments submitted in writing by Member States and conditioning adoption of the draft as the Codex standard are attached to the draft. Interested states can suggest a final approval of the standard or accept the Codex standard with specific comments. Standards approved and published in the CA, and later in EU documents concerning chemical contaminants, specify their maximum levels in the product or amounts (thresholds) determining whether certain actions should be taken (Commission Recommendation 2013).

19.3 REGULATIONS OF THE EU AND OTHER COUNTRIES CONCERNING THE CONTROL OF HAZARDOUS CHEMICALS IN FOOD

The global chain of food supplies, crossing the borders of multiple states and continents, requires close cooperation between governments and producers for the benefit of consumer health as the global food chain becomes longer and increasingly more complex. Food safety is determined by an increasing range of factors, including technical, geographic, or climatic factors, which require specific legal systems. The established legislation concerning the control of hazardous chemicals in food in various countries of the world is varied. What draws particular attention is the European food safety system as compared to, for instance, the United States and other countries, for example, of the South American zone. Food legislation, driven first of all by human health protection, includes interconnected legal norms governing the health quality of food, its manufacturing, and presence on the market. The European food law is based on the Regulation (EC) No 178/2002 of the European Parliament and of the Council of 28 January 2002 laying down the general principles and requirements of food law, establishing the European Food Safety Authority (EFSA) and laying down procedures in matters of food safety (Regulation (EC) No 178/2002). In particular, they concern formal control of food and feed, food labeling, additives, food for special dietary purposes, and food contaminants. Among numerous institutions participating in the food safety program, the primary role is played by the EFSA. The quoted Regulation assumes that no type of food that would entail health risk due to, for example, presence of hazardous chemicals can be placed on the market. The market should be open only to food products that comply with the adopted rules governing food safety.

According to available information, the US food system should be considered different from the model accepted in the EU, both in its institutional aspects and its material and legal form (Picó 2007). Structurally, the system is dispersed, which requires permanent coordination and cooperation between specialized agencies. Two agencies of the highest importance for ensuring food safety are the Food Safety Inspection Service (FSIS) and the Food and Drug Administration (FDA). The Environmental Protection Agency (EPA) is responsible for examination and for drafting regulations concerning remains of pesticides and chemical contaminants in food and feed. The Federal Grain Inspection Service (FGIS) deals with examination of aflatoxins in cereal and rice. Applicable regulations concerning the production and sale of food ensuring its safety on the federal level include about 30 acts, which concern both individual food groups, and select chemical additives and substances applied in the entire food production chain. To generalize, the food safety policy in the United States is based on the scientific evaluation of threads, risk analysis and, if necessary, the precautionary principle (Picó 2007).

South American states—Argentina, Brazil, Paraguay, Uruguay, and Venezuela—cooperate in food safety matters, under an alliance known as Mercosur. The EU is an important trading partner. In 2002, a document was adopted concerning mutual veterinary and phytosanitary principles which, in practice, correspond to international, US, and EU regulations. For instance, with reference to mycotoxins, Mercosur member states have established common principles concerning methods of sampling and analyses, as well as acceptable levels of the sum of four aflatoxins in peanuts, corn, and aflatoxin M_1 in milk. The control of pesticide residues is required for exporting meat, fish, and aquaculture to the United States and the EU.

Several associations operate in the Asia-Pacific region, including economic cooperation of over 20 Asia-Pacific Economic Cooperation (APEC) states, the objective of which is, among others, to ensure food safety. Those states, through the activities of various groups dealing with the risk assessment related to chemical contaminants, aim at harmonization of global regulations (EU and United States) concerning fish, fishery products, and seafood. It should be emphasized that the legislation of the EU, the United States, and many other countries around the world concerning chemical control of hazardous components in food, apart from insignificant organizational aspects, is convergent. The legislation takes into account the primacy of preserving the health safety of food and of consumer interests, enabling global trade in food.

19.4 REGULATIONS CONCERNING FOOD HYGIENE IN THE EU

Food hygiene covers theoretical knowledge and practical principles aiming at providing consumers with health-promoting food. Food hygiene, in its initial period of development, covered only issues of a biological nature. Since the 1960s, the field of food hygiene has been extended to include the need to examine its problems in two equally important aspects—microbiological and chemical, as at both levels multiple new threats have emerged requiring scientific examination and practical application.

As regards the chemical aspects of food hygiene, two directions deserve particular attention today—protection of chemical components in food determining its nutritional value and practice leading to a reduction or even prevention of the occurrence of external, hazardous chemicals in. In 2004, the EU provided a package of four regulations governing food hygiene for use by Member States. Ensuring human health and life in the food-related aspect is the main aim of regulations concerning food safety, included in Regulation No. 852/2004 the European Parliament and the Council of 29 April 2004. These provisions establish hygiene requirements that must be satisfied by food industry operators at all stages of food manufacturing, processing, and sale. Additionally, they impose an obligation to implement and apply quality assurance systems, hazard analysis and critical control points (HACCP), and Good Hygienic Practice (GHP). The Regulation also specifies requirements concerning hygiene at the level of primary production, as well as the requirements for all food sector operators. The Regulation sets forth the principle that food traded in the EU must satisfy all requirements specified in the above-quoted Regulation (Commission Regulation (EC) No 852/2004).

Regulation No 853/2004 specifies provisions governing safety of food of animal origin, for both raw materials and processed food. It establishes the conditions for placing those products on the food market. One of the principal recommendations is the application of appropriate labeling and, above all, providing information about the state where the manufacturing plant is located. The Regulation presents requirements concerning equipment and veterinary supervision over the slaughterhouse, which is required to obtain information concerning food safety principles, including the status of the farm producing the raw material and food of animal origin. Additionally, such food safety information should concern the health status of animals, medicinal products administered to animals, the occurrence of diseases that may affect product safety, and the results of analyses carried out on samples taken from animals (Commission Regulation (EC) No 853/2004).

Another important document is Regulation (EC) No 882/2004 of 29 April 2004 on official controls performed to ensure the verification of compliance with feed and food law, animal health, and animal welfare rules. It includes legal regulations of official food controls, which should be carried out regularly, without previous notification, at each stage of manufacturing, processing, and distribution. The Regulation defines a physical check, covering, among other, taking samples for analysis and laboratory testing, being of particular importance for examining the content of hazardous chemicals in food. The tasks of reference laboratories specified in the Regulation, the requirements related to the equipment, and the qualifications of their employees are also important aspects. Specific rights of authorities exercising official supervision as regards, for example, events of non-compliance with applicable food law regulations, including a decision on suspending or closing a given plant and on issuing an order to withdraw or destroy food or feed, are of particular significance (Commission Regulation (EC) No 882/2004).

Legislation concerning chemical aspects of food hygiene covers procedures ensuring food safety through controlling, among others, the content of heavy metals—Pb, Cd, and Hg—nitrates(III) and (V), PCBs, dioxins, PAHs, and mycotoxins, taking into consideration food consumption structure, consumer preferences, the results of monitoring of presence of chemical food contaminants, as well as established values of daily and weekly intake. The examination is most often applied to milk and dairy products, infant formulae and food for young children, meat and meat products, fish and fishery products, vegetables and fruits, and other foodstuff.

19.5 REGULATIONS ESTABLISHED FOR CONTROLLING HAZARDOUS CHEMICALS IN FOOD

19.5.1 Maximum Level of Pb in Foodstuff

The maximum levels of Pb in foodstuff established by the EU are presented in Tables 19.1 through 19.5.

TABLE 19.1
Maximum Level of Lead (Pb) in Milk and Dairy Products, Infant Formulae, and Drinks for Young Children

Foodstuff	Closer Description	Wet Weight (mg/kg)
Milk and dairy products	Raw milk, heat-treated milk, and milk for manufacture of milk-based products	0.020
Infant formulae	Infant formulae and follow-on formulae	0.050
	Marketed as powder	
	Marketed as liquid	0.10
	Processed cereal-based foods for infants and young children	0.050
Drinks for young children	Drinks labeled and sold as liquids or to be reconstituted following the instructions of the manufacturer, including fruit juices	0.030
	Drinks to be prepared by infusion or decoction	1.50

Source: Commission Regulation (EU) No 2015/1005 of 25 June 2015 amending Regulation (EC) No 1881/2006 as regards the maximum permissible levels of Pb in foodstuff. *Official Journal of the European Union* L 161, 26.6.2015.

TABLE 19.2
Maximum Level of Lead (Pb) in Meat, Meat Products, Offals, Fats, and Oils

Foodstuff	Closer Description	Wet Weight (mg/kg)
Meat and meat products	Meat of bovine animals, pigs, lambs, and poultry	0.10
Offals	Of bovine animals, sheep, pig, and poultry	0.50
Fats and oils	Fats and oils, including milk fat	0.10

Source: Commission Regulation (EU) No 2015/1005 of 25 June 2015 amending Regulation (EC) No 1881/2006 as regards the maximum permissible levels of Pb in foodstuff. *Official Journal of the European Union* L 161, 26.6.2015.

TABLE 19.3
Maximum Level of Lead (Pb) in Fish, Fishery Products, and Seafood

Foodstuff	Closer Description	Wet Weight (mg/kg)
Fish	Muscle meat of fish including fishery products	0.30
Seafood:	Crustaceans: muscle meat from appendages and abdomen. In case of crabs and crab-like crustaceans (*Brachyura* and *Anomura*), muscle meat from appendages.	0.50
	Bivalve mollusks	1.50
	Cephalopods	0.30

Source: Commission Regulation (EU) No 2015/1005 of 25 June 2015 amending Regulation (EC) No 1881/2006 as regards the maximum permissible levels of Pb in foodstuff. *Official Journal of the European Union* L 161, 26.6.2015.

TABLE 19.4
Maximum Level of Lead (Pb) in Vegetables, Fruiting Vegetables, and Fruit

Foodstuff	Closer Description	Wet Weight (mg/kg)
Vegetables	Vegetables excluding leafy brassica, salsify, leafy vegetables and fresh herbs, fungi, seaweed and fruiting vegetables	0.10
	Leafy brassica, salsify, leaf vegetables excluding fresh herbs and the following fungi *Agaricus bisporus* (common mushroom), *Pleurotus ostreatus* (Oyster mushroom), *Lentinula edodes* (Shiitake mushroom)	0.30
Fruiting vegetables	Sweet corn	0.10
	Fruiting vegetables other than sweet corn	0.05
Fruit	Fruit, excluding cranberries, currants, elderberries, and strawberry tree fruit	0.10
	Cranberries, currants, elderberries, and strawberry tree fruit	0.20

Source: Commission Regulation (EU) No 2015/1005 of 25 June 2015 amending Regulation (EC) No 1881/2006 as regards the maximum permissible levels of Pb in foodstuff. *Official Journal of the European Union* L 161, 26.6.2015.

By the Regulations of 2015, it was established that in products produced from the 2016 fruit harvest onward, the maximum level of Pb content should be reduced to 0.015 mg/kg wet weight. The same Regulation set the maximum level of Pb in honey at 0.10 mg/kg wet weight (Commission Regulation (EU) No 2015/1005).

TABLE 19.5
Maximum Level of Lead (Pb) in Juices, Wine, Honey, Cereals, and Pulses

Foodstuff	Closer Description	Wet Weight (mg/kg)
Juices	Fruit juices, concentrated fruit juices as reconstituted and fruit nectars	
	Produced exclusively from berries and other small fruit	0.05
	Juices made from fruit other than berries and small fruits	0.03
Wine	Wine (including sparkling wine, but excluding liqueur wine, cider, perry, and fruit wine, as well in aromatized wines, wine-based drinks, and aromatized wine-product cocktails[a]	0.20
Honey		0.10
Cereals and pulses		0.20
		CR-EU No 1881/2006

Source: Commission Regulation (EU) No 2015/1005 of 25 June 2015 amending Regulation (EC) No 1881/2006 as regards the maximum permissible levels of Pb in foodstuff. *Official Journal of the European Union* L 161, 26.6.2015.

[a] By the Regulations of 2015, it was established that in products produced from the 2016 fruit harvest onward, the maximum level of Pb content should be reduced to 0.015 mg/kg wet weight.

19.5.2 Maximum Levels of Cd in Foodstuff

The maximum levels of Cd in milk and dairy products have not been set in the applicable regulations of the EU. Some EU Member States, including Poland, specify the maximum levels of Pb and Cd in milk and dairy products under a monitoring program for heavy metal content (Wojciechowska-Mazurek et al. 2010, Szkoda et al. 2011). The EU regulations establish the maximum level of Cd in infant formula and food for young children as well as in meat and in products of farm-bred terrestrial animals, in fish and fishery products, as well as in seafood. The maximum limits for Cd content have been also established for vegetables and fruits, and for products made from them, as well as for cereal, rice, and soybean. In recent years, the limits of Cd content have also been applied to cocoa and its products, including chocolate (Commission Regulation (EU) No 488/2014). The maximum levels of Cd in various foods, established by the EU, are presented in Tables 19.6 through 19.10.

In 2014, the maximum levels of Cd in cocoa and chocolate products were established, to be applied as of 2019.

19.5.3 Maximum Levels of Hg in Foodstuff

The examination of Hg content in food products becomes an exceptionally important element in the aspect of food safety and human health protection. The evaluation of

TABLE 19.6
Maximum Level of Cadmium (Cd) in Infant Formulae

Foodstuff	Closer Description	Wet Weight (mg/kg)
Infant formulae and follow-on formulae	Powdered formulae manufactured from cows' milk proteins or protein hydrolysates	0.010
	Liquid formulae manufactured from cows' milk proteins or protein hydrolysates	0.005
	Powdered formulae manufactured from soy protein isolates, alone or in a mixture with cows' milk proteins	0.020
	Liquid formulae manufactured from soy protein isolates, alone or in a mixture with cows' milk proteins	0.010
	Processed cereal-based food and other baby foods for infants and young children	0.040

Source: Commission Regulation (EU) No 488/2014 of 12 May 2014 and Commission Regulation (EC) No 629/2008 of 2 July 2008 amending Commission Regulation (EC) No 1881/2006 as regards the maximum levels of Cd in foodstuff. *Official Journal of the European Union* L 138, 13.5.2014.

TABLE 19.7
Maximum Level of Cadmium (Cd) in Meat and Meat Products

Foodstuff	Closer Description	Wet Weight (mg/kg)
Meat and meat products	Meat (excluding offal) of bovine animals, sheep, pig, and poultry	0.050
	Horse meat, excluding offal	0.20
Offals	Offals such as liver of bovine animals, sheep, poultry, and horses	0.50
	Kidneys of bovine animals, sheep, pig and poultry	1.0

Source: Commission Regulation (EU) No 488/2014 of 12 May 2014 and Commission Regulation (EC) No 629/2008 of 2 July 2008 amending Commission Regulation (EC) No 1881/2006 as regards the maximum levels of Cd in foodstuff. *Official Journal of the European Union* L 138, 13.5.2014.

Hg content in food is made pursuant to the Commission Regulation (Commission Regulation (EU) No 1881/2006), as amended, setting maximum levels for certain contaminants in foodstuff. As results from this Regulation, limits regarding the maximum Hg content are currently set only for select foodstuff in the EU states, that is, for fish and fish products (Table 19.11) (Commission Regulation (EU) No 1881/2006, Commission Regulation (EC) No 565/2008, Commission Regulation (EU) No 420/2011).

TABLE 19.8
Maximum Level of Cadmium (Cd) in Fish, Fishery Products and Seafood

Foodstuff	Closer Description	Wet Weight (mg/kg)
Fish, fishery products and seafood	Muscle meat of fish	0.050
	excluding:	
	Mackerel (*Scomber* species), tuna (*Thunnus* species, *Katsuwonus pelamis*, *Euthynnus* species), bichique *Sicyopterus lagocephalus*)	0.10
	Muscle meat of bullet tuna	0.15
	Muscle meat of anchovy (*Engraulis species*) swordfish (*Xiphias gladius*), sardine (*Sardina pilchardus*)	0.25
Crustaceans	Muscle meat from appendages and abdomen. In case of crabs and crab-like crustaceans (*Brachyura and Anomura*), muscle meat from appendages	0.50
Bivalve mollusks	Bivalve mollusks and cephalopods (without viscera)	1.00

Source: Commission Regulation (EU) No 488/2014 of 12 May 2014 amending Commission Regulation (EC) No 1881/2006 as regards the maximum levels of Cd in foodstuff. *Official Journal of the European Union* L 138, 13.5.2014.

TABLE 19.9
Maximum Level of Cadmium (Cd) in Cereal, Rice, Soy and Vegetables

Foodstuff	Closer Description	Wet Weight (mg/kg)
Cereal, rice, and soy	Cereal grains, excluding wheat and rice	0.10
	Wheat grains and rice grains	
	Wheat bran and wheat germ for direct consumption and for soybeans	0.20
Vegetables	Vegetables and fruit excluding root and tuber vegetables, leafy vegetables, fresh herbs, leafy brassica, stem vegetables, fungi, and seaweed	0.050
	Root and tuber vegetables (excluding celeriac, parsnips, salsify, and horseradish), stem vegetables (excluding celery). For potatoes, the maximum level applies to peeled potatoes	0.10
	Leafy vegetables, fresh herbs, leafy brassica, celery, celeriac, parsnips, salsify, horseradish, and the following fungi: *Agaricus bisporus* (common mushroom), *Pleurotus ostreatus* (Oyster mushroom), *Lentinula edodes* (Shiitake mushroom)	0.20
	Fungi other than the above-mentioned	1.00

Source: Commission Regulation (EU) No 488/2014 of 12 May 2014 amending Commission Regulation (EC) No 1881/2006 as regards the maximum levels of Cd in foodstuff. *Official Journal of the European Union* L 138, 13.5.2014.

TABLE 19.10
Maximum Level of Cadmium (Cd) in Cocoa Powder and Chocolate—(from the 1.01.2019)

Foodstuff	Closer Description	Wet Weight (mg/kg)
Cocoa powder and chocolate products	Milk chocolate with <30 % total dry cocoa solids	0.10
	Chocolate with <50% total dry cocoa solids; milk chocolate with ≥30% total dry cocoa solids	0.30
	Chocolate with ≥50% total dry cocoa solids	0.80
	Cocoa powder sold to the final consumer or as an ingredient in sweetened cocoa powder sold to the final consumer (drinking chocolate)	0.60

Source: Commission Regulation (EU) No 488/2014 of 12 May 2014 amending Commission Regulation (EC) No 1881/2006 as regards the maximum levels of Cd in foodstuff. *Official Journal of the European Union* L 138, 13.5.2014.

TABLE 19.11
Maximum Level of Mercury (Hg) in Fish and Fishery Products

Foodstuff	Closer Description	Wet Weight (mg/kg)
Fish, fishery products	Fish, fishery products	0.50
	Muscle meat of the following fish—anglerfish (*Lophius* species), Atlantic catfish (*Anarhichas lupus*), bonito (*Sarda sarda*), eel (*Anguilla* species), emperor (*Hoplostethus* species), grenadier (*Coryphaenoides rupestris*), halibut (*Hippoglossus hippoglossus*), marlin (*Makaira species*), megrim (*Lepidorhombus species*), mullet (*Mullus species*), pike (*Esox lucius*), plain bonito (*Orcynopsis unicolor*), poor cod (*Tricopterus minutes*), Portuguese dogfish (*Centroscymnus coelolepis*), rays (*Raja species*), redfish (*Sebastes marinus, S. mentella, S. viviparus*), sail fish (*Istiophorus platypterus*), scabbard fish (*Lepidopus caudatus, Aphanopus carbo*), seabream, pandora (*Pagellus* species), shark (all species), snake mackerel or butterfish (*Lepidocybium flavobrunneum, Ruvettus pretiosus, Gempylus serpens*), sturgeon (*Acipenser species*), swordfish (*Xiphias gladius*), tuna (*Thunnus* species, *Euthynnus* species, *Katsuwonus pelamis*)	1.0

Source: Commission Regulation (EC) No 1881/2006 of 19 December 2006 setting maximum levels for certain contaminants in foodstuff. *Official Journal of the European Union* L 364, 20.12.2006.

19.5.4 Maximum Levels of Nitrates(V) and (III) in Foodstuff

Nitrates(V) and (III) are among those hazardous compounds, the maximum level of which is limited both in food of animal origin and of plant origin. At the same time, they are regarded as components naturally occurring in raw materials of plant origin, including many vegetables. In the EU, very strict norms apply as regards the nitrate content in food intended for infants and children. According to the norms assumed, the content of nitrates(V) cannot exceed 200 mg per kg wet weight (Commission Regulation No 1881/2006). In foodstuff intended for infants and young children under three, regulations specifying nitrate levels distinguish between formulae with and without milk. Products of plant origin, including vegetables and potatoes, are subject to particular control. As regards vegetables, particular limits are set for lettuce and spinach, differentiating the period of their harvesting and the method of their cultivation—grown in the open air or grown under cover. Maximum levels of nitrates(V) and (III) have been set more precisely for several types of vegetables (Smoczyński and Pietrzak-Fiećko 1999, Zhong et al. 2002, Regulation of the Minister of Health 1993 and 2003).

The maximum levels of nitrates(V) and (III) in foods, established by the EU, are presented in Tables 19.12 to 19.14.

TABLE 19.12
Maximum Levels of Nitrates(V) and (III) in Milk-Based Products for Infants and Children Under Three, and General-Purpose Milk

Foodstuff	Closer Description	Nitrates(V) mg/kg of the Product	Nitrates(III) mg/kg of the Product
Milk-based products for infants and children under three, and general-purpose milk	Powdered full-fat milk (for production of milk, modified milk, and modified formulae, and in cereal and milk-cereal products—porridges and gruels)	20.0	1.00
	Powdered and liquid modified milk, the maximum content of nitrates(V) expressed as $NaNO_3$	50.0	1.00
	Milk and vegetable products, milk, vegetable and fruit products, milk and fruit products with bananas, cereal, and vegetable products, cereal, vegetable and fruit products with bananas, milk-fruit products and milk, cereal and fruit products with bananas, the maximum level of nitrates(V) expressed as $NaNO_3$	200.0	1.00

Source: Regulation of the Minister of Health of 13 January 2003 on maximum levels of chemical and biological contaminants that may be present in food, food ingredients, allowed additional substances, substances processing aids or on food. Diary of Law the Republic of Poland No 37, 326, 4.03.2003 (in polish).

TABLE 19.13
Maximum Levels of Nitrates(V) and (III) in Non-Milk-Based Products for Infants and Children Under Three

Foodstuff	Closer Description	Nitrates(V) mg/kg of the Product	Nitrates(III) mg/kg of the Product
Non-milk-based products for infants and children under three	Fruit juices excluding bananas, fruit juices with pumpkin and carrot and apple juices without sugar, as well as in fruit products—excluding bananas—expressed as $NaNO_3$	100.0	1.00
	Fruit and vegetables juices and fruit juices with bananas, as well as fruit products with bananas, the maximum level of nitrates(V) expressed as $NaNO_3$	200.0	1.00
	Banana products and banana products with the addition of other fruits (with the greatest share of bananas) and vegetable products, as well as vegetable and vegetable and milk products—the maximum level of nitrates (V) expressed as $NaNO_3$	250.0	1.00
	Preserved meat and poultry containing no less than 40% meat and poultry raw material, the maximum level of nitrates(V) expressed as $NaNO_3$	50.0	1.00

Source: Regulation of the Minister of Health of 13 January 2003 on maximum levels of chemical and biological contaminants that may be present in food, food ingredients, allowed additional substances, substances processing aids or on food. Diary of Law the Republic of Poland No 37, 326, 4.03.2003 (in Polish).

An intensive nitrogen cycle in the environment, forced by heavy nitrogen fertilization, results in significant growth of nitrate content in some vegetables, including lettuce and spinach. Since the nitrate content in vegetables, including, for instance, climatic conditions) its maximum levels in vegetables are differentiated, for example, depending on the season (for example, fresh lettuce harvested from 1 October to 31 March and from 1 April to 30 September–Table 19.14).

A general recommendation was assumed for producers of vegetables (in particular, for lettuce and spinach) to modify their farming methods to meet the maximum levels established by the EU authorities.

19.5.5 Maximum Levels of PCBs in Foodstuff

Out of all 209 PCB congeners, 12 PCB congeners make a very dangerous group, with a structure similar to toxic dioxins. These are four congeners labeled as 77, 81, 126, and 169, without chlorine substitution at the ortho positions, defined as

TABLE 19.14
Maximum Levels of Nitrates(V) and (III) in Products of Plant Origin—Lettuce, Spinach, and Rucola

Foodstuff	Closer Description	Nitrates(V) mg/kg of the Product	Nitrates(III) mg/kg of the Product
Products of plant origin—lettuce, spinach, and rucola	Fresh spinach (*Spinacia oleracea*)	3500	–
	Preserved, deep-frozen, or frozen spinach	2000	
	Fresh lettuce (*Lactuca sativa L.*) grown in the open air, harvested between 1 April and 30 September (except iceberg-type lettuce) expressed as $NaNO_3$	4000	–
	Fresh lettuce grown under cover	3000	
	Fresh lettuce grown under cover and harvested from 1 October to 31 March (except for the iceberg-type lettuce) expressed as $NaNO_3$	5000	
	Fresh lettuce grown under cover	5000	
	Iceberg-type lettuce grown under cover	2500	
	Iceberg-type lettuce grown in the open air	2000	
	Rucola (*Eruca sativa, Diplotaxis sp. Brassica tenuifolia, Sisymbrium tenuifolium*) harvested from 1 October to 31 March	7000	
	Rucola harvested from 1 April to 30 September	6000	

Source: Commission Regulation (EU) No 1258/2011 of 2 December 2011 amending.

non-ortho, and eight labeled as 105, 114, 118, 123, 156, 157, 167, and 189, with only one chlorine atom as mono-ortho substitute, which are referred to as dioxin-like congeners. Other PCB congeners do not exhibit dioxin-like toxicity but have a different toxicological profile. Among those PCB congeners, a group included into the so-called indicator congeners is distinguished, which includes six congeners labeled with the following numbers—28, 52, 101, 138, 153, and 180. Each polychlorinated biphenyl congener with properties similar to dioxins demonstrates a slightly different toxicity level. The introduction of the concept of the so-called toxic equivalency factor (TEF) allows to sum up the toxicity of these different congeners and facilitates risk assessment and regulatory control. This means that quantitative results of analytical tests referring to the total of all PCBs congeners with an effect similar to dioxins posing a toxicological risk are expressed in quantifiable units referred to as Toxic Equivalency Quantities (TEQ) (Commission Regulation (EU) No 1259/2011). Legal regulations establishing the limits of PCB congeners apply to milk and milk products, infant formula, and food intended for infants and young children. Regulations also concern vegetable oils and fats, as well as meat and meat products of farm animals, and fish, fishery products, and marine oils (Commission Regulation

TABLE 19.15
Maximum Levels of Polychlorinated Biphenyls (PCBs) in Milk and Milk Products, and the Food Intended for Young Children

Foodstuff	Closer Description	The Sum of PCBs with Properties Similar to Dioxins (WHO-PCB_TEQ)	The Sum of Indicator PCB
Milk and milk products	Raw milk and dairy products, including milk fat	3.0 pg/g fat	40 ng/g fat
Food intended for young children	Baby food intended for infants and young children	0.1 pg/g wet weight	1.0 ng/g wet weight

Source: Commission Regulation (EU) No 1259/2011 of 2 December 2011 amending Regulation (EC) No 1881/2006 as regards maximum levels for dioxins, dioxin-like PCBs and non dioxin-like PCBs in foodstuff. *Official Journal of the European Union* L 320, 3.12.2011.

(EU) No 1881/2006, 565/2008, 1259/2011 and Commission Recommendation No 2013/711/EU and Commission Recommendation of 11 September 2014).

Table 19.15 presents data on the maximum level of PCBs in milk and milk products, and food intended for young children.

Table 19.16 presents data on the maximum level of PCBs in foodstuff.

19.5.6 Maximum Levels of Dioxins in Foodstuff

Commission Regulation (EU) No 1881 of 19 December 2006 specified the maximum levels of dioxins in foodstuff expressed as TEQ (Commission Regulation (EU) No 1881/2006). The term "dioxins" in the referred Regulation is understood as the group of 75 polychlorinated dibenzo-p-dioxin (PCDD) congeners and 135 polychlorinated dibenzofuran (PCDF) congeners, of which 17 are of toxicological concern. In subsequent years, those regulations were supplemented, and since 2011, they have also been applicable to Poland.

Established regulations concerning maximum levels of dioxins include milk and dairy products, infant formulae, and food intended for infants and young children. Additionally, regulations include vegetable oils and fats, marine oils, and oils of other marine organisms intended for human consumption, as well as meat and meat products of farm animals, fish, fishery products, and marine oils (Commission Regulation (EU) No 1881/2006, 565/2008, 1259/2011, and Commission Recommendation No 2013/711/EU).

The maximum levels of dioxins in foods are presented in Tables 19.17 to 19.19.

19.5.7 Maximum Levels of PAHs in Foodstuff

For many years, there were no clear legal regulations concerning the maximum levels of PAHs in food products. It was believed that there was no basis for determining the PAH content that would not have any adverse effect on the human body.

TABLE 19.16
Maximum Levels of Polychlorinated Biphenyls (PCBs) in Vegetable Oils and Fats, Meat and Meat Products, Fat Separated from the Tissue, Hen Eggs and Egg Products, Muscle Meat of Fish, and Fishery Products

Foodstuff	Closer Description	The Sum of PCBs with Properties Similar to Dioxins (WHO-PCB-TEQ) pg/g fat	Sum of PCB28, PCB52, PCB101, PCB138, PCB153 and PCB180 Ng/g fat
Vegetable oils and fats	Vegetable oils and fats	0.50	40
Meat and meat products	Meat of pigs (excluding edible offals)	0.25	40
	Poultry meat	1.25	40
	Meat of bovine animals and sheep	1.5	40
Liver	Liver of bovine animals, sheep, pigs, poultry, and derived products thereof	5,5	40
Fat separated from the tissue	Of pigs	0.25	40
	Of poultry	1.25	40
	Fat of bovine animals and sheep	1.5	40
Hen eggs	Hen eggs and egg products	2.5	40
Muscle meat of fish and fishery products	Muscle meat of fish and fishery products and products thereof, with the exemption of wild-caught eel, wild-caught fresh water fish, with the exception of diadromous fish species caught in fresh water, fish liver and derived products, and marine oils	3.0	75.0 ng/g wet weight
	Muscle meat of wild-caught fresh water fish, with the exception of diadromous fish species caught in fresh water, and products thereof	3.0	125 ng/g wet weight
	Muscle meat of wild-caught eel (*Anguilla anguilla*) and products thereof	6.5	300 ng/g wet weight
Marine oils.	Marine oil intended for consumption by people, and fish liver and its products	4.25	200

Source: Commission Regulation (EU) No 1259/2011 of 2 December 2011 amending Regulation (EC) No 1881/2006 as regards maximum levels for dioxins, dioxin-like PCBs and non dioxin-like PCBs in foodstuff. *Official Journal of the European Union* L 320, 3.12.2011.

TABLE 19.17
Maximum Levels of Dioxins in Milk, Milk Products, Milk Fat, Food for Young Children, Hen Eggs, and Vegetable Fats

Foodstuff	Closer Description	The Sum of Dioxins (WHO-PCDD/F-TEQ)	The Sum Dioxins and PCB (WHO-PCDD/F-PCB-TEQ
Milk and milk products	Raw milk and in dairy products and milk fat	2.5 pg/g fat	5.5 pg/g fat
Foods for infants and young children		0.1 pg/g wet weight	0.2 pg/g wet weight
Hen eggs	Hen eggs and egg products	2.5 pg/g fat	5.0 pg/g fat
Vegetable oils and fats	Vegetable oils and fats	0.75 pg/g fat	1.25 pg/g fat

Source: Commission Regulation (EU) No 1259/2011 of 2 December 2011 amending Regulation (EC) No 1881/2006 as regards maximum levels for dioxins, dioxin-like PCBs and non dioxin-like PCBs in foodstuff. *Official Journal of the European Union* L 320, 3.12.2011.

TABLE 19.18
Maximum Levels of Dioxins in Meat and Meat Products

Foodstuff	Closer Description	The Sum of Dioxins (WHO-PCDD/F-TEQ) pg/g fat	The Sum Dioxins and PCB (WHO-PCDD/F-PCB-TEQ) pg/g fat
Meat and meat products	Meat of pigs	1.0	1.25
	Poultry meat	1.75	3.0
	Meat of bovine animals and sheep	2.50	4.0
Livers	Livers of terrestrial animals listed above	4.5	10.0
Fat separated from the tissue	Of pigs	1.00	1.25
	Of poultry	1.75	3.0
	Of bovine animals and sheep	2.5	4.0

Source: Commission Regulation (EU) No 1259/2011 of 2 December 2011 amending Regulation (EC) No 1881/2006 as regards maximum levels for dioxins, dioxin-like PCBs and non dioxin-like PCBs in foodstuff. *Official Journal of the European Union* L 320, 3.12.2011.

It was assumed that practically any dose of PAHs had an effect at the DNA level. It was considered necessary to clearly recommend the effective reduction of PAH content in food to a reasonably attainable extent. To minimize the risk of the threat to consumer health, individual states established maximum PAH levels in various types of foodstuff through the introduction of legal acts. In 2001, pursuant to Commission Regulation (EC) No 466/2001 of 8 March 2001, a process of setting maximum levels for certain foreign chemicals in select foodstuff was initiated

TABLE 19.19
Maximum Levels of Dioxins in Muscle Meat of Fish and Fishery Products, and Marine Oils

Foodstuff	Closer Description	Sum of Dioxins (WHO-PCDD/F-TEQ) pg/g Wet Weight	Sum of Dioxins and Dioxin-like PCBs (WHO-PCDD/F-PCB-TEQ) pg/g Wet Weight
Muscle meat of fish and fishery products	Muscle meat of fish and fishery products and products thereof, with the exemption of wild-caught eel, wild-caught fresh water fish, with the exception of diadromous fish species caught in fresh water, fish liver and derived products, marine oils	3.5	6.5
	Muscle meat of wild caught fresh water fish, with the exception of diadromous fish species caught in fresh water, and products thereof	3.5	6.5
	Muscle meat of wild caught eel (*Anguilla anguilla*) and products thereof	3.5	10.0
	Fish liver and its products excluding oils of sea animals	–	20.0
Marine oils	Marine oil intended for consumption by people and fish liver and its products	1.75 pg/g fat	6.0 pg/g fat

Source: Commission Regulation (EU) No 1259/2011 of 2 December 2011 amending Regulation (EC) No 1881/2006 as regards maximum levels for dioxins, dioxin-like PCBs and non dioxin-like PCBs in foodstuff. *Official Journal of the European Union* L 320, 3.12.2011.

(OJ EU L 77 of 16 March 2001). Next, in 2005, pursuant to Commission Regulation EU No. 208/2005 of 4 February 2005, Regulation (EC) No 466/2001 was amended, by introducing Section 7 to the Annex, with the following wording "Polycyclic aromatic hydrocarbons," and thus setting the highest (maximum) levels of benzo(a)pyrene (BaP) in select types of food. In EU Regulation No. 1881/2006 of 19 December 2006, the maximum levels of PAHs have been set, and more precisely of benzoBaP in select foodstuff. By another Regulation No 835/2011 of 19 August 2011, the maximum levels for BaP and the sum of four PAHs, namely BaP, benz(a)anthracene, benzo(b)fluoranthene, and chrysene, have been set for the following groups of foodstuff, as presented in Tables 19.20 to 19.22.

TABLE 19.20
Maximum Levels of PAHs in Oils and Fats, Coconut Oil, Cocoa Beans, and Derived Products

Foodstuff	Closer Description	Benzo(a)Pyrene μg/kg Product	Sum of Benzo(a)Pyrene, Benz(a)Anthracene, Benzo(b)Fluoranthene and Chrysene μg/kg Product
Oils and fats	Excluding cocoa butter and coconut oil	2.0	10.0
Coconut oil	Intended for direct human consumption or use as an ingredient in food	2.0	20.0
Cocoa beans	And derived products	5.0	30.0

Source: Commission Regulation (EU) No 835/2011 of 19 August 2011 amending Regulation (EC) No 1881/2006 as regards maximum levels for polycyclic aromatic hydrocarbons in foodstuff. *Official Journal of the European Union* L 215, 20.8.2011.

TABLE 19.21
Maximum Levels of PAHs in Muscle Meat of Smoked Fish and Smoked Fishery Products

Foodstuff	Closer Description	Benzo(a) Pyrene μg/kg Product	Sum of Benzo(a)Pyrene, Benz(a)Anthracene, Benzo(b)Fluoranthene and Chrysene μg/kg Product
Meat	Smoked meat and smoked meat products	2.0	12.0
Fish	Muscle meat of smoked fish and smoked fishery products, excluding smoked sprats and bivalve mollusks. The maximum level for smoked crustaceans applies to muscle meat from appendages and abdomen. In case of smoked crabs and crab-like crustaceans (*Brachyura* and *Anomura*), it applies to muscle meat from appendages.	2.0	12.0
	Smoked sprats and canned smoked sprats (*Sprattus sprattus*); bivalve mollusks (fresh, chilled, or frozen); heat-treated meat and heat-treated meat products sold to the final consumer	5.0	30.0
	Smoked bivalve mollusks	6.0	35.0

Source: Commission Regulation (EU) No 835/2011 of 19 August 2011 amending Regulation (EC) No 1881/2006 as regards maximum levels for polycyclic aromatic hydrocarbons in foodstuff. *Official Journal of the European Union* L 215, 20.8.2011.

TABLE 19.22
Maximum Levels of PAHs in Processed Cereal-Based Foods and Infant Formulae

Foodstuff	Closer Description	Benzo(a)Pyrene μg/kg Product	Sum of Benzo(a)Pyrene, Benz(a)Anthracene, Benzo(b)Fluoranthene and Chrysene μg/kg Product
Processed cereal-based foods	Processed cereal-based foods and baby foods for infants and young children	1.0	1.0
Infant formula	Infant formulae and follow-on formulae, including infant milk and follow-on milk	1.0	1.0
	Dietary food for special medical purposes intended specifically for infants	1.0	1.0

Source: Commission Regulation (EU) No 835/2011 of 19 August 2011 amending Regulation (EC) No 1881/2006 as regards maximum levels for polycyclic aromatic hydrocarbons in foodstuff. *Official Journal of the European Union* L 215, 20.8.2011.

19.5.8 Maximum Levels of Aflatoxins in Foodstuff

Mycotoxins—hazardous chemicals of biological origin occurring in food—also include aflatoxins produced by some *Aspergillus* species. In view of their already documented toxicity, their content in food and feed should be controlled. Therefore, it is recommended that the maximum levels of aflatoxins should be set, as well as other mycotoxins in foodstuff (ideally, as low as reasonably achievable). This particularly concerns products that are intended for the most sensitive groups of consumers—newborns and young children. Authorities supervising food safety in the EU as well as other states of the world set regulations concerning the maximum levels of aflatoxins in milk, cereals, and nuts at the beginning of the present century. In subsequent regulations, the group of foodstuff was extended by infant formulae, and the maximum levels of aflatoxins in various products of plant origin were changed, including cereals, maize, rice, nuts, dried fruit, and spices. The actual maximum level of aflatoxins in foods is presented in Tables 19.23 to 19.26.

TABLE 19.23
Maximum Levels of Aflatoxins in Raw and Processed Milk, Food for Infants, and Young Children

Foodstuff	Closer Description	B_1 μg/kg	$B_1 + B_2 + G_1 + G_2$ μg/kg	M_1 μg/kg
Raw and processed milk	Milk-based products must be free from aflatoxins $B_1 + B_2 + G_1 + G_2$,	–	–	0.050
Food for infants and young children	Infant formula and follow-on formula, including infant milk and follow-on milk, which cannot contain aflatoxins $B_1 + B_2 + G_1 + G_2$	–	–	0.025
	Processed cereal-based foods and baby foods for infants and young children	0.10	–	0.025
	Dietary foods for special medical purposes intended specifically for infants	0.10	–	0.025

Source: Commission Regulation (EU) No 165/2010 of 26 February 2010 amending Regulation (EC) No 1881/2006 setting maximum levels for certain contaminants in foodstuff as regards aflatoxins. *Official Journal of the European Union* L 50, 27.2.2010.

TABLE 19.24
Maximum Levels of Aflatoxins in Cereals, Maize, Rice, and Nuts

Foodstuff	Closer Description	B_1 μg/kg	$B_1 + B_2 + G_1 + G_2$ μg/kg	M_1 μg/kg
Cereals	All cereals and all products derived from cereals, including processed cereal products, with the exception of maize, rice and processed cereal-based foods	2.0	4.0	–
Maize and rice	Maize and rice to be subjected to sorting or other physical treatment before human consumption or use as an ingredient in foodstuff	5.0	10.0	–
Nuts	Peanuts and in other oilseeds to be subjected to sorting or other treatment before human consumption, except for the above-mentioned nuts intended for crushing for refined vegetable oil production	8.0	15.0	–
	The same nuts intended for direct human consumption or used as an ingredient in foodstuff	2.0	4.0	–

Source: Commission Regulation (EU) No 165/2010 of 26 February 2010 amending Regulation (EC) No 1881/2006 setting maximum levels for certain contaminants in foodstuff as regards aflatoxins. *Official Journal of the European Union* L 50, 27.2.2010.

TABLE 19.25
Maximum Levels of Aflatoxins in Almonds, Pistachios, Apricot Kernels, and Dried Fruit

Foodstuff	Closer Description	B_1 µg/kg	$B_1 + B_2 + G_1 + G_2$ µg/kg	M_1 µg/kg
Almonds, pistachios, and apricot kernels	Treatment before human consumption	12.0	15.0	
	Nuts intended for direct human consumption or use as an ingredient in foodstuff	8.0	10.0	
Dried fruit	Dried fruit and processed products made of dried fruit intended for direct human consumption or used as an ingredient in foodstuff	2.0	4.0	
	Dried fruit subjected to treatment before human consumption	5.0	10.0	

Source: Commission Regulation (EU) No 165/2010 of 26 February 2010 amending Regulation (EC) No 1881/2006 setting maximum levels for certain contaminants in foodstuff as regards aflatoxins. *Official Journal of the European Union* L 50, 27.2.2010.

TABLE 19.26
Maximum Levels of Aflatoxins in Spices

Foodstuff	Closer Description	B_1 µg/kg	$B_1 + B_2 + G_1 + G_2$ µg/kg	M_1 µg/kg
Spices	Spices derived from the Capsicum L. species dried fruit, whole or ground, including chillies, chilli powder, cayenne, and paprika.	5.0	10.0	–
	Additionally, *Piper* spp. and its fruits, including white and black pepper, as well as nutmeg (*Myristyca fragrans*), ginger (*Zingiber officinale*), and turmeric (*Curcuma longa*).			–
	Individual spices and spice mixes containing one or more of the above-mentioned spices.	5.0	10.0	

Source: Commission Regulation (EU) No 165/2010 of 26 February 2010 amending Regulation (EC) No 1881/2006 setting maximum levels for certain contaminants in foodstuff as regards aflatoxins. *Official Journal of the European Union* L 50, 27.2.2010.

19.5.9 Maximum Levels of Ochratoxin A in Foodstuff

The EFSA adopted on 4 April 2006, at the request of the Commission, an updated scientific opinion concerning the content of ochratoxin A in food. On the basis of this opinion, the maximum levels of mycotoxins have been established for cereals, cereal products, dried vine fruit, roasted coffee, wine, grape juice and food for infants and young children. According to EU Commission Regulation No 1881/2006 of 19 December 2006, maximum levels of ochratoxin A have been set for select foodstuff.

The maximum levels of ochratoxin A in foodstuff (Cereals and coffee beans, dried vine fruit, wine and juice and spices) are presented in Table 19.27.

TABLE 19.27
Maximum Levels of Ochratoxin A in Cereals and Coffee Beans, Dried Vine Fruit, Wine, Juice [CR-EU No 1881/2006], and Spices [CR-EU No 105/2010 and CR-EU No 2015/1137]

Foodstuff	Closer Description	µg/kg
Cereals and coffee beans	Unprocessed cereals	5.0
	All products derived from unprocessed cereals and cereals intended for direct human consumption	3.0
	Processed cereal-based food and food for infants and young children	0.50
	Roasted coffee beans and ground roasted coffee	5.0
	Soluble coffee	10.0
Dried vine fruit, wine, and juice	Dried vine fruit—currants, raisins, and sultanas	10.0
	Wine, including sparkling wine and fruit wine (excluding liqueur wine and wine with an alcoholic strength of not less than 15% vol.)	2.0
	The same maximum level of ochratoxin A has been set for grape juice, reconstituted concentrated grape juice, grape nectar, grape must, and concentrated grape must as reconstituted, intended for direct human consumption.	2.0
Spices	*Capsicum* spp. (dried fruits thereof, whole or ground, including chillies, chilli powder, cayenne, and paprika), *Piper* spp. (fruits thereof, including white and black pepper), *Myristica fragrans* (nutmeg), *Zingiber officinale* (ginger), *Curcuma longa* (turmeric). Mixtures of spices containing one or more of the above-mentioned spices	15.0

19.5.10 Maximum Levels of Deoxynivalenol (DON), Zearalenone, and Fumonisins in Foodstuff

Based on scientific opinions and an assessment of the dietary intake, the maximum levels of DON, zearalenone, and fumonisins have been set. They are presented in Tables 19.28 to 19.30.

TABLE 19.28
Maximum Levels of Deoxynivalenol (DON) in Cereals and Cereal-Based Products

Foodstuff	Closer Description	µg/kg
Cereals and cereal-based products	Unprocessed durum wheat, oats, and maize	1750
	Unprocessed cereals other than the above mentioned	1250
	Cereals intended for direct human consumption, cereal flour (including maize flour, maize meal and maize grits, and bran as end product marketed for direct human consumption and germ and dry pasta)	750
	Bread and small bakery wares, pastries, biscuits, cereal snacks, and breakfast cereals	500
	Processed cereal-based food and food for infants and young children	200

Source: Commission Regulation (EC) No 1881/2006 of 19 December 2006 setting maximum levels for certain contaminants in foodstuff. *Official Journal of the European Union* L 364, 20.12.2006.

TABLE 19.29
Maximum Levels of Zearalenone in Foodstuff Cereals and Cereal-Based Products

Foodstuff	Closer Description	µg/kg
Cereals and cereal-based products	Cereals intended for direct human consumption, cereal flour, bran as end product marketed for direct human consumption and germ	75
	Unprocessed cereals other than maize	100
	Unprocessed maize	200
	Maize intended for direct human consumption, maize flour, maize meal, maize grits, maize germ, and refined maize oil	200
	Processed cereal-based food and food for infants and young children	20
	Bread, small bakery wares, pastries, biscuits, cereal snacks, and breakfast cereals	50
	Processed cereal-based food (except for processed maize-based food) and food for infants and young children	20

Source: Commission Regulation (EC) No 1881/2006 of 19 December 2006 setting maximum levels for certain contaminants in foodstuff. *Official Journal of the European Union* L 364, 20.12.2006.

TABLE 19.30
Maximum Levels of Fumonisins in Cereals and Cereal-Based Products

Foodstuff	Closer Description	$B_1 + B_2$ µg/kg
Cereals and cereal-based products	Unprocessed maize	2000
	Maize flour, maize meal, maize grits, maize germ, and refined maize oil	1000
	Maize-based food intended for direct human consumption	400
	Processed maize-based foods and foods for infants and young children	200

Source: CR-EU No 1881/2006.

19.6 LEGAL REQUIREMENTS CONCERNING METHODS OF SAMPLING AND ANALYSIS FOR THE PURPOSES OF CONTROL OF HAZARDOUS CHEMICALS IN FOOD

Standards approved and published in the CA, and afterward in the EU documents, concerning the established maximum levels of hazardous chemicals in food also provide information concerning the methods of sampling and chemical analysis. Legislations of many countries also determine and recommend methods considered necessary and compliant with the principles of the Committee on Methods of Analysis and Sampling. It has been assumed that if two or more methods are considered equal, the standard should consider them as alternatives (Gertig and Duda 2004).

Sampling and methods of analysis for the official control of the levels of Pb, Cd, and Hg in foodstuff are governed by the regulations set forth in the Directive of 2001 (Commission Directive No 2001/22/EC). The established regulations have been improved by EU Commission Regulation No 333 of 2007. This Regulation starts with specification of the methods of sampling—planning, packaging, and labeling. Depending on the chemical properties of hazardous compounds in foodstuff, specific procedures for preparing samples for analyses are described. Additionally, the basic criteria for the choice of a method for analysis of Pb, Cd, and Hg content for foodstuff listed in EU Regulation No 1881/2006 are described. The Regulation defines, among others, such criteria as limit of determination (LOD), limit of quantification (LOQ), as well as precision, recovery, and specificity of the method (e.g., the method should be free of matrix interferences or spectral interference) (Commission Regulation (EU) No 1883/2006).

Sampling and methods of analysis for the official control of nitrates(V) and (III) in foodstuff are governed by the provision specified in the EU Regulation of 2006 (Commission Regulation (EU) No 1883/2006).

Sampling and methods of analysis for the official control of dioxins and dl PCBs in foodstuff are governed by the provision specified in the EU Regulation of 2006 (Commission Regulation (EU) No 1883/2006). Those provisions were extended by ndl-PCBs in the regulation of 2012. This Regulation applies only to sampling and analyzing of the level of dioxins, dl-PCBs, and ndl-PCBs for the purposes of EU Regulation No. (Commission regulation (EU) No 252/2012). Another improvement concerning the methods of sampling and analyzing samples for the purposes of control of dioxin, dl-PCBs, and ndl- PCBs—at the same time repealing Regulation 252/2012—has been introduced through Commission Regulation of 2014 (Commission Regulation (EU) No 252/2012).

Regulation No 333/2007of 28 March 2007 concerns detailed procedures with regard to heavy metals and BaP.

EU Regulation No 333/2007 of 28 March 2007 and Directive of the European Commission No 2005/10/EC of 4 February 2005 specified requirements and performance criteria for analytical methods applied for quantitative determination of BaP and other PAH compounds. This Regulation includes basic criteria for choosing the method of analysis of PAHs for foodstuff listed in EU Regulation No. 1881/2006. The Regulation specifies, among others, such criteria as LOD, LOQ, as well as precision, recovery, and specificity of the method. In case of BaP, what is important is the specificity of the method (the method must be free from matrix interference or spectral interference), LOD, which should be not lower than 0.3 μg/kg, LOQ not lower than 0.9 μg/kg, and recovery—ranging from 50% to 120% (Commission Regulation (EU) No 401/2006).

EU Commission Regulation No 401/2006 specifies the method for taking samples of cereals and cereal products, methods for determining aflatoxins B_1, B_2, G_1 and G_2, and M_1. Pursuant to the quoted regulation, the same sampling method should be applied to the same product for monitoring the mycotoxin level.

19.7 HAZARD CONTROL OF TOXIC AND OTHER HARMFUL COMPOUNDS IN FOODS

Hazard control in relation to harmful compounds in food is maintained by official authorities and the scientific community, which ensures a comprehensive position to ensure public confidence. The nature of the issue is based on risk analysis. Assessment of health risks related to consumer exposure to harmful chemicals aims at describing the relationships between the scale of exposure and the frequency of negative health effects. The results of risk assessment can provide a basis for establishing safe exposure limits for food, but also in relation to occupational and environmental factors. Today, risk analysis is becoming the basis of all food safety strategies. EU regulations indicate the need to apply a three-stage procedure—risk assessment, risk management, and risk communication. Risk assessment should be treated as a scientific stage and the basis for each regulation related to protection of human health protection. The most important security measure for consumers is to establish maximum residue levels (MRLs) of chemicals in specific food products—the components of a daily diet. On a global level, MRL values for food are established through a scientific procedure in the CD system. The basic element in risk assessment is identification of risk and its full characteristics. This consists in identifying biological, chemical, physical, and other factors related to the condition of food that may cause negative health effects in consumers. Risk characteristics are related to a qualitative and quantitative evaluation of the nature of hazardous health effects resulting from the above-mentioned factors, which may occur in food. For chemical factors, what should be established is the relation between the dose and the response.

Stage two—risk management—is a legislative stage carried out within state or international structures. Protection of consumer health is a significant element in risk management carried out by specialized governmental agencies, taking into account the applicable sanitary measures. The objective is to reduce risk and provide protection against its effects. Risk management is understood as undertaking activities aimed at risk identification, evaluation, and control, and the supervision of implemented measures. The third element in risk management is appropriate communication about food-related risks affecting human life. The information obtained through risk analysis must be comprehensively used, not only as regards its dissemination, but with its full inclusion into the risk management process by taking proper decisions. Therefore, risk communication should explain the reasons underlying the decisions taken as part of risk management. An important element of the entire risk assessment process is the need to take into account the prudence principle resulting from the existence of multiple sources of uncertainty and the lack of scientifically approved facts. Therefore, the degree of uncertainty and possible variables in available scientific data should be explicitly included in risk analysis.

It should be emphasized that an early warning system for food risk is an important element of EU policy. In Regulation No. 178/2002, the EU established the European Rapid Alert System for Food and Feed (RASFF). The system enables rapid exchange of necessary information between participants of an official control carried out by respective authorities of EU Member States. It plays a key role in ensuring the free flow of safe and health-promoting food in Europe. Risk evaluation applies to food, materials, and products coming into contact with food and feed. The system also includes information on preventive measures taken in individual EU states. Teams of specialists are appointed to evaluate the risk to consumer health if it is proven that any food product parameters, materials, or products intended to come into contact with food do not comply with applicable regulations. The risks to consumer health that are analyzed most frequently include cases of exceeding the maximum residue limits of chemicals in foodstuff. The system makes it possible to prevent the health effects of hazardous chemicals by taking appropriate actions at all stages in the food chain. The first report on the operation of the RASFF system for 2002–2003 included 454 alert notifications, while in 2008, there were 528 such notifications (Ludwicki and Kostka 2008). In 2013, 3137 alert notifications were given in RASFF. Alert notifications concerning food and feed concerned the presence of pathogenic microorganisms in 204 cases, while in 78 cases, the alerts concerned mycotoxins and 73 concerned heavy metals (Buczkowska et al. 2014). Today, the RASFF system is viewed as a significant element of sanitary—epidemiological supervision of food production and the health protection strategy for the EU population. However, it is necessary to constantly undertake activities toward increasing responsibility and strengthening cooperation between the Member States. It will also be possible to increase the efficiency of control through, for example, extension of research into improvement of analytical methods to determine hazardous compounds and to search for tests for their rapid detection, and consequently, systematic adjustment of EU legislation to potential new threats. What is also indicated is the plausibility of risk evaluation at the stage preceding introduction of a product into the market, which helps prevent health effects by taking measures at an earlier stage of the food chain.

19.8 SUMMARY AND CONCLUSIONS

To summarize, it can be assumed that legislation of many states in the world, as well as states being parties to international agreements, aims at ensuring the conditions for the production of food that ensure health and safe life of humans from birth to natural death. In practice, it requires taking measures for environmental protection and health safety of food. When obtaining plant and animal material directly from the environment, the status of that environment determines the nutritional and health quality of the raw materials. Progressive chemicalization of agriculture, as well as applied raw material processing technologies, has resulted in food that may contain chemical contamination and remains that are potentially hazardous for consumers. This requires the application of good manufacturing practice (GMP) and appropriate quality assurance systems throughout the entire food chain. As it turns out, those efforts do not guarantee that food will be completely free from potentially hazardous or toxic chemicals. Under these circumstances, in order to ensure the health safety of food, it is necessary to monitor it for the presence of hazardous chemicals. At the same time, as a result of the research conducted, measures are being taken to determine the maximum levels of hazardous chemicals in food. Those levels, published in relevant documents of the EU derived from the CA, have become the basis for the official control of food. In addition, a system of undertaking preventive measures and efficient intervention in the emergence of hazardous chemical in food has been established. In extreme situations, this may result in discontinuing production and withdrawing the bad food. This situations lead to drawing the following conclusions:

- International cooperation has led to the development of a system in the form of the CA, the compliance with which helps ensure safe food for customers
- Established regulations of the EU, the United States, and other countries concerning the control of the maximum levels of hazardous chemicals are very similar, which enables global exchange of food products if those regulations are complied with
- The established regulations of the EU concerning food hygiene and the control of potentially hazardous chemicals (heavy metals—Pb, Cd, and Hg), nitrates(V) and nitrates(III), PCBs, dioxins, PAHs, and mycotoxins), with regard to their maximum levels, provide a guarantee that the food present on the market will always be of proper nutritional and health quality

REFERENCES

Buczkowska, M., T. Sadowski, and J. Gadomska. 2014. Early warning system concerning food and feed. *Problems of Hygiene and Epidemiology* 95(3): 550–555. (in Polish).

Codex Alimentarius Commission. 2010. Procedural manual. FAO/WHO Rome, nineteenth edition. ISBN 978-92-5-106493-1.

Commission Directive 2001/22/EC of 8 March 2001 laying down the sampling methods and the methods of analysis for the official control of the levels of lead, cadmium, mercury and 3-MCPD in foodstuffs. *Official Journal of the European Union* L 77, 16.3.2001.

Commission Directive 2005/10/EC of 4 February 2005 laying down the sampling methods and the methods of analysis for the official control of the levels of benzo [a] pyrene in foodstuffs. *Official Journal of the European Union* L 34, 8.2.2005.

Commission Recommendation of 11 September 2014 amending the Annex to Recommendation 2012/711/EC on the reduction of the presence of dioxins, furans and PCBs in feed and food. *Official Journal of the European Union* L 272, 13.9.2014.

Commission Recommendation of 3 December 2013 on the reduction of the presence of dioxins, furans and PCBs in feed and food. (2013/711/EU). *Official Journal of the European Union* L 323, 4.12.2013.

Commission Regulation (EU) No 466/2001 of 8 March 2001 setting maximum levels for certain contaminants in foodstuffs. *Official Journal of the European Communities* L 77, 16.3.2001.

Commission Regulation (EC) No 208/2005 of 4 February 2005 amending Regulation (EC) No 466/2001 as regards polycyclic aromatic hydrocarbons. *Official Journal of the European Union* L 34, 8.2.2005.

Commission Regulation (EC) No 401/2006 of 23 February 2006 laying down the methods of sampling and analysis for the official control of the levels of mycotoxins in foodstuffs. *Official Journal of the European Union* L 70, 9.3.2006.

Commission Regulation (EC) No 1881/2006 of 19 December 2006 setting maximum levels for certain contaminants in foodstuffs. *Official Journal of the European Union* L 364, 20.12.2006.

Commission Regulation (EC) No 1883/2006 of 19 December 2006 laying down methods of sampling and analysis for the official control of levels of dioxins and dioxin-like PCBs in certain foodstuffs. *Official Journal of the European Union* L 364, 20.12.2006.

Commission Regulation (EC) No 333/2007 of 28 March 2007 laying down the methods of sampling and analysis for the official control of the levels of lead, cadmium, mercury, inorganic tin, 3-MCPD and benzo(a)pyrene in foodstuffs. *Official Journal of the European Union* L 88, 29.3.2007.

Commission Regulation (EC) No 629/2008 of 2 July 2008 amending Regulation (EC) No 1881/2006 setting maximum levels certain contaminants in foodstuffs. *Official Journal of the European Union* L 173, 3.8.2008.

Commission Regulation (EC) No 565/2008 of 18 June 2008 amending Regulation (EC) No 1881/2006 setting maximum levels for certain contaminants in foodstuffs as regards the establishment of a maximum level for dioxins and PCBs in fish liver. *Official Journal of the European Union* L 160, 19.6.2008.

Commission Regulation (EC) No 105/2010 of 5 February 2010 amending Regulation No 1881/2006 setting maximum levels for certain contaminants in foodstuffs as regards ochratoxin A. *Official Journal of the European Union* L 35, 6.2.2010.

Commission Regulation (EU) No 165/2010 of 26 February 2010 amending Regulation (EC) No 1881/2006 setting maximum levels for certain contaminants in foodstuffs as regards aflatoxins. *Official Journal of the European Union* L 50, 27.2.2010.

Commission regulation (EU) No 420/2011 of 29 April 2011 amending Regulation (EC) No 1881/2006 setting maximum levels for certain contaminants in foodstuffs. *Official Journal of the European Union* L 111, 30.4.2011.

Commission Regulation (EU) No 835/2011 of 19 August 2011 amending Regulation (EC) No 1881/2006 as regards maximum levels for polycyclic aromatic hydrocarbons in foodstuffs. *Official Journal of the European Union* L 215, 20.8.2011.

Commission Regulation (EU) No 1258/2011 of 2 December 2011 amending Commission Regulation (EC) No 466/2001 of 8 March 2001 setting maximum levels for certain contaminants in foodstuffs. *Official Journal of the European Union* L 320, 3.12.2011.

Commission Regulation (EU) No 1259/2011 of 2 December 2011 amending Regulation (EC) No 1881/2006 as regards maximum levels for dioxins, dioxin-like PCBs and non-dioxin-like PCBs in foodstuffs. *Official Journal of the European Union* L 320, 3.12.2011.

Commission Regulation (EU) No 252/2012 of 21 March 2012 laying down methods of sampling and analysis for the official control of levels of dioxins, dioxin-like PCBs and non-dioxin-like PCBs in certain foodstuffs and repealing Regulation (EC) No 1883/2006. *Official Journal of the European Union* L 84, 23.3.2012.

Commission Regulation (EU) No 488/2014 of 12 May 2014 amending Commission Regulation (EC) No 1881/2006 as regards the maximum levels of cadmium in foodstuffs. *Official Journal of the European Union* L 138, 13.5.2014.

Commission Regulation (EU) No 2015/1005 of 25 June 2015 amending Regulation (EC) No 1881/2006 as regards the maximum permissible levels of lead in foodstuffs. *Official Journal of the European Union* L 161, 26.6.2015.

Commission Regulation (EU) 2015/1137 of 13 July 2015 amending Regulation (EC) No 1881/2006 as regards the maximum level of Ochratoxin A in *Capsicum* spp. Spices. *Official Journal of the European Union* L 185, 14.7.2015.

Council Decision of 17 November 2003 on the accession of the European Community to the Codex Alimentarius Commission (2003/822/EC). *Official Journal of the European Union* L 309, 26.11.2003.

Gertig, H. and G. Duda. 2004. *Food and Health and Law*. Medical Publishing House PZWL: Warsaw (in Polish).

Ludwicki, J.K. and G. Kostka. 2008. Violations of MRLs for pesticide residues in food reported for risk assessment according to RASFF procedures in Poland. *Annals of the National Institute of Hygiene* 59(4): 389–396 (in Polish).

Picó, Y. 2007. *Food Toxicants Analysis Techniques, Strategies and Developments.* Elsevier Amsterdam, NL.

Regulation (EC) No 178/2002 of 28 January 2002 of the European Parliament and of the Council laying down the general principles and requirements of food law, establishing the European Food Safety Authority and laying down procedures in matters of food safety. *Official Journal of the European Union* L 31, 1.2.2002.

Regulation (EC) No 852/2004 of the European Parliament and of the Council of 29 April 2004 on the hygiene of foodstuffs. *Official Journal of the European Union* L 139, 30.4.2004.

Regulation (EC) No 853/2004 of the European Parliament and of the Council of 29 April 2004 laying down specific hygiene rules for food of origin animal. *Official Journal of the European Union* L 226, 25.6.2004.

Regulation (EC) No 882/2004 of the European Parliament and of the Council of 29 April 2004 on official controls performed to ensure compliance with the feed and food law, animal health and animal welfare rules. *Official Journal of the European Union* L 165, 30.4.2004.

Regulation of the Minister of Health of 13 January 2003 on maximum levels of chemical and biological contaminants that may be present in food, food ingredients, allowed additional substances, substances processing aids or on food. Diary of Law the Republic of Poland No 37, 326, 4.03.2003 (in Polish).

Regulation of the Minister of Health and Social Welfare of 8 October 1993 on maximum residues in foodstuffs of chemicals used in cultivation, preservation, storage and transport of plants. Diary of Law the Republic of Poland No. 104, 476 (in polish).

Smoczyński, S. and R. Pietrzak-Fiećko. 1999. Nitrates and nitrites in selected vegetables. *Natural Sci* 3: 333–339.

Szkoda, J., A. Nawrocka, M. Kmiecik, and J. Żmudzki. 2011. Control tests of toxic elements in foods of animal origin. *Environment and Natural Resources* 48: 475–484.

Wojciechowska-Mazurek, M., M. Mania, K. Starska, and M. Opoka. 2010. Cadmium in foodstuffs—the desirability of lowering limits. *Food Industry* 64(2): 45–48 (in Polish).

Zhong, W., C. Hu, and M. Wang. 2002. Nitrates and nitrites in vegetables from north China: content and intake. *Food Addit Contam* 19(12): 1125–1129.

Index

Note: Page numbers followed by f and t refer to figures and tables, respectively.

B

C

D

I

N

O

P

Q

R

U

V

W

X

Y

Z